Advances in Experimental Medicine and Biology

Volume 1269

Advances in Experimental Medicine and Biology provides a platform for scientific contributions in the main disciplines of the biomedicine and the life sciences. This series publishes thematic volumes on contemporary research in the areas of microbiology, immunology, neurosciences, biochemistry, biomedical engineering, genetics, physiology, and cancer research. Covering emerging topics and techniques in basic and clinical science, it brings together clinicians and researchers from various fields.

Advances in Experimental Medicine and Biology has been publishing exceptional works in the field for over 40 years, and is indexed in SCOPUS, Medline (PubMed), Journal Citation Reports/Science Edition, Science Citation Index Expanded (SciSearch, Web of Science), EMBASE, BIOSIS, Reaxys, EMBiology, the Chemical Abstracts Service (CAS), and Pathway Studio.

2019 Impact Factor: 2.450 5 Year Impact Factor: 2.324.

More information about this series at http://www.springer.com/series/5584

Edwin M. Nemoto • Eileen M. Harrison
Sally C. Pias • Denis E. Bragin
David K. Harrison • Joseph C. LaManna
Editors

Oxygen Transport to Tissue XLII

Springer

Editors
Edwin M. Nemoto
Department of Neurosurgery
University of New Mexico
Albuquerque, NM, USA

Sally C. Pias
Department of Chemistry
New Mexico Institute of Mining and
Technology (New Mexico Tech)
Socorro, NM, USA

David K. Harrison
St. Lorenzen, Italy

Eileen M. Harrison
Bozen, Italy

Denis E. Bragin
Lovelace Biomedical Research Institute
Albuquerque, NM, USA

Joseph C. LaManna
Department of Physiology & Biophysics
Case Western Reserve University
School of Medicine
Cleveland, OH, USA

ISSN 0065-2598 ISSN 2214-8019 (electronic)
Advances in Experimental Medicine and Biology
ISBN 978-3-030-48236-7 ISBN 978-3-030-48238-1 (eBook)
https://doi.org/10.1007/978-3-030-48238-1

This Springer imprint is published by the registered company Springer Nature Switzerland AG
The registered company address is: Gewerbestrasse 11, 6330 Cham, Switzerland

Preface

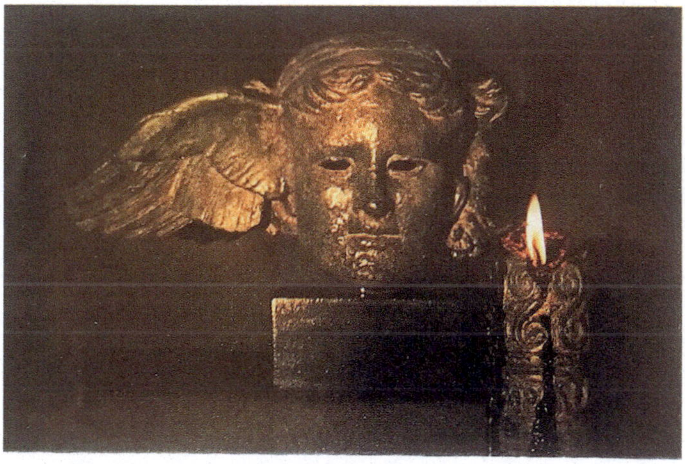

Hypnos and the Flame
(original photograph courtesy of Dr. John W. Severinghaus)

In his foreword to John Nunn's book *Applied Respiratory Physiology*, John Severinghaus, an anesthesiologist and also my postdoctoral mentor as a Fellow at the Cardiovascular Research Institute at the University of California, San Francisco, wrote the following under the title "A Flame for Hypnos."

> The lighted candle respires and we call it flame. The body respires and we call it life. Neither flame nor life are substance, but process. The flame is as different from the wick and wax as life from the body, as gravitation from the falling apple or love from a hormone. Newton taught science to have faith in processes as well as substance-to compute, predict and depend upon an irrational attraction.

Such has been our study of oxygen, the substance in the whole of physiology and clinical medicine from the air we breathe to its consumption at the level of the mitochondrion for the past 47 years since 1973 when the International Society of Oxygen Transport to Tissue (ISOTT) was founded.

Although this 47th Annual meeting of our society began under the duress of a shortened time scale, we were able to host approximately 95 participants to enjoy the sunshine and American Indian Culture here in the Midwest, where art is king. We enjoyed the company and presentations of all the attendees and hope that all had an excellent experience in New Mexico and Albuquerque.

Department of Neurosurgery
University of New Mexico,
Albuquerque, NM, USA

Edwin M. Nemoto

In Memoriam

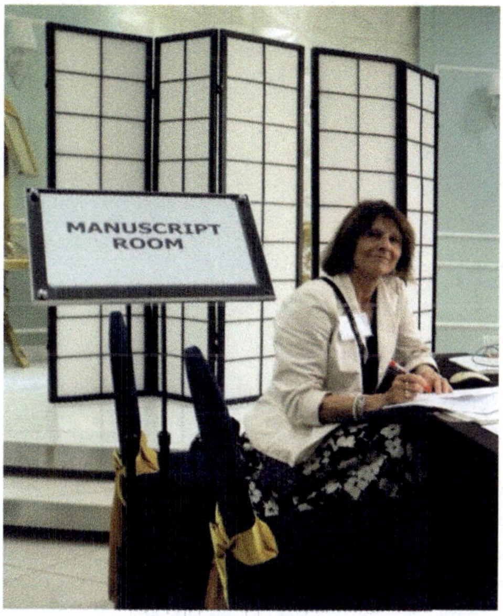

Laraine Visser

"To my loved ones, I thought it might be nice if—later on—in your own time and in a place that you like, you might want to celebrate (my) life. You could do this alone, or with someone else that we shared good times with… with love as always. Laraine "Larry" Visser-Isles".

For well over 20 years Laraine Visser was present at every ISOTT meeting cheerfully sitting at the manuscript desk accepting submissions for the proceedings, offering advice and reminding authors about the other documents the publisher required to accompany their papers. She was also a very lively and popular participant in the meetings' social events. Fifteen years ago she managed to persuade me to volunteer to take on the scientific editing of the book in order to ensure the smooth flow of manuscripts between her, reviewers and the technical editor. This relieved the Principal Editor (the president) from a large amount of work and ensured a consistent standard from year to year.

Her presence at the meeting was only a small part of her contribution, however. Starting straight after the meeting with those manuscripts that had been submitted and continuing for the following 2 or 3 months, she would carefully go through each manuscript, correcting them to ensure that the English was comprehensible. In some cases this required corresponding with the authors to find out exactly what was meant in a particular sentence or paragraph. Her task was to keep her changes to a minimum, but on occasions she went beyond the call of duty and took on the challenge of entirely correcting almost incomprehensible manuscripts. In all of her work she was cheerful and constructive and her sense of humour came over in the many e-mails we exchanged during the editing process.

She was a key element in the team (the "dream team" she called it) that has edited the ISOTT volume for the last 15 years. All of us in ISOTT are grateful for her long service to the society. She will be sorely missed.
On behalf of ISOTT
David Harrison

ISOTT 2019 Awardees

Melvin H Knisely Award
Ting Li
Dietrich Lubbers Award
Kazuki Hotta
Britton Chance Award
Alexander Kalyanov
Bruley Awardees
Gary Angles
Tim Darlington
Min Feng
Thea Huesing
Bhabuk Koirala
Sho Kojima
Jonathan Nguyen
Labiblias Rahman
Mandy Rauschner
Aarti Sethuraman
Eileen Thiessen

ISOTT 2019 Sponsors

Kinesio
Vitech Bio
Clin EPR, LLC, Lyme, NH
Oxford Optronix
Scientica Instrumentation
Hamamatus
Fujifilm
Visualsonics

Contents

Part III Tumor Oxygenation and Modeling

Part I

Oxygen Metabolism and Health Monitoring

Chronic Ketosis Modulates HIF1α-Mediated Inflammatory Response in Rat Brain

1

Aarti Sethuraman, Prahlad Rao, Atul Pranay,
Kui Xu, Joseph C. LaManna,
and Michelle A. Puchowicz

Abstract

Hypoxia inducible factor alpha (HIF1α) is associated with neuroprotection conferred by diet-induced ketosis, but the underlying mechanism remains unclear. In this study, we use a ketogenic diet in rodents to induce a metabolic state of chronic ketosis, as measured by elevated blood ketone bodies. Chronic ketosis correlates with neuroprotection in both aged and following focal cerebral ischemia and reperfusion (via middle cerebral artery occlusion, MCAO) in mouse and rat models. Ketone bodies are known to be used efficiently by the brain, and metabolism of ketone bodies is associated with increased cytosolic succinate levels that inhibits prolyl hydroxylases allowing HIF1α to accumulate. Ketosis also regulates inflammatory pathways, and HIF1α is reported to be essential for gene expression of interleukin 10 (IL10). Therefore, we hypothesized that ketosis-stabilized HIF1α modulates the expression of inflammatory cytokines orchestrating neuroprotection. To test changes in cytokine levels in rodent brain, 8-week-rats were fed either the standard chow diet (SD) or the KG diet for 4 weeks before ischemia experiments (MCAO) were performed and the brain tissues were collected. Consistent with our hypothesis, immunoblotting analysis shows IL10 levels were significantly higher in KG diet rat brain compared to SD, whereas the TNFα and IL6 levels were significantly lower in the brains of KG diet-fed group.

Keywords

Ketone bodies · Hypoxia · Hypoxia inducible factors · Cytokines · Ischemic reperfusion

A. Sethuraman · P. Rao · A. Pranay
Department of Pediatrics, University of Tennessee Health Science Center, Memphis, TN, USA

K. Xu · J. C. LaManna
Department of Physiology & Biophysics, Case Western Reserve University, Cleveland, OH, USA

M. A. Puchowicz (✉)
Department of Pediatrics, University of Tennessee Health Science Center, Memphis, TN, USA

Department of Nutrition, Case Western Reserve University, Cleveland, OH, USA
e-mail: mpuchowi@uthsc.edu

1.1 Introduction

The mechanism through which diet-induced ketosis confers neuroprotection remains unclear despite its clinical applications for over seven decades [1]. Studies have implicated ketosis in modulating metabolic profiles and inflammatory pathways [1–3]. The ketogenic diet (KG) is a high-fat, very-low-carbohydrate diet which results in hepatic production of ketone bodies due

E. M. Nemoto et al. (eds.), *Oxygen Transport to Tissue XLII*, Advances in Experimental Medicine and Biology 1269, https://doi.org/10.1007/978-3-030-48238-1_1

to elevated beta-oxidation of fats by the liver. Ketosis results in elevated blood ketone bodies (beta-hydroxybutyrate and acetoacetate; BHB, AcAc) which are alternate energy substrates to glucose and are known to be well utilized by the brain, especially during glucose sparing conditions [3]. Ketones are beneficial substrates during metabolic derangements of glucose metabolism such as with ischemia/reperfusion injury-induced oxidative stress. The KG diet is a well-established non-pharmacological approach to treat drug-resistant epilepsy in children and has shown promise in treating other neurological conditions such as Alzheimer and stroke [4, 5].

We have consistently reported that ketosis induced by KG diet or by local intraventricular infusions of BHB correlates with neuroprotection following focal cerebral ischemia and reperfusion (via middle cerebral artery occlusion, MCAO) in rat (Fig. 1.1a, modified [2]) and mouse (data not shown), respectively [1, 2]. The metabolic adaptation to chronic ketosis and the mechanistic actions of ketosis in the brain (globally and cellular) are multifactorial but not well understood. Prolyl dehydrogenase (PHD)-mediated oxygen sensing and regulation of hypoxia inducible factors have been well studied, but normoxic regulation of this pathway warrants further study. This study focused on investigating the potential mechanisms associated with normoxic accumulation of hypoxia inducible factor-1 alpha (HIF1α) in diet-induced ketotic rats [1]. Specifically, we investigated the role of KG diet on inflammatory responses as associated with HIF1α stabilization in preconditioned ketotic rat brain. We targeted markers of pro- vs anti-inflammatory cytokines (TNFα and IL6 vs IL10) in cortical brain of ketotic rat to determine potential neuroprotective mechanisms mediated by HIF1α.

1.2 Methods

Animals: Experimental protocols were approved by the Institutional Animal Care and Use Committee (IACUC) at Case Western Reserve University (CWRU). Male: Two separate cohorts of Wistar male rats (8 weeks old) were fed either KG (high fat, carbohydrate restricted; $n = 4$) or standard lab chow (STD; $n = 4$) diets for 4 weeks before performing either focal cerebral ischemia (by MCAO) and infarct measurements or tissue collections (brain and blood), as previously described [1]. Rats were maintained on a 12:12 light-dark cycle with their diets and water available ad libitum. Diet Protocols: ketogenic (KG; 89.5 fat %, 10.4 protein %, 0.1 CHO %; Research

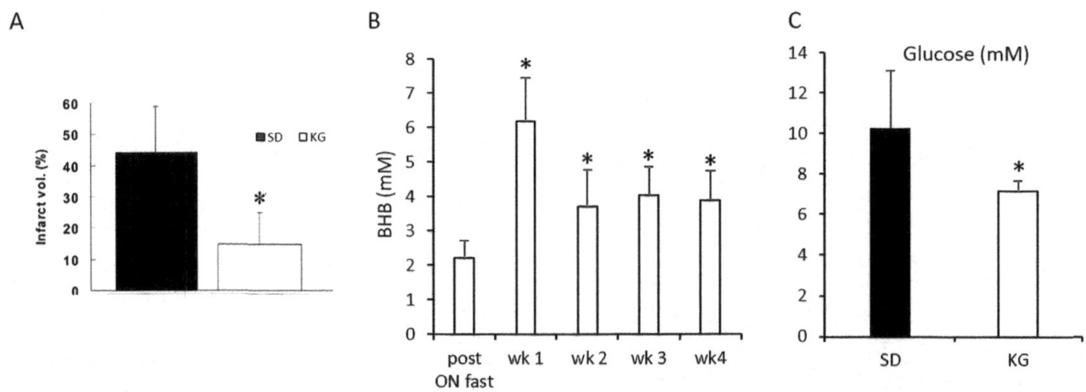

Fig. 1.1 (**a**) Infarct volumes in rat brains following MCAO were significantly lower in KG diet- vs SD diet-fed rats (modified from [2]). (**b**) Blood ketones (BHB) in rats fed with the ketogenic diet were measured with Precision Xtra® handheld keto-monitor. The blood ketone levels in KG-fed rats spiked the first week and stabilized in the following weeks. (**c**) Absolute glucose levels measured in blood plasma using GC-MS analysis show that glucose levels were elevated in the SD as compared to the KG diet-fed rats. The values presented are the mean ± S.E.M. ($n = 4$). * Denotes statistical significance ($p < 0.05$)

Diets, New Brunswick, NJ diet) and standard (STD; 27.5 fat %, 20.0 protein %, 52.6, provided by the CWRU animal facility). Weekly BHB concentrations were analyzed using a keto-meter (Precision Xtra, Abbott, Alameda California) from a small blood sample taken from the tail. *Metabolic Panels (Gas Chromatography Mass Spectrometry [GC-MS]-Based Analysis)*: Absolute glucose concentration (mM) was measured from blood plasma collected. The metabolite derivatives were assayed on an Agilent 5973N-MSD equipped with an Agilent 6890 GC system coupled to a DB-17MS capillary column (30 m × 0.25 mm × 0.25 μm) and operated in electron impact ionization mode [3]. *Western Blot Analysis*: Nuclear protein extracts prepared from cortical brain were immunoblotted using anti-HIF1α and anti-HIF2α antibodies and normalized to TBP, while the cytosolic protein extract was immunoblotted with anti-IL10, anti-IL6, and anti-TNFα and normalized to GAPDH, as previously described [6, 7]. Proteins were detected by chemiluminescence, and densitometric quantification was performed using ImageJ software. *Statistical Analysis*: All values were presented as mean ± SEM. Statistical analyses were performed using GraphPad Prism 7®. The comparison between any two groups was analyzed with a t-test for paired sample, two-tailed. Significance was considered at the level of $p < 0.05$.

1.3 Results

Blood Metabolites in KG and SD Diet-Fed Rats: Blood ketone levels in KG-fed rats spiked in the first week of diet to 6.2 mM and stabilized throughout the remaining weeks to an average of 3.9 mM (Fig. 1.1B). Absolute concentrations of plasma glucose were determined using GC-MS (Fig. 1.1C). Plasma glucose concentrations trended lower (but not statistically significant) in KG compared to SD diet group. *Diet-Induced Ketosis on HIF1α-Mediated Inflammatory Response*: Immunoblotting results (Fig. 1.2) show significantly higher protein levels of HIF1α in cortical brain of KG rats compared to SD group, while HIF2α levels remained unchanged between groups. Consistent with our hypothesis, IL10 levels were significantly higher in KG rat cortical brain compared to SD, while the TNFα and IL6 levels were significantly lower in KG group (Fig. 1.2B).

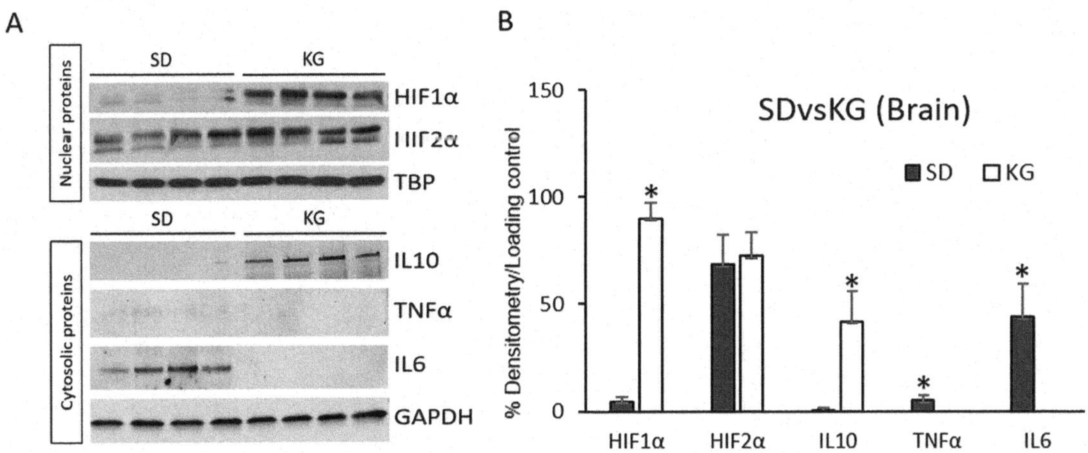

Fig. 1.2 (**a**) Western blot analysis of HIF1α, HIF2α, and cytokines IL10, TNFα, and IL6. HIF1α and HIF2α protein levels were normalized to TATA-box binding protein (TBP) loading control, while IL10, TNFα, and IL6 were normalized to GAPDH. (**b**) HIF2α protein levels remain unchanged, but HIF1α was significantly higher in KG rat brain. Expression of anti-inflammatory cytokine IL10 was significantly higher in KG brain, while no expression of pro-inflammatory cytokines IL6 and TNFα was observed. The values presented are the mean ± S.E.M. ($n = 4$). * Denotes statistical significance ($p < 0.05$)

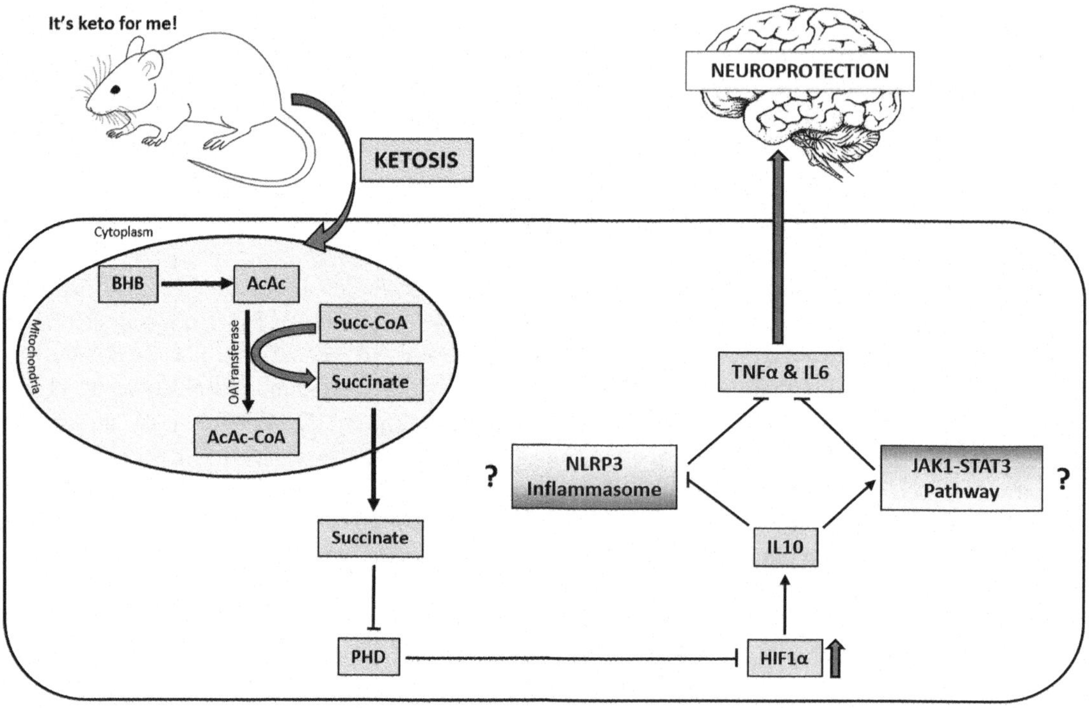

Fig. 1.3 Schematic model of our conclusion and future direction. Utilization of ketone bodies generated by metabolism of ketogenic diet as energy source causes accumulation of succinate on a cellular level in rat brains, which in turn inhibits prolyl hydroxylases resulting in accumulation of HIF1α. IL10, in turn, causes a downregulation of pro-inflammatory cytokines TNFα and IL6, leading to a neuroprotective phenotype. Further studies are needed to delineate the pathways involved in this downregulation (abbreviations used: AcAc, acetoacetate; BHB, β-hydroxybutyrate; CoA, coenzyme A; PHD, prolyl dehydrogenase; and Succ-CoA, succinyl-CoA)

1.4 Discussion

In this study, we show that normoxic stabilization of HIF1α in cortical ketotic rat brain is associated with modification of inflammatory cytokines which could confer neuroprotection following ischemic injury.

Diet-induced stabilization of HIF1α in rodent brain under normoxic ketotic conditions has been previously shown by Puchowicz et al. [1–3]. HIF1α can transcriptionally regulate IL10 levels by direct binding to hypoxia-responsive elements (HREs) on the IL10 promoter [8]. Further, overexpression of IL10 in mice has been associated with a resistance to ischemic injury (MCAO) [9]. Our study brings together ketosis-mediated stabilization of HIF1α and a potential neuroprotective phenotype in rats via IL10-mediated regulation of inflammatory cytokines. The inverse relationship we observe with HIF1α and IL6 levels has also been observed in a study by Schaefer et al. They reported HIF1α protein levels were higher under sustained hypoxia with a significant reduction in both mRNA and protein levels of IL6 [10].

IL10-meditated inflammatory pathways have been extensively studied for its implications in the design of targeted approaches aiming at controlling deleterious inflammation in the brain [11]. Our study connects to IL10-mediated immune regulation through downregulation of pro-inflammatory cytokines. One potential mechanism for this downregulation is via attenuation of the NLRP3 inflammasome as reported by Kanneganti et al. [12], thereby suspending activation of downstream pro-inflammatory cytokines like IL6 and TNFα. Secondly, IL10 receptor activation has been shown to specifically activate the JAK1-STAT3-mediated downregulation of pro-inflammatory cytokines [13]. Further, IL10-JAK1-STAT3 pathway has been described as the negative regulator of inflammation that controls both the degree and duration of inflammation [14].

Figure 1.3 is a scheme of our model system; it depicts the mechanism for HIF1α stabilization by KG diet is through cellular metabolic redox signaling within the mitochondria. Specifically, succinate is an intermediate of ketone body catabolism which is generated at the level of the citric acid cycle following activation of AcAc to AcAc-CoA as coupled to the conversion of succinyl-CoA to succinate via CoA-transferase (OAT). To maintain metabolic redox, succinate is transported out of the mitochondria into cytosol where it acts to inhibit prolyl hydroxylases (PHD), thus resulting in HIF1α accumulation. Lastly, the molecular pathway involved in HIF1α-mediated downregulation of pro-inflammatory cytokines (IL6 and TNFα) is via IL10-mediated attenuation of the NLRP3 inflammasome or via IL10/JAK1/STAT3-mediated transcriptional attenuation. Thus, neuroprotection by ketosis involves modulation of the inflammatory response in the rat brain.

Acknowledgments This study was supported by NIH grant R01 NS 38632; Mouse Metabolic Phenotyping Consortium (*P&F 20497-21, MMPC*).

References

1. Puchowicz MA, Zechel JL, Valerio J et al (2008) Neuroprotection in diet-induced ketotic rat brain after focal ischemia. J Cereb Blood Flow Metab 28(12):1907–1916
2. Xu K, Ye L, Sharma K et al (2017) Diet-induced ketosis protects against focal cerebral ischemia in mouse. Adv Exp Med Biol 977:205–213
3. Zhang Y, Xu K, Kerwin T et al (2018) Impact of aging on metabolic changes in the ketotic rat brain: glucose, oxidative and 4-HNE metabolism. Adv Exp Med Biol 1072:21–25
4. Gasior M, Rogawski MA, Hartman AL (2006) Neuroprotective and disease-modifying effects of the ketogenic diet. Behav Pharmacol 17(5–6):431–439
5. Gibson CL, Murphy AN, Murphy SP (2012) Stroke outcome in the ketogenic state – a systematic review of the animal data. J Neurochem 123(Suppl 2):52–57
6. Sethuraman A, Brown M, Seagroves TN et al (2016) SMARCE1 regulates metastatic potential of breast cancer cells through the HIF1A/PTK2 pathway. Breast Cancer Res 18(1):81
7. Sethuraman A, Brown M, Krutilina R et al (2018) BHLHE40 confers a pro-survival and pro-metastatic phenotype to breast cancer cells by modulating HBEGF secretion. Breast Cancer Res 20(1):117
8. Cai Z, Luo W, Zhan H et al (2013) Hypoxia-inducible factor 1 is required for remote ischemic preconditioning of the heart. Proc Natl Acad Sci U S A 110(43):17462–17467
9. Garcia JM, Stillings SA, Leclerc JL et al (2017) Role of Interleukin-10 in acute brain injuries. Front Neurol 8:244
10. Schaefer E, Wu W, Mark C et al (2017) Intermittent hypoxia is a proinflammatory stimulus resulting in IL-6 expression and M1 macrophage polarization. Hepatol Commun 1(4):326–337
11. Lobo-Silva D, Carriche GM, Castro AG et al (2016) Balancing the immune response in the brain: IL-10 and its regulation. J Neuroinflammation 13(1):297
12. Gurung P, Li B, Subbarao Malireddi RK et al (2015) Chronic TLR stimulation controls NLRP3 inflammasome activation through IL-10 mediated regulation of NLRP3 expression and caspase-8 activation. Sci Rep 5:14488
13. Verma R, Balakrishnan L, Sharma K et al (2016) A network map of Interleukin-10 signaling pathway. J Cell Commun Signal 10(1):61–67
14. Hutchins AP, Diez D, Miranda-Saavedra D (2013) The IL-10/STAT3-mediated anti-inflammatory response: recent developments and future challenges. Brief Funct Genomics 12(6):489–498

2 Event-Related NIRS and EEG Analysis for Mental Stress Monitoring

Labiblais Rahman, Katsunori Oyama, Atsuhiro Tsubaki, and Kaoru Sakatani

Abstract

Mental disorders caused by chronic stress are difficult to identify, and colleagues in the work environment may suddenly report symptoms. Social barriers exist including the financial cost of medical services and the lack of a perceived need for treatment even if potential patients have a desire to receive mental healthcare. Self-report inventories such as the Beck Depression Inventory (BDI-II) and State-Trait Anxiety Inventory (STAI) can assess the emotional valence for mental health assessment, but medical expertise may be required for interpretation of the results. Contingency plans for clinical supervision and referral sources are necessary for sufficient mental healthcare using self-report inventories. On the other hand, the laterality index at rest (LIR) has been proposed for evaluation of the mental stress level from near-infrared spectroscopy (NIRS) data in the prefrontal cortex in the resting state. However, the potential for long-term monitoring has not been investigated with sufficient evaluation results. In this study, feature values were extracted from both NIRS and EEG signals each week for 10 weeks in four young participants with an average BDI-II score of 17.7, i.e., indicative of mild depression. Temporal changes in LIR and heart rate (HR) were compared with STAI-Y1 and BDI-II scores. We found cross-correlations between the time series of LIR and STAI-Y1 within one-week delay. In addition, the time series of LIR was also correlated with BDI-II with one-week delay. Importantly, by annotating the larger changes in LIR and HR on daily life events, the changes in LIR and HR were different depending on the type of life event that affected these moods.

Keywords

NIRS · Mood disorder · Health monitoring · Laterality index at rest

L. Rahman
Graduate School of Computer Science, Nihon University, Tokyo, Japan

K. Oyama (✉)
Department of Computer Science, College of Engineering, Nihon University, Tokyo, Japan
e-mail: oyama.katsunori@nihon-u.ac.jp

A. Tsubaki
Institute for Human Movement and Medical Sciences, Niigata University of Health and Welfare, Niigata, Japan

K. Sakatani
Department of Human and Engineered Environmental Studies, The University of Tokyo, Tokyo, Japan

E. M. Nemoto et al. (eds.), *Oxygen Transport to Tissue XLII*, Advances in Experimental Medicine and Biology 1269, https://doi.org/10.1007/978-3-030-48238-1_2

2.1 Introduction

For health monitoring, near-infrared spectroscopy (NIRS) can be used to monitor the hemodynamic response to mental stress for early detection of unusual changes related to various types of illnesses. Recent studies have identified the prefrontal cortex (PFC) as a key region that is involved in the experience and regulation of emotional responses [1]. State anxiety (STAI-Y1), a subscale of the State-Trait Anxiety Inventory, is one of the useful inventories for tracking changes of the emotional valence for health monitoring. STAI-Y1 ranges between 20 and 80 with 20 questions. STAI-Y1 can be estimated from the laterality index at rest (LIR) of oxyhemoglobin concentration changes using a machine learning algorithm [2]. LIR was originally developed for objective assessment of mental stress levels by measuring changes in the hemoglobin concentration in the bilateral PFCs at rest [3, 4]. LIR can also be applied from the laterality of electroencephalogram (EEG) alpha-band powers in the bilateral PFCs at rest, which is known as frontal alpha asymmetry (FAA). A recent finding from an EEG study is that FAA is conditionally correlated with the Beck Depression Inventory (BDI-II) score [5]. The BDI-II score ranges from 0 to 63 with 21 questions, and each question is assigned with four answers marked as 0 through 3.

However, LIR has rarely been applied for assessment of daily changes in emotional valence, due to the burden of using NIRS equipment or EEG sensors for a long period of time. The values of LIR extracted from the NIRS signals may be physiologically related to FAA and heart rate (HR), although these parameters have not been compared with sufficient conditions. On the other hand, self-report inventories such as STAI-Y1 and BDI-II are difficult to use with continuous monitoring of life events such as stress factors including major disasters and changes in human relations. These self-report inventories are not designed for checking such changes.

The health monitoring approach in this study aims to explore the potential of the periodic use of NIRS for long-term mental stress monitoring. The main contribution of this study is the application of LIR to find unusual changes in emotional valence, including depression risk and anxiety symptoms.

2.2 Methods

In this study, LIR needed to be obtained at an arbitrary time during the resting state. Therefore, calculation of LIR was automated by taking into consideration the temporal change for k seconds in the resting state (Fig. 2.1). Concentration changes in oxyhemoglobin during measurement of the right and left PFCs are assigned the variables $h_r(t)$ and $h_l(t)$, respectively. The values h_{r_min} and h_{l_min} are the minimum values during the measurement for k seconds. LIR for k seconds as the difference between the changes in hemodynamic responses of $h_r(t)$ and $h_l(t)$ is then averaged:

$$\mathrm{LIR} = \frac{1}{k}\sum_{t=0}^{k}\frac{\left(h_r(t)-h_{r\_min}\right)-\left(h_l(t)-h_{l\_min}\right)}{\left(h_r(t)-h_{r\_min}\right)+\left(h_l(t)-h_{l\_min}\right)}$$

FAA is obtained from the difference in EEG alpha power between the right and left frontal regions. In this study, the FAA is averaged during the resting state. Spectral powers between 8 and 12 Hz at the right and left PFCs are assigned to $s_r(t)$ and $s_l(t)$, respectively. In this experiment, $s_r(t)$ denotes averaged alpha power at a discrete time t in the electrode positions of FP2 and F4 over the right hemisphere, whereas $s_l(t)$ is the average alpha power in the electrode positions of FP1 and F3 over the left hemisphere. Each epoch to obtain alpha power is 60 seconds long, and FAA for k seconds is then averaged:

$$\mathrm{FAA} = \frac{1}{k}\sum_{t=0}^{k}\frac{s_r(t)-s_l(t)}{s_r(t)+s_l(t)}$$

In this experiment, we studied four young participants (two males and two females; ages between 23 and 26 with average BDI-II score of 17.7) as shown in Table 2.1, i.e., indicative of mild depression, who participated in this experiment at noon on every Monday, Wednesday, and Friday for

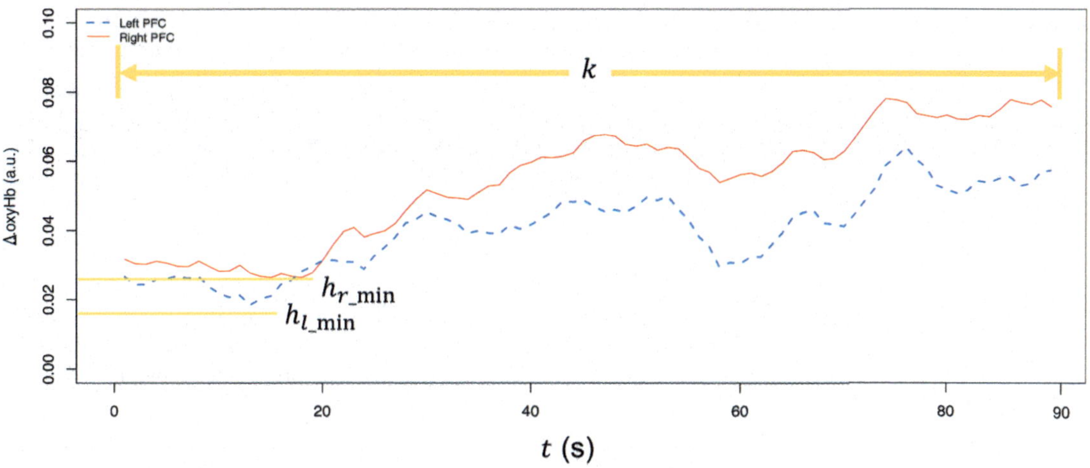

Fig. 2.1 Acquisition of parameters for extraction of the value of LIR

over 10 weeks. We evaluated the emotional valence for each participant using the STAI-Y1 and BDI-II tests. Recordable life events during the experiment, such as "trouble at a holiday party," were collected in their daily journals along with the results of BDI-II and STAI-Y1 tests. Before each measurement, the participants reported their body conditions, e.g., hours of sleep and meal time. We measured the changes in oxyhemoglobin concentration in the bilateral PFCs in the resting condition using a Pocket NIRS (Hamamatsu Photonics K.K., Japan). FAA was measured with Open BCI EEG sensors. Each measurement was conducted as follows: (1) EEG signals were recorded in the resting state with the eyes closed for 90 seconds, (2) then NIRS signals were recorded in the same manner, and (3) the participants filled in the forms of STAI-Y1 and BDI-II and wrote comments in their daily journal. HR data were measured throughout the experiment with smart watches (Fig. 2.2).

2.3 Results

Cross-correlation function (CCF) was employed for correlation analysis on the time series data from the experimental results. In this analysis, cross-correlation was calculated from the weekly changes of LIR, FAA, HR, STAI-Y1, and BDI-II. Note that these weekly changes were standardized by standard deviations to compare their temporal changes. From the experimental results, the changes in LIR and FAA were conditionally correlated with STAI-Y1 and BDI-II scores; however, depending on how the participants answered the self-report inventories, time lags of 1 week can be found as the correlation coefficients in bold shown in Tables 2.2 and 2.3. The changes in HR mostly followed after the changes in LIR and FAA. For example, the change in BDI-II score of Participant 1 is delayed nearly a week from the change in LIR, as shown in Fig. 2.3. Participant 1 had a BDI-II score of 20, which is on the border between mild and moderate depression according to the cutoff value of 20. LIR and FAA fluctuated during the life events such as "Trouble at a holiday party," as shown in Figs. 2.3 and 2.4. On the other hand, similar change patterns can be found after this period.

Participant 1 had a BDI-II score of 20, which is on the border between mild and moderate depression according to the cutoff value of 20. The values of LIR, FAA, and HR fluctuated during life events such as "Trouble at a holiday party." On the other hand, moderate changes were found during the life event "Winter break." Note that the values in Figs. 2.3 and 2.4 are standardized by standard deviations.

Table 2.1 Statistical summary: feature values (Ave. ± SD) obtained

	Age	Sex	LIR	FAA	HR	BDI	STAI Y1	# of sample data
Participant 1	23	F	0.099 ± 0.191	−0.046 ± 0.01	76 ± 16.5	20 ± 8	43.8 ± 5.1	24
Participant 2	26	F	−0.021 ± 0.221	−0.049 ± 0.041	99.4 ± 5.6	13.2 ± 4.5	49 ± 6.4	23
Participant 3	23	M	0.091 ± 0.208	−0.065 ± 0.026	85 ± 5.2	7.1 ± 6.1	43.3 ± 0.8	23
Participant 4	23	M	0.066 ± 0.203	−0.041 ± 0.028	93.9 ± 6.9	30.3 ± 2.2	40.4 ± 2.4	21

Fig. 2.2 Experimental protocol

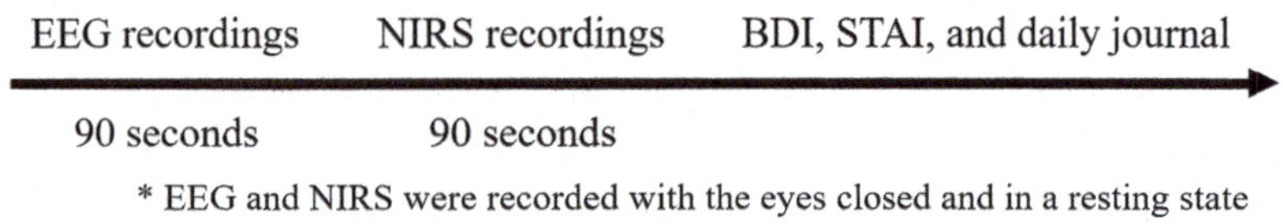

Table 2.2 Cross-correlations with STAI scores with time lags of 1 week

	LIR			FAA			HR		
	lag −1	lag 0	lag 1	lag −1	lag 0	lag 1	lag −1	lag 0	lag 1
Participant 1	0.29	0.22	**0.40**	−0.25	**0.49**	0.04	−0.18	**0.62**	−0.15
Participant 2	**0.57**	−0.52	0.40	**0.39**	−0.83	0.21	−0.24	**0.37**	−0.16
Participant 3	**0.33**	−0.04	−0.13	−0.34	**0.41**	−0.54	−0.63	−0.03	**0.34**
Participant 4	−0.06	0.18	−0.67	−0.32	**0.53**	−0.17	−0.31	**0.55**	−0.05

Table 2.3 Cross-correlations with BDI-II scores with time lags of 1 week

	LIR			FAA			HR		
	lag −1	lag 0	lag 1	lag −1	lag 0	lag 1	lag −1	lag 0	lag 1
Participant 1	**0.54**	−0.06	0.13	−0.13	**0.19**	−0.09	−0.24	**0.66**	−0.08
Participant 2	−0.49	**0.91**	−0.67	−0.18	**0.40**	−0.33	0.03	−0.28	**0.71**
Participant 3	**0.66**	0.19	−0.29	−0.32	−0.14	−0.03	−0.21	−0.05	0.18
Participant 4	−0.13	0.15	0.15	−0.32	0.01	−0.06	−0.15	−0.50	0.16

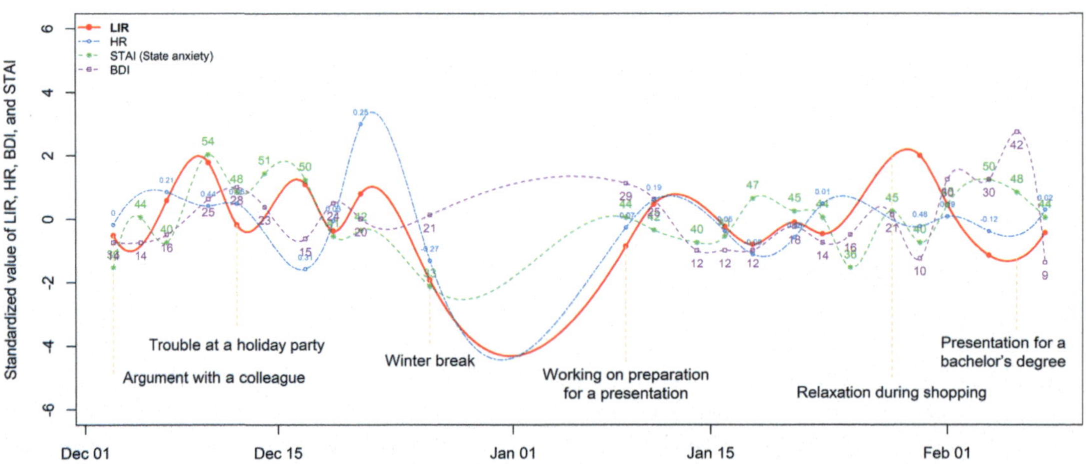

Fig. 2.3 Participant 1: Temporal changes of LIR to be compared with the feature values of HR, STAI-Y1, and BDI-II

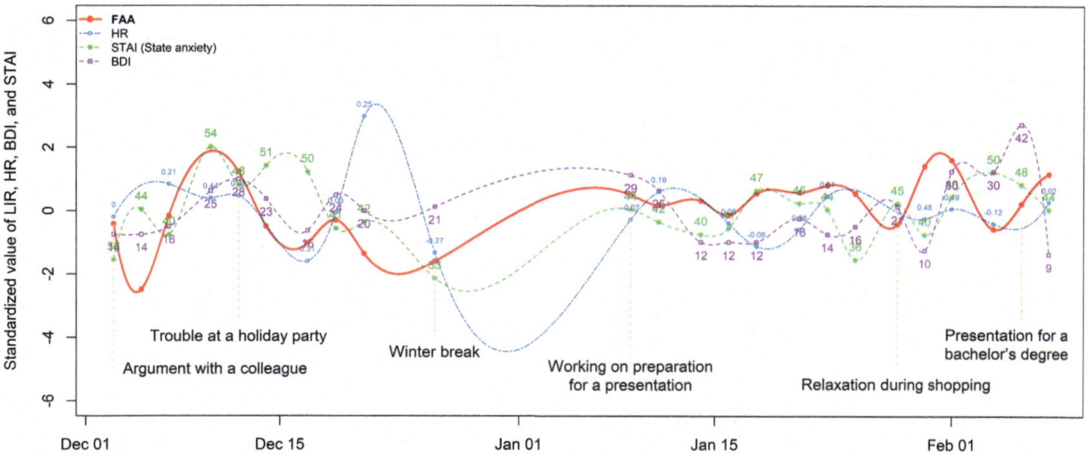

Fig. 2.4 Participant 1: Temporal changes of FAA to be compared with the feature values of HR, STAI-Y1, and BDI-II

2.4 Discussion

The experimental results suggest that both LIR and FAA can be feature values for assessment of daily changes in emotional valence; however, these results require further analysis with sample data obtained over longer periods so that a regression model can be developed to detect unusual change. This study was performed with the assumption that users can easily put on the wearable sensors in the home setting. In this experiment, NIRS signals were recorded just 90 seconds to extract the values of LIR, and we found that 90 seconds of measurement is sufficient in the home setting. Further improvement in the sensor equipment and measurement methods may have a large impact on the success of long-term monitoring.

In this paper, we discussed the applicability of LIR for the assessment of emotional valence. From the experimental result obtained with periodic NIRS recordings, LIR was compared with STAI-Y1 and BDI-II scores. We found cross-correlations between LIR and STAI-Y1 scores and between LIR and BDI scores. These observations provide rich information for the mental stress monitoring.

Future investigations will involve the development of a user-interface system that provides estimated STAI-Y1 and BDI scores for efficient health monitoring. The experimental results also suggest the potential for detection of unusual changes in emotional valence. Optimization of the method may eventually allow early detection of depression risk and anxiety symptoms.

References

1. Balconi M, Grippa E, Vanutelli ME (2015) What hemodynamic (fNIRS), electrophysiological (EEG) and autonomic integrated measures can tell us about emotional processing. Brain Cogn 95:67–76
2. Fukuda Y et al (2014) A Bayesian algorithm for anxiety index prediction based on cerebral blood oxygenation in the prefrontal cortex measured by near infrared spectroscopy. IEEE J Transl Eng Health Med 2:1–10
3. Davidson RJ, Jackson DC, Kalin NH (2000) Emotion, plasticity, cortex, and regulation: perspectives from affective neuroscience. Psychol Bull 126(6):890–909
4. Ishikawa W, Sato M, Fukuda Y, Matsumoto T, Takemura N, Sakatani K (2014) Correlation between asymmetry of spontaneous oscillation of hemodynamic changes in the prefrontal cortex and anxiety levels: a near-infrared spectroscopy study. J Biomed Opt 19(2):027005
5. Allen JJ, Reznik SJ (2015) Frontal EEG asymmetry as a promising marker of depression vulnerability: summary and methodological considerations. Curr Opin Psychol 4:93–97

Simulation Study of Breast Cancer Lipid Changes Affecting Membrane Oxygen Permeability: Effects of Chain Length and Cholesterol

3

Qi Wang, Rachel J. Dotson, Gary Angles, and Sally C. Pias

Abstract

Tumor radiotherapy relies on intracellular oxygen (O_2) to generate reactive species that trigger cell death, yet hypoxia is common in cancers of the breast. De novo lipid synthesis in tumors supports cell proliferation but also may lead to unusually high levels of the 16:1 palmitoleoyl (Y) phospholipid tail, which is two carbons shorter than the 18:1 oleoyl (O) tail abundant in normal breast tissue. Here, we use atomic resolution molecular dynamics simulations to test two hypotheses: (1) the shorter, 16:1 Y, tail of the de novo lipid biosynthesis product 1-palmitoyl,2-palmitoleoyl-phosphatidylcholine (PYPC) promotes lower membrane permeability relative to the more common lipid 1-palmitoyl,2-oleoylphosphatidylcholine (POPC), by reducing oxygen solubility in the interleaflet region, and (2) cholesterol further lessens the permeability of PYPC by reducing overall O_2 solubility and promoting PYPC tail order adjacent to the rigid cholesterol ring system. The simulations conducted here indicate that PYPC has a permeability of 14 ± 1 cm/s at 37 °C, comparable to 15.4 ± 0.4 cm/s for POPC. Inclusion of cholesterol in a 1:1 ratio with phospholipid intensifies the effect of chain length, giving permeabilities of 10.2 ± 0.2 cm/s for PYPC/cholesterol and 11.0 ± 0.6 cm/s for POPC/cholesterol. These findings indicate that PYPC may not substantially influence membrane-level oxygen flux and is unlikely to hinder breast tissue oxygenation.

Keywords

Molecular dynamics simulation · Hypoxia · Cholesterol · De novo lipid · Fatty acid biosynthesis

Q. Wang · R. J. Dotson · G. Angles · S. C. Pias (✉)
Department of Chemistry, New Mexico Institute of Mining and Technology (New Mexico Tech), Socorro, NM, USA
e-mail: sally.pias@nmt.edu

3.1 Introduction

Hypoxia is a common attribute of the tumor microenvironment [1]. Yet, tumor radiotherapy relies on intracellular O_2 to generate reactive oxygen radicals that damage DNA and lead to cell death [2, 3]. Thus, factors affecting the intracellular oxygen content of tumor cells are of interest for predicting and enhancing radiotherapy outcomes. This study addresses the possible influence of de novo fatty acids and cholesterol in breast tumors on intracellular oxygenation. Specifically, atomistic molecular dynamics simu-

E. M. Nemoto et al. (eds.), *Oxygen Transport to Tissue XLII*, Advances in Experimental Medicine and Biology 1269, https://doi.org/10.1007/978-3-030-48238-1_3

lations are used to examine membrane-level effects of lipid chain length and cholesterol on oxygen permeability, as well as solubility and diffusion within model membranes. Atomistic simulations enable precise control over lipid composition, along with subnanometer and picosecond timescale resolution. Prior simulation and experimental studies indicate that lipid compositional variations alter membrane oxygen permeability, as well as the pathway of oxygen diffusion [4–8].

The common membrane phospholipid 1-palm itoyl-2-oleoyl-phosphatidylcholine (POPC), or PC(16:0,18:1), has hydrocarbon tails that are well matched in chain length. Though its two tails differ in the number of carbons, the 16:0 saturated tail extends to roughly the same length as the 18:1 monounsaturated tail. Here, we use a conventional notation that specifies the number of carbons in the tail, *n*, followed by the number of *cis* double bonds, *x*, giving *n*:*x*.

De novo fatty acid biosynthesis is typically upregulated in cancers, and the new fatty acids are used to build membranes for cell proliferation [9]. Products of de novo lipid biosynthesis are unusually abundant in breast cancer cells [10]. In particular, the cell membranes of poor-prognosis breast tumors appear to contain high levels of the 16:1 palmitoleoyl (Y) fatty acyl tail, which can form 1-palmitoyl-2-palmitoleoyl-phosphatidylcholine (PYPC) [9]. The POPC and PYPC lipids are identical in structure, except that the unsaturated tail of PYPC is two carbons shorter than that of POPC. We anticipated that the shorter tail would introduce chain-length mismatch and, therefore, would promote tail interdigitation at the leaflet–leaflet interface. As such, the first hypothesis tested in this study is that the shorter, 16:1 Y, tail of PYPC promotes lower membrane permeability relative to POPC, by reducing oxygen solubility in the interleaflet region.

The study also examines the effects of cholesterol (chol) in combination with PYPC, as cholesterol modifies the free energy landscape of oxygen translocation in POPC and promotes oxygen solubility in the interleaflet region [6]. Cholesterol accounts for 20–40% of the membrane lipid molecules in most cell types and occurs at higher levels in the eye lens [8, 11] and in red blood cells (RBCs). The RBC membrane cholesterol-to-phospholipid ratio is typically 1:1 (50 mol% cholesterol) [12]. We previously found that POPC bilayer O_2 permeability decreases when cholesterol is enriched [6], and this finding is consistent with experiment [8]. The O_2 lipid–water partition coefficient (or relative solubility) is reduced roughly in proportion to the permeability decrease in POPC/chol [13], as predicted by Overton's rule [14]. Cholesterol reduces the solubility of oxygen within the bilayer, as a whole, but increases the solubility locally in the interleaflet region [6]. The second hypothesis tested in this study is that cholesterol further lessens the permeability of PYPC by reducing overall O_2 solubility and promoting PYPC tail order adjacent to the rigid cholesterol ring system.

The oxygen permeability and related properties are studied for PYPC alone and with 50% cholesterol. Comparison is made to POPC alone and with 50% cholesterol. The 50% cholesterol level (1:1 mixing ratio) was chosen because permeability changes were previously observed at and above this level [6, 8].

3.2 Methods

All-atom molecular dynamics (MD) simulations were carried out with graphics processing unit (GPU)-enabled AMBER code, version 14 [15, 16]. The Lipid14 force field, cholesterol extension, and TIP3P water model were applied [17–19]. The pressure was fixed at 1 bar using the Monte Carlo barostat with anisotropic scaling, and the temperature was maintained at 310 K using the Langevin thermostat with a collision frequency of 1 ps^{-1}. Bonds to hydrogen were constrained with SHAKE [6]. The simulation timestep was 2 fs, with coordinates written every 1 ps. Periodic boundary conditions were applied, and particle-mesh Ewald was used to calculate nonbonding interactions, with a cutoff distance of 10 Å.

Four simulation systems were constructed: PYPC, POPC, PYPC/chol (1:1 mixing ratio, or 50 mol% cholesterol), and POPC/chol.

Table 3.1 Simulation system composition (number of molecules or lipids per leaflet), bilayer area, and headgroup-to-headgroup thickness from calculated electron density curves, D_{HH}

System	POPC	Cholesterol	Water	O_2	Area (Å^2)	D_{HH} (Å)
POPC	64/64	0/0	4460	20	4080 ± 90	38.5
PYPC	64/64	0/0	4460	20	3960 ± 80	37.3
POPC/chol	32/32	32/32	4460	20	2690 ± 30	45.5
PYPC/chol	32/32	32/32	4460	20	2640 ± 20	45.8

Compositional details are provided in Table 3.1. As in other recent work, statistical sampling was enhanced by augmenting the O_2 concentration to reach 110–140 mM averaged over the whole system [5, 6]. Equilibration was conducted over 150 ns for the systems without cholesterol and 400 ns for those with cholesterol (to facilitate lipid mixing). Subsequent production simulations of 300 ns were the basis of all data analysis reported. Each system was simulated in duplicate, to enable assessment of convergence and estimation of error. Calculated values are reported as mean ± standard deviation, averaging over both duplicate trajectories and both bilayer leaflets in each trajectory.

The membrane O_2 permeability, P_M, for each system was computed from unrestrained simulations by tracking O_2 half-permeation events, as in our earlier work [6] but with a factor of 2 correction applied to account for O_2 entry via both bilayer leaflets under periodic boundary conditions. The resulting equation,

$$P_M = \frac{\Phi_{esc}}{4N_w}, \tag{3.1}$$

generates P_M by normalizing the frequency of O_2 molecule escapes from the bilayer, Φ_{esc}, by the average O_2 population in the water, N_w. Overton's rule predicts P_M to be directly proportional to a solute's lipid–water partition coefficient, K, and its diffusion coefficient within the membrane, D_M, but inversely proportional to the membrane thickness, h [14]:

$$P_M = \frac{K \cdot D_M}{h}. \tag{3.2}$$

Electron density and bilayer-depth-dependent free energy, $\Delta G(z)$, were calculated as in our earlier work [6]. Briefly, $\Delta G(z)$ was computed as the natural log of the depth-dependent O_2 lipid–water partition coefficient, $K(z)$:

$$\Delta G(z) = -RT \cdot lnK(z), \tag{3.3}$$

where R is the ideal gas constant and T is the simulation temperature.

3.3 Results and Discussion

Figure 3.1 provides images of the PYPC and PYPC/chol model systems, along with several plots of bilayer-depth-dependent properties calculated from the simulations. Included are electron density profiles, relative free energy profiles for O_2 (equivalent to potentials of mean force), and O_2 lipid–water partition coefficient profiles. Electron density is given here as an indicator of physical packing density as a function of the bilayer depth, plotted as distance from the bilayer center. The free energy profile reflects the relative favorability of O_2 occurrence at various depths and, in this study, is equivalent to a normalized log-concentration curve for O_2 (see Eq. 3.3). The partition coefficient profile is a representation of the bilayer-depth-dependent O_2 concentration, normalized to the O_2 concentration in the water layer. Table 3.2 provides bilayer permeability values calculated with Eq. (3.1), along with related physical properties, including a bilayer-average partition coefficient.

Incorporation of cholesterol tightens the packing of the lipids within the bilayer plane and causes the phospholipid tails to lengthen (Fig. 3.1b vs. a). These structural effects are reflected in pronounced changes in the shape of the electron density and free energy profiles (Fig. 3.1c, d), as well as in the lipid order parameter, $<S_{CD}>$ (Table 3.2). Earlier studies found

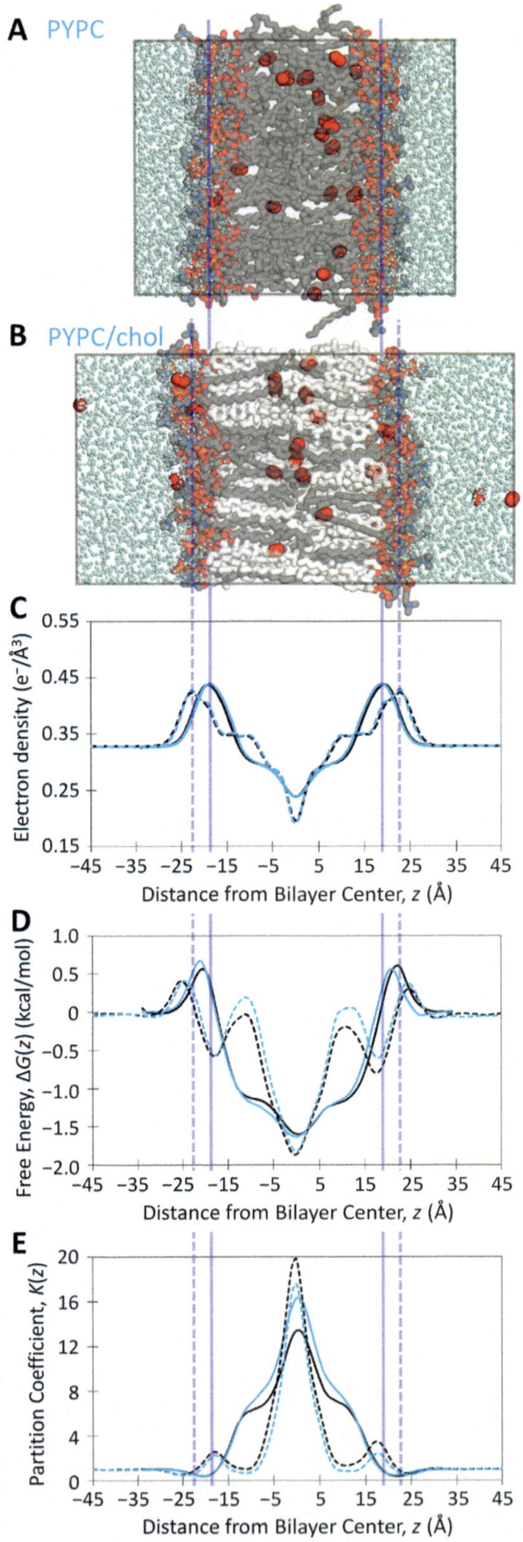

Fig. 3.1 Model lipid bilayer images, together with plots of bilayer-depth-dependent properties. (**a**, **b**) Simulation snapshot images for PYPC and PYPC/chol. Water molecules shown as cyan dots, lipids as gray bonds with headgroups colored by element, O_2 molecules as red spheres, and cholesterol as white bonds; all H atoms omitted for clarity.

Table 3.2 Bilayer physical properties: membrane permeability, P_M, permeation thickness, h, lipid order parameter plateau, $<S_{CD}>$, and average bilayer–water partition coefficient, $<K>$

Bilayer	P_M (cm/s)	h (Å)	P_M/P_w [a]	$<S_{CD}>$ [b]	$<K>$
PYPC	14 ± 1	56	0.31	0.203	5.3 ± 0.4
POPC	15.4 ± 0.4	56	0.33	0.204	5.3 ± 0.5
PYPC/chol	10.2 ± 0.2	62	0.24	0.395	3.5 ± 0.4
POPC/chol	11.0 ± 0.6	62	0.26	0.388	3.8 ± 0.2

[a]Permeability of a water layer of the same thickness as the associated bilayer, from $P_w = D_w/h$, where $D_w = 2.60 \times 10^{-5}$ cm²/s is the experimental diffusion coefficient for O_2 in water at 310 K (see Ref. [6]). Wherever h = 56 Å, P_w = 46 cm/s, and wherever h = 62 Å, P_w = 42 cm/s

[b]Calculated over 16:0 (*sn*-1) tail carbons 4–8, as in Ref. [23]. Standard deviation ~0.006

similar physical changes upon cholesterol incorporation [6, 20, 21]. The bilayer-depth-dependent electron density curves peak in the headgroup regions and are lowest in the bilayer center, regardless of cholesterol content or phospholipid type (Fig. 3.1c). Cholesterol incorporation generates an intensification of electron density along the region spanned by the rigid cholesterol ring system (flat zone starting ca. 17 Å from the bilayer center) and a sharp decrease in electron density around the bilayer center (0 Å).

The electron density profiles are nearly identical for the two phospholipid systems (PYPC and POPC, solid lines) and for the two phospholipid–cholesterol systems (PYPC/chol and POPC/chol, dashed lines). The free energy profiles (Fig. 3.1d) are, likewise, nearly the same for PYPC and POPC. Averaging the partition coefficient over the whole bilayer gives nearly identical values, $<K>$, for POPC and PYPC (Table 3.2).

As such, the free energy and partition coefficient data suggest that the permeability of PYPC should be the same or somewhat higher than that of POPC. Indeed, independent calculation of permeability, P_M, using Eq. (3.1) indicates that PYPC and POPC are equally permeable (Table 3.2). The error ranges of the two P_M values overlap. Both bilayers have permeabilities about one-third the permeability of an unstirred water layer of the same thickness (P_M/P_w in Table 3.2).

The free energy profile for PYPC/chol has more pronounced energy barriers than POPC/chol at the headgroups (ca. 25 Å from the bilayer center) and, more prominently, spanning the rigid cholesterol ring system (ca. 10 Å from the center). The increased magnitude of these barriers would tend to favor reduced permeability for PYPC/chol, relative to POPC/chol. Although the mean permeability of PYPC/chol is ~7% lower than that of POPC/chol, the calculated error ranges just overlap (Table 3.2), suggesting the difference may not be significant. The PYPC/chol free energy well is slightly less deep than that of POPC/chol, reflected in a diminished partition coefficient, $K(z)$, peak for PYPC/chol (Fig. 3.1e).

Depth-dependent diffusion coefficient profiles estimated from O_2 mean-squared displacements did not reveal any differences (data not shown). The bilayer areas and thicknesses, likewise, are similar (Table 3.1). Both cholesterol-rich bilayers have permeabilities about one-fourth the permeability of a water layer of the same thickness (P_M/P_w).

Ongoing work will address in more detail the possible roles of local diffusion coefficients, O_2 molecule residence time within the bilayer, and molecular void ("empty" volume) distribution. Limitations of the current work include imperfect O_2 and lipid force fields, which tend

Fig. 3.1 (continued) (**c**) Electron density profiles. *Legend for all plots:* PYPC (blue solid lines), POPC (black solid lines), PYPC/chol (blue dashed lines), POPC/chol (black dashed lines). Each curve represents one of two duplicate simulation trajectories. Vertical lines indicate the approximate bilayer depths of the headgroup electron density peaks and show corresponding depths among the images and plots for PYPC (solid line) or PYPC/chol (dashed line). (**d**) Relative depth-dependent free energy profiles for O_2, $\Delta G(z)$. (**e**) Depth-dependent O_2 lipid–water partition coefficient, $K(z)$

to exaggerate O_2 lipid–water partitioning and the POPC bilayer thickness [22], as well as a lack of physical experimental data for PYPC and PYPC/chol bilayers. Additionally, the bilayers studied here are highly simplified and lack the variety of lipids as well as proteins present in real biological membranes. Still, we find these simplified models useful for teasing out molecular physical influences on membrane oxygen permeability.

3.4 Conclusions

We have studied the effects of lipid chain length and cholesterol on bilayer O_2 permeability, to discern whether de novo fatty acid biosynthesis in breast tumors can modulate cellular hypoxia. The study indicates that the phospholipid PC(16:0/16:1), or PYPC, does not significantly reduce phospholipid bilayer permeability, relative to the more common lipid POPC. Cholesterol did reduce PYPC permeability by ~20% (after eliminating thickness effects by dividing by the permeability of a water layer of the same thickness). The permeability-reducing effect of cholesterol (at the level of 50 mol%) was equally effective for PYPC and POPC. Assuming that lipid bilayer permeability is a physical determinant of intracellular oxygenation, these findings indicate that increased PYPC abundance in breast tumor cells is unlikely to hinder cellular-level oxygen delivery.

Acknowledgments This work was supported by a gift from the Glendorn Foundation and by the National Institutes of Health under National Institute of General Medical Sciences grant P20GM103451. Lipid bilayer images were generated using PyMOL software [24].

References

1. Semenza GL (2016) The hypoxic tumor microenvironment: a driving force for breast cancer progression. Biochim Biophys Acta 1863:382–391. https://doi.org/10.1016/j.bbamcr.2015.05.036
2. Hou H, Mupparaju SP, Lariviere JP et al (2013) Assessment of the changes in 9L and C6 glioma pO_2 by EPR oximetry as a prognostic indicator of differential response to radiotherapy. Radiat Res 179:343–351. https://doi.org/10.1667/RR2811.1
3. Wondrak GT (2009) Redox-directed cancer therapeutics: molecular mechanisms and opportunities. Antioxid Redox Signal 11:3013–3069. https://doi.org/10.1089/ars.2009.2541
4. De Vos O, Van Hecke T, Ghysels A (2018) Effect of chain unsaturation and temperature on oxygen diffusion through lipid membranes from simulations. Adv Exp Med Biol 1072:399–404
5. Ghysels A, Venable RM, Pastor RW, Hummer G (2017) Position-dependent diffusion tensors in anisotropic media from simulation: oxygen transport in and through membranes. J Chem Theory Comput 13:2962–2976. https://doi.org/10.1021/acs.jctc.7b00039
6. Dotson RJ, Smith CR, Bueche K et al (2017) Influence of cholesterol on the oxygen permeability of membranes: insight from atomistic simulations. Biophys J 112:2336–2347. https://doi.org/10.1016/j.bpj.2017.04.046. PMCID: PMC5474842
7. Angles G, Dotson R, Bueche K, Pias SC (2017) Predicted decrease in membrane oxygen permeability with addition of cholesterol. Adv Exp Med Biol 977:9–14. https://doi.org/10.1007/978-3-319-55231-6_2. PMCID: PMC5673249
8. Widomska J, Raguz M, Subczynski WK (2007) Oxygen permeability of the lipid bilayer membrane made of calf lens lipids. Biochim Biophys Acta 1768:2635–2645. https://doi.org/10.1016/j.bbamem.2007.06.018
9. Hilvo M, Denkert C, Lehtinen L et al (2011) Novel theranostic opportunities offered by characterization of altered membrane lipid metabolism in breast cancer progression. Cancer Res 71:3236–3245. https://doi.org/10.1158/0008-5472.CAN-10-3894
10. Kuhajda FP (2000) Fatty-acid synthase and human cancer: new perspectives on its role in tumor biology. Nutrition 16:202–208. https://doi.org/10.1016/S0899-9007(99)00266-X
11. Mouritsen OG, Zuckermann MJ (2004) What's so special about cholesterol? Lipids 39:1101–1113
12. Jandl JH (1996) Blood: textbook of hematology, 2nd edn. Little, Brown and Company, Boston
13. Dotson RJ, Pias SC (2018) Reduced oxygen permeability upon protein incorporation within phospholipid bilayers. Adv Exp Med Biol 1072:405–411. https://doi.org/10.1007/978-3-319-91287-5_65. PMCID: PMC6202029
14. Missner A, Pohl P (2009) 110 years of the Meyer-Overton rule: predicting membrane permeability of gases and other small compounds. ChemPhysChem 10:1405–1414
15. Salomon-Ferrer R, Götz AW, Poole D et al (2013) Routine microsecond molecular dynamics simulations with AMBER on GPUs. 2. Explicit solvent particle mesh Ewald. J Chem Theory Comput 9:3878–3888. https://doi.org/10.1021/ct400314y
16. Case DA, Berryman JT, Betz RM et al (2015) AMBER 2015. University of California, San Francisco

17. Dickson CJ, Madej BD, Skjevik ÅA et al (2014) Lipid14: the Amber lipid force field. J Chem Theory Comput 10:865–879. https://doi.org/10.1021/ct4010307
18. Madej BD, Gould IR, Walker RC (2015) A parameterization of cholesterol for mixed lipid bilayer simulation within the Amber Lipid14 force field. J Phys Chem B 119:12424–12435. https://doi.org/10.1021/acs.jpcb.5b04924
19. Jorgensen WL, Chandrasekhar J, Madura JD et al (1983) Comparison of simple potential functions for simulating liquid water. J Chem Phys 79:926. https://doi.org/10.1063/1.445869
20. Pan J, Tristram-Nagle S, Nagle JF (2009) Effect of cholesterol on structural and mechanical properties of membranes depends on lipid chain saturation. Phys Rev E 80:021931. https://doi.org/10.1103/PhysRevE.80.021931
21. Ferreira TM, Coreta-Gomes F, Ollila OHS et al (2013) Cholesterol and POPC segmental order parameters in lipid membranes: solid state ^{1}H-^{13}C NMR and MD simulation studies. Phys Chem Chem Phys 15:1976–1989. https://doi.org/10.1039/c2cp42738a
22. Dotson RJ, Shea R, Byrd E, Pias SC. Optimization of an additive molecular oxygen model for membrane simulation studies. In preparation
23. Venable RM, Brown FLH, Pastor RW (2015) Mechanical properties of lipid bilayers from molecular dynamics simulation. Chem Phys Lipids 192:60–74. https://doi.org/10.1016/j.chemphyslip.2015.07.014
24. The PyMOL Molecular Graphics System, Version 1.7.6.5 Schrödinger, LLC

Updated Evaluation of Cholesterol's Influence on Membrane Oxygen Permeability

Rachel J. Dotson, Emily McClenahan, and Sally C. Pias

4

Abstract

There is a surprising gap in knowledge regarding the mechanism of oxygen (O_2) diffusional delivery at the level of tissues and cells. Yet, the effectiveness of tumor radiotherapy, the success of tissue engineering, and healthy metabolism all require ample intracellular oxygen. Tissue-level diffusion takes place in a complex and crowded macromolecular environment. Cholesterol-rich cellular membranes have been thought to reduce oxygen flux. Here, we use atomistic molecular dynamics simulations to update prior estimates of bilayer permeability and related parameters for 1-palmitoyl,2-oleoylphosphatidylcholine (POPC) and POPC/cholesterol bilayers, using a modified O_2 model with improved membrane–water partitioning behavior. This work estimates an oxygen permeability coefficient of 15 ± 1 cm/s for POPC and 11.5 ± 0.4 cm/s for POPC/cholesterol (1:1 molecular ratio) at 37 °C. The permeability of POPC is found to be ~1/3 that of a water layer of similar thickness, and the permeability of POPC/cholesterol is estimated to be 20–30% below that of POPC. Void pathway visualization and free energy data support channeling of oxygen toward the center of cholesterol-incorporating membranes, while partition coefficient data suggest reduced membrane solubility of oxygen due to cholesterol. Further study is needed to understand whether diffusion pathway changes due to cholesterol and other molecular compositional factors influence oxygen availability within tissue.

Keywords

Hypoxia · Tissue engineering · Hydrophobic channeling · Simulation · Void pathways

R. J. Dotson · E. McClenahan · S. C. Pias (✉)
Department of Chemistry, New Mexico Institute of Mining and Technology (New Mexico Tech), Socorro, NM, USA
e-mail: sally.pias@nmt.edu

4.1 Introduction

Oxygen (O_2) diffusion across cellular plasma membranes and among intracellular compartments is required for its delivery to tissues. Oxygen delivery in the diffusive regime is especially important where vessels are occluded, damaged, or shunted and where the vessel population is sparse. Clinical conditions affected by tissue-level oxygen diffusion include, for example, diabetic peripheral tissue hypoxia [1], as well as tumor hypoxia and associated radiotherapy resistance [2, 3]. Cell survival in engineered tissue constructs also depends critically on oxygen diffusion because vessels are generally absent and tissue thicknesses are often in the millimeter range [4].

E. M. Nemoto et al. (eds.), *Oxygen Transport to Tissue XLII*, Advances in Experimental Medicine and Biology 1269, https://doi.org/10.1007/978-3-030-48238-1_4

The rate of diffusive oxygen transport reflects the solubility and diffusion coefficient of O_2 in complex and crowded macromolecular environments. Available diffusion pathways include compositionally complex cellular membranes and protein-crowded cytoplasmic and interstitial fluids. Recent work by our group has focused on clarifying the influence of membrane cholesterol [5] and transmembrane proteins [6] on the kinetics and pathway of oxygen diffusion, using atomistic molecular dynamics simulations. This approach provides atomic resolution insight into the diffusion process, as well as enables calculation of thermodynamic parameters such as free energy.

We previously conducted a simulation study of cholesterol incorporation with the phospholipid 1-palmitoyl,2-oleoylphosphatidylcholine (POPC) [5], which is abundant in eukaryotic plasma membranes. Cholesterol, too, is a normal membrane constituent and typically occurs in the range 20–40% (of the total lipid molecules) in the plasma membranes of most cell types and ~50% in normal red blood cell (RBC) membranes [7, 8]. Our study tested the oxygen permeability effects of 0%, 13%, 25%, 33%, 50%, and 63% cholesterol in combination with POPC. We additionally tested 100% cholesterol bilayers as a mimic of the noncrystalline cholesterol bilayer domain observed in eye lens fiber cells [9].

The accuracy of POPC and POPC/cholesterol oxygen permeability and partition coefficient estimates calculated from the simulations was evaluated through comparison with experimental data [5]. These comparisons enabled identification of a flaw in the O_2 model, resulting in overestimation of the lipid–water partition coefficient by a factor of 2 or 3. Based on Overton's rule (Eq. 4.2, below), this overestimation is expected to result in proportional overestimation of bilayer permeability coefficients.

Here, we provide updated estimates of permeability and related parameters for POPC and POPC/cholesterol (50%), using an O_2 model with improved partitioning behavior [10]. In addition, we visualize dynamic void pathways in POPC and POPC/cholesterol (25% or 50%) bilayers. The 50% cholesterol level mimics the lipid composition of red blood cells [8] and eye lens fiber cells [11], while 25% is toward the lower end of the normal cholesterol range of 20–40% for most cell types [7]. Voids, or transiently "empty" volumes, are thought to facilitate solute transport through lipid bilayers. Several studies have quantified voids in phospholipid and phospholipid/cholesterol bilayers [12–15]. Here, time-continuous void pathways within the bilayers are visualized and discussed in relation to oxygen partitioning and permeability.

4.2 Methods

All-atom molecular dynamics simulations were conducted using graphics processing unit (GPU)-enabled Amber 14 biomolecular simulation software [16, 17]. The Lipid14 and ff14SB force fields were used to model lipids and proteins, respectively, along with the TIP3P water model [18–20]. Parameters for modeling O_2 were developed in-house and were the same as in our earlier work [5], except that some simulations here used an updated oxygen model in which the Lennard–Jones (LJ) well depth, ε, and interparticle distance of minimum potential energy, r_0, were adjusted to match the values used for the ester carbonyl oxygen atom type (*oC*) in the Lipid14 force field [18]. The updated oxygen model is designated O_2–L14LJ. The earlier model used LJ parameters based on the *o* atom type in the GAFF force field [21] and is designated "O_2–GLJ."

To test the effects of cholesterol on oxygen diffusion, simulations were carried out using lipid bilayers composed of the common membrane phospholipid POPC with varying levels of cholesterol incorporation (0%, 25%, or 50%). The simulation system compositions are provided in Table 4.1. Example simulation systems are imaged in Fig. 4.1, in Results and Discussion, which also illustrates the periodic boundary conditions applied in the simulations.

As in our earlier work, the systems were preequilibrated for a minimum of 700 ns [5], and the same preequilibrated bilayers were used as starting structures for simulations with both oxygen models. Each system was simulated in

Table 4.1 Simulation system compositions (number of molecules) and bilayer areas, A_{bil}

System name	POPC	Cholesterol	Water	O_2	A_{bil} (Å^2) Langevin	A_{bil} (Å^2) Berendsen
POPC	128	0	4445	35	4095	4142
25% chol	96	32	4447	33	Not applicable	3241
50% chol	64	64	4449	31	2698	2722

Mean A_{bil} from simulations with Langevin or Berendsen thermostat, standard deviation ≤12 Å^2

duplicate, with two independent 300 ns trajectories used for analysis and error estimation. The current simulations used conditions identical to our earlier work [5], except that the method of temperature regulation was varied here, as noted below. Briefly, the simulations were conducted in the isothermal–isobaric (NPT) ensemble, with the temperature maintained at 310 K (37 °C) and the pressure at 1.0 bar. The simulation time step was 2 fs, and the SHAKE algorithm [22] was used to constrain all bonds to hydrogen. The Monte Carlo barostat was used for pressure control, with volume change attempts every 100 steps. Temperature regulation was achieved using either the Berendsen weak-coupling thermostat [23] with a coupling constant of 1.0 ps, as previously [5], or Langevin dynamics with a collision frequency of 1.0 ps^{-1}.

The lipid bilayer oxygen permeability, P_M, was assessed by explicitly counting the frequency of O_2 molecule escapes from the bilayer at equilibrium, Φ_{esc}, and normalizing that frequency to the average population of O_2 in the water layer, N_w. Given that the goal was to assess permeability for oxygen *crossing* the bilayer (passing through both leaflets), the number of escapes is also scaled by 1/4 to adjust for counting escapes from both bilayer leaflets (1/2) following entry from either leaflet (1/2). The resulting equation incorporates a factor of 2 correction relative to our earlier work [5]:

$$P_M = \frac{\Phi_{esc}}{4N_w}. \tag{4.1}$$

Overton's rule predicts the membrane permeability of a solute to be directly proportional to the membrane–water partition coefficient, K_P, and the diffusion coefficient (diffusivity) within the membrane, D_M, but inversely proportional to the membrane thickness, h [24]:

$$P_M = \frac{K_P \cdot D_M}{h}. \tag{4.2}$$

For a given bilayer, the escape threshold used to obtain Φ_{esc} for Eq. (4.1) was half the thickness of the lipid bilayer, $\pm h/2$, and was determined as in our earlier study [5]. Bilayer-depth-dependent free energy curves, $\Delta G(z)$, were calculated as previously [5]. z is the dimension perpendicular to the plane of the lipid bilayer.

To visualize void pathways across the lipid bilayers, the tunnel analysis software Caver Analyst 1.0 was used [25]. Time series of simulation snapshots from our previous study [5] were analyzed for each bilayer in a series of ten consecutive frames, spaced 1 ps apart. Time-continuous void pathways were identified using a probe radius of 0.75 Å (~1/3 the radius of an O_2 molecule). This small probe radius generated continuous pathways, which were absent with larger probe size. Though we do not interpret the resulting tunnels to represent actual O_2 migration pathways, very small probe radii have been found to generate void volume fraction profiles [12] similar in shape to oxygen concentration curves [5]. Thus, we expect void pathways associated with the 0.75 Å probe to provide some relevant insight.

4.3 Results and Discussion

Figure 4.1 provides simulation snapshot images for the updated oxygen model (O_2–L14LJ) in hydrated bilayers of POPC alone or with 50% cholesterol (top), along with associated bilayer-depth-dependent free energy curves (middle). Void pathways are also imaged for POPC alone and with 25% or 50% cholesterol (bottom). Table 4.2 provides permeability coefficients, P_M, and related biophysical parameters, including

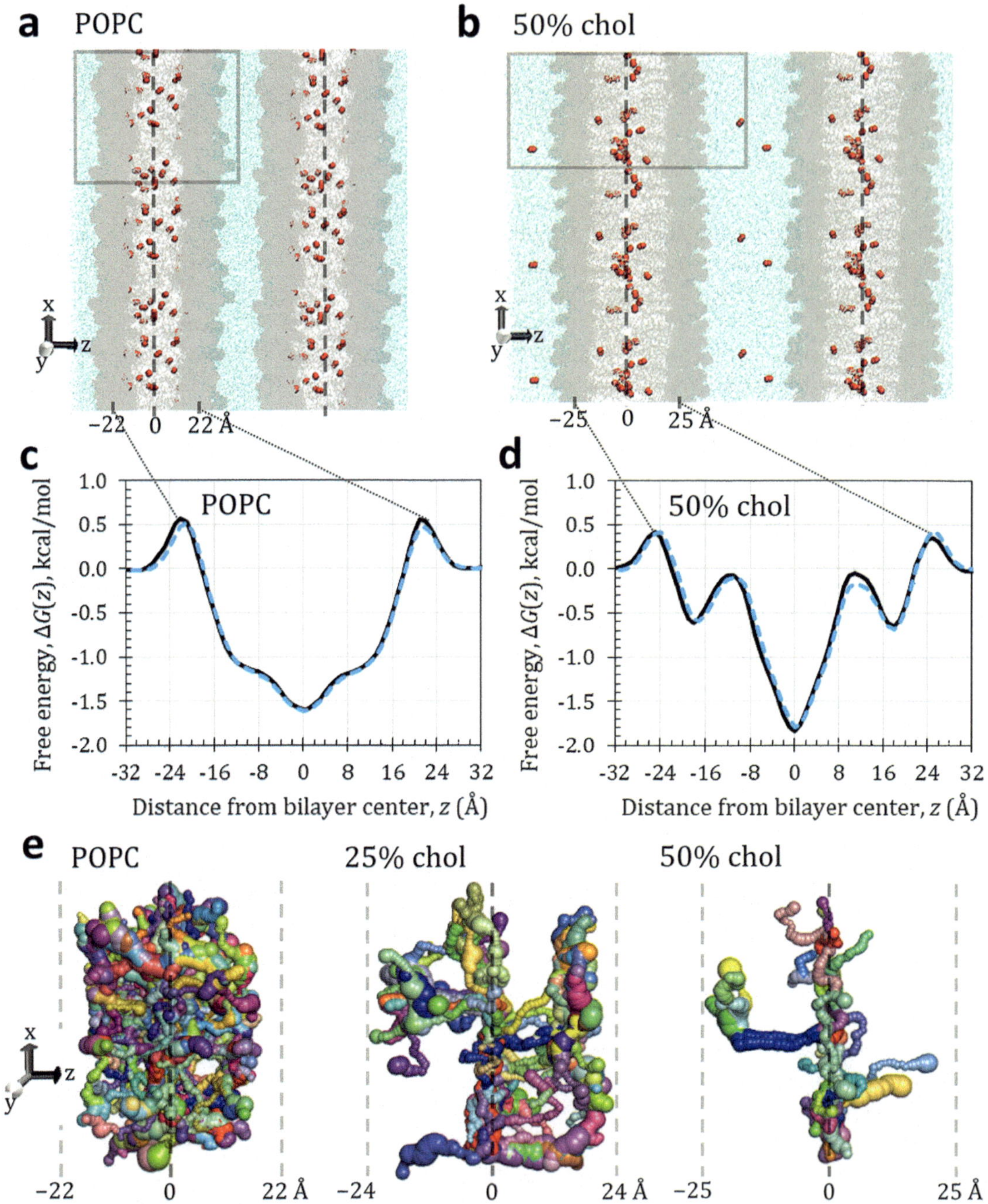

Fig. 4.1 (**a**, **b**) Representative simulation snapshots for POPC and 50% cholesterol, showing the primary simulation box (gray outline) with composition specified in Table 4.1 and adjacent images to illustrate the periodic boundary conditions. The simulation "sees" an infinitely wide bilayer in both *x* and *y* dimensions and an infinite number of membrane and water layers in the *z* dimension. O_2 molecules visualized as red spheres and water as light blue dots. POPC and cholesterol shown in gray (darker areas are POPC headgroups). Labels indicate approximate positions of bilayer center and headgroup-associated free energy barriers. Dashed line indicates bilayer center. (**c**, **d**) Relative bilayer-depth-dependent free energy curves for O_2 in POPC and 50% cholesterol, using the Langevin thermostat (black lines) or the Berendsen thermostat (dotted blue lines). (**e**) Void pathways within each bilayer, oriented as in panel b but displayed at larger scale. Shown are continuous pathways generated from ten consecutive

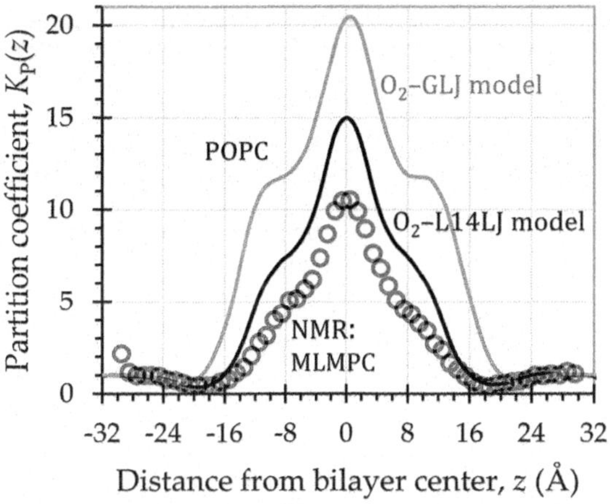

Fig. 4.2 Depth-dependent O_2 lipid–water partition coefficient curves, $K_P(z)$, showing improved partitioning for the updated O_2–L14LJ model (black line), relative to the original O_2–GLJ model (gray line). Circles represent $K_P(z)$ calculated from experimental NMR data [27], for O_2 in MLMPC at 318 K. Simulations used POPC at 310 K, with Langevin temperature control (collision frequency 1.0 ps^{-1}) and the Monte Carlo barostat

lipid–water partition coefficients averaged over all bilayer depths, $<K_P>$. Parameters calculated with the original oxygen model, O_2–GLJ, and the updated model, O_2–L14LJ, are compared. Our earlier work [5] used the weak-coupling Berendsen thermostat [23] to control the simulation temperature. Due to concerns of uneven temperature distribution with this thermostat [26], the current work uses Langevin temperature control preferentially. For completeness, Table 4.2 includes parameters calculated with both thermostats.

First, we note that the simulation snapshot images show concentrating of O_2 molecules toward the bilayer center in the 50% cholesterol system, compared with the POPC system, where the molecules are distributed more evenly throughout the hydrophobic tail region. The free energy curves reflect this shift, showing a narrower and deeper well flanking the bilayer center ($z = 0$ Å). The greater depth of the well in the 50% cholesterol curve indicates greater local lipid–water partitioning of O_2, as the free energy is proportional to the negative logarithm of the local partition coefficient. A similar narrowing is observed in the void-pathway image for 50% cholesterol and, to a lesser extent, for 25% cholesterol, compared with POPC.

The average O_2 lipid–water partition coefficient, $<K_P>$, of 3.3 ± 0.3 for the 50% cholesterol bilayer is lower than that of POPC, at 4.8 ± 0.1 (lower part of Table 4.2, bold type). Regardless of lipid composition, the $<K_P>$ values obtained with the updated O_2–L14LJ oxygen model are ~1.5 times lower than those in our earlier study with the original O_2–GLJ model (upper part of Table 4.2, Ref. [5]).

Figure 4.2 compares the bilayer-depth-dependent partition coefficient, $K_P(z)$, for the original and updated O_2 models with an O_2 partition coefficient curve calculated from experimental nuclear magnetic resonance (NMR) data [27]. It should be noted that the experiment used the phospholipid 1-myristelaidoyl,2-myristoylphosphatidylcholine (MLMPC) at 318 K, while the simulations used POPC at 310 K. Direct correspondence is, thus, not expected. However, the curves should (and do) match in general shape, and the maximum partition coefficient is expected to be similar. The comparison indicates improvement in lipid–water partitioning for O_2–L14LJ, relative to the original O_2–GLJ model.

Our previous study showed that addition of 25% cholesterol to POPC reduced the average lipid–water partition coefficient by 39% but did not reduce the bilayer permeability. An explanation for this result is not readily apparent in our data. It is interesting that the void pathways are substantially fewer in the 25% cholesterol bilayer compared with POPC and are more localized to

Fig. 4.1 (continued) trajectory snapshots spaced 1 ps apart (covering 10 ps of simulation time), using a 0.75 Å probe to identify empty volumes transiently devoid of atoms. Voids large enough to contain the probe are pictured as spheres, which are connected into pathways through occurrence of neighboring voids in consecutive snapshots. Sphere size represents void volume. Locally continuous pathway segments are distinguished by color. Labels and dashed lines indicate approximate bilayer-depth positions in ångströms

Table 4.2 Comparison of permeability and related biophysical parameters calculated with the original and updated O_2 models, at 37 °C with two different simulation thermostats

System	Thermostat	P_M (cm/s)	h (Å)	P_w (cm/s)	P_M/P_w	$<K_P>$
Original oxygen model, O_2–GLJ						
POPC	Berendsen [a]	26 ± 2	56	46	0.57	8.0 ± 0.5
	Langevin	21 ± 3	54	48	0.44	8.6 ± 0.1
25% chol	Berendsen [a]	24 ± 2	60	43	0.56	6.2 ± 0.1
50% chol	Berendsen [a]	21 ± 1	60	43	0.49	5.0 ± 0.0
Updated oxygen model, O_2–L14LJ						
POPC	Berendsen	20.5 ± 0.8	56	46	0.44	4.7 ± 0.4
	Langevin	**15 ± 1**	**54**	**48**	**0.31**	**4.8 ± 0.1**
50% chol	Berendsen	15.6 ± 0.8	60	43	0.36	3.51 ± 0.02
	Langevin	**11.5 ± 0.4**	**60**	**43**	**0.27**	**3.3 ± 0.3**

Values shown as mean ± standard deviation, where applicable. P_M, membrane O_2 permeability coefficient; h, bilayer thickness; P_w, permeability of an unstirred water layer of the same thickness as the respective bilayer, calculated as $P_w = D_w/h$, where $D_w = 2.60 \times 10^{-5}$ cm²/s is the experimental diffusion coefficient for O_2 in water at 37 °C (see Ref. [5]); $<K_P>$, lipid–water partition coefficient averaged over all bilayer depths

[a]Data in these rows from Ref. [5]. P_M values corrected by a factor of 2, as in Eq. (4.1)

subregions of the bilayer. This effect is amplified in 50% cholesterol, where very few void pathways span the leaflets and where the orientation of the pathways is distinctly perpendicular to the bilayer plane. The latter observation is consistent with the finding of Vattulainen and colleagues that cholesterol incorporation led to fewer voids, which were elongated and primarily oriented normal to the bilayer [13].

The Langevin thermostat is known to dampen diffusive motion, by increasing the apparent viscosity of the medium. For O_2, this effect translates to a downward shift of the bilayer-depth-dependent diffusion coefficient curve [10, 28] and an overall reduction of the diffusion coefficient throughout the simulation system. Accordingly, the membrane permeability coefficient values, P_M, are systematically lower for each bilayer simulated with the Langevin thermostat than the same bilayer with the Berendsen barostat (Table 4.2). Assessment of the updated O_2–L14LJ model indicates that the lipid–water partition coefficient remains overestimated (Fig. 4.2 and Ref. [10]). As such, with respect to the permeability coefficient, it appears there may be cancellation of errors due to underestimated diffusion coefficient and overestimated partition coefficient.

With the Langevin thermostat and the updated oxygen model O_2–L14LJ, the permeability is estimated to be 15 ± 1 cm/s for POPC and 11.5 ± 0.4 cm/s for 50% cholesterol (lower part of Table 4.2). These values are consistent in trend with those reported in our earlier study (Berendsen thermostat, upper half of Table 4.2) but are ~1.5 times lower in magnitude. The current permeability values are also consistent with values in another study in this volume for POPC alone and with 50% cholesterol at 37 °C, calculated independently using the updated oxygen model O_2–L14LJ, though the combined results suggest that the error bars should be somewhat wider than estimated in the current study [29].

The ratio P_M/P_w provides a useful, thickness-independent means of comparing the permeabilities of various bilayers. P_w is the permeability of a water layer of the same thickness as a given bilayer and here is calculated using the simulation bilayer thickness, h, combined with an experimental value for the oxygen diffusion coefficient in pure water. P_M/P_w additionally enables evaluation of the permeability of a given bilayer relative to the permeability of unstirred water. With the updated oxygen model, P_M/P_w indicates POPC to have ~1/3 the permeability of a water layer of the same thickness, compared with a somewhat lower value of 0.27 for 50% cholesterol.

4.4 Conclusions

This study provides updated estimates of the transbilayer oxygen permeability of POPC and 50% cholesterol bilayers. The permeability coefficients use a corrected equation and an updated simulation O_2 model, along with the more thermodynamically rigorous Langevin thermostat. The POPC bilayer, at 17 cm/s, is estimated to be about 1/3 as permeable as a water layer of the same thickness, while POPC with 50% cholesterol is estimated to be 20–30% less permeable than POPC. These permeabilities are expected to have a direct influence on transbilayer oxygen flux.

In a tissue-level diffusion scheme dominated by water-based pathways (interstitial fluid and cytoplasm), the membrane permeabilities calculated here would not be rate-limiting [5]. Membrane proteins have not been accounted for here but have been included in our recent work [6]. Their influence is substantial, yet we have no indication, thus far, that even protein-rich membranes would be rate-limiting for aqueous-dominated diffusion. It is important to consider, however, that experimental and theoretical evidence points toward lipid-mediated diffusion pathways [30]. In such a scheme, the radial diffusion coefficient [31] and interleaflet solubility of oxygen would likely play a role in determining the magnitude of oxygen flux to subcellular compartments within tissue. As such, further study of lipid-mediated oxygen diffusion and assessment of the permeability of protein-crowded aqueous fluids and membranes is needed.

Acknowledgments The authors thank Richard Pastor for helpful comments on the manuscript. The research was enabled by an IDeA award from the National Institute of General Medical Sciences of the National Institutes of Health (P20GM103451) and by a gift from the Glendorn Foundation. VMD [32] software was used to generate the simulation system images.

References

1. Cicco G, Giorgino F, Cicco S (2011) Wound healing in diabetes: hemorheological and microcirculatory aspects. Adv Exp Med Biol 701:263–269
2. Multhoff G, Radons J, Vaupel P (2014) Critical role of aberrant angiogenesis in the development of tumor hypoxia and associated radioresistance. Cancers (Basel) 6(2):813–828
3. Hou H, Dong R, Lariviere JP et al (2011) Synergistic combination of hyperoxygenation and radiotherapy by repeated assessments of tumor pO2 with EPR oximetry. J Radiat Res 52(5):568–574
4. Rouwkema J, Koopman BFJM, Van Blitterswijk CA et al (2009) Supply of nutrients to cells in engineered tissues. Biotechnol Genet Eng Rev 26(1):163–178
5. Dotson RJ, Smith CR, Bueche K et al (2017) Influence of cholesterol on the oxygen permeability of membranes: insight from atomistic simulations. Biophys J 112(11):2336–2347
6. Dotson RJ, Pias SC (2018) Reduced oxygen permeability upon protein incorporation within phospholipid bilayers. Adv Exp Med Biol 1072:405–411
7. Mouritsen OG, Zuckermann MJ (2004) What's so special about cholesterol? Lipids 39(11):1101–1113
8. Jandl J, Blood H (1996) Textbook of hematology, 2nd edn. Little, Brown and Company, Boston
9. Raguz M, Mainali L, Widomska J, Subczynski WK (2011) The immiscible cholesterol bilayer domain exists as an integral part of phospholipid bilayer membranes. Biochim Biophys Acta Biomembr 1808(4):1072–1080
10. Dotson RJ, Shea R, Byrd E, Pias SC. Optimization of an additive molecular oxygen model for membrane simulation studies. In preparation
11. Widomska J, Raguz M, Subczynski WK (2007) Oxygen permeability of the lipid bilayer membrane made of calf lens lipids. Biochim Biophys Acta 1768(10):2635–2645
12. Marrink SJ, Sok RM, Berendsen HJC (1996) Free volume properties of a simulated lipid membrane. J Chem Phys 104(22):9090–9099
13. Falck E, Patra M, Karttunen M et al (2004) Impact of cholesterol on voids in phospholipid membranes. J Chem Phys 121:12676–12689
14. Mahinthichaichan P, Gennis RB, Tajkhorshid E (2016) All the O2 consumed by Thermus thermophilus cytochrome ba3 is delivered to the active site through a long, open hydrophobic tunnel with entrances within the lipid bilayer. Biochemistry 55(8):1265–1278
15. Chipot C, Comer J (2016) Subdiffusion in membrane permeation of small molecules. Sci Rep 6:1–14
16. Case DA, Berryman JT, Betz RM et al (2015) AMBER 2015. University of California, San Francisco
17. Salomon-Ferrer R, Götz AW, Poole D et al (2013) Routine microsecond molecular dynamics simulations with AMBER on GPUs. 2. Explicit solvent particle mesh Ewald. J Chem Theory Comput 9(9):3878–3888

18. Dickson CJ, Madej BD, Skjevik ÅA et al (2014) Lipid14: the Amber lipid force field. J Chem Theory Comput 10(2):865–879
19. Maier JA, Martinez C, Kasavajhala K et al (2015) ff14SB: improving the accuracy of protein side chain and backbone parameters from ff99SB. J Chem Theory Comput 11(8):3696–3713
20. Jorgensen WL, Chandrasekhar J, Madura JD et al (1983) Comparison of simple potential functions for simulating liquid water. J Chem Phys 79(2):926
21. Wang J, Wolf RM, Caldwell JW et al (2004) Development and testing of a general Amber force field. J Comput Chem 25(9):1157–1174
22. Ryckaert J-P, Ciccotti G, Berendsen HJC (1977) Numerical integration of the Cartesian equations of motion of a system with constraints: molecular dynamics of n-alkanes. J Comput Phys 23(3):327–341
23. Berendsen HJC, Postma JPM, van Gunsteren WF et al (1984) Molecular dynamics with coupling to an external bath. J Chem Phys 81(8):3684
24. Missner A, Pohl P (2009) 110 years of the Meyer-Overton rule: predicting membrane permeability of gases and other small compounds. Chemphyschem 10(9–10):1405–1414
25. Kozlikova B, Sebestova E, Sustr V et al (2014) CAVER Analyst 1.0: graphic tool for interactive visualization and analysis of tunnels and channels in protein structures. Bioinformatics 30(18):2684–2685
26. Feller SE, Zhang Y, Pastor RW, Brooks BR (1995) Constant pressure molecular dynamics simulation: the Langevin piston method. J Chem Phys 103(11):4613
27. Al-Abdul-Wahid MS, Yu CH, Batruch I et al (2006) A combined NMR and molecular dynamics study of the transmembrane solubility and diffusion rate profile of dioxygen in lipid bilayers. Biochemistry 45(35):10719–10728
28. Gaalswyk K, Awoonor-Williams E, Rowley CN (2016) Generalized Langevin methods for calculating transmembrane diffusivity. J Chem Theory Comput 12(11):5609–5619
29. Wang Q, Dotson RJ, Angles G, Pias SC (2020) Simulation study of breast cancer lipid changes affecting membrane oxygen permeability: effects of chain length and cholesterol. Adv Exp Med Biol
30. Pias SC (2020) Pathways of oxygen diffusion in cells and tissues: hydrophobic channeling via networked lipids. Adv Exp Med Biol 1232:183–190
31. Ghysels A, Venable RM, Pastor RW, Hummer G (2017) Position-dependent diffusion tensors in anisotropic media from simulation: oxygen transport in and through membranes. J Chem Theory Comput 13:2962–2976
32. Humphrey W, Dalke A, Schulten K (1996) VMD – visual molecular dynamics. J Mol Graph 14:33–38

Systems Biology Model of Cerebral Oxygen Delivery and Metabolism During Therapeutic Hypothermia: Application to the Piglet Model

5

Joshua Russell-Buckland, P. Kaynezhad, S. Mitra, G. Bale, C. Bauer, I. Lingam, C. Meehan, A. Avdic-Belltheus, K. Martinello, A. Bainbridge, N. J. Robertson, and I. Tachtsidis

Abstract

Hypoxic ischaemic encephalopathy (HIE) is a significant cause of death and disability. Therapeutic hypothermia (TH) is the only available standard of treatment, but 45–55% of cases still result in death or neurodevelopmental disability following TH. This work has focussed on developing a new brain tissue physiology and biochemistry systems biology model that includes temperature effects, as well as a Bayesian framework for analysis of model parameter estimation. Through this, we can simulate the effects of temperature on brain tissue oxygen delivery and metabolism, as well as analyse clinical and experimental data to identify mechanisms to explain differing behaviour and outcome. Presented here is an application of the model to data from two piglets treated with TH following hypoxic-ischaemic injury showing different responses and outcome following treatment. We identify the main mechanism for this difference as the Q_{10} temperature coefficient for metabolic reactions, with the severely injured piglet having a median posterior value of 0.133 as opposed to the mild injury value of 5.48. This work demonstrates the use of systems biology models to investigate underlying mechanisms behind the varying response to hypothermic treatment.

Keywords

Broadband NIRS · Hypothermia · Systems biology · Piglet · Brain

J. Russell-Buckland (✉) · P. Kaynezhad · G. Bale
C. Bauer · I. Tachtsidis
Department of Medical Physics and Biomedical Engineering, University College London, London, UK
e-mail: j.russell-buckland.15@ucl.ac.uk

S. Mitra · I. Lingam · C. Meehan · A. Avdic-Belltheus
K. Martinello · N. J. Robertson
Institute for Women's Health, University College London, London, UK

A. Bainbridge
Department of Medical Physics and Biomedical Engineering, University College London Hospital, London, UK

5.1 Introduction

Hypoxic-ischaemic encephalopathy (HIE) is a significant cause of death and morbidity amongst neonates with around 700,000 deaths attributed to HIE alone annually [1]. Following neonatal HI injury, infants are treated with therapeutic hypothermia (TH) at a body temperature of 33.5 °C

E. M. Nemoto et al. (eds.), *Oxygen Transport to Tissue XLII*, Advances in Experimental Medicine and Biology 1269, https://doi.org/10.1007/978-3-030-48238-1_5

[2]. However, 45–55% of cases treated with hypothermia end with death or moderate to severe neurodevelopmental disability [1, 3]. During hypothermia, a close neuromonitoring is in place combining clinical electroencephalography (EEG) [4] and broadband NIRS [2, 5] as a research tool in the neonatal unit in University College London Hospital (UCLH). After completion of TH, infants undergo magnetic resonance imaging (MRI) and spectroscopy (MRS) [6]. The collected multimodal data has the potential to provide not only diagnostic and prognostic information but also insights on the mechanisms of the injury.

Our approach to analysis of this multimodal data has been multifaceted, with one key facet being the development and application of a physiology-informed "mathematical model" of the cerebral circulation under a systems biology approach, which is specially designed for the interpretation of bNIRS signals [7–12].

The first model BRAINCIRC was developed in 2005 [7]. This was later simplified and extended to include metabolism in 2008 via the BrainSignals model [8]. This was used to develop the BrainPiglet model [9], with the piglet being a common clinical model of human neonates. BrainPiglet was extended and used to investigate the effect of hypoxic ischaemia in the piglet model in the BrainPigletHI model [10]. Separate to the piglet models, BrainSignals was simplified further in the BrainSignals Revisited (BSRV) model to improve run time [11]. BSRV was extended to include extracerebral blood flow in BSX and looked at the confounding effects of the scalp on measurements [12]. Recently, significant work has been undertaken in developing the "BP Hypothermia" model (BPH1) which extended the BrainPiglet HI model to include temperature as an input [13]. This is needed to properly interpret data collected during therapeutic hypothermia. For example, it has been observed that both cerebral metabolic rate of oxygen ($CMRO_2$) and cerebral blood flow (CBF) in piglets decrease with reduced body temperature [14]. For reliable inferences to be made using systems biology models, they must be able to simulate this behaviour.

We present here an extended version of this model, BP Hypothermia 2 (BPH2), able to incorporate the effect of temperature separately for both metabolic and haemodynamic processes and reactions. This model is then validated against data collected from piglets undergoing TH following HIE.

5.2 Methods

BPH2 follows the same form as the original BP Hypothermia model [14], incorporating the effect of temperature by adapting work by Orlowski et al. [15]. Reaction rates, Michaelis-Menten rate constants and diffusion rates are modified by the quantities

$$k_{i,\mathrm{new}} = k_{i,\mathrm{previous}} \times Q_{10,\mathrm{haemo}}^{\left(T_{\mathrm{new}} - T_{\mathrm{previous}}\right)/10}$$

$$k_{j,\mathrm{new}} = k_{j,\mathrm{previous}} \times Q_{10,\mathrm{met}}^{\left(T_{\mathrm{new}} - T_{\mathrm{previous}}\right)/10}$$

where $Q_{10,\,\mathrm{haemo}}$ is the Q_{10} coefficient for haemodynamic reactions, $Q_{10,\,\mathrm{met}}$ is the Q_{10} coefficient for metabolic reactions, $k_{i,\,*}$ is the reaction rate for the ith haemodynamic reaction and $k_{j,\,*}$ is the reaction rate for the jth metabolic reaction at temperatures T_{new} and T_{previous}. Q_{10} is the temperature coefficient, defined as the ratio of reaction rates measured for the same reaction at two temperatures 10 °C apart. $0 < Q_{10} < 1$ indicates that decreasing temperature increases the reaction rate, whilst $Q_{10} > 1$ indicates that decreasing temperature decreases the reaction rate. Figure 5.1 outlines the structure of this model.

This model was then used to analyse data from two piglets, as shown in Fig. 5.2. Data was collected as per [16], with the piglets' common carotid arteries occluded for a period of around 25 minutes. Following HI, the piglets were treated with TH at 33.5 °C. HbO_2, HHb and CCO data was collected via bNIRS, whilst the thalamic lactate/N-acetyl-aspartate (Lac/NAA) ratio was measured at 24 hours using proton MRS. Piglet LWP475 suffered a mild injury with a 10-minute CCO recovery fraction of

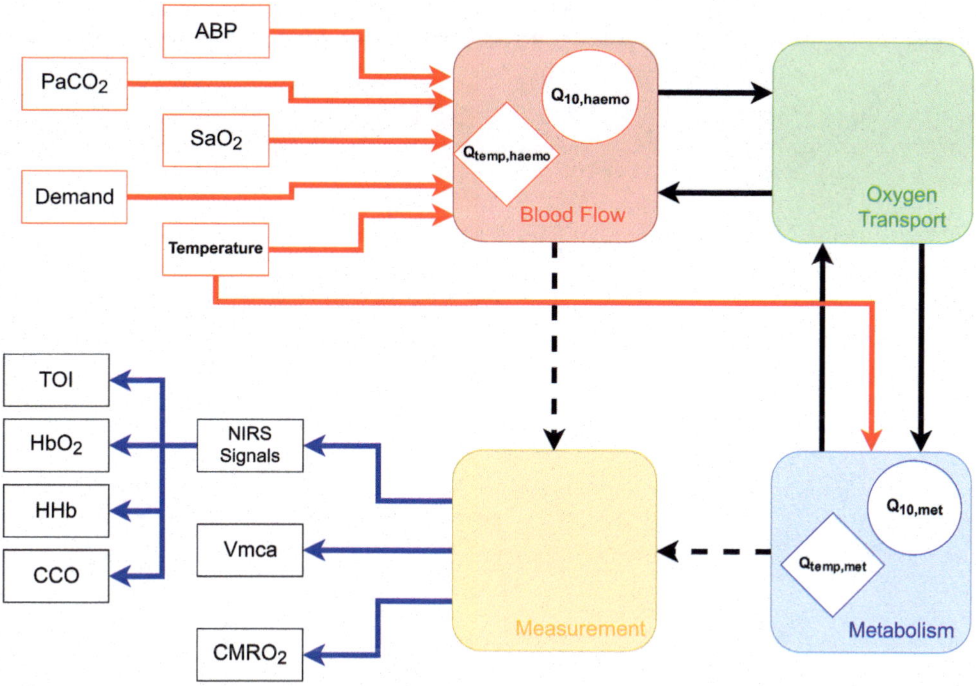

Fig. 5.1 General structure of the BrainPiglet hypothermia 2 model. Model inputs, arterial blood pressure (ABP), arterial oxygen saturation (SaO_2), partial pressure of CO_2 ($PaCO_2$) and demand, and outputs, concentrations of oxyhaemoglobin (HbO_2), deoxyhaemoglobin (HHb) and cytochrome-*c*-oxidase (CCO), tissue oxygenation index (TOI), middle cerebral artery velocity (V_{mca}) and cerebral metabolic rate of oxygen ($CMRO_2$), are shown, as well as each of the four sub-models and the general relations between each. New additions are shown in bold. Temperature is added as an input to the model. Parameter $Q_{10,\ met}$ and temporary variable $Q_{temp,\ met}$ are added to the metabolic compartment, and parameter $Q_{10,\ haemo}$ and temporary variable $Q_{temp,\ haemo}$ are added to the blood flow compartment

122% and a Lac/NAA ratio of 0.21 (Lac/NAA ≥ 0.39 [6] is associated with a poor outcome). Piglet LWP479 suffered a severe injury with a 10-minute CCO recovery fraction of 69% and a 24-hour Lac/NAA ratio of 1.03. Both piglets received TH with piglet LWP475 responding typically, as per [13], with increased HbO_2, decreased HHb and decreased CCO, whilst piglet LWP479 responded atypically with an "inverted" response in the bNIRS signals. Model analysis was performed using the BayesCMD framework [17].

Before performing model fitting, it is necessary to reduce the model down to manageable number of parameters. This is done using sensitivity analysis (SA) in order to identify parameters that control the majority of the behaviour we are attempting to simulate. We used the Morris method, summarising model output by the normalised root-mean-square error (NRMSE) between simulation and measured data. This was performed twice per model, once substituting the NRMSE value of failed runs with zero and once replacing it by 10,000,000. This was done to try and find a balance between including sensitive parameters that may produce failed runs and only selecting parameters that overwhelmingly cause failed runs. Failed runs should not be ignored completely as the reason a run fails is likely to be due to an invalid value for a highly sensitive parameter. Parameter count was reduced from an original count of 234 to a fitted count of 11, with this parameters shown in Table 5.1.

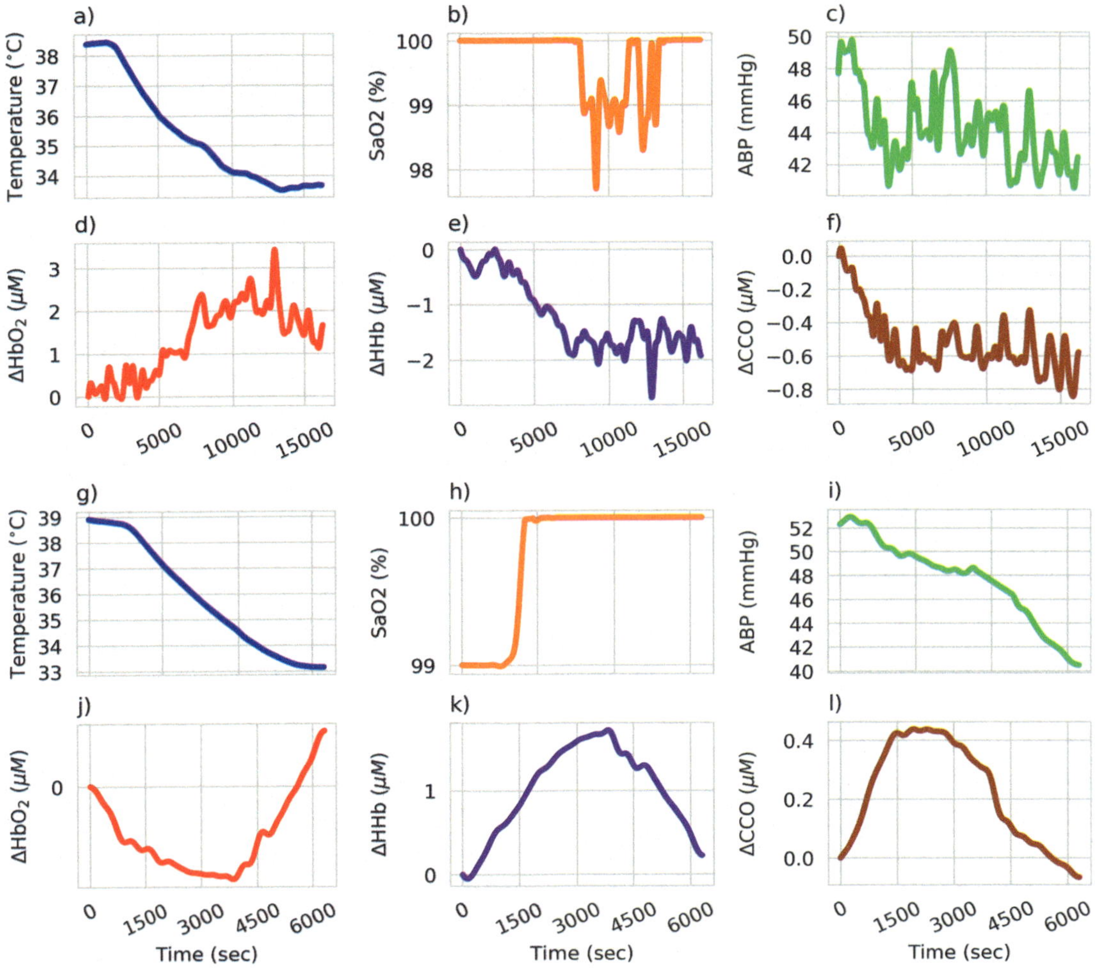

Fig. 5.2 Data for piglets LWP475 (**a–f**) and LWP479 (**g–l**). Measured data for piglets LWP475 and LWP479, showing the piglet response to hypothermia across measurable quantities

5.3 Result

Following this, posterior parameter distribution fitting was performed using approximate Bayesian computation via a rejection algorithm with a total of 50,000,000 samples. Each parameter was given an uninformative uniform prior distribution. The top 0.01% of parameter samples, based on NRMSE, were used to generate posterior distributions for each piglet giving a posterior of 5000 samples. These are shown in Fig. 5.3 with piglet LWP475 shown in blue and piglet LWP479 in orange. A distinct difference between the parameter spaces of the two piglets is clearly visible for $Q_{10,\,\mathrm{met}}$, $Q_{10,\,\mathrm{haemo}}$, normal oxidised fraction of Cu_A ($a_{\mathrm{frac},\,n}$) and the normal total concentration of HbO_2 binding sites in blood ($X_{\mathrm{tot},\,n}$), with $Q_{10,\,\mathrm{met}}$ showing the most obvious and potentially important disparity. For further information about $a_{\mathrm{frac},\,n}$ and $X_{\mathrm{tot},\,n}$, see Table 5.1 and [10].

Figure 5.4 shows the posterior predictive distributions for each piglet generated by sampling repeatedly from the posterior distributions shown in Fig. 5.3. The posterior predictive distributions are shown in blue and include a 95% confidence interval, whilst data is shown in green. The model simulations show good agreement with the measured data with only a small time lag between the model and data for the CCO signal in piglet LWP479. Importantly, the model can correctly reproduce the overall behaviour of the system in both piglets suggesting that the posterior distri-

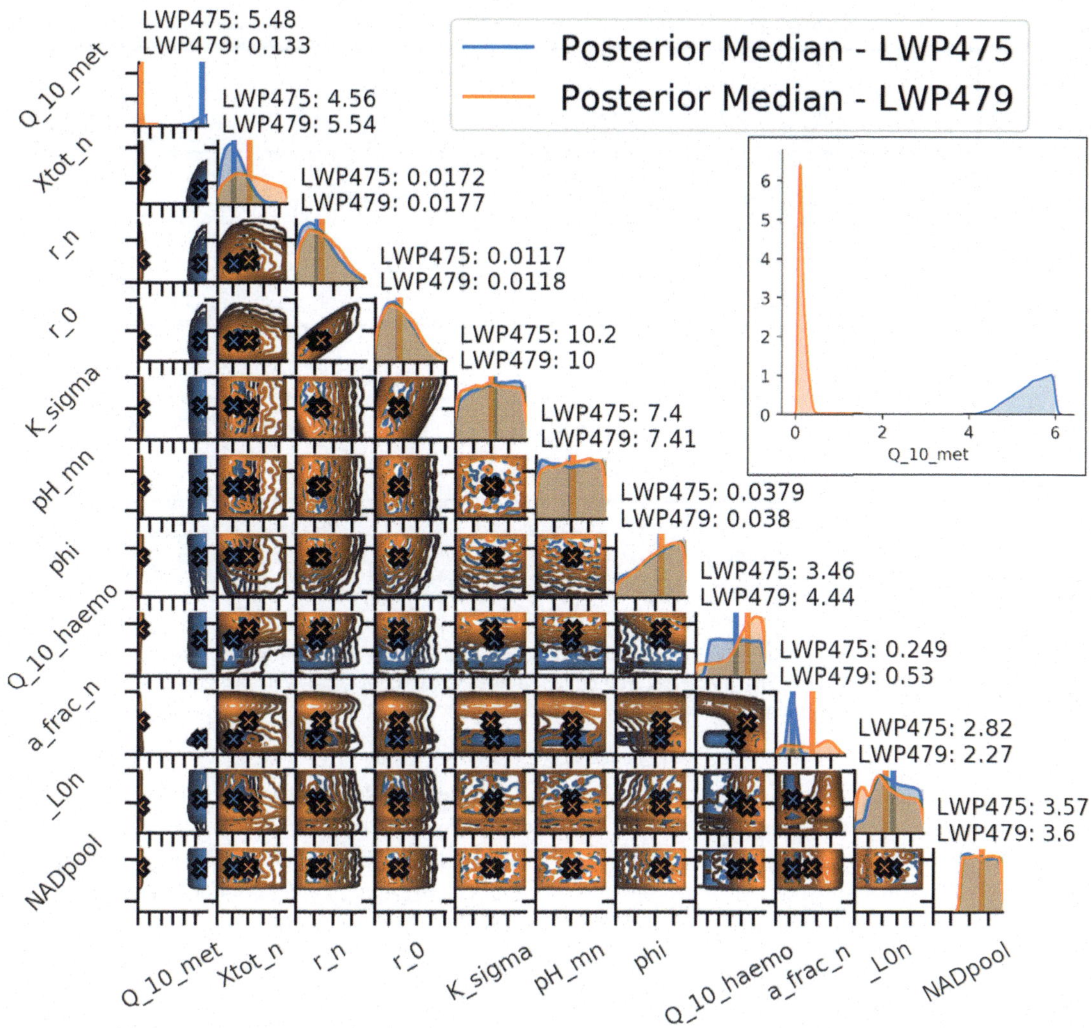

Fig. 5.3 Posterior parameter distributions. Posterior distributions of parameters with those for piglet LWP475 shown in blue and those for piglet LWP479 shown in orange. Inset are the marginal distributions for parameter $Q_{10,\ met}$. A distinct difference in the parameter value between the two piglets is clearly visible, with piglet LWP479 having a distribution of values well below 1. For more information about specific parameters, please see Table 5.1

butions produced in Fig. 5.3 are reasonably good indications of the mechanisms behind the difference in the measured responses to hypothermia.

5.4 Discussion

We have successfully expanded our model of hypothermia in the piglet brain to incorporate different temperature effects on metabolic and haemodynamic reactions. Additionally, this has been achieved without introducing excessive complexity into the model, adding only one new parameter as compared to the previous BPH1 model – Q_{10} is split into $Q_{10,met}$ and $Q_{10,haemo}$. This model has then been validated against data collected from two piglets suffering the same injury to differing levels of severity. Not only was this able to validate the new model but it was also able to provide some insight into the different haemodynamic and metabolic behaviour seen in both piglets.

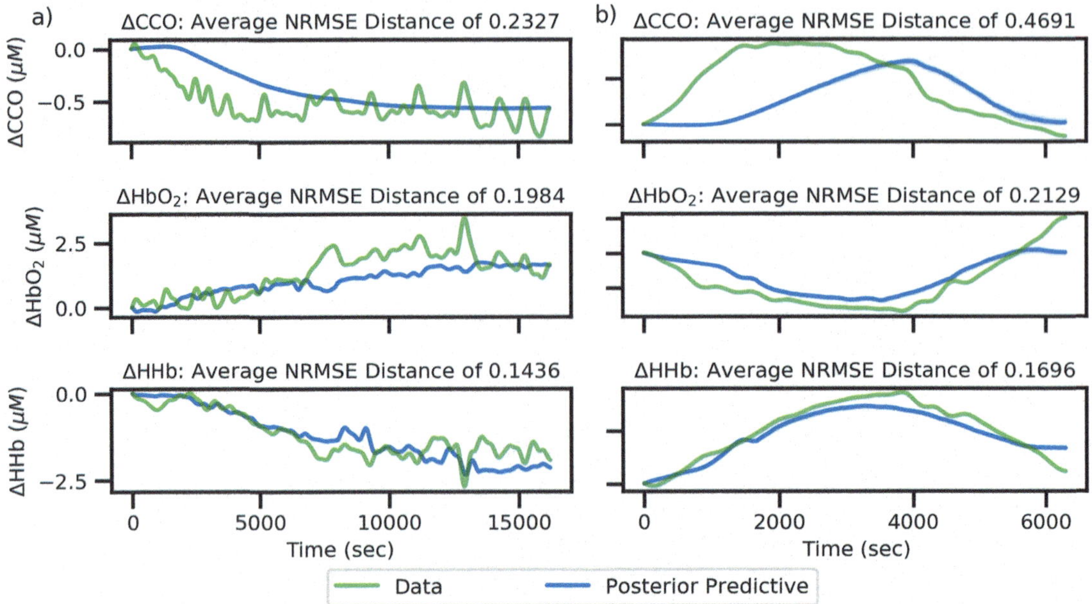

Fig. 5.4 Posterior predictive distributions for piglet LWP475 (**a**) and LWP479 (**b**). The posterior predictive distributions show good agreement between model (blue) and data (green) in both piglets, with the model able to reproduce overall large-scale behaviours

Table 5.1 Final model parameters as selected by sensitivity analysis

Symbol	Description	Default value
Q_10_met	Temperature coefficient for metabolic reactions	2.23
Q_10_haemo	Temperature coefficient for haemodynamic reactions	2.23
Xtot_n	Normal total haemoglobin concentration	5.4 mM
r_n	Normal blood vessel radius	0.0187 cm
r_0	Special radius in the elastic tension relationship	0.0126 cm
K_sigma	Parameter controlling sensitivity of σ_e to vessel radius	10
pH_mn	Normal mitochondrial pH	7.4
phi	Oxygen concentration at half-maximal saturation	0.036 mM
a_frac_n	Normal oxidised fraction Cu_A	0.67
_L0n	Normal concentration of lactate in the cytoplasm	3.0 mM
NADpool	Total mitochondrial NAD and NADH concentration	3.0 mM

Piglet LWP475 suffered a mild injury, as indicated by both its typical response to hypothermia, as per [13], and its Lac/NAA ratio of 0.21. The $\boldsymbol{Q_{10,met}}$ and $\boldsymbol{Q_{10,haemo}}$ values obtained by fitting are all above 1 indicating that decreasing temperature does decrease reaction rates for both haemodynamic and metabolic reactions. In contrast, piglet LWP479 suffered a severe injury and exhibited an atypical response to hypothermia. The HbO2, HHb and CCO signals all produce behaviour opposite to that seen in piglet LWP475. Model analysis then showed that this is likely to be due to a breakdown in how the metabolic reactions responded to hypothermia, with $\boldsymbol{Q_{10,met}}$ values all within a narrow distribution well below 1, with a median value of 0.133. Thus, for this piglet, hypothermia will increase metabolic reaction rate rather than decrease it, but haemodynamic reaction rate will react "typically", reducing with temperature. A small time lag is seen between measured data and predictive posterior distribution, which may be due to the model reduction removing a parameter necessary to control this behaviour. Improvement of the model reduction process may help with this.

Whilst it is not possible to draw clinical conclusions from these results yet, the different parameter spaces for these two piglets does potentially highlight issues with treating all HIE injuries in the same way. Findings here suggest that in certain circumstances the initial injury may impact on how the various reactions and processes respond to cooling and that this change in response may be the opposite of that desired. Further work will look at applying these methods and models to understanding data collected from human neonates that have suffered HIE.

References

1. Hassell KJ, Ezzati M, Alonso-Alconada D et al (2015) New horizons for newborn brain protection: enhancing endogenous neuroprotection. Arch Dis Child Fetal Neonatal Ed 100:F541–F552
2. Bale G, Mitra S, de Roever I et al (2019) Oxygen dependency of mitochondrial metabolism indicates outcome of newborn brain injury. J Cereb Blood Flow Metab 39(10):2035–2047
3. Gluckman P, Wyatt J, Azzopardinna D et al (2005) Selective head cooling with mild systemic hypothermia after neonatal encephalopathy: multicentre randomized trial. Lancet 365(9460):663–670
4. Murray D, Boylan GB, Ryan AC et al (2009) Early EEG findings in hypoxic-ischemic encephalopathy predict outcomes at 2 years. Pediatrics 124:e459–e467
5. Bale G, Mitra S, Meek J et al (2014) A new broadband near-infrared spectroscopy system for in vivo measurements of cerebral cytochrome-c-oxidase changes in neonatal brain injury. Biomed Opt Express 5(10):3450–3466
6. Mitra S, Kendall GS, Bainbridge A et al (2019) Proton magnetic resonance spectroscopy lactate/N--acetylaspartate within 2 weeks of birth accurately predicts 2-year motor, cognitive and language outcomes in neonatal encephalopathy after therapeutic hypothermia. Arch Dis Child Fetal Neonatal Ed 104:F424–F432
7. Banaji M, Tachtsidis I, Delpy D, Baigent S (2005) A physiological model of cerebral blood flow control. Math Biosci 194(2):125–173
8. Banaji M, Mallet A, Elwell CE, Nicholls P, Cooper CE (2008) A model of brain circulation and metabolism: NIRS signal changes during physiological challenges. PLoS Comput Biol 4(11):e1000212
9. Moroz T, Banaji M, Robertson NJ, Cooper CE, Tachtsidis I (2012) Computational modelling of the piglet brain to simulate near-infrared spectroscopy and magnetic resonance spectroscopy data collected during oxygen deprivation. J R Soc Interface 9(72):1499–1509
10. Caldwell M, Moroz T, Hapuarachchi T et al (2015) Modelling blood flow and metabolism in the preclinical neonatal brain during and following hypoxic-ischaemia. PLoS One 10:e0140171
11. Caldwell M, Hapuarachchi T, Highton D et al (2015) BrainSignals revisited: simplifying a computational model of cerebral physiology. PLos One 10:e0126695
12. Caldwell M, Scholkmann F, Wolf U, Wolf M, Elwell C, Tachtsidis I (2016) Modelling confounding effects from extracerebral contamination and systemic factors on functional near-infrared spectroscopy. NeuroImage 143:91–105
13. Russell-Buckland J, Tachtsidis I (2020) Developing a model to simulate the effect of hypothermia on cerebral blood flow and metabolism. Adv Exp Med Biol 1232:299–306
14. Ehrlich MP, McCullough JN, Zhang N et al (2002) Effect of hypothermia on cerebral blood flow and metabolism in the pig. Ann Thorac Surg 73:191–197
15. Orlowski P, McConnell FK, Payne S (2014) A mathematical model of cellular metabolism during ischemic stroke and hypothermia. IEEE Trans Biomed Eng 61(2):484–490
16. Kaynezhad P, Mitra S, Bale G, Bauer C, Lingam I, Meehan C, Avdic-Belltheus A, Martinello K, Bainbridge A, Robertson NJ, Tachtsidis I (2019) Quantification of the severity of hypoxic ischemic brain injury in a neonatal preclinical model using miniature broadband-NIRS measurements of cytochrome-c-oxidase. Neurophotonics 6(4):045009
17. Russell-Buckland J, Barnes CP, Tachtsidis I (2019) A Bayesian framework for the analysis of systems biology models of the brain. PLoS Comput Biol 15(4):e1006631

6 Effect of Adrenaline on Cerebral Blood Oxygenation Measured by NIRS in a Rat Asphyxia Cardiac Arrest Model

Yu Okuma, Tsukasa Yagi, Tai Yin, Takeyuki Kiguchi, Taku Iwami, Lance B. Becker, and Koichiro Shinozaki

Abstract

Adrenaline is an important pharmacologic treatment during cardiac arrest (CA) for resuscitation. Recent studies suggest that adrenaline increases the likelihood of return of spontaneous circulation (ROSC) but does not contribute to improving neurological outcomes of CA. The mechanisms have not been elucidated yet. A bimodal increase in mean arterial pressure (MAP) is observed after adrenaline injection in rodent CA models [17]. In this study, we focused on alteration of systemic arterial pressure in conjunction with the measurement of cerebral blood oxygenation (CBO) such as oxyhemoglobin (Oxy-Hb), deoxyhemoglobin (Deoxy-Hb), and tissue oxygenation index (TOI) by near-infrared spectroscopy (NIRS). Male Sprague–Dawley rats were used. We attached NIRS between the nasion and the upper cervical spine. Rats underwent 10-minute asphyxia to induce CA. Then, cardiopulmonary resuscitation (CPR) was started, followed by a 20 μg/kg of bolus adrenaline injection at 30 seconds of CPR. This injection accelerated the first increase in MAP, and ROSC was observed with an abrupt increase in CBO. Interestingly, the second increase in MAP, once it exceeded a certain value, was accompanied by paradoxical decreases of Oxy-Hb and TOI, while Deoxy-Hb increased. Based on this finding, we compared Oxy-Hb, Deoxy-Hb, and TOI at the first MAP $\approx$ 100 mmHg and the second MAP $\approx$ 100 mmHg. The average of Oxy-Hb and TOI from the 13 animals significantly decreased at the second increase in MAP over 100 mmHg, while Deoxy-Hb significantly increased. NIRS identified a decrease in Oxy-Hb after ROSC. These findings may be a clue to understanding the mechanism of how and why adrenaline alters the neurological outcomes of CA post-resuscitation.

Keywords

Cardiac arrest · Adrenaline · Cerebral blood oxygenation (CBO) · Near-infrared spectroscopy (NIRS) · Autoregulation

Y. Okuma (✉) · T. Yagi · T. Yin · L. B. Becker
K. Shinozaki
Feinstein Institute for Medical Research, Northwell Health System, Manhasset, NY, USA

T. Kiguchi · T. Iwami
Kyoto University Health Service, Kyoto, Japan

6.1 Introduction

The 2015 International Liaison Committee on Resuscitation (ILCOR) Advanced Life Support (ALS) Guidelines [1] recommended the use of

E. M. Nemoto et al. (eds.), *Oxygen Transport to Tissue XLII*, Advances in Experimental Medicine and Biology 1269, https://doi.org/10.1007/978-3-030-48238-1_6

intravenous adrenaline during resuscitation after cardiac arrest (CA), while recent studies have revealed that adrenaline increased the likelihood of return of spontaneous circulation (ROSC) but did not contribute to improving the neurological outcomes in CA [2, 3]. The mechanisms have not been elucidated yet. A bimodal increase in mean arterial pressure (MAP) is observed after adrenaline injection in rodent CA models [4]. There are a few studies that evaluated the cerebral blood oxygenation (CBO) by near-infrared spectroscopy (NIRS) in swine, but there is no study focused on the relationship between CBO by NIRS and the bimodal increasing in MAP observed in rodent CA models [5]. In this study, we focused on this alteration of the systemic arterial pressure in conjunction with the measurement of cerebral blood oxygenation (CBO) such as oxyhemoglobin (Oxy-Hb), deoxyhemoglobin (Deoxy-Hb), and tissue oxygenation index (TOI) by near-infrared spectroscopy (NIRS). We also tested the effects of adrenaline on both MAP and CBO in sham animals.

6.2 Methods

6.2.1 Animal Preparation

The details of the methods for a rat asphyxia CA model have been described previously [6, 17]. In brief, 12 adult male Sprague–Dawley rats (450–550 g, Charles River Laboratories) were anesthetized with 4% isoflurane (Isothesia, Butler-Schein AHS) and intubated with a 14-gauge plastic catheter (Surflo, Terumo Medical Corporation). Animals were mechanically ventilated. Anesthesia was maintained with isoflurane 2% at a fraction of inspired O_2 (FIO_2) of 0.3. The left femoral artery was cannulated (sterile polyethylene-50 catheter inserted for 20 mm) for continuous arterial pressure monitoring. A temperature probe was placed in the esophagus for continuous temperature monitoring. The core temperature was maintained at 36.5 ± 1.0 °C during the surgical procedure. The left femoral vein was cannulated with a polyethylene-50 catheter, which was advanced into the inferior vena cava for drug infusion. We attached NIRS (NIRO-200NX, Hamamatsu Photonics, Japan) from the nasion to the upper cervical spine of the rats. The distance between the emission and the detection probes was 3 cm. We examined the mean arterial pressure (MAP), end-tidal carbon dioxide ($ETCO_2$), and Oxy/Deoxy-Hb and TOI. The NIRS device records the oxygen saturation level (TOI) and the changes in concentration of Oxy-Hb and Deoxy-Hb in real time (100 Hz). Data averaged every 20 seconds were used. After instrumentation setup, neuromuscular blockade was achieved by slow intravenous administration of 2 mg/kg of vecuronium bromide (Hospira, USA). Asphyxia was induced in the rats by switching off the ventilator and CA occurred 3–4 minutes after asphyxia started. We defined CA as a MAP below 20 mmHg; CA was completely untreated during 10 minutes of CA. Mechanical ventilation was restarted at an FIO_2 of 1.0, and manual cardiopulmonary resuscitation (CPR) was delivered to CA animals. Chest compressions were performed at a rate of 240–300 per minute. At 30 seconds after the beginning of CPR, a 20 μg/kg bolus of adrenaline was given to animals through the venous catheter. Following ROSC, defined as a systolic blood pressure above 60 mmHg, CPR was discontinued. If ROSC did not occur by 5 minutes of CPR, resuscitation was terminated. In order to evaluate the dynamics of CBO in post-CPR, we assessed Oxy-Hb, Deoxy-Hb, and TOI 20 seconds before and after the time when MAP reached 100 mmHg. MAP always increased twice after the injection of adrenaline in post-CPR. Six rats underwent sham surgeries including vecuronium and adrenaline administrations but without asphyxia or CPR. The sham animals had one peak of increased MAP after the injection of adrenaline.

6.2.2 Statistical Analysis

Data are shown as mean and SD. The Mann–Whitney U test was used for continuous variables. One-way analysis of variance (ANOVA) was used for the group comparison with post hoc analysis of the Tukey test. We also presented the results of our multiple parameters. All statistical analyses were performed with JMP (version 10.1 software; SAS Institute, Cary, NC, USA). P-values less than 0.05 were considered significant.

6.3 Results

Figure 6.1 shows the trend of MAP, heart rate, TOI, Oxy-Hb, Deoxy-Hb, and EtCO2 in a CA animal and a sham animal. In CA animals, the first peak of increased MAP was observed at ROSC, and it was always followed by the second slow peak of MAP that occurred approximately 10 minutes after ROSC. In CA animals, there was a significant difference in the trend of CBO between the first and the second peak of increased MAP. When animals achieved ROSC and MAP reached 100 mmHg for the first time, Oxy-Hb and TOI increased but Deoxy-Hb decreased. However, when MAP reached 100 mmHg for the second time, Oxy-Hb and TOI decreased but Deoxy-Hb increased. This CBO alteration pattern at the second peak was considered paradoxical compared to that of the first peak ($n = 6$). In sham animals, the CBO alteration when MAP increased to 100 mmHg was the paradoxical pattern, in which Oxy-Hb and TOI decreased and Deoxy-Hb increased as MAP increased (Fig. 6.2).

6.4 Discussion

In the present study, we found significantly different patterns of CBO between the first and the second increase in MAP after CPR. The phenomenon of CBO alteration at the second peak of MAP after CPR was similar to that of the effect of adrenaline on sham animals.

It has been accepted that higher Oxy-Hb and rSO2(TOI) suggests improvement in brain function [7, 8]. Because of this, adrenaline is considered damaging to the brain since it paradoxically decreases blood perfusion into the brain. Likewise, after cardiac arrest, adrenaline may decrease brain oxygenation post-CA [5], and it could be harmful even though it is considered necessary for CPR [2, 3].

Adrenaline is referred to as a double-edged sword because it has a beneficial effect on the heart by promoting resuscitation but also has a harmful effect on blood flow to the brain, which in turn is considered to deteriorate neurological outcomes. The mechanisms of altering CBO, the cerebral blood flow (CBF), and the microcirculation have been poorly understood [3, 9, 10]. A previous study indicated that adrenaline might increase and stabilize CBF under isoflurane [11]. Given our findings that Oxy-Hb and TOI decreased after adrenaline administration, adrenaline might affect the microcirculation in a different way from that for CBF. Previous studies indicated that the vasoactive tone might be incompetent after prolonged CA, resulting in reduced cerebrovascular resistance and increased

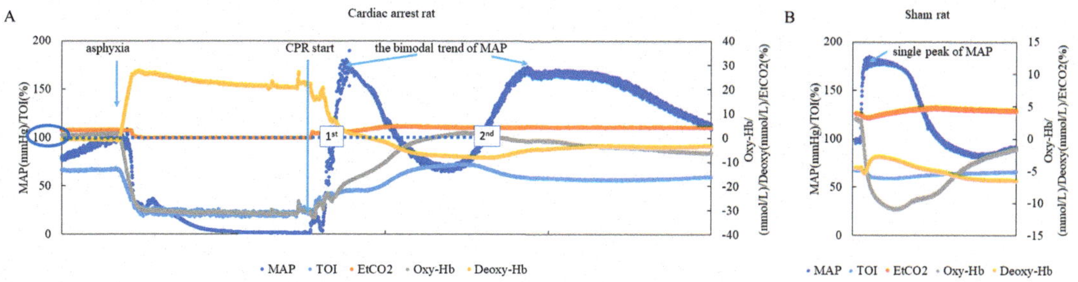

Fig. 6.1 The representative changes in mean arterial pressure (MAP), heart rate, end-tidal carbon dioxide ($EtCO_2$), and cerebral blood oxygenation (CBO) including oxyhemoglobin (Oxy-Hb), Deoxy-Hb, and tissue oxygenation index (TOI) in (**a**) a cardiac arrest rat and (**b**) a sham rat. Bimodal peaks in MAP were seen in cardiac arrest, while single peak was observed in sham

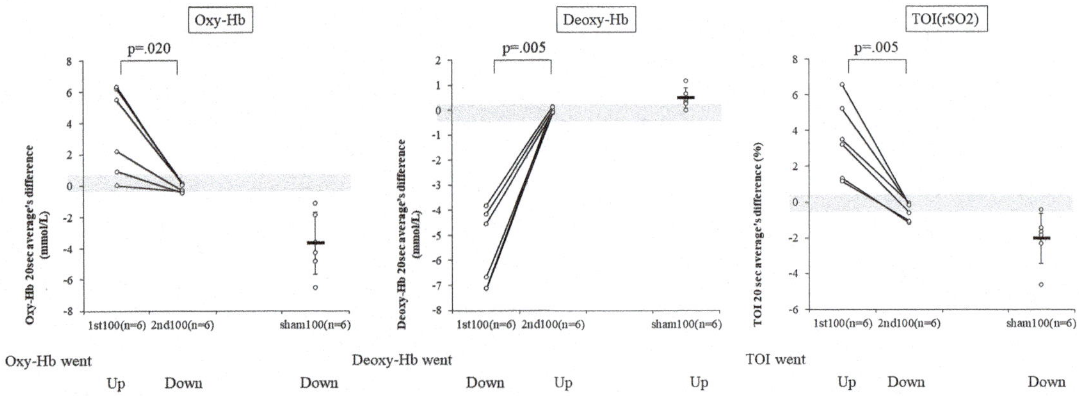

Fig. 6.2 The dynamic trend's comparison of cerebral blood oxygenation (CBO) including oxyhemoglobin (Oxy-Hb), Deoxy-Hb, and tissue oxygenation index (TOI) when mean arterial pressure (MAP) reached 100 mmHg after adrenaline injection in sham model (sham100) and at the first time (first 100) and at the second time (second 100) in cardiac arrest model. rSO2, regional cerebral tissue oxygen saturation

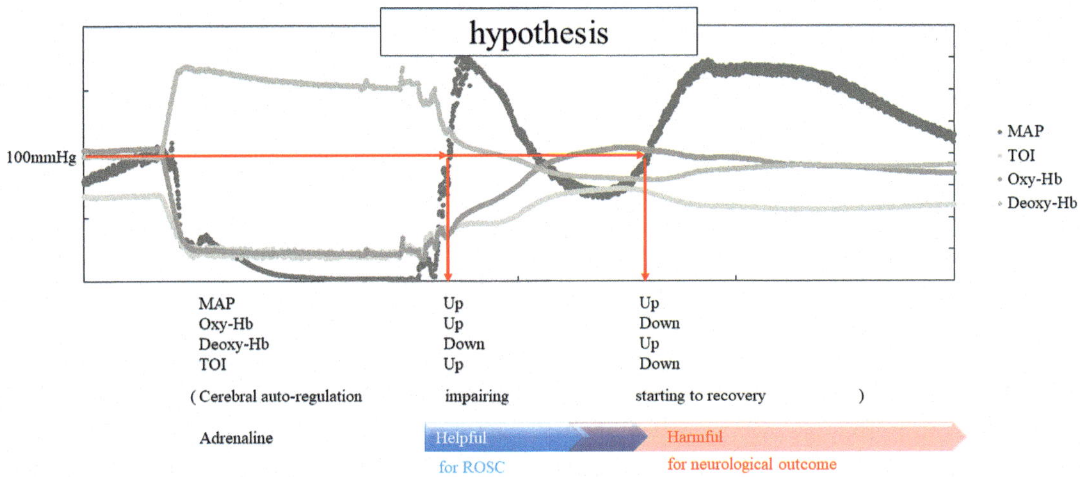

Fig. 6.3 Our hypothesis of adrenaline's effect. MAP, mean arterial pressure; Oxy-Hb, oxyhemoglobin; Deoxy-Hb, deoxyhemoglobin; TOI, tissue oxygenation index; ROSC, return of spontaneous circulation

cerebral microcirculation [12, 13]. Therefore, a linear relationship between MAP and CBO is plausible under conditions of severely devastated cerebral autoregulation as was seen at ROSC [14, 15]. The mechanism that explains the second peak of increased MAP is not clear, but as heart rate also indicated, it may originate from a delayed release of endogenous catecholamine and/or an activation of the sympathetic nervous system that changes the microcirculatory autoregulation [4].

Based on these hypothetical mechanisms and the findings in the present study, we hypothesized that the administration of adrenaline would affect the cerebral microcirculation and CBO (Fig. 6.3), which may depend on the status of cerebral autoregulation. CA is a time-sensitive disorder so autoregulation in the cerebral microcirculation is heavily impacted by the time after resuscitation [16]. As the cerebral autoregulation recovers, the effect of adrenaline on the cerebral microcirculation alters, and it in turn changes the effect on CBO, which may have a harmful effect on the neurological outcomes.

The current study includes several limitations. First, we did not show a correlation between the

CBO by NIRS and the CBF. It is necessary to monitor CBF, but due to technical difficulties in small animal models, further work will be required to better define the relationship of CBO with CBF using larger animal models. Second, the next study needs to examine the effect of exogenous and endogenous adrenaline, which may include additive effects after CA.

6.5 Conclusion

NIRS identified a decrease in Oxy-Hb after ROSC. This phenomenon might be a clue to help understand the mechanism of how and why adrenaline interferes with the improvement of neurological outcomes in post-CA.

References

1. Link MS, Berkow LC, Kudenchuk PJ et al (2015) Part 7: adult advanced cardiovascular life support: 2015 American Heart Association guidelines update for cardiopulmonary resuscitation and emergency cardiovascular care. Circulation 132:S444–S464
2. Hagihara A, Hasegawa M, Abe T et al (2012) Prehospital epinephrine use and survival among patients with out-of-hospital cardiac arrest. JAMA 307:1161–1168
3. Perkins GD, Ji C, Deakin CD, Quinn T et al (2018) A randomized trial of epinephrine in out-of-hospital cardiac arrest. N Engl J Med 379:711–721
4. Neumar RW, Bircher NG, Sim KM et al (1995) Epinephrine and sodium bicarbonate during CPR following asphyxial cardiac arrest in rats. Resuscitation 29:249–263
5. Ristagno G, Tang W, Huang L et al (2009) Epinephrine reduces cerebral perfusion during cardiopulmonary resuscitation. Crit Care Med 37:1408–1415
6. Shinozaki K, Becker LB, Saeki K et al (2018) Dissociated oxygen consumption and carbon dioxide production in the post-cardiac arrest rat: a novel metabolic phenotype. J Am Heart Assoc 7(13):e007721. https://doi.org/10.1161/jaha.117.007721
7. Hallacoglu B, Sassaroli A, Fantini S et al (2011) Cerebral perfusion and oxygenation are impaired by folate deficiency in rat: absolute measurements with noninvasive near-infrared spectroscopy. J Cereb Blood Flow Metab 31:1482–1492
8. Nosrati R, Lin S, Ramadeen A et al (2017) Cerebral hemodynamics and metabolism during cardiac arrest and cardiopulmonary resuscitation using hyperspectral near infrared spectroscopy. Circ J 81:879–887
9. Sigal AP, Sandel KM, Buckler DG et al (2019) Impact of adrenaline dose and timing on out-of-hospital cardiac arrest survival and neurological outcomes. Resuscitation 139:182–188
10. Gough CJR, Nolan JP (2018) The role of adrenaline in cardiopulmonary resuscitation. Crit Care 22:139
11. Myburgh JA, Upton RN, Grant C et al (2002) The cerebrovascular effects of adrenaline, noradrenaline and dopamine infusions under propofol and isoflurane anaesthesia in sheep. Anaesth Intensive Care 30:725–733
12. Lee SK, Vaagenes P, Safar P et al (1989) Effect of cardiac arrest time on cortical cerebral blood flow during subsequent standard external cardiopulmonary resuscitation in rabbits. Resuscitation 17:105–117
13. van den Brule JMD, van der Hoeven JG, Hoedemaekers CWE (2018) Cerebral perfusion and cerebral autoregulation after cardiac arrest. Biomed Res Int 2018:4143636
14. Nishizawa H, Kudoh I (1996) Cerebral autoregulation is impaired in patients resuscitated after cardiac arrest. Acta Anaesthesiol Scand 40:1149–1153
15. Tsuji M, Saul JP, du Plessis A et al (2000) Cerebral intravascular oxygenation correlates with mean arterial pressure in critically ill premature infants. Pediatrics 106:625–632
16. Weisfeldt ML, Becker LB (2002) Resuscitation after cardiac arrest: a 3-phase time-sensitive model. JAMA 288:3035 3038
17. Okuma Y, Shinozaki K, Yagi T et al (2019) Combination of cardiac and thoracic pump theories in rodent cardiopulmonary resuscitation: a new method of three-side chest compression. Intensive Care Med Exp 7(1)

Two Consecutive Invasive Surgeries Utilizing Zymogen Protein C (ZPC) That Enhanced Patient Safety and Reduced Costs

7

Duane F. Bruley, J. M. Abdallah, M. B. Streiff, S. E. Reeg, C. C. Hasty, K. C. Bruley, M. Duncan, R. Duncan, E. E. Thiessen, M. B. White, and S. B. Bruley

Abstract

This case report describes a major surgical procedure for a protein C-deficient, hypercoagulable patient who underwent two back-to-back invasive surgeries, hip replacement, and spinal stenosis correction. The patient, an 84-year-old male with a history of deep vein thromboses (DVT) and pulmonary emboli (PE), was treated pre-, peri-, and postoperatively with zymogen protein C (ZPC-Baxter, International) and recovered without clotting or increased bleeding. During the procedure, the patient was not administered any other anticoagulants. There have now been several case reports on different patients with unrelated teams in various locations worldwide using zymogen protein C during surgical procedures. Thus, this procedure is becoming a viable choice for patients with a high probability of clotting during and after invasive surgery. This case focuses on accomplishing safer surgery and reducing costs, by using less ZPC while accomplishing two surgeries in one procedure. As a result, this procedure might be useful for many medical situations where acquired protein C deficiency could be a problem (e.g., sepsis, pregnancy, etc.). This approach may have greater application to medical conditions other than protein C deficiency, where clotting and inflammation can become issues.

Keywords

Patient safety · Reduced costs · Zymogen protein (ZPC) · Invasive surgeries · Hypercoagulable

D. F. Bruley (✉) · K. C. Bruley · E. E. Thiessen
M. B. White · S. B. Bruley
Synthesizer, Inc., Ellicott City, MD, USA

J. M. Abdallah · S. E. Reeg · C. C. Hasty · M. Duncan · R. Duncan
Vidant Medical Center, East Carolina University, Greenville, NC, USA

M. B. Streiff
Johns Hopkins Medical Institutions, Baltimore, MD, USA

7.1 Introduction

This paper presents a major case highlighting the benefits of utilizing zymogen protein C (ZPC) pre-, peri-, and postoperatively for major invasive surgery involving a protein C-deficient patient. The patient is an 84-year-old man who has previously experienced DVTs, lung emboli, and super-

E. M. Nemoto et al. (eds.), *Oxygen Transport to Tissue XLII*, Advances in Experimental Medicine and Biology 1269, https://doi.org/10.1007/978-3-030-48238-1_7

ficial thrombophlebitis in previous invasive surgeries. The procedure described here involves a total hip replacement immediately followed by spinal stenosis correction. Although the use of perioperative ZPC is still rare, other cases have been previously reported. As reported by Bruley and Streiff, the use of ZPC is unique in its ability to achieve safer anticoagulation [1]. The authors refer to ZPC as nature's "silver bullet" because the anticoagulation activity is available only when and where it is needed and the half-life in the body is much shorter for activated protein C (APC), which results in local anticoagulation without causing bleeding anywhere in the body. All other anticoagulants, natural or manufactured, can cause bleeding even when dosing is carefully monitored. In fact, many professionals in the healthcare and pharmaceutical industries define an anticoagulant as a drug that "does" cause bleeding. This results in a large financial burden on the healthcare industry. Most importantly, patients can die due to internal and external bleeds created or enhanced by presently administered anticoagulants. The prevention and lysis of clots (both are functions of APC) allows normal blood flow and therefore results in the required tissue oxygenation for cell function and survival. After an extensive literature search, it appears that the first use of perioperative ZPC was reported in 1994 by Toupance et al. [2]. In this case, a hereditary PC-deficient patient who had been on chronic hemodialysis was considered for renal transplantation. The authors suggested that chronic uremia and hemodialysis might inhibit the anticoagulant characteristics of blood factors such as protein C, protein S, or antithrombin III, as well as administered heparin. Therefore, in the perioperative period, the authors used human protein C concentrate [3, 4] in addition to standard anticoagulant therapy to prevent thrombosis during and after the transplantation.

There have been several more recent papers published on the use of processed ZPC via immunoaffinity chromatography (Ceprotin, Baxter International Inc., first approved for use in the USA on March 30, 2007). The first paper that was published presented the hypothesis that the use of perioperative protein C during hip replacement would provide greater safety for the patient [5]. This hypothesis was tested and published with outstanding results [6]. The subject was a 73-year-old male who had previous histories of superficial thrombophlebitis, deep vein thrombosis (DVT), and serious lung emboli. The patient underwent the procedure with no clots or bleeds and recovered fully.

Another clinical outcome involved a 75-year-old male with a history of blood clotting that developed a serious internal bleed following a colonoscopy in which a large flat polyp was removed near the cecum [7]. This procedure was done without ZPC (Ceprotin), and the bleed occurred 10 days later at which time the patient was hospitalized for 6 days. Soon after admission, the patient was placed on ZPC, while the doctors worked to locate the bleed. The gastroenterologist did a colonoscopy to determine and repair the problem area. He successfully placed three endoclamps that resolved the bleed. The procedure was successful, and the patient recovered without any clotting or extra bleeding.

A highly invasive and complex surgery was performed on a 77-year-old male with protein C deficiency and a history of clotting and bleeding problems [8]. The patient had been diagnosed after experiencing painless jaundice with bile duct cancer and complications in other organs (liver). The procedure performed was a pancreaticoduodenectomy for pancreatic cancer. The patient was at very high risk for clotting problems. Therefore, it was decided to use a perioperative ZPC (Ceprotin) procedure. Considering the complexity and extent of the surgery, it is significant that there were no clotting or bleeding issues with the procedure.

Another case report involves an 81-year-old male with a hematological history that put him at very high risk for clotting and bleeding complications [9]. He first experienced blood clots due to a hernia surgery in 1964 and was hospitalized for 16 days postsurgery with life-threatening DVTs and lung emboli. This patient was determined later to be protein C deficient at the 38% level. He experienced eight other serious clotting episodes due to other surgeries or traumas. This medical history represents a projected 100% probability of developing a blood clot in the reported surgery. However, ZPC (Ceprotin) was administered perioperatively, and the patient underwent the procedure without any hematological complications.

7.2 Case Presentation

The main goal of this paper is to highlight a very complex case involving successive total hip replacement and spinal surgery on an 84-year-old male with a history of deep vein thromboses, emboli, and superficial thrombophlebitis. The patient suffers from protein C deficiency (heterozygote) and is on chronic anticoagulation therapy (warfarin). His clotting history and other medical indicators for clotting put him at a 100% probability of developing a medical complication due to clotting during or after surgery. Because of the potential complications in this case and the high cost of ZPC, it was decided to perform both surgeries back-to-back and to use pre-, peri-, and postoperative ZPC along with standard anticoagulation therapy (with only ZPC being used during the surgery). This case highlights the amazing success of the perioperative use of zymogen protein C to prevent blood clotting without bleeds.

Patient Z was admitted for consecutive hip and back surgery on January 26, 2016. Team A performed the right total hip arthroplasty, and under the same ZPC regime, this was followed immediately by a second procedure to address the lumbar spinal stenosis, performed by Team B. Patient Z had a baseline protein C activity of 34% which makes him highly prone to blood clotting phenomena, particularly during invasive surgery. The protocol for ZPC (Ceprotin, Baxter, International) was 7500 units IV at 11 pm, the night before surgery, and then 4500 units IV approximately every 6 hours. The surgery took place on January 27, 2016, from 8 am to 12 pm. Ceprotin (4500 units) was administered at 4 am and 12 pm on the day of surgery and then every 6 hours until January 29 at 6 pm. The morning of the surgery, his protein C activity was 148%. Protein C activity was drawn before each administration of ZPC. On January 29 at 10 pm, the first dose of Lovenox at 80 mg every 12 hours was started. The Lovenox was administered through 7:50 pm on February 10, 2016. (Note: 1 dose of Lovenox was withheld at 10 pm due to excessive hip drain output.) On January 31, he was transfused with 2 units of packed red blood cells (PRBC) for anemia and then transferred to rehab and finally discharged to his home on February 11. During Lovenox use, Coumadin was started at 5 mg/day beginning February 2, at 4 pm, and ended on February 5 at 10:30 am and 6 mg/day at 4 pm and ended on February 8 at 9 am and then put on 7.5 mg/day beginning on February 8, 4 pm, and ending on February 11 at 11:30 am (see Table 7.1). The patient completed both surgeries and recovery with no clotting complications and remains on warfarin therapy indefinitely.

7.3 Discussion

Autoprothrombin IIA was first noted and named by Seeger in 1960 [10]. Stenflo later isolated and named it protein C [11]. Zymogen protein C (ZPC), the inactive form of protein C, is a vitamin K-dependent glycoprotein circulating in plasma. The zymogen is converted to the active form via the thrombin-thrombomodulin complex attached to the endothelial cell surfaces as well as other cell components in the blood. The activation requires binding of the GLA residues on membrane phospholipids, along with its cofactor protein S. The active form of protein C (APC) deactivates factors Va and VIIIa [12]. It has also been suggested that APC enhances fibrinolysis by inhibiting plasminogen activation inhibitor (PAI). Natural or acquired deficiencies of ZPC can lead to thrombosis (blood clots) that are known to occur mainly on the venous side of the circulatory system. After many years of scientific and basic research, ZPC and APC have been used in the clinical setting, particularly to prevent thrombosis in protein C-deficient patients and for cases of sepsis. While boluses of APC can sometimes complicate the bleeding process, because of the natural process of activation of ZPC in the body, ZPC has no such complications [1]. It is speculated that many other medical procedures

Table 7.1 ZPC administration and protein C blood level

Time ZPC level measured	ZPC level (%, ref. 65–135%)	Time PC bolus administered	ZPC bolus administered (units)	Notes
1/26/16: 10:55 pm	34	1/26/16: 11:00 pm	7500	Baseline pre-op PC
1/27/16: 3:56 am	148	1/27/16: 4:00 am	4500	
1/27/16: 8:00 am				Surgery
1/27/16: 11:56 am	145	1/27/16: 12:00 pm	4500	
1/27/16: 5:28 pm	145	1/27/16: 5:28 pm	4500	
1/27/16: 10:10 pm	>200	1/28/16: 12:00 am	4500	
1/28/16: 3:42 am	>200	1/28/16: 6:00 am	4500	
1/28/16: 10:21 am	>200	1/28/16: 12:00 pm	4500	
1/28/16: 4:32 pm	>200	1/28/16: 6:00 pm	4500	
		1/29/16: 12:00 am	4500	
1/29/16: 4:40 am	>200	1/29/16: 6:00 am	4500	
1/29/16: 11:05 am	>200	1/29/16: 12:00 pm	4500	
1/29/16: 4:39 pm	>200	1/29/16: 8:13 pm	4500	Last bolus
1/29/16: 11:22 pm	>200			
1/30/16: 4:50 am	196			

and pathologies could benefit from the biological properties of ZPC. However, studies are expensive and complicated, making it difficult to perform case studies so gathering data requires funding to complete. Time will tell following further research and case reports.

Based on the approximate shelf value of $34.40/unit of Ceprotin, this surgery for ZPC alone cost approximately $134,160. Considering that the patient's ZPC level during that time may have risen above 200% of normal, it is important to find the optimal safe dose to minimize the expense of ZPC.

Alternatively, it is important to continue research and development to establish improved bioprocessing strategies that will reduce production costs of ZPC. One approach that shows promise is the replacement of immunoaffinity chromatography (IAC) with immobilized metal affinity chromatography (IMAC) [13–16]. It is estimated that this approach could reduce product costs by a factor of 500–1000. Other possible approaches might include the use of mini-antibodies (mini-Mab) leading to the development of inexpensive ligands to reduce the PC production cost [17]. Additionally, the use of transgenic animals has been demonstrated to produce less expensive blood proteins [18]. Although less attractive from an economic point of view, further investigation of recombinant DNA technology via bioreactors is another possibility. Because of the need to reduce the cost of important life-saving blood proteins, it is encouraged that research and development be funded and promoted in this arena.

This was a very complicated surgery that would normally result in clotting complications, considering the patient's medical indicators. The patient suffers from protein C deficiency (heterozygote) and is on chronic anticoagulation therapy (warfarin). This clotting history and other medical indicators for clotting put the patient at an extremely high probability of developing a superficial thrombophlebitis (STP), a deep vein thrombus (DVT), and/or a pulmonary embolus (PE) during or after surgery. Because of these potential clotting complications in this case, it was decided to use pre-, peri-, and postoperative ZPC along with standard anticoagulation therapy. The result was that the total estimated blood loss for the surgeries was 550 cc, which is normal. There were no blood clots during or after the surgery.

This paper presents an important example of improving safety for a complex surgery using ZPC. The strategy has great benefits for protein C-deficient patients and could find use in a variety of medical procedures. This case helps to validate the importance of ZPC in effecting safer surgery in high-risk patients. It also supports the mechanism of ZPC acting as an anticoagulant without causing bleeding. Most importantly, this paper contributes clinical results indicating that smaller amounts of expensive ZPC can be used to achieve the same satisfactory results. More clinical studies must be completed to target the optimum levels of ZPC with respect to cost and effectiveness. These case studies are rare because of the cost of each experiment and the difficulty in getting a willing patient along with a surgeon, hematologist, and medical team to carry out the procedure. Whatever it takes, the world needs a safe anticoagulant that will not result in costly bleeds and mortality. This example is a step in the process to achieve this goal.

References

1. Bruley DF, Streiff MB (2013) Nature's "silver bullet" for anticoagulation: mechanism of zymogen protein C to activated protein C. Adv Exp Med Biol 765:15–21
2. Toupance O, Nguyen P, Brandt B et al (1994) Prevention of vascular thrombosis by human purified protein C concentrate in a patient with familial PC deficiency undergoing renal transplantation. Transpl Int 7:144–145
3. Dreyfus M, Magny JF, Bridey F et al (1991) Treatment of homozygous protein C deficiency and neonatal purpura fulminans with a purified protein C concentrate. N Engl J Med 325:1565–1568
4. Schwarz HP, Schramm W, Dreyfus M (1990) Monoclonal antibody purified protein C concentrate: initial clinical experience. In: Bruley DF, Drohan WN (eds) Protein C and related anticoagulants. Gulf Publishing, Houston
5. Bruley DF (2009) Zymogen protein C concentrate for safer heterozygote surgery, I am a guinea pig! Adv Exp Med Biol 645:115–121
6. Bruley DF, Mears SC, Streiff MB (2010) Safer surgery using zymogen protein C concentrate. Adv Exp Med Biol 662:439–445
7. Bruley DF, Jagannath SB, Streiff MB (2011) Zymogen protein C to prevent clotting without bleeding during invasive medical procedures. Adv Exp Med Biol 701:91–97
8. Bruley DF, Schulick RD, Streiff MB (2013) Pancreaticoduodenectomy using perioperative zymogen protein C to help prevent blood clotting: a trilogy on increased patient safety. Adv Exp Med Biol 789:299–307
9. Bruley DF et al (2016) A compelling case for the use of perioperative zymogen protein C for increased patient safety. Adv Exp Med Biol 923:15–21
10. Mammen EF, Thomas WR, Seegers WH (1960) Activation of purified prothrombin to autoprothrombin I or autoprothrombin II (platelet cofactor II or autoprothrombin II-A). Thromb Diath Haemorrh 5:218–249
11. Stenflo J (1976) A new vitamin K-dependent protein. Purification from bovine plasma and preliminary characterization. J Biol Chem 251(2):355–363
12. Marlar RA, Kleiss AJ, Griffin JH (1982) Mechanism of action of human activated protein C, a thrombin-dependent anticoagulation enzyme. Blood 59:1067–1072
13. Wu H, Bruley DF (1999) Homologous blood protein separation using immobilized metal affinity chromatography: protein c separation from prothrombin with application to the separation of facto IX and prothrombin. Biotechnol Prog 15(5):928–931
14. Wu H, Bruley DF (2002) Chelator, metal ion and buffer studies for protein c separation. Comp Biochem Physiol A Mol Integr Physiol 132(1):213–220
15. Thiessen EE, Bruley DF (2003) Theoretical studies of IMAC interfacial phenomena for the production of protein C. Adv Exp Med Biol 540:183–190
16. Porath J (1992) Immobilized metal ion affinity chromatography. Protein Expr Purif 3(4):263–281
17. Korah LK, Ahn DG, Kang KA (2003b) Mini-antibody production process for the purification of protein C. Adv Exp Med Biol 510:127–131
18. Velander WH, Lubon H, Drohan WN (1997) Transgenic livestock as drug factories. Sci Am 276(1):70–74

Scanning Tissue Oxygen Needle Probe

8

S. Ashkenazi, D. Cho, and C. W. Song

Abstract

A new device designed to scan oxygen partial pressure along a line in a biological tissue is described in this paper. The probe is housed in a stainless-steel needle. As opposed to other devices for oxygen scanning in tissue, the new probe does not require mechanical translation of the needle in the tissue. The probe includes an active sensing area along the needle shaft that can be scanned optically by an internal optical fiber. This feature allows for repeated scans of tissue oxygen along a line without translating the needle with respect to the tissue, thus avoiding tissue damage associated with needle motion. First, we describe the design of the device including its sensing mechanism, mechanical design, optical configuration, and signal processing. We then move on to describe the results of the device characterization and testing. Finally, we conclude by discussing possible applications of the device in research and in clinical diagnoses and treatment monitoring.

Keywords

Tissue oxygen scanning · Phosphorescence · Oxygen sensor · pO_2 profile

8.1 Introduction

Oxygen plays a critical role in tissue viability and function in almost all living forms and particularly in mammalians. It is essential for cellular metabolism and proliferation. Measuring tissue oxygen is therefore of prime interest in both research and clinical diagnoses and treatments. Current tools for direct measurement of partial pressure in tissue can be categorized into three types: (1) imaging modalities based on oxygen-sensitive contrast agents, (2) implantable oxygen sensors, and (3) needle-mounted oxygen probes. Imaging modalities including electron paramagnetic resonance (EPR) [1] and photoacoustic lifetime imaging [2] provide detailed spatial information of tissue oxygen distribution using 2D images. These methods, however, are limited in penetration depth and require injection of contrast agents that are, currently, not approved by the FDA for use in tissue oxygen imaging. Implantable sensors use dye encapsulation to avoid the need to directly stain

S. Ashkenazi (✉)
Department of Biomedical Engineering, University of Minnesota, Minneapolis, MN, USA

A-Scan LLC, Minneapolis, MN, USA
e-mail: ashke003@umn.edu; shai@ascan-llc.com

D. Cho · C. W. Song
Department of Therapeutic Radiology-Radiation Oncology, University of Minnesota, Minneapolis, MN, USA

E. M. Nemoto et al. (eds.), *Oxygen Transport to Tissue XLII*, Advances in Experimental Medicine and Biology 1269, https://doi.org/10.1007/978-3-030-48238-1_8

the tissue. Oxygen partial pressure (pO_2) in the vicinity of the sensor is measured by diffusion of oxygen into the sensor and establishing a state of equilibrium between the sensor and its immediate vicinity. These sensors, therefore, measure the volume average of tissue pO_2 in a single region [3]. Needle sensors use a sensing tip mounted at the tip of a syringe needle. Their use is mainly in research [4]; however, several oxygen needle probes have been approved for clinical applications [5].

In many cases of clinical interest, the distribution of oxygen in tissue is nonhomogeneous. Gradients in tissue oxygen can form due to pathologies such as wounds, cancer tumor, vascular disease, and diabetes-induced capillary damage. Spatially resolved pO_2 information is therefore crucial for understanding pathology-related physiological processes. This need has led researchers to construct and use mechanical scanning devices to move needle probes in a tissue in order to measure a depth profile of the tissue pO_2 [6]. A major drawback of such an approach is the excessive damage to the tissue resulting from repeat translation of the needle in the tissue. Another limitation of mechanical needle scanning is the need to re-establish a steady state in the tissue with respect to stress, interstitial fluid flow, and oxygen tension. This sets a very low limit to the scan velocity, often making this technique impractical.

Here, we describe a new approach to the problem of tissue pO_2 scanning. A new oxygen needle probe design, based on internal optical scanning, allows for repeated pO_2 scans along the line formed by the needle shaft without moving the needle. The design solves the problem of excessive tissue damage because only one needle penetration is required before repeated scans can be performed. The rate of scan is not limited by the need to re-establish a steady state at every scan position.

In the second section, we will describe the mechanical and optical design of the needle probe. In the third section, we will describe experimental results that characterize performance such as accuracy, temporal step response, and spatial step response. In the last section, we will discuss the potential use of the new device in research and in clinical applications.

8.2 Sensor Design

8.2.1 Oxygen Sensing by Phosphorescence

Optical sensing of pO_2 generally relies on measuring oxygen-dependent phosphorescence of photosensitizer dyes. These dyes typically have high quantum yield for intersystem crossing, allowing efficient photoexcitation of the first triplet state (T1). The rate of relaxation back to the ground state depends on oxygen concentration because of energy transfer occurring through collision with oxygen molecules. The decay rate depends on oxygen partial pressure according to Stern-Volmer equation [7] as follows:

$$\alpha_1 = \alpha_0 + k_{O2}\, p \tag{8.1}$$

where α_0 is the phosphorescence decay rate at zero oxygen conditions, α_1 is the decay rate at oxygen partial oxygen p, and k_{O2} is the quenching rate coefficient. Following a short pulse optical excitation of a photosensitizer dye, phosphorescence intensity can be described by the following expression:

$$I(t) = I_{PH} \exp(-\alpha_1 t) \tag{8.2}$$

where I_{PH} is the initial phosphorescence intensity immediately after the excitation pulse. By measuring the temporal decay of the phosphorescence and fitting the measured data points to an exponential function, the decay rate can be extracted. Equation (8.1) is then used to evaluate the oxygen partial pressure. The parameters α_0 and k_{O2} are obtained by a preliminary two-point calibration procedure.

8.2.2 Needle Probe Optical Scanner Design

Needle-mounted oxygen optical probes make use of the above sensing mechanism to sense oxygen at a tip of a syringe needle where a sensing dye, embedded in a polymer matrix, is deposited. An optical fiber is used to deliver excitation light to the sensing material and to collect phosphorescence light for analysis. These devices are useful mainly in research where they are used in applications such as new material development, tissue engineering, and preclinical studies.

Needle oxygen probes are extremely useful for a single-point measurement. Measuring spatial distribution of oxygen can only be performed by using mechanical scanning devices to translate the needle tip along a line within the tissue volume. This approach is far from optimal. It is slow, it generates tissue damage which might greatly affect the measurement results, and it is often impractical to scan more than once.

Having these limitations in mind, we have designed a probe that can repeatedly scan tissue oxygen along a line with no relative motion between the probe and tissue. This is achieved by depositing an oxygen-sensitive dye along the outer surface of a long glass capillary. A fiber optics having a side-firing tip is used to excite and collect phosphorescence light. The fiber is positioned inside the glass capillary and can be translated along the capillary axis. The fiber tip can effectively illuminate and collect light from a localized region on the outer surface of the capillary having a typical size of 0.2 mm. By translating the fiber tip along the length of the capillary, a line scan is formed. The capillary is housed in a stainless-steel tube for mechanical protection. The stainless-steel tubing has an elongated opening along its length to allow contact between the surrounding tissue and the sensor dye layer on the outer surface of the capillary. A schematic diagram of the needle probe structure is shown in Fig. 8.1.

8.3 Simulation Study

The scanner directly measures the pO_2 distribution within the dye/polymer active layer. Since it is a thin layer in contact with the tissue, it is expected that the spatial pO_2 profile in the sensing layer accurately reflects the pO_2 profile in the tissue. However, the diffusivity and solubility of oxygen is different in the sensing layer and the tissue. This difference in oxygen transport properties can lead to measurement errors. A computer simulation study has been performed to test this source of error in pO_2 profile measurement.

A finite element model of tissue has been generated using COMSOL software (COMSOL). The model mimics oxygen transport in tissue by including localized sources (blood capillaries) and distributed oxygen consumption (metabolic active cells). The consumption is further divided into a normal tissue region and a cancer-mimicking region having a higher metabolic rate. The model is cylindrically symmetric and does not attempt to emulate a realistic physiological structure. The model generates a nonuniform oxygen distribution along the symmetry axis. The model also includes a scanning needle structure positioned along the symmetry axis. An oxygen concentration profile is evaluated with and without a polymer active layer along the needle axis. The model results for pO_2 distribution, pO_2 profile along the probe's active layer, and the error introduced due to placement of the active layer are shown in Fig. 8.2.

The simulation results show that, in the specific model example, the error in the pO_2 profile measurement introduced by the modified oxygen transport of the active sensing layer is smaller than 0.6 mmHg. This relatively low error is a

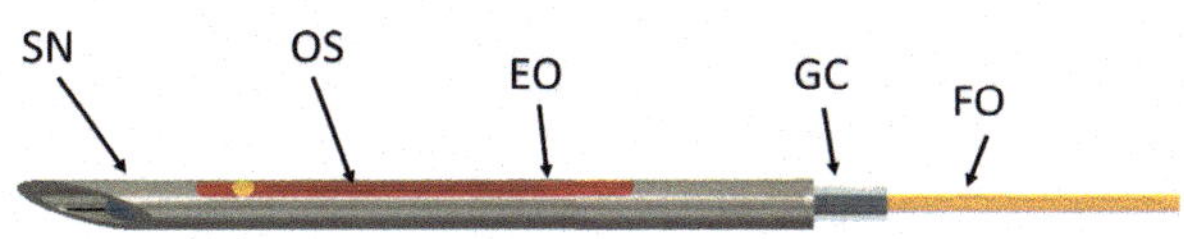

Fig. 8.1 Internal optical scanner needle probe design includes a stainless-steel needle housing of 0.46 mm diameter (SN), elongated opening (EO) milled through the needle wall, and an inner glass capillary (GC), allowing optical sensing by a moveable inner optical fiber (FO). The oxygen sensing layer (OS) is deposited on the outer surface of the capillary. The sensing layer is in physical contact with the tissue. The glass capillary acts as an optical window for the probing optical fiber

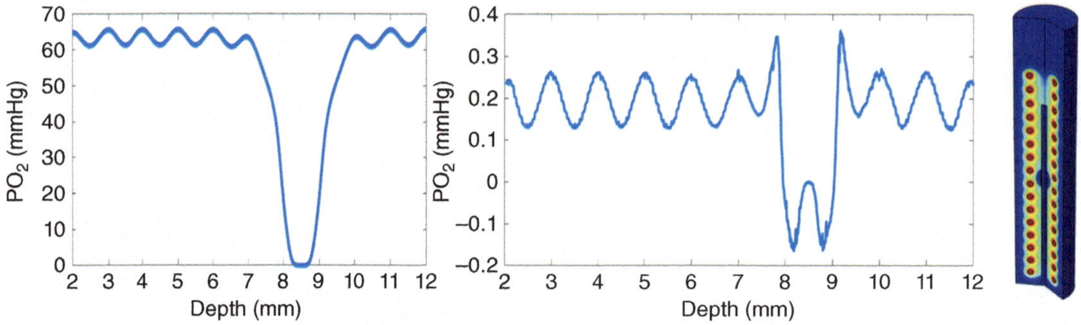

Fig. 8.2 Numerical simulation of a scanning needle in tissue. The tissue model includes a blood vessel (constant pO_2), a periodic array of normal cells (regions of oxygen consumption), and a single region of cancer tissue (high oxygen consumption). *Left*: Oxygen distribution in the tissue along the outer side of the needle is evaluated with no polymer sensing layer. The profile shows periodic pO_2 modulation around the normal cells and a sharp drop to hypoxic level at the cancer region. *Middle*: The same profile was then evaluated with introduction of a polymer sensing layer. The difference between the two profiles is shown. *Right*: 3D depiction of the simulation model

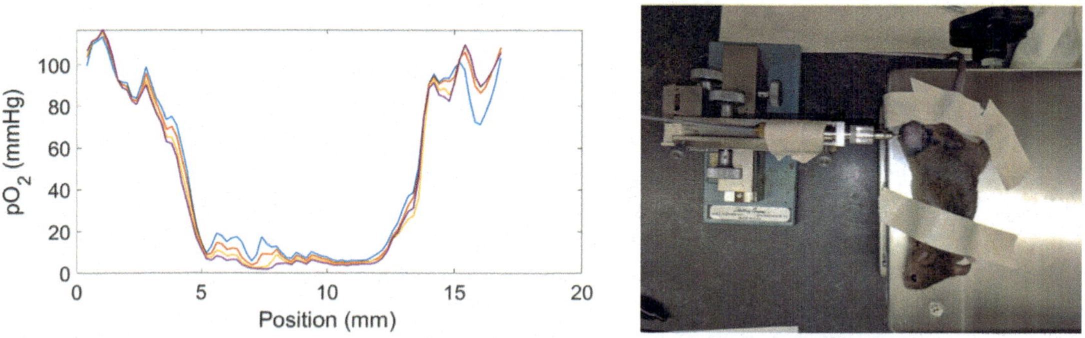

Fig. 8.3 *Right*: A cancer model mouse bearing a tumor on its hind limb positioned on a height-adjustable platform. A scanning needle mounted on an XYZ stage is inserted through the tumor tissue. *Left*: Several scan profiles, measured at 3-minute intervals showing decreasing pO_2 level and stabilization after 12 minutes

result of limited lateral diffusion in the active layer due to its small thickness and lower diffusivity (relative to tissue).

8.4 In Vivo Pilot Study

The pO_2 scanning needle probe and a dedicated driver system have been applied to measure pO_2 profiles in mice cancer models. The model used is FSaII fibrosarcoma of C3H mice grown subcutaneously in the hind limb. Tumors were grown to a size of 6–8 mm. Before scanning, the mice were anesthetized by ketamine/xylazine injection. A scanning needle was inserted through a cut in the skin, penetrating through the bulk of the tumor. Scans were also acquired in healthy muscle tissue of the other hind limb for comparison. Precise and stable insertion was accomplished by affixing the mouse to a lab jack and mounting the scanning needle on an XYZ translation stage. Typical results are shown in Fig. 8.3.

8.5 Conclusions

A scanning tissue oxygen probe has been developed to allow multiple-point measurement along a shaft of the needle probe. Measuring pO_2 at different points along the needle is accomplished by internal fiber-optic scanning, thus avoiding mechanical translation of the needle with respect to the tissue. This mechanism allows for repeated line scans while significantly reducing measurement artifact associated with tissue damage and oxygen redistribution due to needle motion.

References

1. Elas M et al (2006) Electron paramagnetic resonance oxygen images correlate spatially and quantitatively with Oxylite oxygen measurements. Clin Cancer Res 12(14):4209–4217
2. Shao Q, Ashkenazi S (2015) Photoacoustic lifetime imaging for direct in vivo tissue oxygen monitoring. J Biomed Opt 20(3):036004
3. Montero-Baker MF et al (2015) The First-in-Man 'Si Se Puede' Study for the use of micro-oxygen sensors (MOXYs) to determine dynamic relative oxygen indices in the feet of patients with limb-threatening ischemia during endovascular therapy. J Vasc Surg 61:1501–1510.e1
4. Griffiths JR, Robinson SP (1999) The OxyLite: a fibre-optic oxygen sensor. Br J Radiol 72(859):627–630
5. Dings J, Meixensberger J, Jäger A, Roosen K (1998) Clinical experience with 118 brain tissue oxygen partial pressure catheter probes. Neurosurgery 43(5):1082–1094
6. Vaupel P, Schlenger K, Knoop C, Höckel M (1991) Oxygenation of human tumors: evaluation of tissue oxygen distribution in breast cancers by computerized O2 tension measurements. Cancer Res 51(12):3316–3322
7. Boaz H, Rollefson GK (1950) The quenching of fluorescence. Deviations from the Stern-Volmer law. J Am Chem Soc 72(8):3435–3443

9 Transcranial Photobiomodulation of Clearance of Beta-Amyloid from the Mouse Brain: Effects on the Meningeal Lymphatic Drainage and Blood Oxygen Saturation of the Brain

Oxana Semyachkina-Glushkovskaya, M. Klimova, T. Iskra, D. Bragin, A. Abdurashitov, A. Dubrovsky, A. Khorovodov, A. Terskov, I. Blokhina, N. Lezhnev, V. Vinnik, I. Agranovich, A. Mamedova, A. Shirokov, N. Navolokin, B. Khlebsov, V. Tuchin, and J. Kurths

Abstract

Here, we demonstrate the therapeutic effects of transcranial photobiomodulation (tPBM, 1267 nm, 32 J/cm^2, a 9-day course) in mice with the injected model of Alzheimer's disease (AD) associated with accumulation of beta-amyloid (Aβ) in the brain resulting in neurocognitive deficit vs. the control group (CG) (the neurological severity score (NNS), AD 3.67 ± 0.58 vs. CG 1.00 ± 0.26%, $p < 0.05$) and mild cerebral hypoxia (AD 72 ± 6% vs. CG 97 ± 2%, $p < 0.001$). The course of tPBM improved neurocognitive status of mice with AD (NNS, AD 2.03 ± 0.14 vs. CG 1.00 ± 0.26, vs. 2.03 ± 0.14, $p < 0.05$) due to stimulation of clearance of Aβ from the brain via the meningeal lymphatic vessels (the immunohistochemical and confocal data) and an increase in blood oxygen saturation of the brain tissues (the pulse oximetry data) till 85 ± 2%, $p < 0.05$. These results open breakthrough strategies for non-pharmacological therapy of AD and clearly demonstrate that tPBM might be a promising

O. Semyachkina-Glushkovskaya (✉) · M. Klimova · T. Iskra · A. Abdurashitov · A. Dubrovsky · A. Khorovodov · A. Terskov · I. Blokhina · N. Lezhnev · V. Vinnik · I. Agranovich · A. Mamedova · V. Tuchin
Saratov State University, Saratov, Russia

D. Bragin
Lovelace Biomedical Research Institute, Albuquerque, NM, USA

University of New Mexico School of Medicine, Departments of Neurology and Neurosurgery, Albuquerque, NM, USA

A. Shirokov · B. Khlebsov
Institute of Biochemistry and Physiology of Plants and Microorganisms, Russian Academy of Sciences, Saratov, Russia

N. Navolokin
Saratov State Medical University, Saratov, Russia

J. Kurths
Saratov State University, Saratov, Russia

Humboldt University, Physics Department, Berlin, Germany

Potsdam Institute for Climate Impact Research, Potsdam, Germany

E. M. Nemoto et al. (eds.), *Oxygen Transport to Tissue XLII*, Advances in Experimental Medicine and Biology 1269, https://doi.org/10.1007/978-3-030-48238-1_9

therapeutic target for preventing or delaying AD based on stimulation of oxygenation of the brain tissues and activation of clearance of toxic molecules via the cerebral lymphatics.

Keywords

Transcranial photobiomodulation · Alzheimer's disease · Clearance of beta-amyloid · Blood oxygen saturation of the brain · Meningeal lymphatic drainage

9.1 Introduction

Alzheimer's disease (AD) is an incurable neurodegenerative disorder, which is characterized by widespread accumulation of Aβ plaques resulting in the progressive development of dementia [1]. In 2013, 6.8 million people in the USA had been diagnosed with dementia, among which 5 million had a diagnosis of AD. This number is expected to double by 2050 due to the increased aging population [2]. Currently, there are no pharmacological medications for an effective therapy of AD [3]. Therefore, the non-pharmacological approaches for treatment of AD will be a priority in the next couple of decades. Recently, it has been discovered that meningeal lymphatic (MLV) dysfunction may be an aggravating factor in AD pathology and augmentation of MLV function was proposed as a therapeutic target for prevention of age-associated neurological diseases [4]. The transcranial photobiomodulation (tPBM) might be a promising method for stimulation of lymphatic clearance of Aβ and therapy of AD. The PBM known as low-level laser therapy was proposed more than 50 years ago [5]. The PBM is based on shining red lasers (600–700 nm) or near-infrared light (760–1200 nm) onto the head via the intact scalp and skull. The light penetrates into the brain where it is absorbed by specific chromophores that stimulates generation of adenosine triphosphate and nitric oxide with an increase in energetic and metabolic capacities of the brain tissues [5]. A number of reviews have focused on application of tPBM for treatment of AD and depression [6, 7], traumatic brain injuries, and stroke [8]. tPBM reduces Aβ-mediated hippocampal neurodegeneration and memory impairments in rodents, inhibits Aβ-induced brain cell apoptosis, and causes a reduction in Aβ plaques in the cerebral cortex [9]. Here, we tested our hypothesis that tPBM will stimulate clearance of Aβ from the brain of mice with AD via the activations of cerebral lymphatic drainage and an increase of energy metabolism of the brain tissues.

9.2 Methods

The experiments were performed in the following groups: (1) control group including the intact mice, (2) sham-treated mice, (3) untreated mice with AD without tPBM, and (4) mice with AD that received tPBM over 9 days, $n = 10$ in each group in all sets of experiments.

To induce AD in mice, we used the injection of Aβ (1–42) peptide (1 μL, 200 μmol) in the CA1 field of the hippocampus bilaterally (Fig. 9.1-III). The neurobehavioral status of the mice was obtained by the neurological severity score (NSS). The object recognition test was used for memory evaluation.

A fiber Bragg grating wavelength locked high-power laser diode (LD-1267-FBG-350, Innolume, Dortmund, Germany) emitting at 1267 nm (32 J/cm^2) was used for tPBM [10]. The mice were recovered after the surgery procedure of injection of Aβ 3 days. Afterward, mice were treated by tPBM for 9 days each second day under inhalation anesthesia (1% isoflurane at 1 L/min N_2O/O_2 – 70:30). The mice, with shaved heads, were fixed in stereotaxic frame and irradiated in the area of the frontal cortex using the sequence of: 17 min – irradiation, 5 min – pause over 61 min.

A custom-made laser speckle contrast imaging (LSCI) system was used to monitor relative cerebral blood flow (rCBF). The blood oxygen saturation (SpO2) in the brain was monitored using a pulse oximeter (model CMS60D, Contec Medical Systems Co., Ltd., Qinhuangdao, China). Oxyhemoglobin saturation is presented as a percentage of HbO2 vs. the total Hb in the blood. The mouse's head was fixed in stereotaxic frame, and then the optode was placed on the lateral aspect of the skull

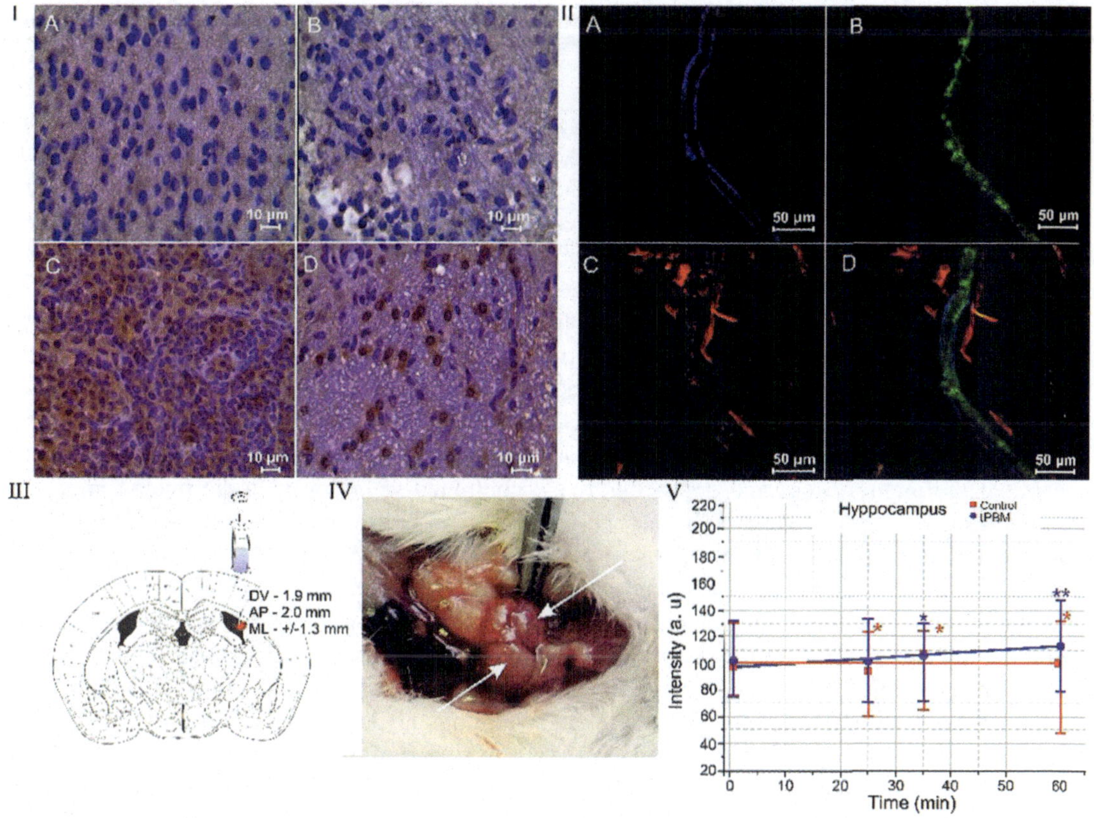

Fig. 9.1 tPBM effects on distribution of Aβ deposition in the mouse brain and clearance of Aβ via MLVs: (I) ICH imaging of Aβ depositions (brown color) in the brain tissues in the control group (a), in the sham-treated group (b), in the mice with AD, (c) and in mice with AD after tPBM (d); (II) the clearance of Aβ (green color) via MLVs (blue color): (a) MLV labeled by LYVE-1, (b) the presence of fluorescent Aβ in MLVs, (c) the cerebral venous vessels (red color) labeled by CD31, and (d) the merged image from a, b, and c; (III) stereotaxic coordinates of intrahippocampal injection of Aβ (1–42) peptide in mice; (IV) anatomical position of dcLNs on the neck of mouse; (V) OCT data of rate of accumulation of GNRs in dcLNs in untreated mice (black line) and in mice that received tPBM (red line) after GNR injection into the hippocampus. $*p < 0.05$ vs. basal level; $n = 10$ in each group

close to right and left branches of the sagittal sinus. The recording of the brain saturation was performed during 15 min.

For histological analysis of Aβ depositions in the cortex, we used the protocol for the immunohistochemical (IHC) analysis with anti-Aβ antibody (1:500; Abcam, ab182136, Cambridge, USA).

Gold nanorods (GNRs) coated with thiolated polyethylene glycol (5 μL at a rate of 0.1 μL/min, diameter and length of 16 ± 3 nm and 92 ± 17 nm) were injected in the hippocampus. Afterward, optical coherence tomography (OCT, Thorlabs GANYMEDE) (central wavelength 930 nm, spectral band 150 nm, axial resolution 4.4 μm in water, and maximal imaging depth 2.7 mm) imaging of deep cervical nodes (dcLNs) was performed for 1 h in each mouse. The GNR was used with a concentration of 500 μg/mL and the injected dose of 5 μL containing 2.5 μg Au. The GNR content in dcLNs was evaluated by atomic absorption spectroscopy (AAS) using a spectrophotometer (Thermo Scientific Inc., Waltham, Massachusetts, USA).

The confocal imaging of the clearance of fluorescent Aβ (HiLyte Fluor 647-conjugated amyloid-β42 at 0.05 μg mL^{-1}, AnaSpec, Inc.) via MLVs was performed using the method of brain meninx dissection and antibodies for labeling of lymphatic (LYVE-1) and cerebral (CD31) endothelium (1:500; Santa Cruz Biotechnology, Santa Cruz, USA) with further confocal microscopy of the dura mater (Olympus, Japan).

9.3 Results

9.3.1 The Effects of tPBM on the Level of Aβ in the Mouse Brain with AD

In the first step, we demonstrated the effectiveness of using the injected model of AD in mice. Figure 9.1-Ic illustrates significant accumulation of Aβ plaques in the hippocampus after intrahippocampal injection of Aβ (1–42). There were no Aβ plaques in the brain tissues in the sham-treated and control groups (CG) (Fig.9.1-Ia and b). The behavior analysis demonstrated the memory loss and neurocognitive failure in mice with AD. The NSS scale, which included the tests of mono-/hemiparesis, startle reflex, round stick balancing, and beam walk, uncovered significant neurological and memory deficit in mice with AD compared with CG (AD 3.67 ± 0.58 vs. CG 1.00 ± 0.26, $p < 0.05$). The object recognition test was used for additional evaluation of neurocognitive status of mice with AD. Two identical objects (cubes) were placed in a cage for 10 min. Then one cube was changed to an object unfamiliar earlier (ball). The time for recognition of new object was faster in CG (7 s) vs. AD (25 s), i.e., this test revealed a memory deficit in AD vs. CG. tPBM course reduced the accumulation of Aβ deposition in the brain tissues compared with untreated mice (Fig. 9.1-Id). The tPBM also improved NNS (AD 2.03 ± 0.14 vs. CG 1.00 ± 0.26, $p < 0.05$) including performance of startle reflex, round stick balancing, and beam walk in mice with AD vs. untreated mice with AD. tPBM improved memory of mice with AD. Indeed, the time for recognition of new object in mice with AD was reduced to 17 s.

9.3.2 Mechanisms of Therapeutic Effects of tPBM in Mice with AD

The study of the mechanisms of therapeutic effects of tPBM showed that tPBM increased the cerebral blood oxygen saturation in both healthy mice and animals with AD. Indeed, SpO_2 was elevated after a single application of tPBM in CG (102 ± 2% vs. 97 ± 2%) and after a 9-day course of tPBM (tPBM 104 ± 3% vs. the untreated control 97 ± 2%), but these changes were not statistically significant. The mice with AD demonstrated a significant decrease in SpO_2 compared with CG (AD 72 ± 6% vs. CG 97 ± 2%, $p < 0.001$). After 9 days of tPBM, we observed an increase in SpO_2 in mice with AD vs. the untreated mice (AD + tPBM: 85 ± 2% vs. AD 72 ± 6%, $p < 0.001$). However, despite a tendency to normalization of the cerebral blood oxygen saturation after tPBM, the level of SpO_2 continued to be lower in the treated mice with AD than in healthy mice (AD + tPBM 85 ± 2% vs. CG + tPBM 102 ± 2%, $p < 0.05$ and vs. CG 97 ± 2%, $p < 0.05$).

LSCI data did not reveal any changes in rCBF in mice with AD compared with the control group as well as after tPBM in both healthy and AD mice (0.37 ± 0.02 0.34 ± 0.02 before and after tPBM in CG; 0.35 ± 0.07 and 0.37 ± 0.09 before and after tPBM in mice with AD).

The elimination of Aβ from the brain of mice with AD after tPBM was accompanied by clearance of Aβ via MLVs. Figure 9.1-II illustrates the presence of fluorescent Aβ in MLVs in mice with AD after a tPBM course. These data are consistent with our previous results demonstrating clearance of molecules, which crossed the opened blood-brain barrier, via MLVs [11]. We hypothesized that the presence of Aβ in MLVs might be due to stimulation of the lymphatic drainage function by tPBM. To test this idea, we analyzed the effect of tPBM on the clearance of GNRs from the hippocampus (the place of injection of Aβ) into dcLN (Fig. 9.1-III–V). Figure 9.1-I–V illustrates that tPBM significantly increased the rate of GNR accumulation in dcLN compared with the intact mice (0.369 ± 0.009 vs. 0.029 ± 0.002, $p < 0.001$). The results of AAS confirmed OCT data and showed a higher level of GNRs in dcLN after tPBM group vs. untreated group (29.3 ± 1.9 vs. 1.8 ± 0.1, $p < 0.001$).

9.4 Conclusions

The results clearly demonstrate that a 9-day course of tPBM (1267 nm, 32 J/cm^2) reduces Aβ plaques in the brain of mice with AD and stimulates the clearance of Aβ via MLVs. The possible mechanism underlying tPBM-mediated stimulation of lymphatic clearance of Aβ might be tPBM improvement of oxygen consumption of the brain structures including the lymphatic system. The increase in oxygen saturation leads to an enhancement of mitochondrial production of adenosine triphosphate that stimulates lymphatic contractility resulting in an increased drainage and clearing functions of the meningeal lymphatic system. tPBM has a high potential to be applied in routine clinical practice as a promising novel non-pharmacological method for therapy of AD.

Acknowledgments This study was supported by grants from Russian Science Foundation 18-75-10033 (Immunohistochemical analysis) and 19-15-00201 (measurement of rCBF, SpO_2); 20-15-00090 (measurement of lymphatic drainage) and the RF Governmental grant 075-15-2019-1885 (Confocal analysis of lymphatic clearance of beta-amyloid). DB was supported by NIH R01 NS112808.

References

1. Santini Z, Koyanagi A, Tyrovolas S et al (2015) Social network typologies and mortality risk among older people in China, India, and Latin America: a 10/66 Dementia Research Group population-based cohort study. Soc Sci Med 147:134–143
2. Ubhi K, Masliah E (2012) Alzheimer's disease: recent advances and future perspectives. J Alzheimers Dis 33(Suppl 1):S185–S194
3. Dunkel P, Chai C, Sperlágh B et al (2012) Clinical utility of neuroprotective agents in neurodegenerative diseases: current status of drug development for Alzheimer's, Parkinson's and Huntington's diseases, and amyotrophic lateral sclerosis. Expert Opin Investig Drugs 21(9):1267–1308
4. Da Mesquita S, Louveau A, Vaccari A (2018) Functional aspects of meningeal lymphatics in ageing and Alzheimer's disease. Nature 560(7717):185–191
5. Hamblin M, Ferraresi C, Huang Y-Y, Freitas L, Carroll J (2018) Low-level light therapy: photobiomodulation. SPIE Press, Bellingham
6. Hennessy M, Hamblin M (2016) Photobiomodulation and the brain: a new paradigm. J Opt 19(1):013003
7. Chang J, Ren Y, Wang R et al (2018) Transcranial low-level laser therapy for depression and Alzheimer's disease. Neuropsychiatry (London) 8(2):477–483
8. Naeser M, Hamblin M (2011) Potential for transcranial laser or LED therapy to treat stroke, traumatic brain injury, and neurodegenerative disease. Photomed Laser Surg 29(7):443–446
9. Lu Y, Wang R, Dong Y et al (2017) Low-level laser therapy for beta amyloid toxicity in rat hippocampus. Neurobiol Aging 49(1):165–182
10. Zinchenko E, Navolokin N, Shirokov A et al (2019) Pilot study of transcranial photobiomodulation of lymphatic clearance of beta-amyloid from the mouse brain: breakthrough strategies for non-pharmacologic therapy of Alzheimer's disease. Biomed Opt Express 10(8):4003–4017
11. Semyachkina-Glushkovskaya O, Chehonin V, Borisova E et al (2017) Photodynamic opening of the blood-brain barrier and pathways of brain clearing. J Biophotonics 11(8):e201700287

Near-Infrared Spectroscopy Might Help Prevent Onset of Cerebral Hyperperfusion Syndrome

10

Yu Okuma, Nobuyuki Hirotsune, Koichiro Shinozaki, Tsukasa Yagi, Yasuhito Kegoya, Yuta Sotome, Yuki Matsuda, Yu Sato, Tomoyuki Tanabe, Kenichiro Muraoka, and Shigeki Nishino

Abstract

Cerebral hyperperfusion syndrome (CHS) is a rare but fatal perioperative complication after surgical correction of carotid stenosis. Despite numerous treatment options for preventing CHS, it does occur in some patients. We developed the outlet gate technique (OGT), in which the embolic balloon was deflated gradually in accordance with the ratio of oxygen saturation measured by a brain oximeter of the ipsilateral brain region to that in the contralateral region. Between June 2017 and May 2018, 39 patients with carotid stenosis underwent endovascular carotid revascularization procedures; of these, 20 underwent the procedure with the OGT. CBO was measured five times in those 20 patients: before the procedure, with the embolic protection device (EPD) on, with the EPD off, during the procedure, and after the procedure. Preventive treatment options were used more frequently in these patients, and although their surgical status seemed more complicated, perioperative complications were not increased. There were almost significant differences between CBO values except between those during and after the procedure with the OGT. This showed that the OGT allowed for stabilization of the CBO and thus has the potential to prevent CHS.

Keywords

Cerebral hyperperfusion syndrome (CHS) · Carotid artery stenting (CAS) · Outlet gate technique (OGT) · Cerebral blood oxygenation (CBO) · Near-infrared spectroscopy (NIRS)

Y. Okuma (✉)
Feinstein Institute for Medical Research, Northwell Health System, Manhasset, NY, USA

Department of Neurological Surgery, Hiroshima City Hiroshima Citizens Hospital, Hiroshima, Japan

N. Hirotsune · Y. Kegoya · Y. Sotome · Y. Matsuda · Y. Sato · T. Tanabe · K. Muraoka
Department of Neurological Surgery, Hiroshima City Hiroshima Citizens Hospital, Hiroshima, Japan

K. Shinozaki · T. Yagi · S. Nishino
Feinstein Institute for Medical Research, Northwell Health System, Manhasset, NY, USA

10.1 Introduction

Cerebral hyperperfusion syndrome (CHS) is an uncommon sequela of carotid endarterectomy or carotid artery stenting (CAS), occurring in only a small percentage of patients after carotid revascularization (from <1% to 3%). After surgical

E. M. Nemoto et al. (eds.), *Oxygen Transport to Tissue XLII*, Advances in Experimental Medicine and Biology 1269, https://doi.org/10.1007/978-3-030-48238-1_10

correction of the carotid stenosis, autoregulation of cerebral blood flow may be lost, and, as a result, the dilated vessels may be unable to vasoconstrict sufficiently to protect the capillary bed [1]. CHS is probably the cause of most postoperative intracerebral hemorrhages and seizures in the first day after CAS and 1 week after carotid endarterectomy. Thus, surgeons must monitor the changes in perfusion volume in the acute phase.

Recently, in order to have the new surgical option preventing immediate CHS, we devised the outlet gate technique (OGT), in which the embolic balloon was deflated step by step in accordance with the ratio of ipsilateral regional cerebral oxygen saturation (rSO_2) to contralateral rSO_2, rSO2 ratio, measured by a brain oximeter, which was actively introduced in the treatment of patients with high surgical risks.

10.2 Methods

10.2.1 Patient Preparation

Our institutional review board approved this retrospective study (28–17). All patients provided informed consent for us to use their data. Thirty-nine patients with high-grade carotid stenosis underwent CAS or staged angioplasty (SAP) between June 2017 and May 2018. We performed OGT or conventional CAS on the basis of preoperative examination findings, including those of digital subtraction angiography and perfusion imaging studies (magnetic resonance imaging or single-photon emission computed tomography (SPECT) or both). We commonly used quantitative SPECT by iodine-123-labeled N-isopropyl-4-iodoamphetamine with or without acetazolamide challenge for the imaging studies. We considered decreased cerebrovascular reactivity or cerebral basal flow as risk factors for CHS, because this reflected the loss of cerebral blood flow autoregulation and the low-flow vascular bed. We also paid attention to angiographic findings such as slow distal washout and poor collateral flow. When meeting one or more of the criteria as described above, the four attending neurosurgeons that included three senior fellows and one fellow, all certified by the Japanese Society for Neuroendovascular Therapy, discussed whether patients should undergo OGT or not.

Patients received dual antiplatelet medication, beginning at least 1 week before the procedure. According to individual risk, we used conventional prevention options such as preoperative injection of edaravone (a free radical scavenger), total anesthesia, strict control of blood pressure, deep sedation with ventilator, and SAP [1]. Systemic heparinization was established for both OGT and conventional SAP/CAS. During procedures with the OGT, bilateral rSO_2 was always monitored with INVOS (5100C Cerebral/Somatic Oximeter; Medtronics, Minneapolis). Data of rSO_2 averaged every 20 seconds were used. The ratio of ipsilateral rSO_2 to contralateral rSO_2, rSO2 ratio was used for perioperative evaluation; these were measured at five times: before the procedure, during inflation of the embolic protection device (EPD), during the first reperfusion after EPD deflation, during gradual reperfusion with the OGT, and after the procedure.

In procedures with and without the OGT, an 8-French balloon guiding catheter or a 6-French long sheath was inserted into the femoral artery, and the tip was placed at the common carotid artery. In both procedures, we used the EPD whenever possible. If it could not be used, we used proximal protection and navigated a micro-guide wire distal to the stenosis and performed angioplasty with a semicompliant balloon 2–4 mm in diameter when inflated. In the procedures with the OGT, we deflated the distal or proximal embolic protection balloon gradually in accordance with the dynamic change in rSO2 ratio. If the ratio changed, following the rSO2 ratio, we also inflated the balloon slightly and waited 2–4 minutes before attempting to deflate it again. In both procedures, we always performed 10-minute delayed carotid angiography to evaluate whether significant recoil or dissection occurred and intracranial angiography to evaluate the improvement in cerebral perfusion [2] (Fig. 10.1).

After surgery, imaging studies, such as magnetic resonance imaging and SPECT, were performed within 3 days. Patients who had undergone SAP then underwent CAS 2–4 weeks later if results of perfusion imaging studies indi-

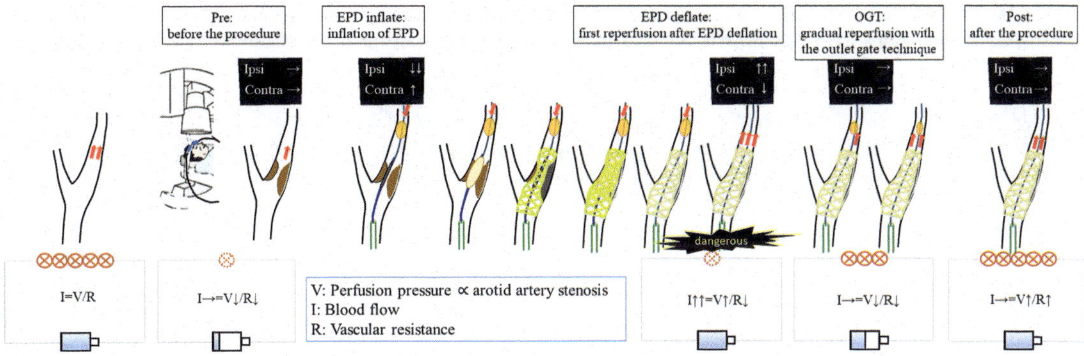

Fig. 10.1 The description block diagram of the outlet gate technique (OGT). Cerebral autoregulation tries to maintain relatively stable cerebral blood flow as possible. Generally, blood flow is determined by vascular resistance and perfusion pressure. Severe internal carotid artery stenosis makes the perfusion pressure go down. In order to maintain the blood flow, autoregulation makes the vascular resistance go down at the minimum. So if surgical carotid revascularization makes perfusion pressure go up immediately, autoregulation cannot catch up and the capillary bed collapses. This is considered as the principal mechanism of cerebral hyperperfusion syndrome. In order to let autoregulation and vascular resistance adapt, we wanted perfusion pressure to increase gradually. This was the concept of the outlet gate technique. Ipsi, ipsilateral; contra, contralateral

cated the need for CAS. We defined periprocedural ischemic stroke, including intracerebral hemorrhage, as well as acute myocardial infarction, permanent complications, and death from any cause as adverse events.

10.2.2 Statistical Analysis

We report the data as means ± standard deviations. We used Fisher's exact test for categorical variables and the Mann–Whitney *U* test for continuous variables. We also used repeated-measures analysis of variance and post hoc analysis with Bonferroni's test. All statistical analyses were performed with EZR software (Saitama Medical Center, Jichi Medical University, Saitama, Japan), and we used R-Commander software (The R Foundation for Statistical Computing, Vienna), designed to add statistical functions frequently used in biostatistics [3]. *P* values less than 0.05 were considered significant.

10.3 Results

Of the 44 patients who underwent elective endovascular carotid revascularization procedures, 5 were excluded from our analysis because continuous mechanical thrombectomy was also carried out. Twenty patients who were determined to be at high risk for CHS were scheduled for OGT (the "OGT group"), and the other 19 patients underwent conventional CAS procedures (the "CAS group").

Baseline characteristics and operative components in the OGT and CAS groups are shown in Table 10.1. General anesthesia was induced approximately six times more frequently in the OGT group (65.0%) than in the CAS group (10.5%; $P = 0.0002$). Edaravone was preoperatively administered approximately five times more commonly in the OGT group (70.0%) than in the CAS group (15.8%; $P = 0.0002$). SAP was performed only in some patients in the OGT group (20.0%; $P = 0.1060$). The operative time was significantly longer for the OGT group (77.7 ± 39.1 minutes) than for the CAS group (42.1 ± 9.9 minutes; $P < 0.0001$). However, there were no significant differences between the two groups with regard to either the number of lesions detected on postoperative diffusion-weighted imaging or postoperative permanent complications.

Intraoperative changes in rSO2 ratio in the OGT group are depicted in Fig. 10.2. The rSO2 ratio changed so remarkable that values were significantly different from one measurement to the next: before the procedure, mean rSO2 ratio was 0.97 ± 0.07; during EPD inflation, 0.87 ± 0.08; during the first reperfusion after EPD deflation, 1.09 ± 0.08; during gradual reperfusion with the

Table 10.1 The baseline characteristics and operative components in patients who underwent surgery with the outlet gate technique (OGT) and in patients who underwent the conventional carotid artery stenting procedure (CAS)

	CAS (*n* = 19)	OGT (*n* = 20)	*P* value
Age (years old)	76.6 ± 5.3	77.3 ± 4.7	0.9098
Male	73.7%	95.0%	0.0915
Symptomatic	47.4%	55.0%	0.7524
Pre-edaravone	15.8%	70.0%	0.0002
General anesthesia	10.5%	65.0%	0.0002
SAP	0%	20.0%	0.1060
Time (minutes)	42.1 ± 9.9	77.7 ± 39.1	<0.0001
DWI positive	47.4%	20.0%	0.0959
Permanent complication	5.3%	0%	0.4872

Pre-edaravone, preoperative administration of edaravone; SAP, staged angioplasty; symptomatic, symptomatic lesion; time, operative time; DWI positive, lesion detected on postoperative diffusion-weighted imaging

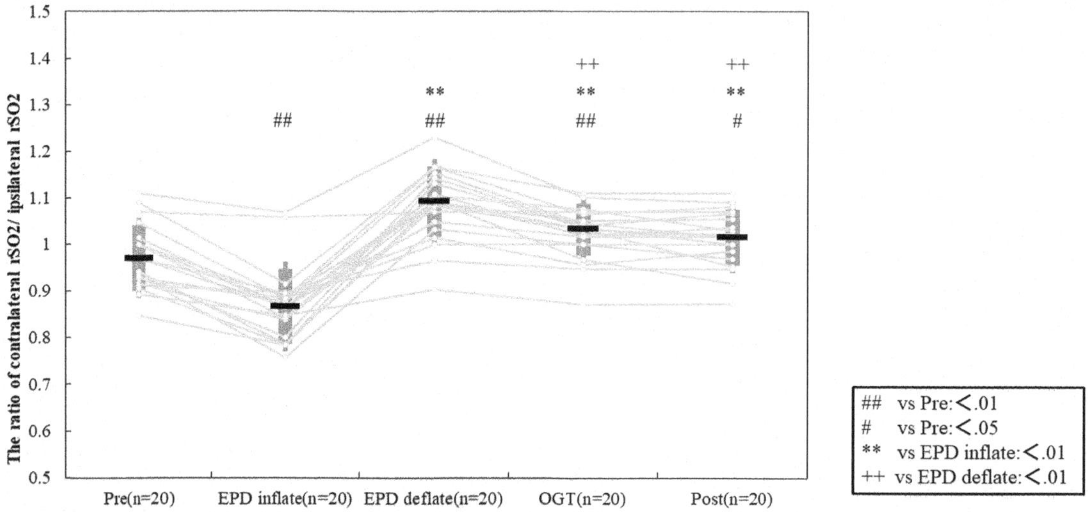

Fig. 10.2 Intraoperative changes in the ratio of ipsilateral regional cerebral oxygen saturation (rSO_2) to contralateral rSO_2, rSO2 ratio CBO. Pre, before the procedure; EPD, embolic protection device; EPD inflate, inflation of EPD; EPD deflate, first reperfusion after EPD deflation; OGT, gradual reperfusion with the outlet gate technique; post, after the procedure. The results are presented as means ± standard deviations. ##$P < 0.01$ compared with pre. #$P < 0.05$ compared with pre. **$P < 0.01$ compared with EPD inflate. ++$P < 0.01$ compared with EPD deflate

OGT, 1.03 ± 0.06; and after the procedure, 1.02 ± 0.06. On the other hand, there was no significant difference between the rSO2 ratio value during gradual reperfusion with the OGT and the rSO2 ratio value after the procedure.

10.4 Discussion

OGT was performed in complicated cases in which cerebral basal flow was severely impaired by internal carotid artery stenosis; affected patients were judged to be at high risk for CHS. Therefore, prevention treatment options such as preoperative administration of edaravone and induction of general anesthesia were used more often in the OGT group. In addition, we deflated the embolic balloon slowly and gradually in accordance with the rSO2 ratio change, and so the OGT necessitated a longer operative time. Nevertheless, OGT did not increase postoperative complications. The monitoring by NIRS indicated that OGT enabled rSO2 ratio to stabilize sooner than it would have otherwise. Additionally, we considered that using OGT was able to lead rSO2 ratio stabilized, so the rSO2 ratio value did not change from gradual reperfusion with the OGT to after the procedure.

Based on the oxygen extraction fraction hemispheric ratio which is commonly used in positron emission tomography (PET), we used the ratio of ipsilateral rSO2 to contralateral rSO2. It is because PET has already been reliable as the method of quantitative evaluation of cerebral blood flow and oxygen metabolism [4, 5].

CHS is one of the most serious potential complications after carotid revascularization, sometimes resulting in acute intracranial hemorrhage that is fatal or produces significant neurological sequelae [1].

Previous studies have revealed the efficacy of SPECT in diagnosing CHS [6], but SPECT is also a complicated, time-consuming procedure. Moreover, another study indicated that CHS occurred significantly earlier after CAS (within 2 hours) than after carotid endarterectomy (peak incidence, on the sixth postoperative day) [7]. Patients who are in danger of CHS during CAS must be identified. rSO2 ratio monitoring with NIRS seemed to be reliable for predicting CHS during CAS [2].

After fatalities during CAS, SAP, a new protocol of carotid angioplasty for patients deemed to be at high risk for CHS, was developed [8]. SAP provides effective revascularization to avoid CHS, but a recent multicenter study in Japan revealed that the incidence of CHS events in patients at high risk remained 4.4%, although the patients underwent almost all prevention treatment options [9]. We therefore paid attention to additional intraoperative procedures and eventually devised the OGT.

This study had several limitations. First, the criteria for determining the risk for CHS remain unclear. Further study is necessary to establish appropriate selection criteria for OGT. Second, there was not a healthy control group. The next study needs to reveal the rSO2 ratio in a healthy group. Third, the sample size was too small to determine the efficiency of OGT in preventing CHS. However, this study also showed that the incidence of periprocedural ischemic events after OGT was not more frequent than that after CAS or SAP. A prospective study, including randomized controlled trials, is needed to confirm the safety of the OGT, to verify its potential for preventing immediate CHS, and to overcome the limitations of this study.

10.5 Conclusion

The OGT, in which stepwise reperfusion is performed with reference to rSO2 ratio values, as measured by NIRS, is a new surgical option that has the potential to prevent immediate CHS and is relatively safe.

References

1. van Mook WN, Rennenberg RJ, Schurink GW et al (2005) Cerebral hyperperfusion syndrome. Lancet Neurol 4:877–888. https://doi.org/10.1016/s1474-4422(05)70251-9
2. Matsumoto S, Nakahara I, Higashi T et al (2009) Near-infrared spectroscopy in carotid artery stenting predicts cerebral hyperperfusion syndrome. Neurology 72:1512–1518. https://doi.org/10.1212/WNL.0b013e3181a2e846
3. Kanda Y (2013) Investigation of the freely available easy-to-use software "EZR" for medical statistics. Bone Marrow Transplant 48:452–458. https://doi.org/10.1038/bmt.2012.244
4. Grubb JRL (1998) Importance of hemodynamic factors in the prognosis of symptomatic carotid occlusion. JAMA 280:1055. https://doi.org/10.1001/jama.280.12.1055
5. Carlson AP, Yonas H, Chang YF et al (2011) Failure of cerebral hemodynamic selection in general or of specific positron emission tomography methodology?: Carotid Occlusion Surgery Study (COSS). Stroke 42:3637–3639. https://doi.org/10.1161/strokeaha.111.627745
6. Hosoda K, Kawaguchi T, Ishii K et al (2003) Prediction of hyperperfusion after carotid endarterectomy by brain SPECT analysis with semiquantitative statistical mapping method. Stroke 34:1187–1193. https://doi.org/10.1161/01.str.0000068781.31429.be
7. Ogasawara K, Sakai N, Kuroiwa T et al (2007) Intracranial hemorrhage associated with cerebral hyperperfusion syndrome following carotid endarterectomy and carotid artery stenting: retrospective review of 4494 patients. J Neurosurg 107:1130–1136. https://doi.org/10.3171/jns-07/12/1130
8. Yoshimura S, Kitajima H, Enomoto Y et al (2009) Staged angioplasty for carotid artery stenosis to prevent postoperative hyperperfusion. Neurosurgery 64:ons122–ons128; discussion ons128–129. https://doi.org/10.1227/01.neu.0000334046.41985.bb
9. Hayakawa M, Sugiu K, Yoshimura S et al (2019) Effectiveness of staged angioplasty for avoidance of cerebral hyperperfusion syndrome after carotid revascularization. J Neurosurg:1–11. https://doi.org/10.3171/2018.8.jns18887

Part II

Oxygen Measurement and Modeling

11 Online Assessment of Hemodynamics in the Suctioned Volume of Biological Tissue by an Embedded Near-Infrared Spectroscopy Sensor

Chenyang Gao and Ting Li

Abstract

Cupping therapy is a promising method to cure or reduce symptoms of some diseases including muscle pain/tenderness/fatigue. Although the applications of cupping therapy have a thousand-year history in traditional Chinese medicine and have been spread to other countries in recent years, cupping therapy is something like a black box, and the unskilled user can hardly control it due to the absence of physiological observations. In this study, we developed a NIRS instrument with three probes to detect the blood-oxygen level of the skin tissue where the cupping therapy is being carried out. Each probe includes two detection channels. One of the probes is embedded in the cup to monitor the hemodynamic parameters in the cupping site, and the other two probes are placed outside, surrounding the cupping site. Using this monitor, we can observe the changes in oxy-hemoglobin ([HbO2]), deoxy-hemoglobin ([Hb]), and total hemoglobin ([tHb]), as well as the heart rate, calculated from the change curves of [HbO2] during cupping therapy in real time. Therefore, the doctor or other users can see the impact of cupping on the tissues to which it is applied which should facilitate the development and understanding of the application of cupping.

Keywords

Cupping therapy · Near-infrared spectroscopy · Hemodynamic parameter · Optical probe

11.1 Introduction

Cupping therapy, as a traditional Chinese healthcare method, has been used to relieve muscle pain and improve general health [1–3]. Its principle therapy is based on the low negative pressure inside the cup that creates suction on the skin, which can induce local stasis of blood in the area covered by the cup. Cupping therapy has a history of more than a thousand years, and its detailed mechanism has been described in Reference [4].

According to the previous studies, cupping therapy can cause changes in hemodynamic parameters including [HbO2], [Hb], and [tHb] in the tissue near to the cupping site [5]. However, there was no effective method to detect the inner cup tissue's physiological parameters, which potentially would be very helpful to users to understand the effect of cupping therapy. The in-site regional hemodynamic change in response to

C. Gao · T. Li (✉)
Institute of Biomedical Engineering, Chinese Academy of Medical Sciences & Peking Union Medical College, Tianjin, P. R. China
e-mail: liting@bme.cams.cn; liting@uestc.edu.cn

E. M. Nemoto et al. (eds.), *Oxygen Transport to Tissue XLII*, Advances in Experimental Medicine and Biology 1269, https://doi.org/10.1007/978-3-030-48238-1_11

cupping therapy is more important than that of the out-site reported previously, because the in-site tissue hemodynamic is much more directly related to the cupping therapeutic effect. Meanwhile, the information from hemodynamic parameters can help practitioners to control the protocol of cupping therapy.

Near-infrared spectroscopy (NIRS) offers a noninvasive, relatively inexpensive method for hemodynamic measurements which have been validated in many shown to be useful for many medical [6–8]. Compared to other measurements such as PET and fMRI, NIRS places fewer limitations on the subjects and the environment and is less susceptible to interference such as from motion artifacts [9, 10]. In recent years, NIRS has been widely used in clinical and theoretical research [11, 12]. Therefore, in order to provide a relatively complete picture of the cupping therapeutic effect, we developed a NIRS system to monitor the hemodynamic alternations in and around the cupping site during cupping therapy.

11.2 Materials and Methods

A diagram of the NIRS system is shown in Fig. 11.1. The NIRS acquisition system includes three modules: the LED drive module, a data collection module, and a main control circuit. We utilized the TLC5916 to drive multi-wavelength LEDs (760 and 850 nm) for lighting in turn. The data collection module includes an AD8916 with eight input channels to convert the analog signal to a digital signal. The main control circuit is designed for controlling the other modules and communication with the host computer software. The sampling rate is set to be 5 Hz.

The NIRS system includes three probes. One of them was embedded into a cup chosen from a conventional cupping kit, and the other two probes were located near to the cupping site. Each probe comprises two detectors and one light source with two wavelengths integrated into the LED. The probe was designed as a circle with a diameter of 3.5 cm so it can be easily embedded in the cup. The distance between detector and light source is set to be 3 cm. The light emission from the LED can penetrate through tissue of up to 1.5 cm depth and be collected by the detectors. The surface of the probe was covered by black rubber to make it comfortable when attached to the skin.

The probe embedded into the cup is shown in Fig. 11.2. The probe was attached to the control circuit with wires which pass through a drilled hole on the side wall of the cup. The hole was then sealed with chemical glue to avoid air leakage. During the experiment, the probe was attached to the skin of the participant with medical double-sided tape.

The digital signal was sent by the NIRS acquisition system to the host software programed by LabVIEW. In the software, raw data of light

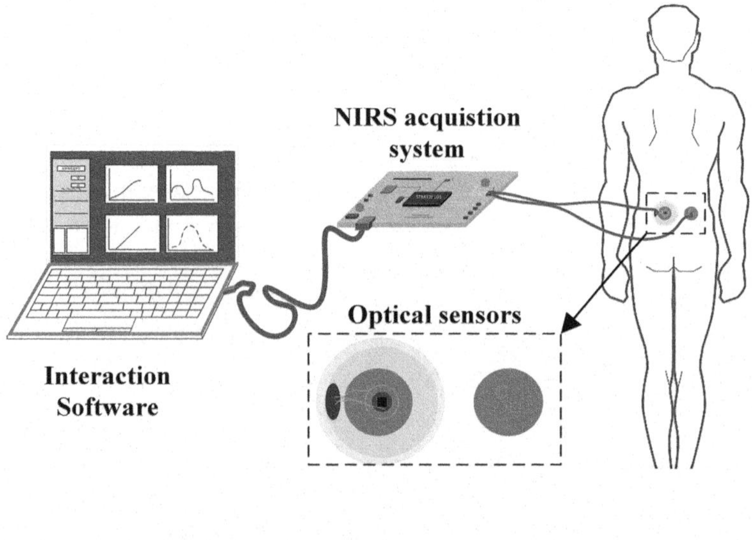

Fig. 11.1 Diagram of the NIRS system

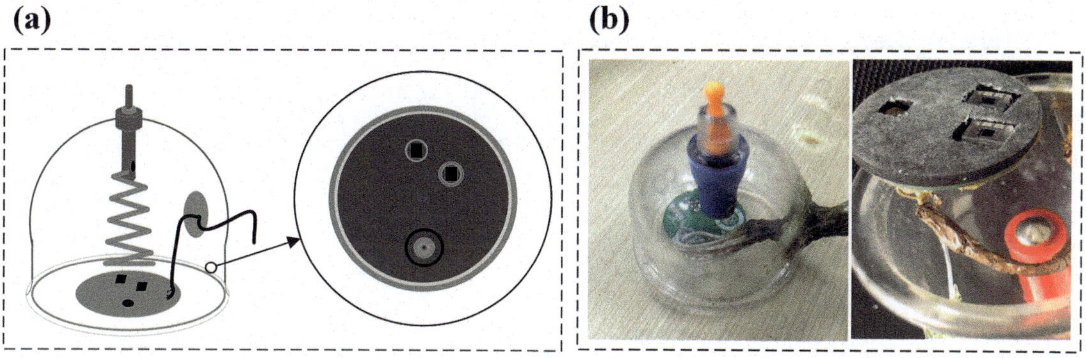

Fig. 11.2 (**a**) Diagram of the probe embedded in the cup. (**b**) Photos of the probe embedded in the cup

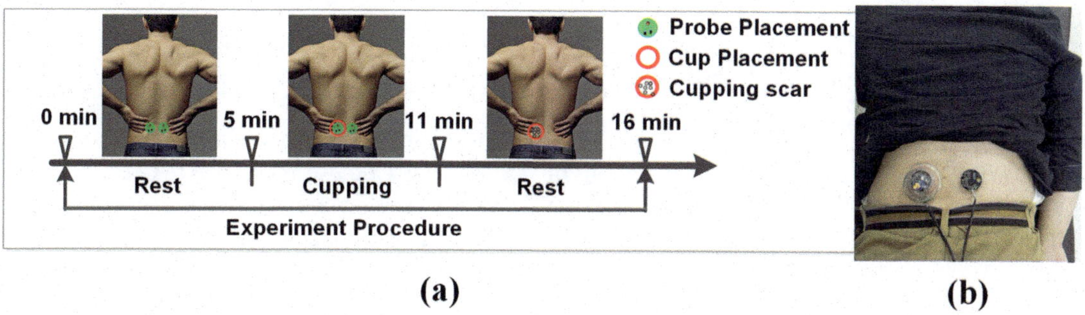

Fig. 11.3 The experiment designs. (**a**) Timeline of the measurement. (**b**) A subject under treatment

intensity was converted into changes of hemodynamic parameters by a modified Beer-Lambert law [6]. The hemodynamic curves of six channels were displayed in the software and saved in a file named by the user. Before the curves were displayed, an online removal of baseline shift was carried out.

We utilized the NIRS monitor on ten healthy subjects (seven males, aged 19–26 years, mean: 22.6 years) to test the ability of in vivo detection. The experiment protocol includes a 5-minute baseline measurement, an 8-minute cupping treatment, and a 6-minute recovery measurement (Fig. 11.3). We chose the acupoint of the kidney as the testing spot because cupping therapy at the acupoint of kidney can effectively relieve the symptoms of lumbago. For each treatment, the pressure inside the cup was kept constant at 0.075 ± 0.005 MPa.

11.3 Results

We tested the electrical performance parameter of the NIRS monitor including dark noise and long-term stability. The dark noise including circuit noise and background noise represents the minimum optical signal which can be detected by the NIRS monitor. Before dark noise testing, we put the probe on an optical phantom and switched off the LEDs. Then we wrapped the probe and phantom in black cloth to keep background light out. The testing lasted 10 minutes, and we calculated the mean value of 10-minute signals as the dark noise. The dark noise is 7 mV. Long-term stability is a key parameter for a detecting system. As in the dark noise testing, we just switched on the LEDs and let the system operate properly. The testing lasted 30 minutes, and we calculated the test data's coefficient of variation (standard

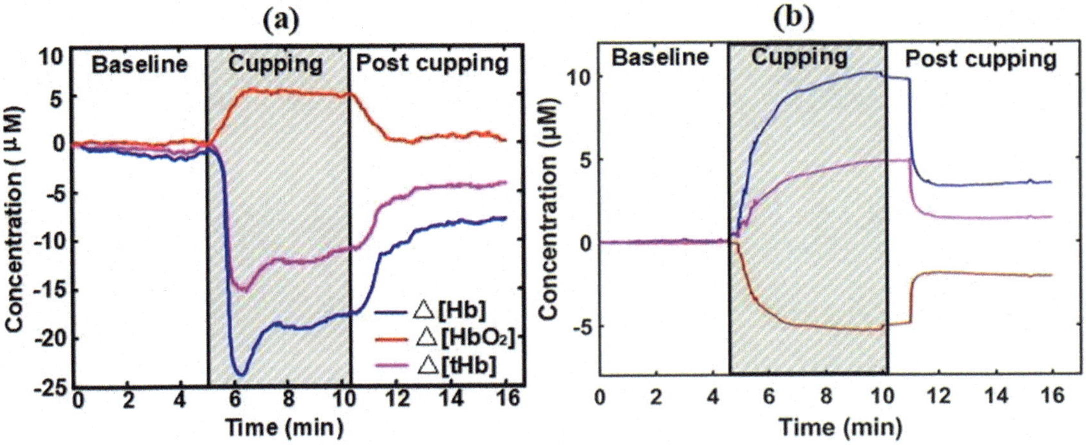

Fig. 11.4 Alterations of hemodynamic parameters averaged across ten subjects during cupping therapy. (**a**) Signals from the channel outside the cup. (**b**) Signals from channel embedded in the cup

deviation divided by mean value) as the long-term stability. The coefficient of variation of 30 minutes is 2.7%. The testing results indicate that the system can detect hemodynamic changes in tissue.

The changes of [HbO2] and [Hb] (Δ[HbO2] and Δ[Hb]) are calculated from the light intensity variations using the modified Beer-Lambert law. The changes in [tHb] (Δ[tHb]) are calculated by Δ[tHb] = Δ[HbO2] + Δ[Hb]. The results from the inner cup and outside cup channels are shown in Fig. 11.4. Significant hemodynamic changes ($p < 0.05$, paired t-test with FDR correction) occurred during cupping therapy, and the results from the inner and outside cup were opposite, indicating the redistribution of blood oxygen due to the cupping treatment.

11.4 Discussion

The hemodynamic alternations in and around the cupping site are in conformity with the actual physiological state. During the cupping stage, the low air pressure blocked the blood flow from the surrounding area into the cupping site. Therefore, the [HbO2] declines, and the [Hb] increases because of consumption of oxygen. In addition, the capillaries are slightly damaged by the low air pressure, which is helpful in triggering the tissues to activate self-repair and accelerate the "new superseding the old" according to the theory of traditional Chinese medicine (TCM) [13]. This can be an explanation for why the [tHb] increased. For the outside channels, the [HbO2] was blocked in the surrounding tissue, suggesting that cupping therapy helps the surrounding tissues to receive more oxy-hemoglobin and the surrounding tissues with the enriched oxygen level can rebuild themselves and recover from the painful state faster. In the post-cupping stage, the hemodynamic alternations are sustained (significant varied from the baseline, $p < 0.05$, paired t-test with FDR correction), which may reasonably be considered as a residual effect of the treatment.

The in vivo testing results show the NIRS monitor can detect the hemodynamic changes during the cupping therapy in and around the cupping site. We found significant hemodynamic alternations during and after cupping therapy, which can be used to evaluate the out-site regional hemodynamic therapeutic effects for cupping therapy in rehabilitation departments and in health care.FundingThis study was supported by the National Key R&D Program of China (No. 2018YFC2001100), National Natural Science Foundation of China (No. 81971660), the program of China Scholarships Council (No. 201908110204), Beijing Major Science and Technology Projects (No. Z191100010618004), Tianjin Special Branch Plan High Level Innovation Team Grant, Tianjin Key Project

Grant (18JCZDJC32700), and the Fundamental Research Funds for the Central Universities (3332019101).

References

1. Liu W, Piao S, Meng X, Wei L (2013) Effects of cupping on blood flow under skin of back in healthy human. World J Acupunct Moxibustion 23:50–52
2. Cao H, Liu J, Lewith GT (2010) Traditional Chinese medicine for treatment of fibromyalgia: a systematic review of randomized controlled trials. J Altern Complement Med 16:397–409
3. Chi LM, Lin LM, Chen CL, Wang SF, Lai HL, Peng TC (2016) The effectiveness of cupping therapy on relieving chronic neck and shoulder pain: a randomized controlled trial. Evid Based Complement Alternat Med 2016:7358918
4. Chirali IZ (2014) Traditional Chinese medicine cupping therapy. Elsevier
5. Li T, Li Y, Lin Y, Li K (2017) Significant and sustaining elevation of blood oxygen induced by Chinese cupping therapy as assessed by near-infrared spectroscopy. Biomed Opt Express 8:223–229
6. Scholkmann F, Kleise S, Metz AJ, Zimmermann R, Mata Pavia J, Wolf U, Wolf M (2011) A review on continuous wave functional near-infrared spectroscopy and imaging instrumentation and methodology. NeuroImage 85:6–27
7. Munk N, Symons B, Shang R, Cheng R, Yu G (2012) Noninvasively measuring the hemodynamic effects of massage on skeletal muscle: a novel hybrid near-infrared diffuse optical instrument. J Bodyw Mov Ther 16:22–28
8. Mancini DM, Bolinger H, Li H, Kendrick K, Chance B, Wilson JR (1994) Validation of near-infrared spectroscopy in humans. J Appl Physiol 77:2740–2747
9. Villringer A, Chance B (1997) Non-invasive optical spectroscopy and imaging of human brain function. Trends Neurosci 20:435–442
10. Hoshi Y (2007) Functional near-infrared spectroscopy: current status and future prospects. J Biomed Opt 12:062106
11. Pan B, Huang X, Li T (2019) Noninvasive and sensitive optical assessment of brain death. J Biophotonics 12(3):e201800240
12. Li T, Lin Y, Zhong F, Gao Y (2018) Longtime driving induced cerebral hemodynamic elevation and behavior degradation as assessed by functional near-infrared spectroscopy and a voluntary attention test. J Biophotonics 11:e201800160
13. Hong SH, Liu LM, Guo Y (2012) Research progress on the mechanism of cupping therapy. Henan Tradit Chin Med 32:261–262

12 Skeletal Muscle Deoxygenation and Its Relationship to Aerobic Capacity During Early and Late Stages of Aging

Shun Takagi, Ryotaro Kime, Norio Murase, Masatsugu Niwayama, Shizuo Sakamoto, and Toshihito Katsumura

Abstract

The aim of this study was to compare muscle O_2 dynamics during exercise among elderly (n = 10, age: 73 ± 3 years), middle-aged (n = 9, age: 50 ± 6 years), and young (n = 10, age: 25 ± 3 years) adults. The subjects performed ramp bicycle exercise until exhaustion. Muscle O_2 saturation (SmO_2) and relative changes from rest in oxygenated hemoglobin/myoglobin (Δoxy-Hb/Mb), deoxygenated hemoglobin/myoglobin (Δdeoxy-Hb/Mb), and total hemoglobin concentration (Δtotal-Hb) were monitored continuously at the vastus lateralis muscle by near-infrared spatial resolved spectroscopy. At given absolute workloads, SmO_2 and Δoxy-Hb/Mb were significantly lower in elderly than the other groups, while Δdeoxy-Hb/Mb, Δtotal-Hb, and pulmonary O_2 uptake (VO_2) were similar among the three groups. In contrast, there were no significant differences in muscle O_2 dynamics during submaximal exercise between middle-aged and young subjects. Muscle O_2 dynamics may be relatively preserved in early stages of aging, although muscle deoxygenation is enhanced in late stages of aging, probably due to reduced convective O_2 supply. Moreover, change in SmO_2 was significantly positively correlated with peak VO_2 in the elderly, while a significant negative relationship was observed in middle-aged and young subjects. In late stages of aging, diminished peak VO_2 may be caused by attenuated convective O_2 transport, while reduced peak VO_2 can be explained by lowered muscle O_2 extraction in early stages of aging.

Keywords

Muscle O_2 extraction · Convective O_2 transport · Elderly adults · Middle-aged adults · Young adults

S. Takagi (✉)
Faculty of Health and Sports Science, Doshisha University, Kyoto, Japan
e-mail: shtakagi@mail.doshisha.ac.jp

R. Kime · N. Murase · T. Katsumura
Department of Sports Medicine for Health Promotion, Tokyo Medical University, Tokyo, Japan

M. Niwayama
Department of Electrical and Electronic Engineering, Shizuoka University, Shizuoka, Japan

S. Sakamoto
Faculty of Sport Sciences, Waseda University, Tokyo, Japan

12.1 Introduction

Near-infrared spectroscopy (NIRS) variables reflect the balance between O_2 utilization and supply in skeletal muscle. Some previous studies

E. M. Nemoto et al. (eds.), *Oxygen Transport to Tissue XLII*, Advances in Experimental Medicine and Biology 1269, https://doi.org/10.1007/978-3-030-48238-1_12

reported that leg blood flow was reduced in the elderly during submaximal cycling exercise, compared to young subjects [1], and the enhancement of muscle deoxygenation measured by NIRS in the elderly was mainly explained by reduced convective O_2 transport [2, 3]. However, to date, the time course of aging on microcirculation and metabolism in skeletal muscle during exercise is not fully understood.

Recent studies demonstrated that minor muscle deoxygenation was observed in subjects with lower systemic aerobic capacity (i.e., peak oxygen uptake (VO_2)), compared to age-matched subjects who had higher peak VO_2 in young [4] and in a mixed group of middle-aged and elderly [5]. However, aging also attenuated peak VO_2, and this reduction appears to start as early as the age of 30 years [6]. Because aging potentially reduces convective O_2 supply [1], there remains a possibility that blunted muscle deoxygenation may not be related to lowered peak VO_2, especially in elderly people. The aim of this study was to investigate the muscle O_2 dynamics during cycling exercise and their relationship to aerobic capacity in elderly, middle-aged, and young subjects.

12.2 Methods

12.2.1 Subjects

Elderly (ELD, $n = 10$; age 73 ± 3 yrs (range: 65–80 yrs), mean ± SD), middle-aged (MID, $n = 9$; age 50 ± 6 yrs (range: 45–60 yrs), and young (YNG, $n = 10$, age 25 ± 3 yrs (range: 20–30 yrs) adults participated in the study (Table 12.1). Height, body weight, and body mass index (BMI) were matched between groups. All subjects were nonobese, as evaluated by BMI. None had cardiovascular disease or diabetes mellitus, nor had been involved in any type of endurance training for at least 12 months before enrollment in the study. This study was approved by the institutional ethics committee. All subjects were informed of the purpose of the study and written consent was obtained.

12.2.2 Experimental Design

The subjects performed 10 W/min (ELD and MID), 15 W/min (ELD and MID), or 20 W/min (MID and YNG) ramp cycling exercise until exhaustion (Strength Ergo 8, Fukuda-Denshi, Japan). Pulmonary O_2 uptake (VO_2) was monitored continuously throughout the exercise (AE310S, Minato Medical Science, Japan). Relative changes from rest in oxygenated hemoglobin/myoglobin concentration (Δoxy-Hb/Mb: an indicator of the balance between O_2 supply and utilization), deoxygenated hemoglobin/myoglobin concentration (Δdeoxy-Hb/Mb: an indicator of the balance between O_2 unloading in the muscle and blood outflow from the muscle), total hemoglobin concentration (Δtotal-Hb: an indicator of blood volume), and muscle O_2 saturation (SmO_2: an indicator of the balance between O_2 supply and utiliza-

Table 12.1 Physical characteristics of subjects

	ELD ($n = 10$)	MID ($n = 9$)	YNG (n = 10)
Age (years)	73 ± 3*#	50 ± 6*	25 ± 3
Men/women	8/2	7/2	8/2
Height (cm)	165.2 ± 9.0	166.5 ± 7.2	169.2 ± 10.5
Body weight (kg)	64.6 ± 10.1	66.2 ± 11.7	64.2 ± 9.7
BMI (kg/m^2)	23.6 ± 3.2	23.7 ± 2.9	22.3 ± 2.3
Fat layer thickness at vastus lateralis (mm)	4.4 ± 1.8	4.8 ± 1.7	4.3 ± 1.9
Peak VO_2 (mL/kg/min)	20.7 ± 3.4*#	29.7 ± 10.5*	45.4 ± 7.3

All data are given as mean ± SD. Significantly different versus young subjects (*$p < 0.05$). Significantly different versus middle-aged subjects (#$p < 0.05$)

tion, which is less sensitive to changes in blood volume than oxy-Hb/Mb) were measured at the vastus lateralis muscle in the left leg by near-infrared spatial resolved spectroscopy (NIR_{SRS}) [7]. The NIR_{SRS} data were averaged over the last 10 s at rest, every 20 W, and at peak exercise. Immediately after peak exercise, all subjects exercised at 10 W for 3 min. During the recovery time of re-saturation, the half-recovery time of SmO_2 (T1/2reoxy) was determined as the time for 50% reoxygenation of SmO_2 from the exhaustion level to the peak level. The measurement site in the vastus lateralis was defined as 30% of the length between the patella and the greater trochanter, above the patella, as defined previously [2].

The probe of the NIR_{SRS} system (Hb12–4, Astem Co., Japan) consisted of one light-emitting diode using two-wavelength (770 and 830 nm) and two photodiode detectors, and the optode distances were 20 and 30 mm. Fat layer thickness at the measurement site was measured by using an ultrasound device (LogiQ3, GE-Yokokawa Medical Systems, Japan), and the light scattering effect of the fat layer on NIR_{SRS} data was corrected by normalizing measurement sensitivity [8].

12.2.3 Statistical Analysis

All data are given as means ± standard deviation (SD). Differences in physical variables, variables at peak exercise, and T1/2reoxy among the three groups were analyzed by 1-way analysis of variance (ANOVA). To compare changes in muscle O_2 dynamics during submaximal exercise between groups, a 2-way repeated-measures ANOVA was used, with group and power output as factors. Because one subject could not exercise at more than 64 W, ANOVA was limited to rest, 20, 40, and 60 W. Where appropriate, the Bonferroni post hoc test was performed. For all statistical analyses, significance was accepted at $p < 0.05$.

12.3 Results

Figure 12.1 represents muscle O_2 dynamics with power output increasing. During submaximal exercise, there was a significant interaction for SmO_2 ($p < 0.05$), and Δoxy-Hb/Mb ($p < 0.05$). As a result, SmO_2 ($p < 0.05$) and Δoxy-Hb/Mb ($p < 0.1$) were significantly lower in ELD than the other groups. In contrast, no significant differences in SmO_2 and Δoxy-Hb/Mb were observed between MID and YNG. There were no significant interactions or main effects of group in Δdeoxy-Hb/Mb and Δtotal-Hb during submaximal exercise. At peak exercise, significantly lower Δoxy-Hb/Mb was found in ELD than in MID and YNG. ΔDeoxy-Hb/Mb and Δtotal-Hb were similar between ELD and MID, though these variables were lower in ELD and MID than in YNG. Although SmO_2 at peak exercise was not significantly different among groups, ΔSmO_2 (values at peak exercise minus values at resting) was significantly lower in MID than YNG. No significant differences in ΔSmO_2 were observed between ELD and MID and between ELD and YNG. T1/2reoxy was significantly longer in ELD (38 ± 11 s, $p < 0.05$) than the other groups, while no significant difference was observed between MID (27 ± 8 s) and YNG (22 ± 4 s). Figure 12.2 displays typical reoxygenation response during recovery in representative subjects.

At a given absolute workload, VO_2 was not significantly different between the three groups. In contrast, peak VO_2 was significantly lower in ELD than MID and YNG, while ELD represented lower peak VO_2, compared with MID. Similarly, peak power output was significantly lower in ELD compared with MID and YNG, and significant differences were also observed between MID and YNG. There were no significant differences in the group in fat layer thickness at the measurement site (Table 12.1).

ΔSmO_2 was significantly negatively related to peak VO_2 in MID ($r = -0.84$, $p < 0.05$) and YNG ($r = -0.70$, $p < 0.05$). In contrast, a significant

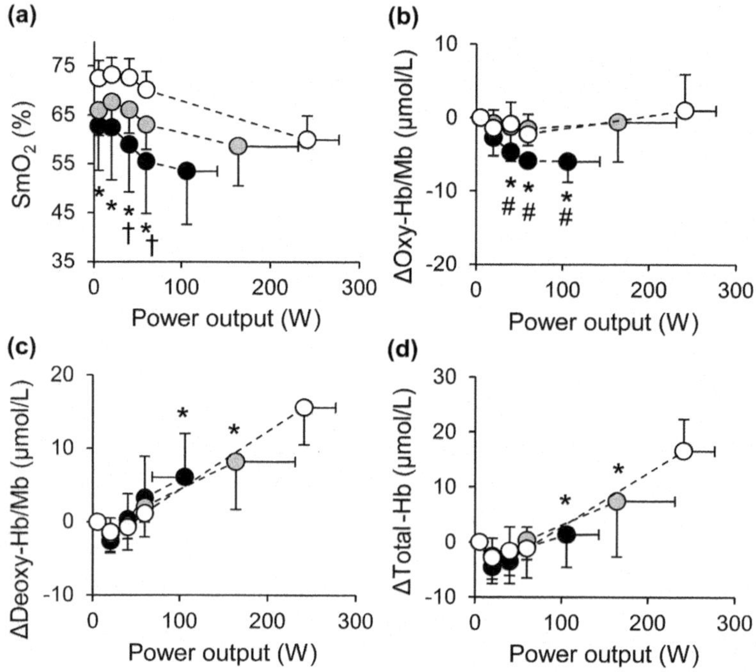

Fig. 12.1 Changes in muscle O_2 saturation (SmO_2: **a**), oxygenated hemoglobin/myoglobin (Δoxy-Hb/Mb: **b**), deoxygenated hemoglobin/myoglobin (Δdeoxy-Hb/Mb: **c**), and total hemoglobin (Δtotal-Hb: **d**) concentration during exercise in elderly (ELD, black), middle-aged (MID, gray) and young (YNG, white) subjects. Significantly different versus YNG (*p < 0.05). Significantly different versus MID (†p < 0.1, #p < 0.05). Symbols indicating a significant difference between power outputs have been omitted for the sake of clarity

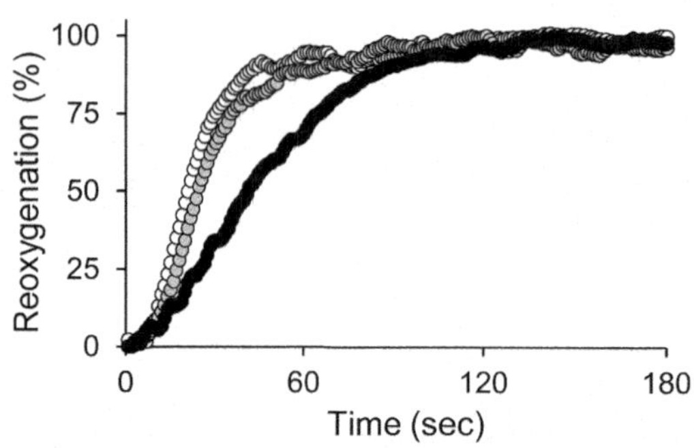

Fig. 12.2 Representative reoxygenation response of muscle O_2 saturation (SmO_2) during recovery in the elderly (ELD, black), middle-aged (MID, gray), and young (YNG, white) subjects. SmO_2 values were normalized so that 0% represents the lowest value and 100% represents the highest value during recovery. Half-recovery time of SmO_2 (T1/2reoxy) of representative subjects in ELD, MID, and YNG were 42, 25, and 22 s, respectively

positive relationship was found in ELD ($r = 0.77$, $p < 0.05$) (Fig. 12.3a). Similarly, Δdeoxy-Hb/Mb at peak exercise tended to be positively related to peak VO_2 in MID ($r = 0.65$, $p = 0.06$) and YNG ($r = 0.55$, $p < 0.1$), while there was significantly negative association with peak VO_2 in ELD ($r = -0.68$, $p < 0.05$) (Fig. 12.3b). Only in ELD, a significant negative relationship was observed between T1/2reoxy and peak VO_2 ($r = -0.73$, $p < 0.05$).

12.4 Discussion

We compared muscle O_2 dynamics during submaximal cycling exercise in elderly, middle-aged, and young subjects to test the effect of early and late stages of aging. At given absolute workloads, significantly lower SmO_2 and Δoxy-Hb/Mb were observed in ELD than in MID (40–60 W), while Δtotal-Hb, which is an index of blood volume, was similar in all groups. These results indicate that, though the present study is of cross-sectional nature, we found that muscle deoxygenation and O_2 extraction were enhanced in late stages of aging. Because VO_2 was similar between ELD and MID, an enhancement of mus-

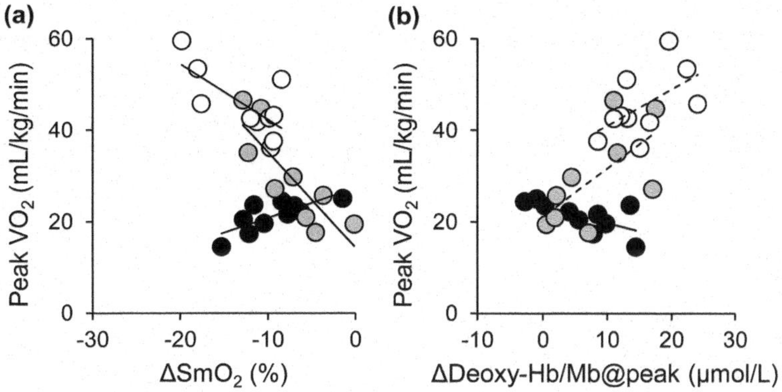

Fig. 12.3 Relationship between muscle deoxygenation and aerobic capacity in elderly (ELD, black), middle-aged (MID, gray), and young (YNG, white) subjects. (**a**) Change in muscle O_2 saturation from rest to peak exercise (ΔSmO_2) and peak VO_2. (**b**) Change in deoxygenated hemoglobin/myoglobin from rest to peak exercise (Δdeoxy-Hb/Mb@peak) and peak VO_2

cle deoxygenation may have been accelerated by reduction of muscle O_2 supply in late stages of aging. Notably, no significant differences in muscle O_2 dynamics were observed between MID and YNG. Therefore, the balance between O_2 supply and utilization in muscle may be relatively preserved during submaximal exercise in early stages of aging. Taken together, our findings lead us to speculate that the impact of aging on muscle O_2 dynamics during exercise may be different between the early and late stages of aging. Ideally, we should match physical activity among three groups to investigate the impact of biological aging without the effects of inactivity. Even though it is generally difficult to match physical activity between elderly and young subjects, further studies are needed.

Significantly higher ΔSmO_2 and lower peak VO_2 and Δdeoxy-Hb/Mb at peak exercise were observed in MID compared to YNG, and we confirmed the relationships between blunted muscle deoxygenation and lowered peak VO_2 in MID and YNG, as seen in previous studies [4, 5]. Though muscle blood flow was not measured directly in this study, these results suggest that lowered peak VO_2 can be partly explained by lowered muscle O_2 extraction in the early stages of aging. In contrast, both ΔSmO_2 and Δdeoxy-Hb/Mb at peak exercise were not significantly different between ELD and MID, while peak VO_2 was significantly impaired in ELD, compared to MID. Moreover, the higher muscle deoxygenation was associated with the low peak VO_2 in ELD, in contrast to the other groups. SmO_2 is an indicator of muscle O_2 supply and utilization, and Δdeoxy-Hb/Mb is basically reflected by O_2 unloading and blood outflow from the muscle [7]. Therefore, the similarities in ΔSmO_2 and Δdeoxy-Hb/Mb between ELD and MID can be interpreted as diminished muscle O_2 supply and consequently attenuated blood outflow from the muscle in late stages of aging. In addition, reduced peak VO_2 in ELD may be attributed to reduced convective O_2 supply, rather than diffusive O_2 transport. Slower reoxygenation and its relationship to low peak VO_2 in ELD may support these interpretations. Our findings newly demonstrated that the relationship between muscle deoxygenation and peak VO_2 may be different between the early and late stages of aging.

In conclusion, the effects of aging on muscle O_2 dynamics may depend on the phase of aging. Because VO_2 was similar during submaximal exercise among the groups, convective O_2 transport may have been compromised, especially in the late stages of aging. Moreover, in the late stages of aging, diminished peak VO_2 was mainly caused by attenuated convective O_2 transport, rather than diffusive O_2 transport, while reduced peak VO_2 was partly explained by lowered muscle O_2 extraction in the early stage of aging.

Acknowledgments The authors are grateful for revision of this manuscript by Andrea Hope. This work was supported in part by JSPS KAKENHI Grant Number 19 K20092 to Shun Takagi.

References

1. Koch DW, Newcomer SC, Proctor DN (2005) Blood flow to exercising limbs varies with age, gender, and training status. Can J Appl Physiol 30(5):554–575
2. Takagi S, Kime R, Murase N et al (2013) Aging affects spatial distribution of leg muscle oxygen saturation during ramp cycling exercise. Adv Exp Med Biol 789:157–162
3. Costes F, Denis C, Roche F et al (1999) Age-associated alteration of muscle oxygenation measured by near infrared spectroscopy during exercise. Arch Physiol Biochem 107(2):159–167
4. Boone J, Barstow TJ, Celie B et al (2016) The interrelationship between muscle oxygenation, muscle activation, and pulmonary oxygen uptake to incremental ramp exercise: influence of aerobic fitness. Appl Physiol Nutr Metab 41(1):55–62
5. Takagi S, Murase N, Kime R et al (2014) Skeletal muscle deoxygenation abnormalities in early post-myocardial infarction. Med Sci Sports Exerc 46(11):2062–2069
6. Fleg JL, Lakatta EG (1988) Role of muscle loss in the age-associated reduction in VO_2 max. J Appl Physiol (1985) 65(3):1147–1151
7. Takagi S (2016) Skeletal muscle oxygen dynamics and peak aerobic capacity. J Phys Fitness Sports Med 5(5):379–383
8. Niwayama M, Suzuki H, Yamashita T et al (2012) Error factors in oxygenation measurement using continuous wave and spatially resolved near-infrared spectroscopy. J Jpn Coll Angiol 52:211–215

Near-Infrared Spectroscopy (NIRS) of Muscle HbO_2 and MbO_2 Desaturation During Exercise

13

Edwin M. Nemoto

Abstract

Continuous noninvasive monitoring of muscle oxygenation has important clinical applications for muscle disorders such as compartmentation syndrome, fibromyalgia, deep vein thrombosis, malignant hyperthermia, and the assessment of training in athletic performance. NIRS has precisely such potential and has been used to detect deep venous thrombosis, evaluate athletic performance, and assess limb reperfusion and revascularization. The aim of this study was to examine the relationship between muscle hemoglobin oxygen (HbO_2) and myoglobin (MbO_2) desaturation using NIRS combined with venous blood sampling and HbO_2 desaturation during forearm muscle exercise. Eleven normal subjects were studied, with informed consent and an IRB-approved protocol. A NIRS sensor (INVOS4100, Somanetics, Corp.) was applied on the volar aspect of the forearm. The subjects exercised their forearm by clenching and relaxing their fist while observing the oximeter and driving the reading to specified levels from 90% to 15% (minimum possible reading). Venous blood samples were withdrawn for measurement of blood gases and oxygen saturation (IL-Co-Oximeter). RSO_2 (%) vs VO_2 Sat showed a two-component HbO_2 desaturation suggesting representation of venous HbO_2 desaturation and perhaps myoglobin oxygen (MBO_2) desaturation. Subtraction of the linear venous HbO_2 curve from the two-component curve suggests MbO_2 desaturation at venous hemoglobin oxygen saturation of about 10–20%. *Conclusions:* The kinetics of desaturation during exercise revealed two components representing HbO_2 and MbO_2 deoxygenation. The data show that MbO_2 represents approximately 40% of the NIRS signal and the balance or 60% to HbO_2.

Keywords

Exercise · Hemoglobin · Myoglobin · Muscle · Near infrared spectroscopy

13.1 Introduction

The differences between hemoglobin (Hb) and myoglobin (Mb) oxygen saturation curves are well known where hemoglobin, with four heme groups, works in a cooperative manner resulting in a sigmoid oxygen desaturation curve, whereas myoglobin, with one heme oxygen binding site, displays a monophasic rectangular hyperbola [1].

E. M. Nemoto (✉)
Department of Neurosurgery, University of New Mexico, Albuquerque, NM, USA
e-mail: enemoto@salud.unm.edu

E. M. Nemoto et al. (eds.), *Oxygen Transport to Tissue XLII*, Advances in Experimental Medicine and Biology 1269, https://doi.org/10.1007/978-3-030-48238-1_13

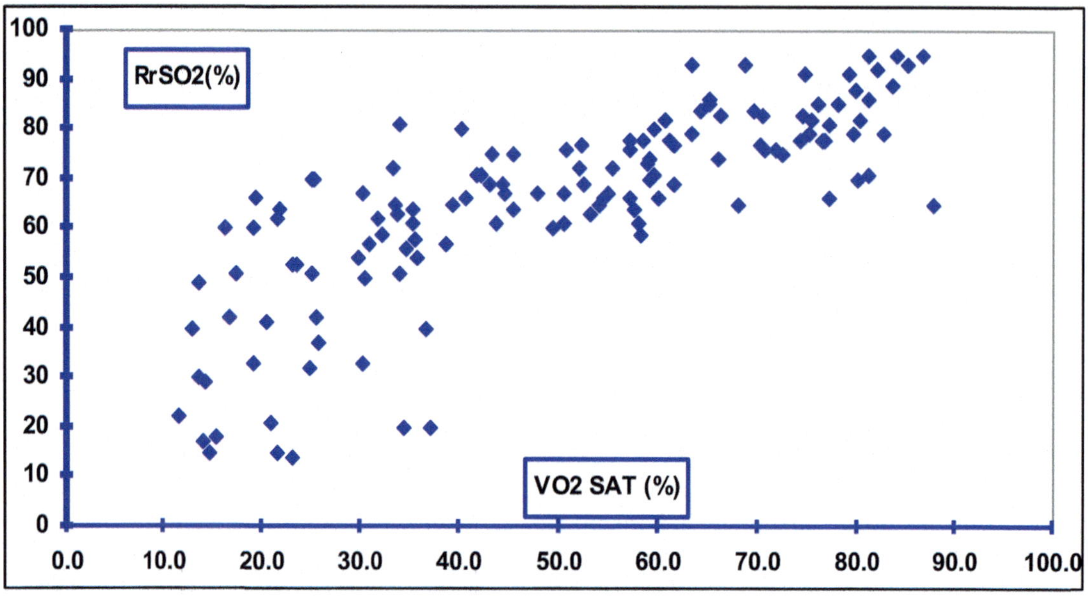

Fig. 13.1 A plot of RSO_2% versus venous oxygen (VO_2%) during forearm exercise suggests a two-component relationship and perhaps the sum of HbO_2 + MbO_2 desaturation kinetics

These result in differences in the HbO_2 and MbO_2 desaturation curves. Although many studies have been done on the desaturation of HbO_2 and MbO_2 using near-infrared spectroscopy (NIRS), [2–5] none have described the oxygen desaturation of Hb and Mb in exercising muscle. Our aim in this study was to determine whether we would be able to differentiate HbO_2 and MbO_2 desaturation in exercising muscle.

13.2 Material and Methods

Eleven normal subjects were studied, with informed consent and an IRB-approved protocol. A 22 ga Intracath was inserted retrograde into the antecubital vein draining the region over which the NIRS sensor (INVOS4100, Somanetics, Corp.) was applied on the volar aspect of the forearm. A baseline rSO2 reading was obtained with simultaneous venous blood sampling with the arm held at the level of the heart. The forearm was raised above the head, and a second reading was obtained with simultaneous sampling of venous blood for blood gas and oxygen saturation measurements.

The subjects were asked to exercise their forearm by clenching and relaxing their fist while observing the oximeter and driving the reading to specified levels from 90% to 15% (minimum possible reading). At each level, a venous blood sample was withdrawn for measurement of blood gases and oxygen saturation (IL-Co-Oximeter).

13.3 Results (Figs. 13.1, 13.2, and 13.3)

13.4 Discussion and Conclusions

Our results show, for the first time, that NIRS detects both HbO_2 and MbO_2 desaturation during exercise as compared to muscle venous blood oxygen saturation. Separation of the MbO_2 desaturation curve from HbO_2 saturation shows that MbO_2 saturation remains unchanged until venous O_2 saturation decreases below 40% and below this MbO_2 rapidly desaturates to 0–10% O_2 saturation with values ranging between 40% and 50% as reported in human gastrocnemius [6].

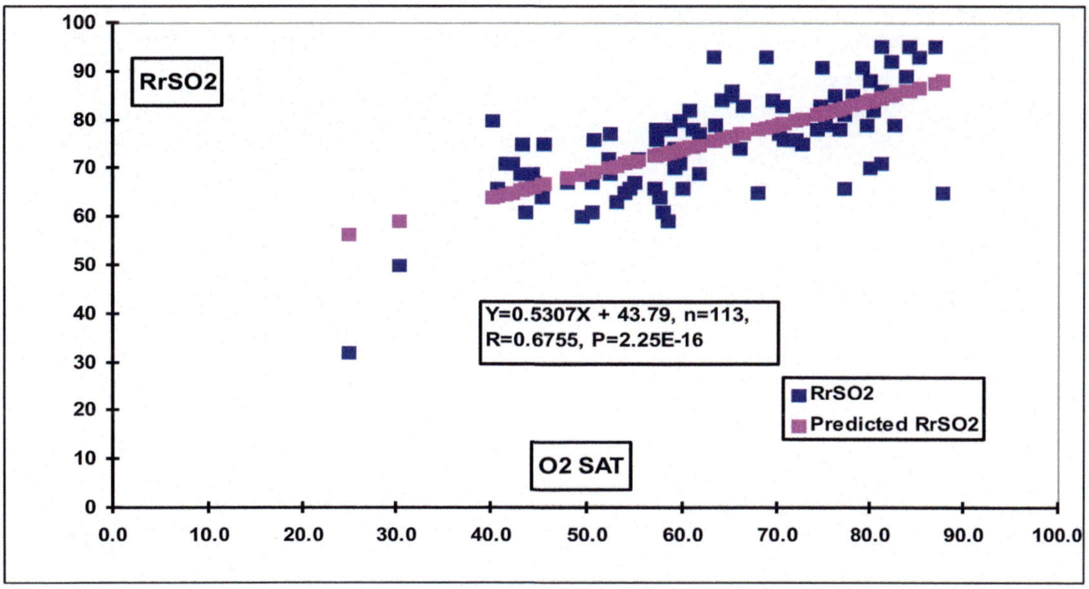

Fig. 13.2 Linear regression analysis and subtraction of the linear component of the composite curve shows a highly significant linear correlation coefficient

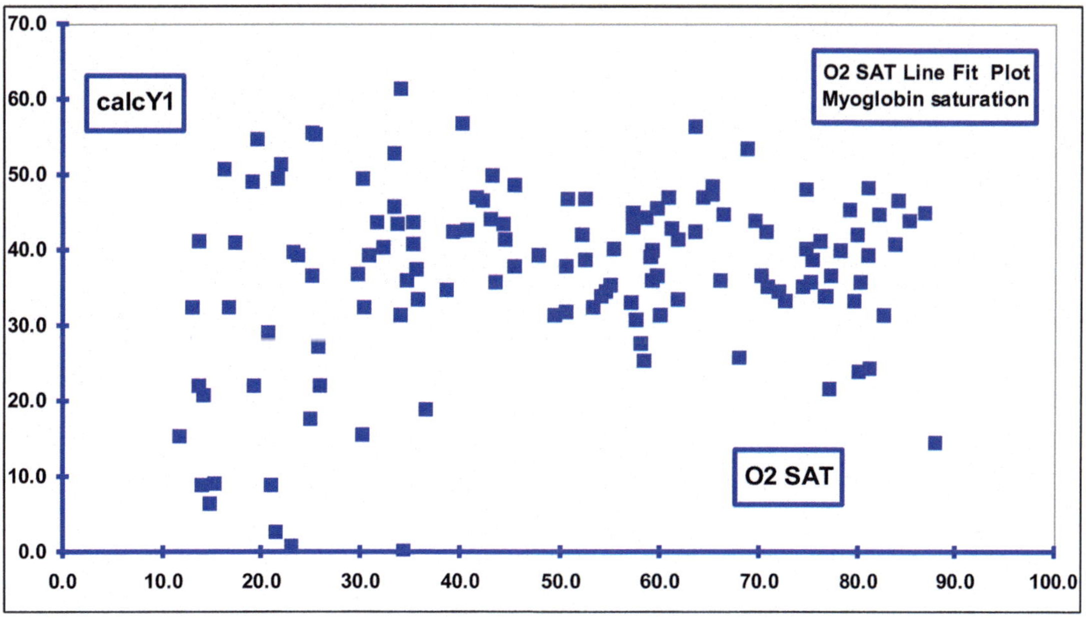

Fig. 13.3 Subtraction of oxyhemoglobin from the two-component desaturation curve shows full saturation of myoglobin at venous hemoglobin oxygen saturation of about 10–20%

References

1. https://www.andrew.cmu.edu/course/03-231/LecF05/Lec12/Lec12.pdf
2. Szmedra L, Im J, Nioka S et al (2001) Hemoglobin/myoglobin oxygen desaturation during Alpine skiing. Med Sci Sports Exerc 33(2):232–236
3. Ferreira LF, Koga S, Barstow TJ (2007) Dynamics of noninvasively estimated microvascular O2 extraction during ramp exercise. J Appl Physiol (1985) 103(6):1999–2004
4. Arakaki LS, Schenkman KA, Ciesielski WA et al (2013) Muscle oxygenation measurement in humans by noninvasive optical spectroscopy and Locally Weighted Regression. Avnal Chim Acta 785:27–33
5. Grassi B, Pogliaghi S, Rampichini S et al (2003) Muscle oxygenation and pulmonary gas exchange kinetics during cycling exercise on-transitions in hum ans. J Appl Physiol 95(1):149–158
6. Molé PA, Chung Y, Tran TK et al (1999) Myoglobin desaturation with exercise intensity in human gastrocnemius. Am J Phys 277(1):R173–R180

14 Relationship Between Corticosteroid Dose and Muscle Oxygen Consumption in Recipients of Hematopoietic Stem-Cell Transplantation

Shinichiro Morishita, Tatsushi Wakasugi, Katsuji Kaida, Yusuke Itani, Kazuhiro Ikegame, Hiroyasu Ogawa, Yoshihiro Fujimori, and Kazuhisa Domen

Abstract

Introduction: After hematopoietic stem-cell transplantation (HSCT), patients exhibit decreased muscle strength and muscle oxygen consumption. Furthermore, total corticosteroid dose affects the reduction in muscle strength after HSCT. However, to date, no studies have investigated the relationship between corticosteroid dose and muscle oxygen consumption and saturation in these patients. The purpose of this study was to investigate the relationship between steroid dose and deoxyhemoglobin (ΔHHb) and muscle oxyhemoglobin saturation (ΔSmO_2) in patients undergoing HSCT. *Methods:* This study included 17 men with hematologic disease who underwent allogeneic HSCT. We evaluated ankle dorsiflexor muscle force, ΔHHb, and ΔSmO_2 in skeletal muscles by near-infrared spectroscopy (NIRS) in patients before and after HSCT. *Results:* Peak ankle dorsiflexion, ΔHHb, and ΔSmO_2 decreased significantly after transplantation as compared to measurements taken before transplantation ($p < 0.01$). The change in peak ankle dorsiflexion from before to after HSCT was not significantly correlated with total steroid dose. However, ΔHHb and ΔSmO_2 from before to after HSCT were significantly correlated with total steroid dose ($p < 0.01$). *Conclusion*: This study showed that higher corticosteroid doses are associated with diminished skeletal muscle O_2 consumption and skeletal muscle O_2 demand relative to supply. Therefore, rehabilitation staff, nurses, and physicians should take note of these findings in patients undergoing HSCT. Moreover, physiotherapists should be carefully measuring muscle oxidative metabolism on skeletal muscle when planning physical exercise in such patients.

S. Morishita (✉)
Institute for Human Movement and Medical Science, Niigata University of Health and Welfare, Niigata, Japan

Department of Physical Medicine and Rehabilitation, Hyogo College of Medicine, Nishinomiya, Japan
e-mail: morishita@nuhw.ac.jp

T. Wakasugi · Y. Itani
Department of Rehabilitation Medicine, Hyogo College of Medicine Hospital, Nishinomiya, Japan

K. Kaida · K. Ikegame · H. Ogawa · Y. Fujimori
Division of Hematology, Department of Internal Medicine, Hyogo College of Medicine, Nishinomiya, Japan

K. Domen
Department of Physical Medicine and Rehabilitation, Hyogo College of Medicine, Nishinomiya, Japan

E. M. Nemoto et al. (eds.), *Oxygen Transport to Tissue XLII*, Advances in Experimental Medicine and Biology 1269, https://doi.org/10.1007/978-3-030-48238-1_14

Keywords

Corticosteroid · Muscle oxygen consumption · Near-infrared spectroscopy · Hematopoietic stem-cell transplantation · Rehabilitation

14.1 Introduction

Allogeneic hematopoietic stem-cell transplantation (allo-HSCT) is a potentially curative treatment for patients with hematological malignancy [1] and is increasingly used to treat hematopoietic diseases worldwide [2]. Patients with hematological malignancies who undergo HSCT exhibit decreased muscle strength after transplantation compared to that before HSCT [3–5]. HSCT patients often experience decreased muscle strength due to decreased physical activity and body weight, which may be exacerbated by chemotherapy [3–5]. Our previous research demonstrated a relationship between total corticosteroid dose and the decrease in muscle strength in patients after HSCT [6]. Additionally, after HSCT, recipients exhibit significant decreases in muscle oxygen consumption, as evidenced by changes in deoxyhemoglobin (ΔHHb) and blood flow to the skeletal muscle according to near-infrared spectroscopy (NIRS) [7], which can be used for noninvasive assessment of muscle oxygenation and hemodynamic parameters during exercise [8]. Furthermore, in another previous study, we showed that there is a relationship between muscle oxyhemoglobin saturation (ΔSmO_2) and muscle strength in allo-HSCT recipients [9]. From these findings, we hypothesized that corticosteroid dose may have an effect on muscle oxygen consumption and saturation in HSCT recipients. However, to date, no studies investigating such a relationship have been performed. The purpose of this study was to investigate the relationship between steroid dose and HHb and SmO_2 in patients undergoing HSCT.

14.2 Methods

14.2.1 Participants

In this prospective observational study, we investigated the relationship between steroid dose, ankle dorsiflexor muscle force, ΔHHb, and ΔSmO_2 in skeletal muscles using NIRS in patients who underwent allo-HSCT at the Hyogo College of Medicine Hospital, Japan, between January 2010 and March 2012. Seventeen patients met our inclusion criteria and were enrolled in the study. Ethical approval for the study was obtained from the Institutional Committee on Human Research of the Hyogo College of Medicine. Female patients were excluded because women have higher subcutaneous fat than men and the accurate NIRS measurement of muscle oxygenation is influenced by subcutaneous fat. Written informed consent was obtained from each patient prior to participation. The following information was collected from the medical records: age, sex, height, body weight, underlying hematological diagnosis, stem-cell source, conditioning, and total steroid dose. Patient evaluation was performed 3 weeks before and 6 weeks after transplantation. Consequently, 17 hematological malignancy patients were included in this study (Table 14.1).

14.2.2 Experimental Procedure

NIRS was used to determine muscle oxygen consumption during exercise in allo-HSCT patients. Muscle utilization of the oxidative metabolic system is represented by NIRS as concentration changes in oxy-Hb (O_2Hb), HHb, and total-Hb volume ($tHb = O_2Hb + HHb$). HHb can be used to quantify muscle oxygen extraction [10]. SmO_2 is represented by NIRS as concentration changes in O_2Hb, HHb, and tHb, according to the following formula: $SmO_2 = O_2Hb/tHb \times 100$. SmO_2 reflects the dynamic balance of O_2 supplied by the microcirculation and O_2 consumption by the

Table 14.1 Demographic and clinical characteristics of HSCT patients ($n = 17$)

Characteristics		Median (range)
Age (in years)		41 (26–63)
Sex	Male	17 (100)
		Mean (SD)
Height (cm)		173.5 (6.9)
Body weight (kg)		64.3 (8.5)
Diagnosis (n)	Acute leukemia	6
	Malignant lymphoma	8
	Myelodysplastic syndrome	2
	Chronic myelogenous leukemia	1
Stem-cell source (n)	Peripheral blood stem cell	11
	Bone marrow	2
	Cord blood	4
Conditioning (n)	Myeloablative	3
	Reduced intensity	14
Steroid dose	Yes	17
Total corticosteroid dose (mg/kg)		54.7 (25.4)

HSCT hematopoietic stem-cell transplantation

muscle. We used tibialis anterior (TA) muscles to monitor muscle oxygen extraction and Hb dynamics. A dynamometer (System 4; Biodex Medical Systems, USA) was used to measure ankle dorsiflexor muscle force (units = N). All participants were instructed to perform three 5-s maximum voluntary contractions (MVCs). The highest peak torque value was measured for repeated isometric contraction tasks. All participants performed a repeated isometric contraction task at 50% of MVC with the right leg. The workload performed was adjusted to 50% MVC of ankle dorsiflexion at a 50% duty cycle for 180 s (90 times). Task failure was defined when two consecutive contractions did not reach the target.

14.2.3 NIRS Measurements

A laser tissue blood oximeter (BOM – L1TRW Omega Wave, Japan) was used to measure concentration changes in O2Hb, HHb, and tHb. The NIRS signals were continuously stored at 10 Hz using Power Lab (AD Instruments, Nagoya, Japan) on a personal computer and analyzed using Lab Chart software (AD Instruments, Nagoya, Japan). The SmO_2 amplitude (ΔSmO_2) was the difference between the minimum SmO_2 value during contractions and the resting SmO_2 value (Fig. 14.1a). Higher ΔSmO_2 values indicate greater O_2 demand relative to supply. The HHb parameter measured the relative change from contraction onset (HHb max). The ΔHHb value was determined as the difference between the maximum HHb value during contractions and the resting value (Fig. 14.1b). A higher ΔHHb value indicates increased muscle oxygen consumption [11].

14.2.4 Statistical Analysis

A paired t-test was used to compare peak ankle dorsiflexion, ΔHHb, and ΔSmO_2 before and after transplantation. Pearson's chi-squared test was used to evaluate the relationship between the total steroid dose and the changes in peak ankle dorsiflexion, ΔHHb, and ΔSmO_2 from before to after HSCT. Statistical analyses were performed using SPSS 21.0 (SPSS Japan Inc., Tokyo, Japan), with results considered statistically significant at $p < 0.05$.

14.3 Results

The median age of the patients in this study was 41 years, and all (100%) patients were men. Patients' hematological diseases included malignant lymphoma, acute leukemia, myelodysplastic syndrome, and chronic myelogenous leukemia. Three patients received myeloablative conditioning, and 14 patients received reduced intensity conditioning. The mean total steroid dose was 54.7 mg/kg (Table 14.1). Peak ankle dorsiflexion, ΔHHb, and ΔSmO_2 decreased significantly after transplantation as compared to measurements taken before transplantation ($p < 0.01$; Table 14.2). The change in peak ankle dorsiflexion from before to after HSCT was not

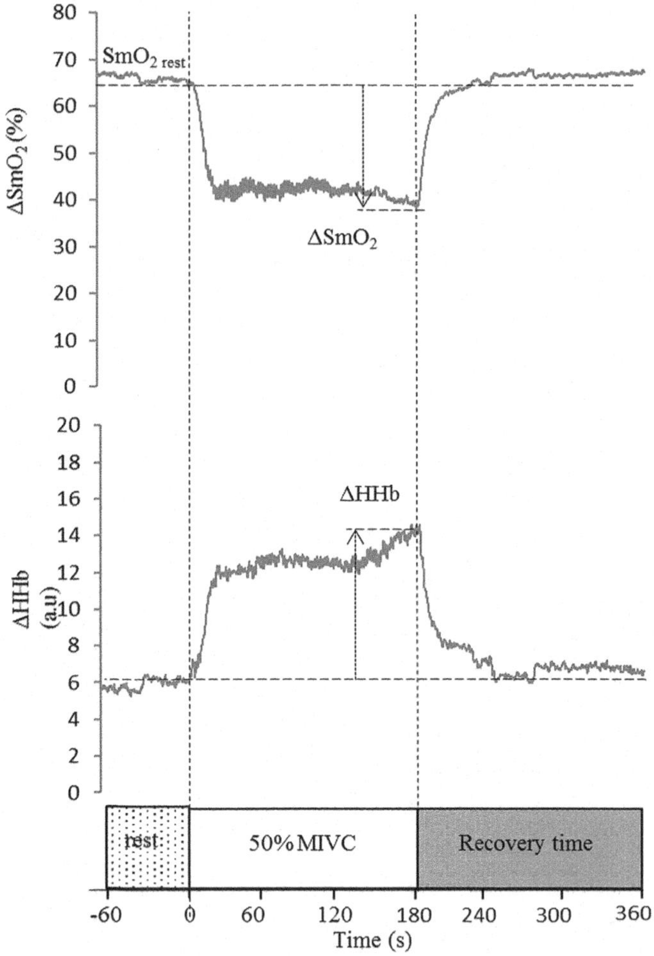

Fig. 14.1 NIRS measurements. Typical raw data of NIRS parameters in the tibialis anterior muscle—oxy-hemoglobin saturation (ΔSmO_2) and deoxyhemoglobin (HHb)—during repeated isometric contractions at 50% maximal voluntary contraction (50% MVC). The vertical dotted lines delimit the duration of the contractions. SmO_2 rest SmO_2 resting average value, ΔSmO_2 oxyhemoglobin saturation amplitude, ΔHHb Δdeoxyhemoglobin amplitude

Table 14.2 Comparison of ankle dorsiflexion scale and NIRS parameters of patients pre- and post-HSCT

	Before HSCT			After HSCT			
Variables	Mean	95% CI lower	Upper	Mean	95% CI lower	Upper	*P*-value
Peak ankle dorsiflexion (Nm)	26.1	21.8	30.4	14.8	12.3	17.3	<0.001
NIRS							
ΔHHb (a.u)	4.9	3.4	6.4	2.5	1.7	3.3	0.006
ΔSmO_2 (%)	−21.5	−16.7	−26.4	−10.4	−7.6	−13.1	<0.001

NIRS near-infrared spectroscopy, *HSCT* hematopoietic stem-cell transplantation, *a.u* arbitrary units, *ΔHHb* maximum de-oxy hemoglobin amplitude, ΔSmO_2, minimum muscle O_2Hb saturation amplitude, *CI* confidence interval significantly correlated with total steroid dose. However, ΔHHb and ΔSmO_2 from before to after HSCT were significantly correlated with total steroid dose ($p < 0.01$; Fig. 14.2a–c).

14.4 Discussion

In the present study, there were significant decreases in peak ankle dorsiflexion, ΔHHb, and ΔSmO_2 after HSCT compared to values measured before transplantation. Thus, HSCT recipients exhibited decreased lower TA muscle strength and muscle O_2 consumption. This is consistent with the results of previous studies showing significant decreases in lower extremity muscle strength after HSCT [3, 5]. Our prior study showed that the O_2 supply was not changed after HSCT [9]. Moreover, this current study showed that ΔHHb was decreased significantly after transplantation. Together, these results suggest that skeletal muscle oxygenation suffers from

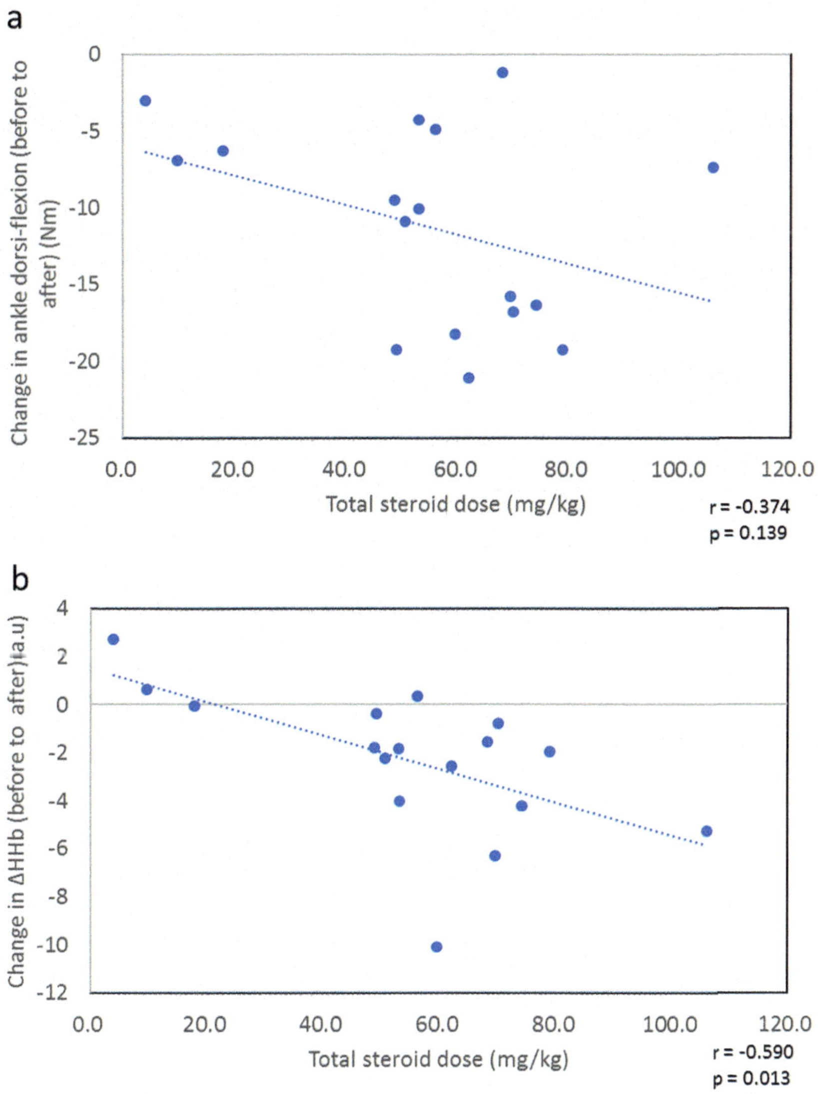

Fig. 14.2 Correlations between steroid dose and skeletal muscle and NIRS parameters. Scatterplots illustrating the relationship between the total steroid dose and skeletal muscle and NIRS parameters. (**a**) Total steroid dose and ankle dorsiflexion, (**b**) total steroid dose and ΔHHb, (**c**) total steroid dose and ΔSmO_2

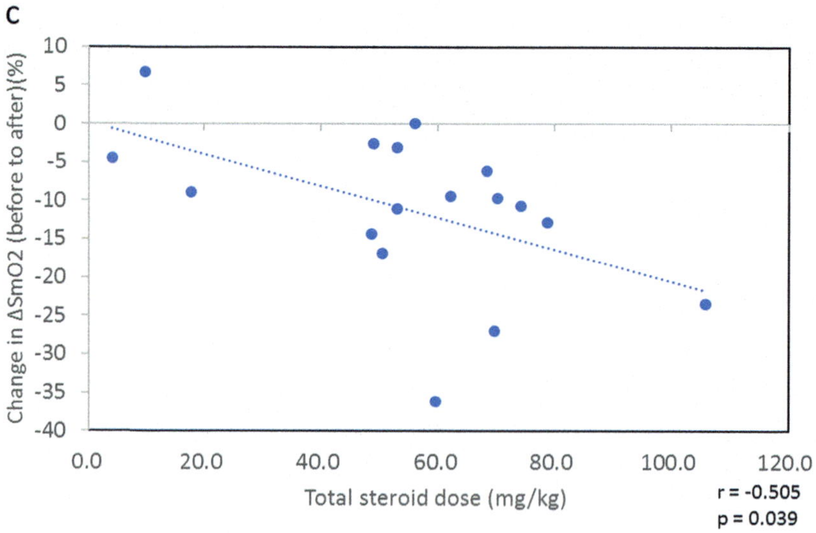

Fig. 14.2 (continued)

impaired oxygen extraction due to mitochondrial dysfunction rather than reduced oxygen supply due to microcirculation following allo-HSCT. To date, the underlying causes of such decreases in muscle strength and O_2 consumption have been unclear. We hypothesized that the oxidative metabolism of skeletal muscle may be altered by corticosteroid treatment after HSCT. Therefore, we investigated the relationship between corticosteroid dose and the change in ΔHHb and ΔSmO_2 from before to after HSCT. The results showed that changes in ΔHHb and ΔSmO_2 were significantly correlated with total corticosteroid dose. These findings suggest that patients treated with higher corticosteroid doses exhibit diminished skeletal muscle O_2 consumption. A previous report showed that corticosteroids have direct catabolic effects on skeletal muscles that can lead to reductions in muscle protein synthesis and protein catabolism [12]. Moreover, other studies have demonstrated that glucocorticoids induce oxidative stress in skeletal muscle [13]. Thus, corticosteroids may induce oxidative stress and reduce muscle protein synthesis after HSCT, leading to reductions in skeletal muscle O_2 consumption. This knowledge may help clinicians to better plan exercises to improve patients' muscle strength and enable appropriate evaluation of physical therapy effects.

In conclusion, recipients of HSCT exhibit decreased lower TA muscle strength and muscle O_2 consumption. Furthermore, the current study demonstrated that higher corticosteroid doses are associated with diminished skeletal muscle O_2 consumption. Therefore, rehabilitation staff, nurses, and physicians should take note of these findings as it pertains to patients undergoing HSCT. Moreover, physiotherapists should carefully measure muscle oxidative metabolism on skeletal muscle when planning physical exercise in such patients.

Acknowledgments This study was supported by a Grant-in-Aid for Exploratory Research from the Niigata University of Health and Welfare, Japan.

References

1. Copelan EA (2006) Hematopoietic stem-cell transplantation. N Engl J Med 354:1813–1826
2. Pidala J, Djulbegovic B, Anasetti C, Kharfan-Dabaja M, Kumar A (2011) Allogeneic hematopoietic cell transplantation for adult acute lymphoblastic leukemia (ALL) in first complete remission. Cochrane Database Syst Rev:CD008818
3. Morishita S, Kaida K, Yamauchi S et al (2017) Relationship of physical activity with physical function and health-related quality of life in patients having undergone allogeneic haematopoietic stem-cell transplantation. Eur J Cancer Care (Engl) 26

4. Takekiyo T, Dozono K, Mitsuishi T et al (2015) Effect of exercise therapy on muscle mass and physical functioning in patients undergoing allogeneic hematopoietic stem cell transplantation. Support Care Cancer 23:985–992
5. Ishikawa A, Otaka Y, Kamisako M et al (2018) Factors affecting lower limb muscle strength and cardiopulmonary fitness after allogeneic hematopoietic stem cell transplantation. Support Care Cancer 27:1793–1800
6. Morishita S, Kaida K, Yamauchi S et al (2013) Relationship between corticosteroid dose and declines in physical function among allogeneic hematopoietic stem cell transplantation patients. Support Care Cancer 21:2161–2169
7. Morishita S, Wakasugi T, Kaida K et al (2018) Fatigue, muscle oxygen consumption and blood flow to the skeletal muscle after allogeneic hematopoietic stem cell transplantation. Adv Exp Med Biol 1072:293–298
8. Hamaoka T, McCully KK, Quaresima V, Yamamoto K, Chance B (2007) Near-infrared spectroscopy/imaging for monitoring muscle oxygenation and oxidative metabolism in healthy and diseased humans. J Biomed Opt 12:062105
9. Wakasugi T, Morishita S, Kaida K et al (2018) Impaired skeletal muscle oxygenation following allogeneic hematopoietic stem cell transplantation is associated with exercise capacity. Support Care Cancer 26:2149–2160
10. Grassi B, Quaresima V (2016) Near-infrared spectroscopy and skeletal muscle oxidative function in vivo in health and disease: a review from an exercise physiology perspective. J Biomed Opt 21:091313
11. duManoir GR, DeLorey DS, Kowalchuk JM, Paterson DH (2010) Kinetics of VO2 limb blood flow and regional muscle deoxygenation in young adults during moderate intensity, knee-extension exercise. Eur J Appl Physiol 108:607–617
12. Liu D, Ahmet A, Ward L et al (2013) A practical guide to the monitoring and management of the complications of systemic corticosteroid therapy. Allergy Asthma Clin Immunol 9:30
13. You JM, Yun SJ, Nam KN, Kang C, Won R, Lee EH (2009) Mechanism of glucocorticoid-induced oxidative stress in rat hippocampal slice cultures. Can J Physiol Pharmacol 87:440–447

15 Relationship Between the Borg Scale Rating of Perceived Exertion and Leg-Muscle Deoxygenation During Incremental Exercise in Healthy Adults

Shinichiro Morishita, Atsuhiro Tsubaki, Kazuki Hotta, Sho Kojima, Daichi Sato, Akihito Shirayama, Yuki Ito, and Hideaki Onishi

Abstract

Introduction: The Borg scale rating of perceived exertion is a reliable indicator and widely used to monitor and guide exercise intensity. We aimed to evaluate the relationships between the Borg scale score and oxygenated hemoglobin (O2Hb) and deoxygenated hemoglobin (HHb) concentrations in the leg muscle as measured by near-infrared spectroscopy (NIRS) during cardiopulmonary exercise testing (CPET) in healthy adult men. We also investigated the relationships between the Borg scale score and the work rate (WR), heart rate (HR), oxygen uptake (VO_2), and minute ventilation (VE). Methods: Participants comprised 12 healthy men. Cardiopulmonary and NIRS parameters were assessed during each minute of CPET and at the end of the test. Results: The Borg scale score was significantly correlated with cardiopulmonary parameters including WR, HR, VO_2, and VE during CPET (Rs = 0.87–0.95; $p < 0.05$). Furthermore, the Borg scale score was significantly correlated with NIRS parameters including O2Hb and HHb levels during CPET (Rs = −0.48 and 0.45, respectively; $p < 0.05$). Discussion: The Borg scale score is significantly correlated with cardiopulmonary parameters (WR, HR, VO_2, and VE), as well as with leg-muscle oxygenation parameters as assessed by NIRS, during CPET in healthy adults. The correlation coefficients obtained from NIRS parameters were lower than those of cardiopulmonary parameters. Conclusions: The Borg scale score might better reflect cardiopulmonary responses than muscle deoxygenation during exercise. These results can aid in the planning of rehabilitation programs for healthy adults.

S. Morishita (✉) · A. Tsubaki · K. Hotta · H. Onishi
Institute for Human Movement and Medical Science, Niigata University of Health and Welfare, Niigata, Japan

Department of Physical Therapy, Faculty of Rehabilitation, Niigata University of Health and Welfare, Niigata, Japan
e-mail: morishita@nuhw.ac.jp

S. Kojima
Institute for Human Movement and Medical Science, Niigata University of Health and Welfare, Niigata, Japan

D. Sato · A. Shirayama · Y. Ito
Department of Physical Therapy, Faculty of Rehabilitation, Niigata University of Health and Welfare, Niigata, Japan

E. M. Nemoto et al. (eds.), *Oxygen Transport to Tissue XLII*, Advances in Experimental Medicine and Biology 1269, https://doi.org/10.1007/978-3-030-48238-1_15

Keywords

Borg scale · Rating of perceived exertion · Near-infrared spectroscopy · Cardiopulmonary exercise testing · Exercise

15.1 Introduction

Previous studies have shown that the deoxygenated hemoglobin (HHb) concentration in leg muscles as measured by near-infrared spectroscopy (NIRS) is increased, relative to the work rate, during ramp-incremental cycle ergometry in healthy adults [1] and patients with heart failure [2]. Similarly, other studies have shown that leg-muscle HHb levels gradually increase with increased exercise intensity, while leg-muscle oxygenated hemoglobin (O_2Hb) levels gradually decrease, during cardiopulmonary exercise testing (CPET) in patients with chronic obstructive pulmonary disease (COPD) [3].

Furthermore, the rating of perceived exertion (RPE) using the Borg scale with the 0–10 category-ratio scale (CR-10) is considered a reliable indicator and is widely used to monitor and guide exercise intensity [4]. The Borg scale can represent extreme intensities of activity. The Borg scale score is significantly correlated with oxygen uptake (VO_2), heart rate (HR), and work rate, which gradually increases during CPET in healthy adults [5]. We hypothesized that the Borg scale score is related to leg-muscle O_2Hb and HHb levels during CPET, which, to date, has not been investigated. Therefore, the purpose of this study was to investigate the relationships between the Borg scale score and leg-muscle O_2Hb and HHb levels on NIRS during CPET in healthy men. We also investigated the relationships between the Borg scale score and the work rate, heart rate (HR), oxygen uptake (VO_2), and minute ventilation (VE).

15.2 Methods

15.2.1 Participants

Twelve healthy male volunteers (mean age, 20.8 ± 0.5 years; mean height, 172.9 ± 7.8 cm; mean body weight, 64.6 ± 9.0 kg) participated in this study. None of the participants exhibited symptoms of neurological or cardiovascular disease, and all were free from medication at the time of the study. Each participant provided written informed consent after receiving information regarding the potential risks, study objectives, measurement techniques, and benefits associated with the study. This study was approved by the Ethics Committee of Niigata University of Health and Welfare (Approval No. 18124-190116) and was conducted in accordance with the ethical standards of the 1964 Declaration of Helsinki and its later amendments or comparable ethical standards.

15.2.2 Experimental Procedure

Participants performed CPET with ramp-exercise protocols to determine the VO_2 and VE. The protocol consisted of a 4-minute rest, 4-minute warm-up, cardiopulmonary exercise, and 2-minute cooldown. A ramp program with an incremental increase in workload of 20 watts/minute on a stationary bicycle (Aerobike 75XLIII; Konami, Tokyo, Japan) with electrocardiography (ECG) (DS-7520, Fukuda Denshi, Tokyo, Japan) and an exhaled gas analyzer (AE-310S; Minato Medical Science, Osaka, Japan) were used. All participants were instructed to maintain a cadence of 50 rotations per minute (rpm) during CPET. Exhaustion was defined as follows [6]: (1) a plateau in VO_2; (2) a respiratory exchange ratio >1.1; (3) HR values near the age-predicted maximal heart rate, calculated as 220 − (0.65 × age); and (4) a decrease in the cycling cadence to <50 rpm, despite strong verbal encouragement. The highest value obtained for VO2 was considered the VO2 peak. We evaluated the HR (using ECG), work rate (in watts), and VO_2 and VE (using an exhaled gas analyzer) for each minute of CPET and at the end of the exercise test. Additionally, the anaerobic thresholds (ATs) during CPET were determined using the V-slope method [7]. All participants were asked "how hard do you feel you are working" using the Borg scale; responses were recorded every minute. The Borg CR-10 scale, which comprises a rating between 0 (nothing at all) and 10 (very very strong) [8], was used in this study.

15.2.3 NIRS Measurements

NIRS was used to determine muscle oxygen consumption during CPET. We evaluated O_2Hb and HHb levels for each minute of CPET and at the end of the exercise test. O_2Hb and HHb levels were measured in the left vastus lateralis muscle using NIRS (OMEGAFLOW BOM-L1 TRW, OMM Corp., Tokyo, Japan). The probe and detector were set in an optically dense rubber holder to ensure stability in their relative positions. They were secured to the thigh using adhesive tape in order to minimize motion artifacts and contamination of the signal by ambient light. The HHb level can be used to quantify muscle oxygen extraction [9]. O_2Hb and HHb parameters are presented as the relative change from those at rest.

15.2.4 Statistical Analysis

The Pearson's chi-squared test was used to evaluate the relationships between the Borg scale score and the work rate, HR, VO_2, VE, and O_2Hb and HHb levels during CPET. Statistical analyses were performed using SPSS 21.0 (SPSS Japan Inc., Tokyo, Japan), with statistical significance set at $p < 0.05$.

Table 15.1 Subjects' characteristics ($n = 12$)

Characteristics	
Age, years	
Mean (SD)	20.8 (0.5)
Height, cm	
Mean (SD)	172.9 (7.8)
Body weight, kg	
Mean (SD)	64.6 (9.0)
Cardiopulmonary exercise testing	
At rest	
Borg scale	0 (0–0)
Work rate (watts)	0 (0)
HR (beat/minute)	76.8 (15.9)
VO_2 (ml/kg/min)	3.9 (0.3)
VE (L)	8.7 (1.3)
Anaerobic threshold (AT)	
Borg scale	2 (1–4)
Work rate (watts)	98.5 (27.1)
HR (beat/minute)	127.3 (10.3)
VO_2 (ml/kg/min)	18.8 (4.9)
VE (L)	27.3 (6.5)
O_2Hb (a.u)	−0.09 (0.15)
HHb (a.u)	0.04 (0.12)
End of test (maximum)	
Borg scale	7 (4–10)
Work rate (watts)	184.3(36.4)
HR (beat/minute)	179.1 (12.8)
VO_2 (ml/kg/min)	32.5 (5.9)
VE (L)	64.9 (20.1)
O_2Hb (a.u)	−0.03 (0.13)
HHb (a.u)	−0.05 (0.18)

SD standard deviation, *HR* heart rate, *VO2* oxygen uptake, *VE* minute ventilation, *O2Hb* oxygenated hemoglobin, *HHb* deoxygenated hemoglobin concentration

15.3 Results

All participants completed CPET (Table 15.1). The Borg scale score was significantly correlated with the work rate, HR, VO_2, and VE during CPET (Rs = 0.87–0.95, $p < 0.05$) (Fig. 15.1a–d). Furthermore, the Borg scale score was significantly correlated with leg-muscle O_2Hb and HHb levels during CPET (Rs = −0.48 and 0.45, respectively; $p < 0.05$) (Fig. 15.1e, f).

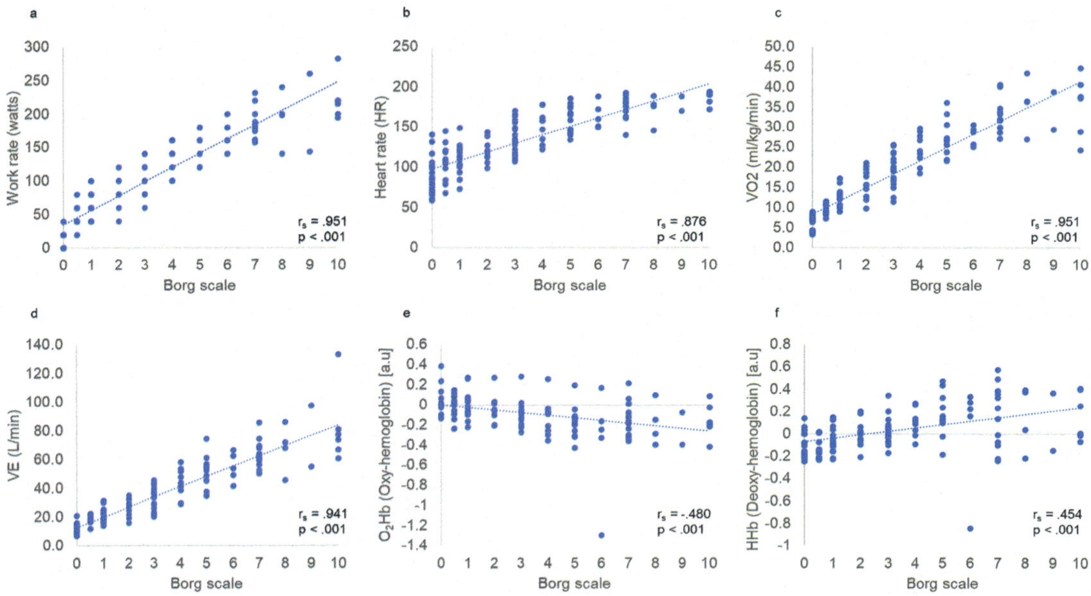

Fig. 15.1 Relationships between the Borg scale rating of perceived exertion and physiological outcomes and O_2Hb and HHb levels during cardiopulmonary exercise testing. Scatterplots illustrating the relationships between the Borg scale score and physiological and NIRS parameters every minute during cardiopulmonary exercise testing for each subject are shown. (a) Work rate, (b) heart rate, (c) VO_2, (d) VE, (e) O_2Hb, (f) HHb. VO_2 oxygen uptake, VE minute ventilation, O_2Hb oxygenated hemoglobin, HHb deoxygenated hemoglobin concentration, NIRS near-infrared spectroscopy

15.4 Discussion

In the present study, the Borg scale score was significantly correlated with physiological parameters, such as the HR, VO_2, and VE, which gradually increased with the work rate during CPET in healthy adults. Additionally, the Borg scale score was significantly correlated with leg-muscle O_2Hb and HHb levels, as assessed by NIRS, during CPET. Our previous study showed that the Borg scale score was significantly correlated with the HR and work rate during CPET in patients with hematological malignancy [10]. Thus, the Borg scale score is correlated to cardiorespiratory function during exercise, as assessed by HR, VO_2, and VE. Another study showed that the Borg scale score is related to leg-muscle fatigue during the incremental exercise test [11]. Furthermore, the Borg scale score represents whole-body fatigue and lower-muscle fatigue during squat lifting [12]. However, in the current study, the correlation coefficients for the relationships between the Borg scale and leg-muscle O_2Hb and HHb levels were lower than those for the relationships between the Borg scale score and the work rate, HR, VO_2, and VE during CPET. Thus, the Borg scale score might better reflect central cardiovascular and respiratory function than leg-muscle oxygen consumption during exercise. Furthermore, the Borg scale may more suitably represent whole-body fatigue than local-muscle fatigue during exercise.

In conclusion, the Borg scale score is significantly correlated with the work rate and physiological parameters (HR, VO_2, and VE) during CPET in healthy adults. Although the Borg scale score is also significantly correlated with leg-muscle O_2Hb and HHb levels during CPET, as assessed by NIRS, these correlation coefficients were lower than those for the physiological parameters. Thus, the Borg scale score may more suitably represent whole-body fatigue than local-muscle fatigue during exercise.

Acknowledgments This study was supported by a Grant-in-Aid for Exploratory Research from the Niigata University of Health and Welfare, Japan.

References

1. Inglis EC, Iannetta D, Murias JM (2017) The plateau in the NIRS-derived [HHb] signal near the end of a ramp incremental test does not indicate the upper limit of O. Am J Physiol Regul Integr Comp Physiol 313:R723–R729
2. Barroco AC, Sperandio PA, Reis M, Almeida DR, Neder JA (2017) A practical approach to assess leg muscle oxygenation during ramp-incremental cycle ergometry in heart failure. Braz J Med Biol Res 50:e6327
3. Tabira K, Horie J, Fujii H et al (2012) The relationship between skeletal muscle oxygenation and systemic oxygen uptake during exercise in subjects with COPD: a preliminary study. Respir Care 57:1602–1610
4. Borg G (1998) Borg's perceived exertion and pain scales: human kinetics. Human Kinetics, Champaign, IL
5. Zamunér AR, Moreno MA, Camargo TM et al (2011) Assessment of subjective perceived exertion at the anaerobic threshold with the Borg CR-10 scale. J Sports Sci Med 10:130–136
6. Rupp T, Thomas R, Perrey S, Stephane P (2008) Prefrontal cortex oxygenation and neuromuscular responses to exhaustive exercise. Eur J Appl Physiol 102:153–163
7. Hopker JG, Jobson SA, Pandit JJ (2011) Controversies in the physiological basis of the 'anaerobic threshold' and their implications for clinical cardiopulmonary exercise testing. Anaesthesia 66:111–123
8. Borg GA (1982) Psychophysical bases of perceived exertion. Med Sci Sports Exerc 14:377–381
9. Muthalib M, Millet GY, Quaresima V, Nosaka K (2010) Reliability of near-infrared spectroscopy for measuring biceps brachii oxygenation during sustained and repeated isometric contractions. J Biomed Opt 15:017008
10. Morishita S, Wakasugi T, Tanaka T et al (2018) Changes in Borg scale for resistance training and test of exercise tolerance in patients undergoing allogeneic hematopoietic stem cell transplantation. Support Care Cancer 26:3217–3223
11. Borg E, Borg G, Larsson K, Letzter M, Sundblad BM (2010) An index for breathlessness and leg fatigue. Scand J Med Sci Sports 20:644–650
12. Ahmad I, Kim JY (2018) Assessment of whole body and local muscle fatigue using electromyography and a perceived exertion scale for squat lifting. Int J Environ Res Public Health 15:784

Effects of Exercise Training on Cardiac and Skeletal Muscle Functions in Patients with Chronic Heart Failure

16

Tsubasa Watanabe, Norio Murase, Ryotaro Kime, Yuko Kurosawa, Sayuri Fuse, and Takafumi Hamaoka

Abstract

The primary symptom in patients with chronic heart failure (CHF) is exercise intolerance. Previous studies have reported that reduced exercise tolerance in CHF can be explained not only by cardiac output (a central factor) but also by reduced skeletal muscle aerobic capacity (a peripheral factor). Although exercise training in CHF improves exercise tolerance, few studies have evaluated the effects of exercise training on each specific central and peripheral factor in CHF. The aim of this study was to investigate the central and peripheral aerobic functions in CHF and the effects of exercise training in CHF on cardiac output and skeletal muscle deoxygenation during exercise. We assessed peak oxygen uptake (VO_2) during cardiopulmonary exercise testing, peak cardiac output (CO) using noninvasive hemodynamic monitoring, and muscle oxygen saturation (SmO_2) using near-infrared spectroscopy (NIRS). Patients with CHF were trained for 12 weeks and performed ramp cycling exercise until exhaustion before and after the exercise training. Peak VO_2, peak CO, and SmO_2 changes from rest to peak exercise (ΔSmO_2) were significantly lower in CHF than those in healthy subjects. As a result of exercise training, peak oxygen uptake in patients with CHF was improved and positively associated with change in ΔSmO_2. In contrast, there was no change in peak cardiac output. The results of this study indicate that both cardiac and skeletal muscle functions in patients with CHF were lower than those in healthy subjects. Further, the results suggest that the improvement of exercise capacity in patients with CHF by exercise training was related to the improved utilization of oxygen (a peripheral factor) in skeletal muscle.

Keywords

Chronic heart failure · Cardiac rehabilitation · Exercise capacity · Skeletal muscle · Near-infrared spectroscopy

16.1 Introduction

Patients with chronic heart failure (CHF) have been reported to show reduced exercise capacity. According to Fick's law, exercise capacity consists of cardiac output (CO) (a central factor) and skeletal muscle oxygen utilization (a peripheral factor). Many previous studies have reported that reduced exercise tolerance in CHF can be

T. Watanabe (✉) · N. Murase · R. Kime · Y. Kurosawa · S. Fuse · T. Hamaoka
Department of Sports Medicine for Health Promotion, Tokyo Medical University, Tokyo, Japan
e-mail: hhspj139@ybb.ne.jp

E. M. Nemoto et al. (eds.), *Oxygen Transport to Tissue XLII*, Advances in Experimental Medicine and Biology 1269, https://doi.org/10.1007/978-3-030-48238-1_16

explained not only by CO but also by reduced skeletal muscle aerobic capacity [1–4]. It has been established that exercise training can improve physiological function and reduce mortality in patients with CHF [1]. Although exercise training in CHF improved exercise tolerance, the effects of exercise training on each specific central and peripheral factor in CHF are not fully understood. The purpose of this study was to assess both the central and peripheral aerobic functions in CHF and the effects of exercise training in CHF on CO and skeletal muscle deoxygenation during exercise.

16.2 Methods

16.2.1 Subjects

Nine patients with CHF and eight age-, height-, and weight-matched subjects without CHF as controls (CON) participated in this study. Their physical and clinical characteristics are shown in Table 16.1. Three patients had old myocardial infarction, two patients had hypertensive cardiomyopathy, and the other patients had, respectively, alcoholic cardiomyopathy, hypertrophic cardiomyopathy, valvular disease, and thyroid dysfunction. All patients had received standard treatments for heart failure and participated in cardiac rehabilitation at Tokyo Medical University Hospital one to three times a week for 12 weeks. Cardiac rehabilitation consisted of continuous cycling training at individual anaerobic threshold, stretching exercises, and resistance training. All patients carried out exercise testing before and after cardiac rehabilitation (CHF_{pre} represents the data before exercise training, and CHF_{post} represents the data after exercise training). The study design and protocols were approved by the institutional review boards of Tokyo Medical University (SH2407), in accordance with the ethical principles contained in the Declaration of Helsinki. All subjects were informed of the purpose and disposition of this study, and written informed consent was obtained.

Table 16.1 Physical and clinical characteristics and medication profiles

	CHF ($n = 9$)	CON ($n = 8$)
Age (yr)	59 ± 14	58 ± 11
Height (cm)	164.5 ± 6.9	170.7 ± 6.8
Weight (kg)	66.3 ± 18.7	70.7 ± 8.8
BMI (kg/m^2)	24.3 ± 5.3	24.2 ± 2.6
BNP (pg/ml)	453.1 ± 390.7	13.8 ± 12.1
Medication (%)		
β-blocker	100	0
Calcium channel antagonist	22.2	0
ACE inhibitor or Angiotensin II receptor antagonist	100	12.5
Diuretics	100	0
Hypertension (%)	100	25
Dyslipidemia (%)	55.6	62.5
Diabetes (%)	44.4	12.5

16.2.2 Exercise Testing

All subjects performed a symptom-limited (leg fatigue or dyspnea) incremental exercise test on an upright electromechanical cycling ergometer (Strength Ergo 8; Fukuda-Denshi, Tokyo, Japan) using a ramp protocol (10 W/min for CHF after a 3-min warm-up at 10, 15, or 20 W/min for CON after a 3-min warm-up at 15 or 20 W). A 12-lead ECG (ML-9000 Stress Test system, Fukuda-Denshi, Tokyo, Japan) was monitored continuously during exercise, and HR was determined by the RR interval. To assess pulmonary oxygen uptake, breath-by-breath gas exchange data were continuously measured (AE300S; Minato Medical Science, Osaka, Japan) during exercise and averaged every 10 seconds.

16.2.3 CO Measurement

During exercise, an impedance cardiography device (Physioflow; Manatec Biomedical, Macheren, France) was employed to measure CO. The instrument uses changes in transthoracic impedance in response to an administered electrical current during cardiac ejection to calculate stroke volume [5].

16.2.4 Skeletal Muscle Oxygenation Measurement

During exercise testing, muscle oxygen saturation (SmO_2) was continuously measured at the belly of the vastus lateralis (VL) muscle in the left leg, which plays the main role in cycling exercise, using near-infrared spectroscopy (NIRS). The measurement site in the VL was defined as 30% of the length between the patella and the greater trochanter above the patella. We defined ΔSmO_2 (SmO_2 at warming up minus SmO_2 at peak exercise) as the utilization of oxygen in skeletal muscle.

16.2.5 Statistical Analysis

All data are expressed as means ± standard deviation (SD). Differences in peak VO_2, peak CO, and ΔSmO_2 were compared between CHF and CON using an unpaired t-test. To assess the effects of exercise training on peak VO_2, peak CO, and ΔSmO_2 in CHF, a paired t-test was used. Pearson's correlation coefficient was used to examine relationship between the change of peak VO_2 and the change of ΔSmO_2 after exercise training. All statistical analyses were executed by IBM SPSS Statistics (version 25, IBM Corporation, USA). For all statistical comparisons, the level of significance was set at $p < 0.05$.

16.3 Results

16.3.1 Comparison Between CHF_{pre} and CON

Peak VO_2 (CHF, 18.4 ± 3.8 ml/kg/min; CON, 30.3 ± 12.8 ml/kg/min; $p = 0.035$) was significantly lower in CHF than that in CON. Moreover, peak CO (CHF, 9.5 ± 3.6 L/min; CON, 17.1 ± 4.9 L/min; $p = 0.005$) and ΔSmO_2 (CHF, 4.5 ± 7.0%; CON, 16.2 ± 7.3%; $p = 0.008$) were significantly lower in CHF than that in CON.

16.3.2 Comparison Between CHF_{pre} and CHF_{post}

Peak VO_2 (CHF_{pre}, 18.4 ± 3.8 ml/kg/min; CHF_{post}, 23.6 ± 8.6 ml/kg/min; $p = 0.04$) and ΔSmO_2 (CHF_{pre}, 4.5 ± 7.0%; CHF_{post}, 12.0 ± 5.8%; $p = 0.02$) were significantly increased by exercise training (Fig. 16.1a, b). However, there was no significant difference in peak CO (CHF_{pre}, 9.2 ± 3.4 L/min; CHF_{post}, 9.2 ± 3.5 L/min; $p = 0.99$) before and after exercise training (Fig. 16.1c). There was a significant correlation between the change of peak VO_2 and the change of ΔSmO_2 after exercise training (Fig. 16.2). One patient's result was excluded, because the observed data was irregular. This irregularity or motion artifact might have been caused by a positional shift of the NIRS probe across the skin surface during exercise.

16.4 Discussion

Many previous studies have reported that CO and/or skeletal muscle oxygen utilization in CHF patients were reduced [3]. However, the mechanisms of exercise intolerance in CHF patients are still under discussion. Fukuda et al. indicated that peak CO was lower in CHF patients with exercise intolerance than in normal subjects [5]. Additionally, previous research reported that skeletal muscle abnormalities may be a crucial contributor to exercise intolerance [3]. The present study demonstrated that exercise capacity (peak VO_2), a central factor (peak CO), and a peripheral factor (ΔSmO_2) were significantly lower in CHF than those in CON. In contrast, Wilson et al. have shown that in CHF patients, the cardiac response to exercise declined and skeletal muscle oxygenation was significantly greater than in normal subjects [6]. These results stand in contrast to the results of the present study. The difference may be due to the degree and/or duration of CHF. Physical inactivity, malnutrition, hypoperfusion, and hypoxia can induce skeletal muscle abnormalities in CHF. The degree and/or duration of these events may play an important role in skeletal muscle abnormalities in CHF. Although there was no mention of the dura-

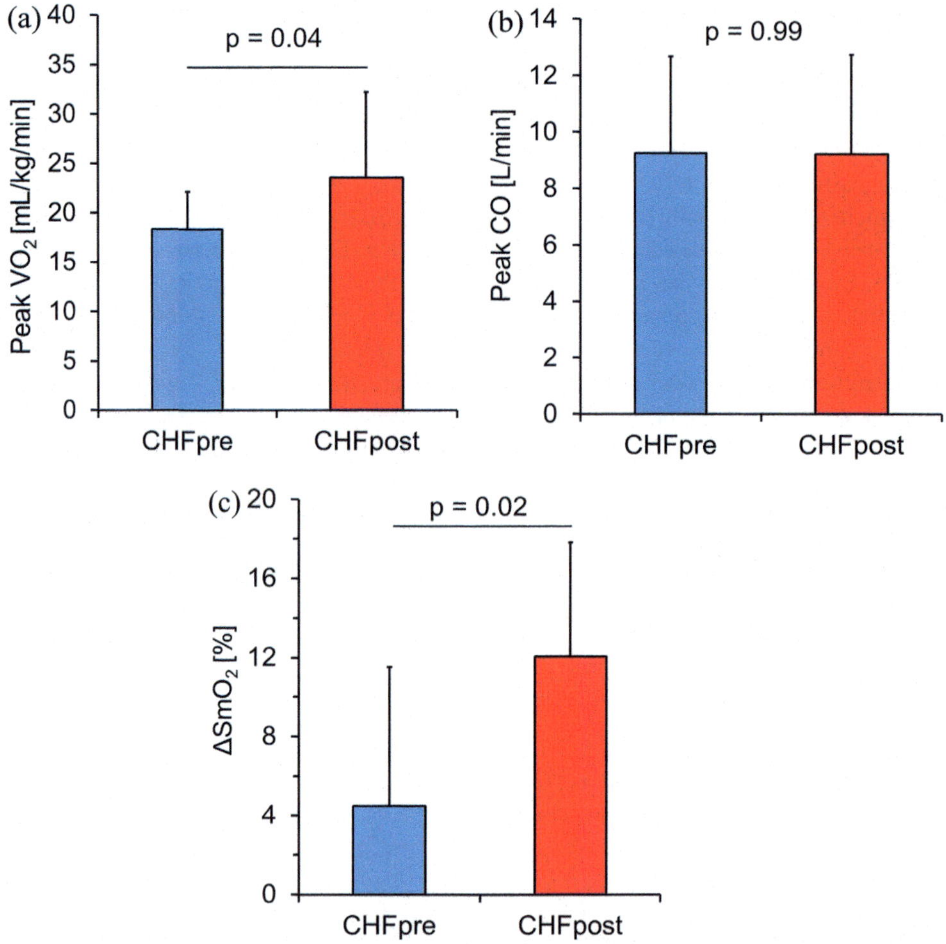

Fig. 16.1 Effects of exercise training on peak VO_2 (**a**), peak CO (**b**), and ΔSmO_2 (**c**) in CHF patients

Fig. 16.2 Relationship between the change of peak VO_2 and the change of ΔSmO_2 after exercise training

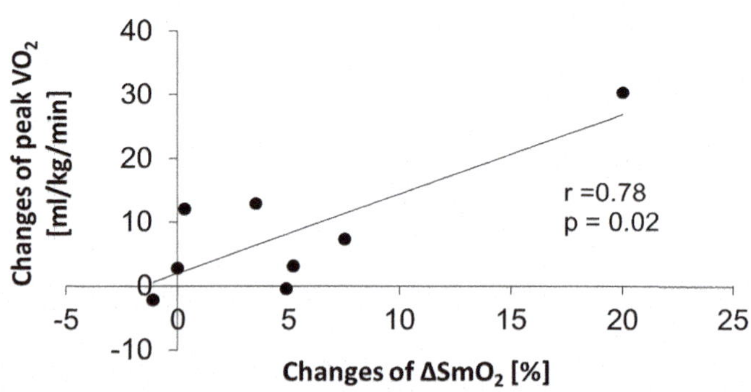

tion of disease in the study by Wilson, we hypothesize that the degree and/or duration of disease in the present study may be more serious and/or longer than in the study by Wilson et al. Further research is needed to clarify the mechanisms of exercise intolerance. Exercise training is an important part of heart failure treatment and improves mortality in CHF patients. In previous research, though CO was increased by cardiotonic agents, there was no effect on exercise capacity in CHF patients [7], which suggests that exercise capacity in CHF patients was improved by exercise training without amelioration of CO. Several studies have stated that the improvement of skeletal muscle function by exercise training significantly affected exercise capacity in CHF patients [3]. The present study is the first report that measured and evaluated CO and ΔSmO_2 simultaneously during exercise in CHF patients. We found that exercise capacity in patients with CHF was improved by exercise training, although there was no change in peak CO. We further discovered that exercise training enhanced the utilization of oxygen in skeletal muscle, and the enhancement is likely to cause an improvement of exercise capacity in patients with CHF. Esposito et al. pointed out that exercise training encouraged morphologic improvement (increased percent oxidative fiber, skeletal muscle capillarity, and mitochondrial volume density) [8]. The valuable changes of skeletal muscle can contribute to improvement in exercise tolerance in patients with CHF.

16.5 Conclusion

Both cardiac and skeletal muscle functions in patients with CHF were lower than those in healthy subjects. Our findings indicate that the improvement of exercise capacity in patients with CHF by exercise training was related to the improved utilization of oxygen in skeletal muscle.

Acknowledgments This work was supported by JSPS KAKENHI Grant Number 16KO1735.

References

1. Hirai DM, Musch TI, Poole DC (2015) Exercise training in chronic heart failure: improving skeletal muscle O_2 transport and utilization. Am J Physiol Heart Circ Physiol 309:1419–1439
2. Anker SD, Ponikowski P, Varney S et al (1997) Wasting as independent risk factor for mortality in chronic heart failure. Lancet 349:1050–1053
3. Tucker WJ, Haykowsky MJ, Seo Y, Stehling E, Forman DE (2018) Im-paired exercise tolerance in heart failure: role of skeletal muscle morphology and function. Curr Heart Fail Rep 15(6):323–331
4. Okita K, Kinugawa S, Tsutsui H (2013) Exercise intolerance in chronic heart failure – skeletal muscle dysfunction and potential therapies. Circ J 77:293–300
5. Taira F, Akihiro M, Miwa K et al (2012) Cardiac output response to exercise in chronic cardiac failure patients. Int Heart J 53(5):293–298
6. Wilson JR, Mancini DM, McCully K, Ferraro N, Lanoce V, Chance B (1989) Noninvasive detection of skeletal muscle underperfusion with near-infrared spectroscopy in patients with heart failure. Circulation 80:1668–1674
7. Maskin CS, Forman R, Sonnenblick EH, Frishman WH, LeJemtel TH (1983) Failure of dobutamine to increase exercise capacity despite hemodynamic improvement in severe chronic heart failure. Am J Cardiol 51:177–182
8. Esposito F, Reese V, Shabetai R, Wagner PD, Richardson RS (2011) Isolated quadriceps training increased maximal exercise capacity in chronic heart failure: the role of skeletal muscle convective and diffusive oxygen transport. J Am Coll Cardiol 58(13):1353–1362

Reduced Scattering Coefficient During Incremental Exercise Is Constant Without Being Affected by Changes in Muscle Oxygenation or Hemodynamics

17

Tasuki Endo, Ryotaro Kime, Sayuri Fuse, Norio Murase, Yuko Kurosawa, and Takafumi Hamaoka

Abstract

Previous studies have reported that the reduced scattering coefficient (μ_s') in the vastus lateralis changes during ramp-incremental exercise due to blood volume changes or accumulation of metabolic by-products. We aimed to clarify the influences of deoxygenation and blood volume changes during exercise on μ_s' dynamics in subjects with various aerobic capacities. Twenty-three healthy young men participated in this study. All subjects performed a ramp-incremental cycling exercise until exhaustion and were divided into two groups: lower (Low: $n = 12$; peak pulmonary oxygen uptake per kg of fat-free mass (VO_{2peak}), 54.2 ± 5.3 mL/kg/min) and higher aerobic capacity group (High: $n = 11$; VO_{2peak}, 69.7 ± 5.2 mL/kg/min) by median of VO_{2peak}. Deoxygenated hemoglobin and myoglobin concentrations (deoxy[Hb + Mb]) and total [Hb + Mb] (total[Hb + Mb]) in the vastus lateralis were monitored during the exercise by three-wavelength (760, 800, and 830 nm) time-resolved NIRS. Similarly, μ_s' at each wavelength was continuously monitored. With increasing exercise intensity, deoxy[Hb + Mb] and total[Hb + Mb] significantly increased in both groups, and the average values of the peak amplitudes of deoxy[Hb + Mb] and total[Hb + Mb] during exercise showed a 106.4% increase and a 17.9% increase from the start of the exercise, respectively. Furthermore, the peak amplitude of total[Hb + Mb] was significantly greater in High. Conversely, there were no changes in μ_s' at any wavelength during exercise and no differences between two groups, suggesting that the great deoxygenation and blood volume changes during incremental exercise have little effect on μ_s' dynamics.

Keywords

Reduced scattering coefficient · Muscle oxygenation · Near-infrared time-resolved spectroscopy · Ramp-incremental cycling exercise · Skeletal muscle microcirculation

T. Endo · R. Kime (✉) · S. Fuse · N. Murase · Y. Kurosawa · T. Hamaoka
Department of Sports Medicine for Health Promotion, Tokyo Medical University, Tokyo, Japan
e-mail: zxc06104@nifty.com

E. M. Nemoto et al. (eds.), *Oxygen Transport to Tissue XLII*, Advances in Experimental Medicine and Biology 1269, https://doi.org/10.1007/978-3-030-48238-1_17

17.1 Introduction

Near-infrared spectroscopy is a noninvasive optical technique for measuring muscle tissue oxygen saturation and, indirectly, changes in muscle blood volume and muscle oxygen consumption [1]. In particular, continuous wave NIRS (NIR_{CWS}), which is a relatively low-cost and compact NIRS device, is widely used in clinical and sports medicine fields. Since NIR_{CWS}, which is operated based on the modified Beer-Lambert law, assumes that the extended optical path length and the light losses due to scattering are constant, oxygenation and hemodynamics evaluated by NIR_{CWS} are qualitative. However, recent studies have reported inconstant reduced scattering coefficient (μ_s') during exercise measured by frequency-domain NIRS or time-resolved NIRS (NIR_{TRS}) [2, 3], which can quantitatively measure changes in muscle oxygenation, blood volume, and μ_s' [1]. If μ_s' is inconstant during exercise, muscle oxygenation and hemodynamics evaluated by NIR_{CWS} should be inaccurate and interpreted incorrectly. Furthermore, although muscle deoxygenation during incremental exercise is greater in individuals with high aerobic capacity [4] and μ_s' during exercise increases due to muscle deoxygenation and/or blood volume increase [2], it is not clear whether greater deoxygenation and/or blood volume changes during exercise induce greater μ_s' changes. Thus, the aim of this study was to clarify μ_s' dynamics during incremental exercise in subjects with various aerobic capacities using NIR_{TRS}.

17.2 Methods

Twenty-three healthy men participated in this study (age, 21 ± 2 years; height, 173.9 ± 6.3 cm; weight, 63.0 ± 5.7 kg). After explanation of experimental protocols and risks of participation, the subjects gave written informed consent to participate. This study was approved by the local ethics committee of Tokyo Medical University (number 2016-173).

All subjects were asked to avoid alcohol and intense exercise for 24 h before the exercise and performed a ramp-incremental cycling exercise, which consisted of a 1-min rest, a 1-min unload pedaling, and increasing workloads by 20 W/min until exhaustion (pedal frequency at 60 rpm), in the upright position on a cycle ergometer (Strength Ergo 8, FUKUDA DENSHI, Japan). After the cycling exercise, the subjects were divided into low aerobic capacity group (Low) and high aerobic capacity group (High) by median of peak pulmonary oxygen uptake (VO_{2peak}) normalized by fat-free mass determined by bio-impedance analysis (InBody 720, InBody Japan, Japan). VO_2 was monitored by a breath-by-breath gas exchange measurement system (AE310S, Minato Medical Science, Japan).

Absolute deoxygenated hemoglobin and myoglobin concentrations (deoxy[Hb + Mb]), total [Hb + Mb] (total[Hb + Mb]), and μ_s' at 760, 800, and 830 nm wavelengths ($\mu_s'_{760}$, $\mu_s'_{800}$, $\mu_s'_{830}$, respectively) were continuously measured by NIR_{TRS} (TRS-21, Hamamatsu Photonics K.K., Japan). The principle of this system has been described in previous studies [5, 6]; briefly, the absorption coefficient (μ_a) and the μ_s' were determined by analytical solutions calculated from fitting the temporal light intensity profiles of measured reflectance light to the photon diffusion equation convolved the instrument response function. In addition, the μ_a allows calculation of absolute deoxy[Hb + Mb] and total[Hb + Mb]. The data sampling rate was 0.16 Hz (ten data per minute). All NIR_{TRS} parameters were resampled to values of every 10% relative intensity to peak workloads (100%W_{max}) for each subject. The relative values were calculated from the average of the last three data before the data closest to the intensity. The NIR_{TRS} measurement site was the belly of the right vastus lateralis, and the NIR_{TRS} probe distance between the source and the detector was 3 cm. Fat layer thickness at the measurement site was measured by an ultrasound device (Vscan Dual Probe, GE Healthcare, Japan).

All data are presented as mean ± standard deviation (SD). To compare the differences in physical characteristics and the peak amplitude of NIR_{TRS} parameters between groups, an unpaired *t* test was used. Changes in NIR_{TRS} parameters during exercise were analyzed by a two-way repeated-measures analysis of variance with group and exercise intensity as factors. The Bonferroni post hoc test was performed to determine specific significant differences. Pearson's correlation coefficient was used to determine correlations between VO_{2peak} and the peak amplitudes of deoxy[Hb + Mb] and total[Hb + Mb] during exercise (Δdeoxy[Hb + Mb] and Δtotal[Hb + Mb], respectively) and between the peak amplitudes and μ_s' at each wavelength ($\Delta\mu_s'_{760}$, $\Delta\mu_s'_{800}$, and $\Delta\mu_s'_{830}$). All statistical analyses were performed by IBM SPSS Statistics (version 25, IBM Corporation, USA), and $P < 0.05$ was accepted as the level of significance.

Table 17.1 Physical characteristics in subjects divided into low aerobic capacity group (Low) and high aerobic capacity group (High) by the median of peak pulmonary oxygen uptake (VO_{2peak})

	Low ($n = 12$)	High ($n = 11$)
Age (years)	22 ± 3	21 ± 1
Height (m)	1.76 ± 0.06	1.72 ± 0.07
Weight (kg)	64.0 ± 5.4	61.9 ± 6.0
Fat-free mass (FFM, kg)	57.2 ± 4.9	55.7 ± 5.1
VO_{2peak} (mL/kgFFM/min)	54.2 ± 5.3	69.7 ± 5.2**
Fat layer thickness (mm)	3.6 ± 0.8	3.5 ± 0.6

Values are expressed as mean ± SD. **Significant difference from Low ($P < 0.01$)

17.3 Results

Physical characteristics in Low and High groups are presented in Table 17.1. No significant differences between groups were found except for peak VO_2.

Changes in deoxy[Hb + Mb] and total[Hb + Mb] during exercise are shown in Fig. 17.1a, b. There was a significant interaction between group × exercise intensity for total[Hb + Mb] ($P < 0.01$) but not for deoxy[Hb + Mb]. Moreover, the significant main effects for group ($P = 0.03$) and exercise intensity ($P < 0.01$) were found in deoxy[Hb + Mb]. Deoxy[Hb + Mb] in High was significantly higher than in Low throughout incremental exercise. In comparing every 10% changes, deoxy[Hb + Mb] significantly and gradually increased to 80%W_{max} (all $P < 0.01$). However, there were no significant differences in Δdeoxy[Hb + Mb] between groups (Low, 35.4 ± 15.2 μM; High, 45.9 ± 15.7 μM; $P = 0.12$). Total[Hb + Mb] in High at each intensity was significantly higher than in Low (all $P < 0.01$). The changes in Low significantly and gradually increased to 40%W_{max} (0–20%W_{max}, both $P = 0.03$; 20–40%W_{max}, both $P < 0.01$). Furthermore, total[Hb + Mb] in High also increased from 10% to 70%W_{max} (10–60%W_{max}, all $P < 0.01$; 60–70%W_{max}, $P = 0.03$), while the changes significantly decreased from 80% to 100%W_{max} (both $P < 0.01$). Additionally, Δtotal[Hb + Mb] was significantly greater in High than Low (30.6 ± 7.9 μM vs. 20.3 ± 9.6 μM, $P = 0.01$). VO_{2peak} was significantly related to Δtotal[Hb + Mb] ($r = 0.50$, $p = 0.01$).

Figure 17.1c–e displays the changes in $\mu_s'_{760}$, $\mu_s'_{800}$, and $\mu_s'_{830}$ during exercise. For all wavelengths μ_s', there were no significant group × exercise intensity interactions and no significant main effects for group or exercise intensity. In addition, no differences in $\Delta\mu_s'$ in the same range of Δdeoxy[Hb + Mb] ($\Delta\mu_s'_{760}$, $P = 0.59$; $\Delta\mu_s'_{800}$, $P = 0.83$; $\Delta\mu_s'_{830}$, $P = 0.65$) and Δtotal[Hb + Mb] ($\Delta\mu_s'_{760}$, $P = 0.24$; $\Delta\mu_s'_{800}$, $P = 0.44$; $\Delta\mu_s'_{830}$, $P = 0.29$) between groups were found. However, interestingly, Δdeoxy[Hb + Mb] and Δtotal[Hb + Mb] were slightly but significantly correlated with $\Delta\mu_s'_{760}$ (Fig. 17.2a, d, respectively), $\Delta\mu_s'_{800}$ (Fig. 17.2b, e, respectively), and $\Delta\mu_s'_{830}$ (Fig. 17.2c, e, respectively).

17.4 Discussion and Conclusions

In this study, we demonstrated that μ_s' at 760, 800, and 830 nm wavelengths measured by NIR_{TRS} were constant throughout the incremental exercise, in contrast to the significant increases in deoxy[Hb + Mb] and total[Hb + Mb]. Furthermore, large deoxygenation or blood volume changes during exercise have little effect on μ_s' dynamics. As described in a previous study [2], muscle deoxygenation measured by NIR_{CWS} may be overestimated if μ_s' during exercise

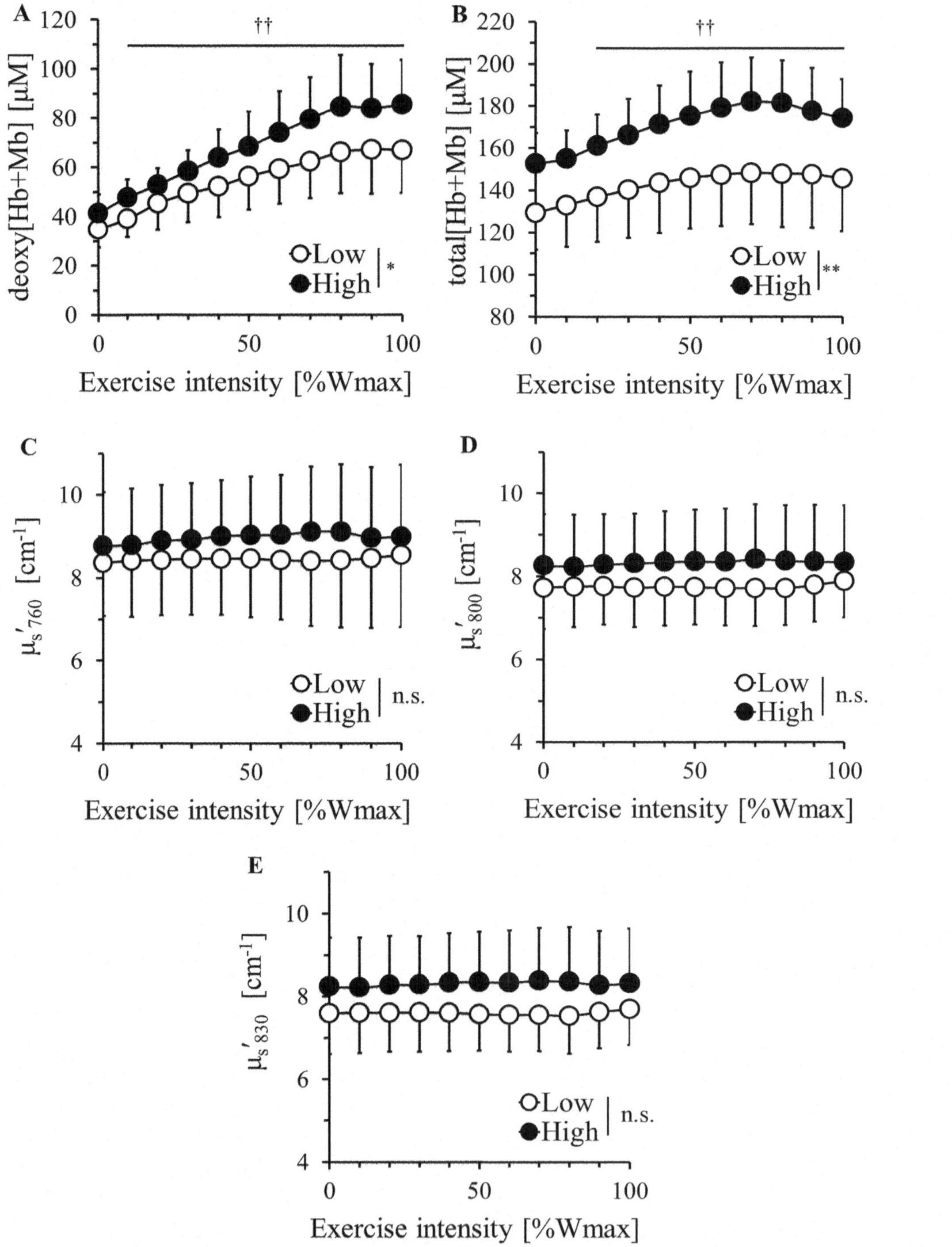

Fig. 17.1 Changes in deoxy[Hb + Mb] (**a**), total[Hb + Mb] (**b**), and reduced scattering coefficient (μ_s') at 760 (**c**), 800 (**d**), and 830 nm (**e**) in the vastus lateralis muscle during ramp-incremental cycling exercise in subjects with low (Low, open circles) and high aerobic capacity (High, closed circles) groups. Values are expressed as mean ± SD. There were significant differences between Low and High groups at each exercise intensity (*$P < 0.05$, **$P < 0.01$) and significant differences from 0% peak workloads (0%Wmax) in both groups (††$P < 0.01$). To simplify the figures, symbols indicating significant differences between exercise intensities within groups (except for comparisons of 0%Wmax and the other intensities) have been omitted

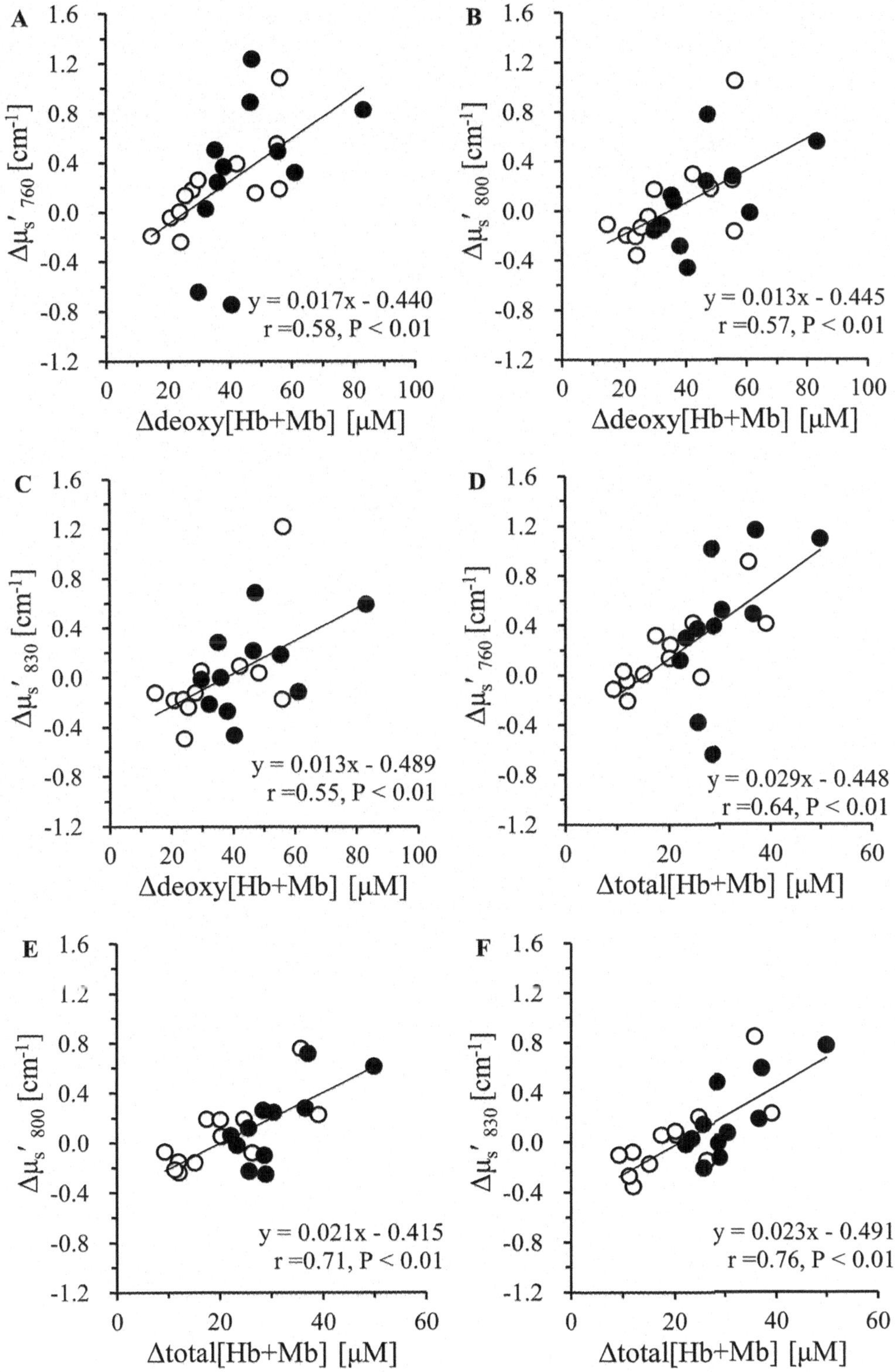

Fig. 17.2 Correlations between the peak amplitudes of deoxy[Hb + Mb] during exercise (Δdeoxy[Hb + Mb]) and μ_s' at each wavelength ($\Delta\mu_s'_{760}$, $\Delta\mu_s'_{800}$, and $\Delta\mu_s'_{830}$) in same range of Δdeoxy[Hb + Mb] (**a**–**c**) and the peak amplitudes of total[Hb + Mb] during exercise (Δtotal[Hb + Mb]) and $\Delta\mu_s'_{760}$, $\Delta\mu_s'_{800}$, and $\Delta\mu_s'_{830}$ in same range of total[Hb + Mb] (**d**–**f**) in subjects with low (open circles) and high aerobic capacity (closed circles)

increases due to blood volume increase or accumulation of metabolic by-products, such as lactate. In our results, however, there were no changes in μ_s' near 40–60%Wmax, where blood lactate starts increasing [7] and no differences in μ_s' dynamics between Low and High. Moreover, since the major lactate absorbance peaks are located in 2050 to 2400 nm [8] and there are no differences in the absorption spectrum at 600–1100 nm wavelengths even when lactate concentration changes more than 200 times [9], increased lactate levels in blood or muscle tissue during exercise may not affect μ_s' dynamics.

In addition, Δdeoxy[Hb + Mb] or Δtotal[Hb + Mb] was significantly related to $\Delta\mu_s'$ at each wavelength. The average changes in Δdeoxy[Hb + Mb] and Δtotal[Hb + Mb] were 40.4 μM (106.4% increases from 0%W_{max}) and 25.2 μM (17.9% increases from 0%W_{max}), respectively, whereas the average changes in $\Delta\mu_s'$ calculated from the linear regression equations were slight changes from 0%W_{max} (0.5–3.3% increase). The Δtotal[Hb + Mb] suggests increased total hemoglobin concentration (i.e., increased red blood cells), since total myoglobin concentration should remain unchanged during exercise. Therefore, these correlations imply that increased total hemoglobin (and deoxy[Hb + Mb]) during maximal cycling exercise has little effect on μ_s', though a red blood cell is generally considered to be light scattering [10, 11]. A further study demonstrated that μ_s' decreased during exercise (from 8.54 cm^{-1} to 8.36 cm^{-1}, a slight but statistically significant decrease by 2.1%) [3]. Our data showing that $\Delta\mu_s'$ was negative in some subjects partially agreed with the previous result (Fig. 17.2). Further studies are needed to interpret those correlations or to clarify the differences from previous results [2, 3].

In conclusion, there were no changes in μ_s' at 760, 800, and 830 nm wavelengths measured by NIR_{TRS} during incremental cycling exercise and no differences in μ_s' dynamics between subjects with various aerobic capacities.

Acknowledgments The authors are grateful to Andrea Hope for revision of this manuscript. We also thank Mikiko Anjo and Ayaka Kime (Tokyo Medical University, Japan) for their helpful technical assistance. This study was supported by JSPS KAKENHI Grant Number 16 K01735.

References

1. Hamaoka T, McCully KK (2019) Review of early development of near-infrared spectroscopy and recent advancement of studies on muscle oxygenation and oxidative metabolism. J Physiol Sci 69(6):799–811. https://doi.org/10.1007/s12576-019-00697-2
2. Ferreira LF et al (2007) Effects of assuming constant optical scattering on measurements of muscle oxygenation by near-infrared spectroscopy during exercise. J Appl Physiol 102:358–367
3. Ganesan G et al (2016) Cerebral and muscle tissue oxygenation during incremental cycling in male adolescents measured by time-resolved NIRS. Pediatr Exerc Sci 28(2):275–285
4. Okushima D et al (2016) Greater VO_{2peak} is correlated with greater skeletal muscle deoxygenation amplitude and hemoglobin concentration within individual muscles during ramp-incremental cycle exercise. Physiol Rep 4(23):e13065
5. Patterson MS et al (1989) Time resolved reflectance and transmittance for the non-invasive measurement of tissue optical properties. Appl Opt 28(12):2331–2336
6. Chance B et al (1989) Time-resolved spectroscopy of hemoglobin and myoglobin in resting and ischemic muscle. Anal Biochem 174(2):698–707
7. Faude O et al (2009) Lactate threshold concepts: how valid are they? Sports Med 39(6):469–490
8. Lafrance D et al (2003) Measurement of lactate in whole human blood with near-infrared transmission spectroscopy. Talanta 60:635–641
9. Horosh M et al (2017) Broadband infrared spectroscopy for non-contact measurement of neurological disease biomarkers in cerebrospinal fluid. Appl Spectrosc 71(3):496–506
10. Paunescu LA et al (2001) In vitro correlation between reduced scattering coefficient and hemoglobin concentration of human blood determined by near-infrared spectroscopy. Proc SPIE 4250:319–326
11. Bosschaart N et al (2014) A literature review and novel theoretical approach on the optical properties of whole blood. Lasers Med Sci 29:453–479

Changes in the Laterality of Oxygenation in the Prefrontal Cortex and Premotor Area During a 20-Min Moderate-Intensity Cycling Exercise

18

Atsuhiro Tsubaki, Shinichiro Morishita, Kazuki Hotta, Yuta Tokunaga, Weixiang Qin, Sho Kojima, and Hideaki Onishi

Abstract

A recent study based on near-infrared spectrometry (NIRS) showed that a single session of moderate-intensity exercise increases the cortical oxyhemoglobin (O_2Hb) level. However, changes in the laterality of O_2Hb throughout such exercises remain unknown. In the present study, we evaluated changes in the laterality of O2Hb in the prefrontal cortex (PFC) and premotor area (PMA) during moderate-intensity cycling for 20 min. Twelve healthy volunteers performed the exercise at 50% of the maximal oxygen consumption after a 3-min rest period. O_2Hb levels in the right (R-) and left (L-) PFC and PMA were measured using multichannel NIRS and averaged every 5 min during the exercise period, and the laterality index (LI) for each 5-min period was calculated. LI for PFC showed significant changes in each period (first, second, third, and fourth periods: −0.40 ± 0.21, −0.03 ± 0.12, 0.14 ± 0.15, and 0.16 ± 0.10, respectively; $p < 0.05$), whereas that for PMA showed no significant changes (−0.07 ± 0.09, 0.23 ± 0.08, 0.17 ± 0.12, and 0.19 ± 0.09, respectively; $p = 0.12$). These findings suggest that the laterality of cortical oxygenation in PFC of healthy, young individuals changes during moderate-intensity exercise for 20 min, thus providing an insight into the mechanisms underlying exercise-induced improvements in brain function.

Keywords

Oxyhemoglobin · Laterality · Prefrontal cortex · Moderate-intensity exercise · Near-infrared spectroscopy

18.1 Introduction

Long-term moderate-intensity exercise improves not only physical fitness but also brain function [1, 2]. Recent studies showed that a single session of moderate-intensity exercise improved cognitive function in young and elderly individuals, with these improvements related to changes in the oxyhemoglobin (O_2Hb) level in the prefrontal cortex (PFC) [3, 4]. Moreover, our previ-

A. Tsubaki (✉) · S. Morishita · K. Hotta · Y. Tokunaga · W. Qin · S. Kojima · H. Onishi
Institute for Human Movement and Medical Sciences, Niigata University of Health and Welfare, Kita Ward, Niigata, Japan
e-mail: tsubaki@nuhw.ac.jp

E. M. Nemoto et al. (eds.), *Oxygen Transport to Tissue XLII*, Advances in Experimental Medicine and Biology 1269, https://doi.org/10.1007/978-3-030-48238-1_18

ous study based on near-infrared spectroscopy (NIRS) showed that cortical oxygenation increased during a 20-min moderate-intensity cycling exercise, with the changes differing among brain regions [5, 6]. However, changes in the laterality of O_2Hb throughout the exercise period remain unknown.

Accordingly, the aim of the present study was to evaluate changes in the laterality of O_2Hb in PFC and the premotor area (PMA) during moderate-intensity cycling for 20 min. The hypothesis was that the laterality of O_2Hb changes during moderate-intensity exercise for 20 min.

18.2 Methods

18.2.1 Participants

This study was approved by the Ethics Committee of Niigata University of Health and Welfare and conformed to the standards outlined in the Declaration of Helsinki. Healthy, young volunteers without any symptoms of neurological, medical, or cardiovascular disease were recruited (Table 18.1). None of the participants were taking any medication at the time of the study, and all of them provided written informed consent after receiving information regarding the potential risks, study objectives, measurement techniques, and benefits associated with the study.

18.2.2 Experimental Procedure

The individual exercise workload was determined on the basis of the maximal oxygen consumption (VO_2max) during an incremental cycling protocol (Aerobike 75XLII; Combi, Tokyo, Japan). Measurements of VO_2max were obtained before the main experiment on the basis of published recommendations [7]. Exhaustion was defined by a plateau in oxygen consumption (VO_2), a respiratory exchange ratio of >1.1, a heart rate value close to the age-predicted maximal heart rate, and a drop in the cycling cadence [8].

Table 18.1 Characteristics of healthy, young volunteers for a study on changes in the laterality of oxyhemoglobin in the prefrontal cortex and premotor area during a 20-min moderate-intensity exercise

Number	12
Age (years)	21.2 ± 0.7
Sex (female/male)	9/3
Height (cm)	161.1 ± 8.2
Weight (kg)	53.3 ± 11.7
VO_2max (mL/kg/min)	30.2 ± 7.1

Values are presented as mean ± standard deviation
VO_2max: maximal oxygen consumption

The main experiment required the participants to observe a 3-min rest period before performing a constant work rate exercise at a workload of 50% VO_2max on a cycle ergometer. This was followed by a 15-min rest period. NIRS signals, skin blood flow (SBF), and the mean arterial pressure (MAP) were continuously measured during the experiment.

18.2.3 NIRS Measurements

A multichannel NIRS imaging system (OMM-3000; Shimadzu Co., Kyoto, Japan) with multiple continuous wavelengths (780, 805, and 830 nm) was used to detect changes in O_2Hb, deoxyhemoglobin (HHb), and total hemoglobin (THb) levels at a sampling rate of 130 ms, on the basis of the modified Beer-Lambert law [9]. The NIRS optodes consisted of 12 light-source fibers and 12 detectors, which provided 24-channel simultaneous recording. The optodes were arranged in a 4 × 6 pattern in a multichannel probe holder, and a 30-mm interoptode distance was set for the measurement of cortical tissue oxygenation. The Cz position of the international 10–20 system was used to ensure consistent optode placement for all participants. Regions of interest (ROIs) included the right (R-) and left (L-) PFC and PMA (Fig. 18.1).

18.2.4 Blood Pressure and SBF Measurements

Beat-to-beat MAP was recorded at the left middle finger using the volume clamping method with a finger photoplethysmograph (Finometer; Finapres Medical Systems, Amsterdam, the

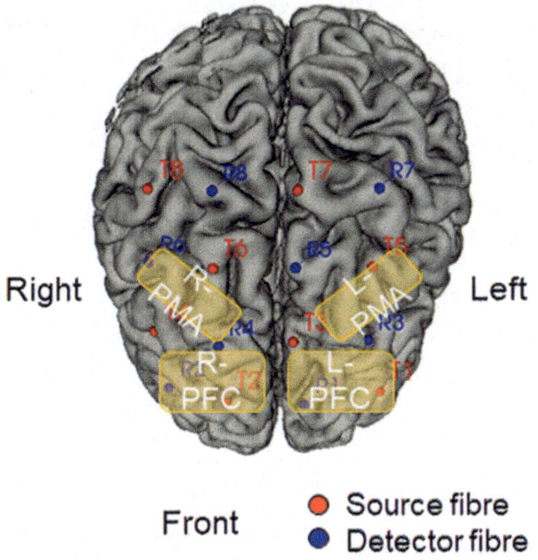

Fig. 18.1 Placement of optodes for near-infrared spectroscopy and the relevant regions of interest for a study on changes in the laterality of oxyhemoglobin in the prefrontal cortex and premotor area during a 20-min moderate-intensity exercise. R-PFC right prefrontal cortex, L-PFC left prefrontal cortex, R-PMA right premotor area, L-PMA left premotor area

Netherlands). Changes in SBF were measured at the forehead using a laser Doppler blood flow meter (Omegaflow FLO-CI; Omegawave Inc., Osaka, Japan). Analog data were converted to digital data using an A/D converter (PowerLab; AD Instruments, Australia) at a sampling rate of 1000 Hz.

18.2.5 Statistical Analysis

SBF and MAP were down-sampled by adopting the sampling rate used for NIRS monitoring. For the measurement of temporal changes, the average O_2Hb, HHb, and THb levels for each ROI, SBF, and MAP were expressed as changes from the average values obtained during the pre-exercise rest phase. O_2Hb levels were averaged every 5 min during the exercise period, and the laterality index (LI) for each 5-min period was calculated as follows: (R-PFC HbO_2 level − L-PFC HbO_2 level)/(R-PFC HbO_2 level + L-PFC HbO_2 level). A positive LI indicates that the increase in HbO_2 in R-PFC is greater than that in L-PFC, whereas a negative LI indicates the opposite [10–12]. One-way analysis of variance was used for LI comparisons, and a p-value of <0.05 was considered statistically significant. All statistical analyses were performed using SPSS version 12 (IBM, IL, USA).

18.3 Results

The temporal changes in O_2Hb, HHb, and THb are shown in Fig. 18.2, while those in SBF and MAP are shown in Fig. 18.3. O_2Hb levels in both PFC and PMA increased during the first 10 min and were maintained over the latter half of the exercise period. LI for PFC showed significant changes in each period (first, second, third, and fourth periods: −0.40 ± 0.21, −0.03 ± 0.12, 0.14 ± 0.15, and 0.16 ± 0.10, respectively; $F(3, 44) = 3.008$, $p < 0.05$), whereas that for PMA showed no significant changes (−0.07 ± 0.09, 0.23 ± 0.08, 0.17 ± 0.12, and 0.19 ± 0.09, respectively; $F(3, 44) = 2.044$, $p = 0.12$).

18.4 Discussion

In the present study, we evaluated changes in the laterality of O_2Hb in PFC and PMA during a 20-min session of moderate-intensity cycling in healthy, young volunteers, with the findings indicating a shift from right dominance to left dominance in PFC and no changes in PMA.

First, we confirmed that O_2Hb changes, not SBF or MAP changes, represented changes in cortical oxygenation. Previous studies have reported that changes in O_2Hb reflect changes in cortical activation [13, 14]. Moreover, SBF or MAP changes have been found to affect O_2Hb signals [15, 16]. If these systemic changes have a strong influence on O_2Hb, a bilateral difference in O_2Hb changes in PFC may not be observed.

We found that the laterality of O_2Hb in PFC changed from right dominance to left dominance during the 20-min session of moderate-intensity exercise. This result indicates that the role of PFC changes during such exercises. R-PFC has been reported as one of the regions involved in sympathetic regulation [17], and L-PFC plays an important role for executive function in healthy young subjects [3].

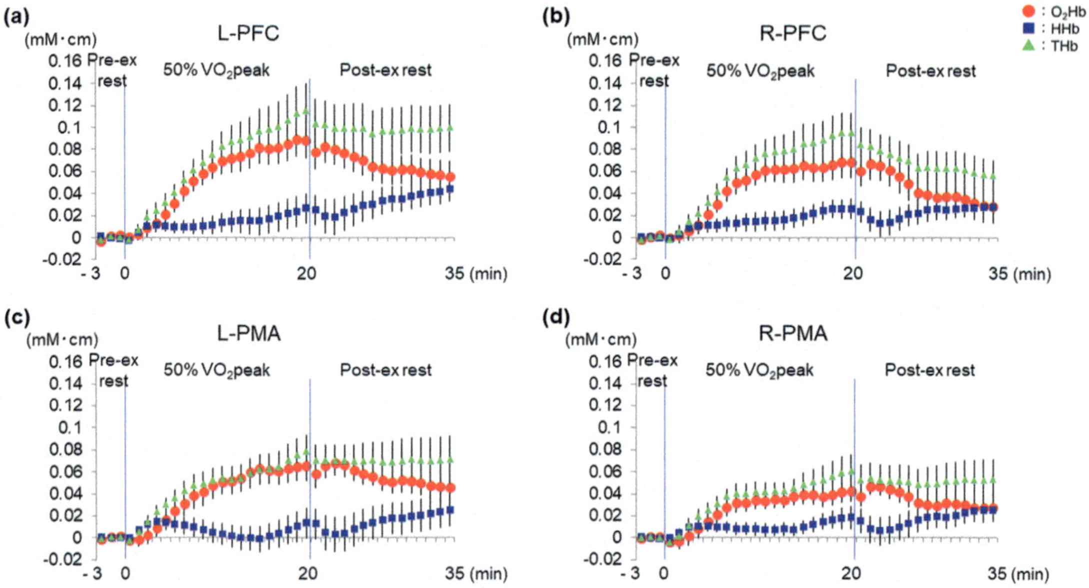

Fig. 18.2 Temporal changes in the average oxyhemoglobin (O_2Hb), deoxyhemoglobin (HHb), and total hemoglobin (THb) levels in the prefrontal cortex and premotor area during a 20-min moderate-intensity exercise. Values are presented as mean ± standard error of the mean (SEM). (**a**) Left prefrontal cortex (L-PFC). (**b**) Right prefrontal cortex (R-PFC). (**c**) Left premotor area (L-PMA). (**d**) Right premotor area (R-PMA)

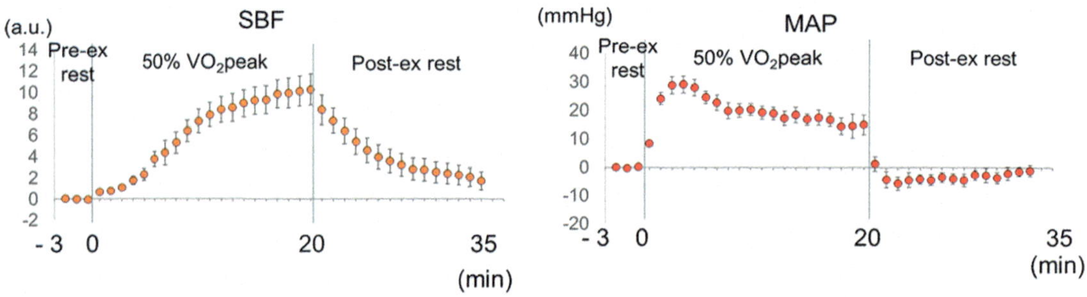

Fig. 18.3 Temporal changes in the average skin blood flow (SBF) and average mean arterial pressure (MAP) during a 20-min moderate-intensity exercise. Values are presented as mean ± standard error of the mean (SEM)

On the other hand, the laterality of O_2Hb in PMA showed no changes during the 20-min exercise period. PMA plays a role in the preparation of movement for control and posture [18]. For maintenance of the sitting position on a cycling ergometer, PMA might maintain the activation through the exercise.

In conclusion, the findings of the present study suggest that the laterality of cortical oxygenation in PFC of healthy, young individuals changes during moderate-intensity exercise for 20 min. Few studies have examined acute changes in the laterality of cerebral oxygenation during exercise; therefore, our findings may provide a valuable insight into the mechanisms underlying exercise-induced improvements in brain function.

Acknowledgments This study was supported by a Grant-in-Aid for Scientific Research (C) from the Japan Society for the Promotion of Science (15K01433) and a Grant-in-Aid for Exploratory Research from Niigata University of Health and Welfare (H30B19).

References

1. Raichlen DA, Alexander GE (2017) Adaptive capacity: an evolutionary neuroscience model linking exercise, cognition, and brain health. Trends Neurosci 40(7):408–421
2. Hillman CH, Erickson KI, Kramer AF (2008) Be smart, exercise your heart: exercise effects on brain and cognition. Nat Rev Neurosci 9(1):58–65
3. Yanagisawa H, Dan I, Tsuzuki D et al (2010) Acute moderate exercise elicits increased dorsolateral prefrontal activation and improves cognitive performance with Stroop test. NeuroImage 50(4):1702–1710
4. Hyodo K, Dan I, Suwabe K et al (2012) Acute moderate exercise enhances compensatory brain activation in older adults. Neurobiol Aging 33(11):2621–2632. https://doi.org/10.1016/j.neurobiolaging.2011.12.022
5. Tsubaki A, Morishita S, Tokunaga Y et al (2018) Changes in cerebral oxyhaemoglobin levels during and after a single 20-minute bout of moderate-intensity cycling. Adv Exp Med Biol 1072:127–131. https://doi.org/10.1007/978-3-319-91287-5_20
6. Tsubaki A, Morishita S, Tokunaga Y et al (2020) Effect of exercise duration on post-exercise persistence of oxyhemoglobin changes in the premotor cortex: a near-infrared spectroscopy study in moderate-intensity cycling exercise. Adv Exp Med Biol 1232:193–199
7. American Thoracic Society; American College of Chest Physicians (2003) ATS/ACCP statement on cardiopulmonary exercise testing. Am J Respir Crit Care Med 167(2):211–277. https://doi.org/10.1164/rccm.167.2.211
8. Rupp T, Perrey S (2008) Prefrontal cortex oxygenation and neuromuscular responses to exhaustive exercise. Eur J Appl Physiol 102(2):153–163. https://doi.org/10.1007/s00421-007-0568-7
9. Boas DA, Gaudette T, Strangman G et al (2001) The accuracy of near infrared spectroscopy and imaging during focal changes in cerebral hemodynamics. NeuroImage 13(1):76–90. https://doi.org/10.1006/nimg.2000.0674
10. Murayama Y, Hu L, Sakatani K (2016) Relation between prefrontal cortex activity and respiratory rate during mental stress tasks: a near-infrared spectroscopic study. Adv Exp Med Biol 923:209–214. https://doi.org/10.1007/978-3-319-38810-6_28
11. Basso Moro S, Bisconti S, Muthalib M et al (2014) A semi-immersive virtual reality incremental swing balance task activates prefrontal cortex: a functional near-infrared spectroscopy study. NeuroImage 85:451–460. https://doi.org/10.1016/j.neuroimage.2013.05.031
12. Ohyanagi H, Tsubaki A, Morishita S et al (2018) Changes in the prefrontal cortex oxygenation levels during cycling in the supine and upright positions. Adv Exp Med Biol 1072:133–137. https://doi.org/10.1007/978-3-319-91287-5_21
13. Miyai I, Tanabe HC, Sase I et al (2001) Cortical mapping of gait in humans: a near-infrared spectroscopic topography study. NeuroImage 14(5):1186–1192. https://doi.org/10.1006/nimg.2001.0905
14. Obrig H, Wolf T, Doge C et al (1996) Cerebral oxygenation changes during motor and somatosensory stimulation in humans, as measured by near-infrared spectroscopy. Adv Exp Med Biol 388:219–224
15. Miyazawa T, Horiuchi M, Komine H et al (2013) Skin blood flow influences cerebral oxygenation measured by near-infrared spectroscopy during dynamic exercise. Eur J Appl Physiol 113(11):2841–2848. https://doi.org/10.1007/s00421-013-2723-7
16. Minati L, Kress IU, Visani E et al (2011) Intra- and extra-cranial effects of transient blood pressure changes on brain near-infrared spectroscopy (NIRS) measurements. J Neurosci Methods 197:283–288
17. Beissner F, Meissner K, Bar KJ et al (2013) The autonomic brain: an activation likelihood estimation meta-analysis for central processing of autonomic function. J Neurosci 33:10503–10511. https://doi.org/10.1523/JNEUROSCI.1103-13.2013
18. Leff DR, Orihuela-Espina F, Elwell CE et al (2011) Assessment of the cerebral cortex during motor task behaviours in adults: a systematic review of functional near infrared spectroscopy (fNIRS) studies. NeuroImage 54(4):2922–2936. https://doi.org/10.1016/j.neuroimage.2010.10.058

Relationship Between Decrease of Oxygenation During Incremental Exercise and Partial Pressure End-Tidal Carbon Dioxide: Near-Infrared Spectroscopy Vector Analysis

19

Sho Kojima, Shinichiro Morishita, Kazuki Hotta, Weixiang Qin, Toshinori Kato, Katsunori Oyama, and Atsuhiro Tsubaki

Abstract

A previous study considered that a decrease in cerebral oxyhemoglobin (O_2Hb) immediately before maximal exercise during incremental exercise is related to cerebral blood flow (CBF) and partial pressure end-tidal carbon dioxide ($P_{ET}CO_2$). This study aimed to investigate the relationship between O_2Hb, $P_{ET}CO_2$, and the estimated value of cerebral blood volume (CBV) with cerebral oxygen exchange (COE) by using vector analysis. Twenty-four healthy young men participated in this study. They performed the incremental exercise (20 W/min) after a 4-min rest and warm-up. The O_2Hb and deoxyhemoglobin (HHb) in the prefrontal cortex (PFC) were measured using near-infrared spectroscopy (NIRS). The $P_{ET}CO_2$ was measured using a gas analyzer. The O_2Hb, HHb, and $P_{ET}CO_2$ were calculated as the amount of change (ΔO_2Hb, ΔHHb, and $\Delta P_{ET}CO_2$) from an average 4-min rest. Changes in the CBV (ΔCBV) and COE (ΔCOE) were estimated using NIRS vector analysis. Moreover, the respiratory compensation point (RCP), which relates to the O_2Hb decline, was detected. The Pearson correlation coefficient was used to establish the relationships among ΔO_2Hb, $\Delta P_{ET}CO_2$, ΔCBV, and ΔCOE from the RCP to maximal exercise. The $\Delta P_{ET}CO_2$ did not significantly correlate with the ΔO_2Hb ($r = 0.03$, $p = 0.88$), ΔCOE ($r = -0.19$, $p = 0.36$), and ΔCBV ($r = -0.21$, $p = 0.31$). These results showed that changes in the $\Delta P_{ET}CO_2$ from the RCP to maximal exercise were not related to changes in the ΔO_2Hb, ΔCOE, and ΔCBV. Therefore, we suggested that the decrease of O_2Hb immediately before maximal exercise during incremental exercise may be related to cerebral

S. Kojima (✉) · A. Tsubaki
Graduate School of Health and Welfare, Niigata University of Health and Welfare, Niigata, Japan

Institute for Human Movement and Medical Sciences, Niigata University of Health and Welfare, Niigata, Japan
e-mail: hpm18008@nuhw.ac.jp

S. Morishita · K. Hotta · W. Qin
Institute for Human Movement and Medical Science, Niigata University of Health and Welfare, Niigata, Japan

T. Kato
Department of Brain Environmental Research, KatoBrain Co., Ltd., Tokyo, Japan

K. Oyama
Department of Computer Science, College of Engineering, Nihon University, Tokyo, Japan

E. M. Nemoto et al. (eds.), *Oxygen Transport to Tissue XLII*, Advances in Experimental Medicine and Biology 1269, https://doi.org/10.1007/978-3-030-48238-1_19

oxygen metabolism by neural activity increase, not decrease of CBF by the $P_{ET}CO_2$.

Keywords

Incremental load exercise · Near-infrared spectroscopy · Prefrontal cortex oxygenation · Partial pressure end-tidal carbon dioxide · NIRS vector analysis

19.1 Introduction

Near-infrared spectroscopy (NIRS) can measure cortical neural activity from oxyhemoglobin (O_2Hb) and deoxyhemoglobin (HHb) [1, 2]. Previous studies have reported a decrease in O_2Hb in the prefrontal cortex (PFC) immediately before maximal exercise during incremental exercise [3, 4]. It was considered that the decrease in O_2Hb was caused by the decrease of cerebral blood flow (CBF) or an increase of cerebral oxygen metabolism due to cerebral neural activity [1, 2]. In addition, previous studies reported that the decrease of CBF was related to the decrease of partial pressure end-tidal carbon dioxide ($P_{ET}CO_2$) [3–5]. Therefore, it was considered that the decrease of O_2Hb immediately before maximal exercise during incremental exercise was caused by the decrease of CBF related to $P_{ET}CO_2$. However, total hemoglobin (O_2Hb+HHb), which indicates cerebral blood volume (CBV), increases with HHb [6, 7]. The HHb increases by oxygen metabolism of cortical neural activity [1]. Thus, the decrease of O_2Hb during incremental exercise may reflect more of oxygen metabolism than the decrease of CBF. Therefore, we have hypothesized that changes of $P_{ET}CO_2$ immediately before maximal exercise during incremental exercise do not correlate with O_2Hb and CBV. Recent studies have developed methods where NIRS vector analysis can estimate the CBV and the cerebral oxygen exchange (COE) from a change in O_2Hb and HHb [8, 9]. This study aimed to investigate the correlation of $P_{ET}CO_2$ with O_2Hb, the estimated value of the CBF, and the COE by using NIRS vector analysis.

19.2 Methods

19.2.1 Participants and Procedures

Twenty-four healthy young male volunteers (mean age 20.7 ± 0.4 years, height 172.2 ± 5.9 cm, weight 64.8 ± 9.9 kg) were recruited among students enrolled at the Niigata University of Health and Welfare for this study. Participants had no history of neurological or orthopedic disorders. Each participant received oral and written descriptions of the objectives, measurement techniques, and risks and benefits of the investigation. All participants consented to inclusion in the study. The study was approved by the Ethics Committee of Niigata University of Health and Welfare (approval number: 18082–181010) and was conducted in accordance with the Declaration of Helsinki.

Participants were instructed to not consume alcohol and caffeine 24 h before the experiment. They were allowed to consume food until 3 h before the experiments. Moreover, food and drink intakes were restricted altogether 3 h before the experiment and immediately after the experiment. The incremental exercise was performed by pedaling with a cycle ergometer (Aerobike 75XLII; Combi, Tokyo, Japan). Participants performed incremental loading, corresponding to 20 watts/min, after 4 min of rest and 4 min of warming up. Pedaling speed was maintained at 50–60 rpm. All participants completed the incremental exercise and discontinued the exercise if they experienced dyspnea or leg fatigue. Parameters measured were O_2Hb, HHb, $P_{ET}CO_2$, and skin blood flow (SBF), and these were measured from rest to the end of the exercise.

19.2.2 Cortical Oxygenation

Cortical O_2Hb, HHb, and THb were measured with a multichannel NIRS imaging system (LABNIRS, Shimadzu Co., Kyoto, Japan) during incremental exercise. We instructed participants to reduce head motion during the experiment. Measurements used eight source probes and eight detector probes (Fig. 19.1); a total of 24 channels

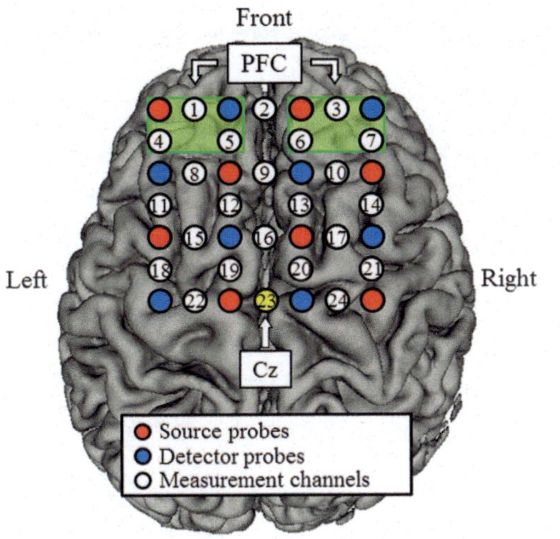

Fig. 19.1 Locations of the source and detector probes and measurement channels. PFC prefrontal cortex, Cz the vertex position

were used. The 24-channel was placed parallel to the vertex (Cz) position of the international 10–20 system. The Cz position of the international 10–20 system was used to ensure consistent placement of optodes in all participants. The probe distance was set at 30 mm. Measurement was performed at a sampling interval of 130 ms. The regions of interest were PFC, and the PFC used channels 1, 3, 4, 5, 6, and 7. Artifacts of head motion were filtered by a band-pass filter.

19.2.3 $P_{ET}CO_2$ and SBF

Changes in the oxygen uptake (VO_2), carbon dioxide output (VCO_2), minute ventilation (VE), partial pressure end-tidal oxygen ($P_{ET}O_2$), and $P_{ET}CO_2$ were measured using a gas analyzer (AE-310, Minato Medical Science, Osaka, Japan) during incremental exercise. The O_2Hb decline immediately before maximal exercise was reported to relate to the respiratory compensation point (RCP). To determine the RCP, we measured the VO_2, VCO_2, VE, and $P_{ET}O_2$. The RCP was determined based on previously reported methods [10]. Changes in the SBF were measured at the forehead using a laser-tissue blood flow oxygen monitor (Omegaflow, FLO-Cl, Omega Wave Inc., Osaka, Japan). Analog data were converted to digital data using an A/D converter (PowerLab, AD Instruments, Australia) at a 130-Hz sampling rate.

19.2.4 Statistical Analysis

The O_2Hb, HHb, $P_{ET}CO_2$, and SBF were calculated as the values of change (ΔO_2Hb, ΔHHb, $\Delta P_{ET}CO_2$, and ΔSBF) from an average 4-min rest. Changes in CBV (ΔCBV) and COE (ΔCOE) were estimated subsequently using ratios of change in ΔO_2Hb and ΔHHb based on previously reported NIRS vector analysis [8, 9]. All parameters measured at rest and warm-up were shown as mean values calculated at 4 min, and each parameter measured during incremental exercise was shown as the average value calculated every tenth of the individual's exercise time period from initiation to the endpoint. Subsequently, the ΔO_2Hb, ΔHHb, $\Delta P_{ET}CO_2$, ΔSBF, ΔCBV, and ΔCOE were calculated by the average values over 5 seconds at the RCP and maximal exercise point (MAX). The correlation between each parameter was decided using the Pearson correlation coefficient for the values of changes from RCP to MAX (e.g., ΔO_2Hb at MAX − ΔO_2Hb at RCP). Statistical analyses were performed using SPSS 21.0 (SPSS Japan Inc., Tokyo, Japan), with statistical significance set at $p < 0.05$.

19.3 Results

The ΔO_2Hb moderately increased with incremental load and decreased before 100%. The ΔHHb, ΔTHb, ΔCBV, and ΔSBF moderately increased with incremental load until 100%. The $\Delta P_{ET}CO_2$ first increased with incremental load and then decreased from 60% to 100%. The ΔCOE moderately decreased with incremental load and increased from 90% to 100% (Fig. 19.2).

The $\Delta P_{ET}CO_2$ significantly correlated with ΔHHb ($r = -0.43$, $p < 0.05$) and did not significantly correlate with ΔO_2Hb ($r = 0.03$, $p = 0.88$), ΔCOE ($r = -0.19$, $p = 0.36$), and ΔCBV ($r = -0.21$, $p = 0.31$) (Fig. 19.3). The ΔSBF did not significantly correlate with ΔO_2Hb ($r = -0.11$, $p = 0.62$) and ΔHHb ($r = 0.23$, $p = 0.27$) (Fig. 19.4).

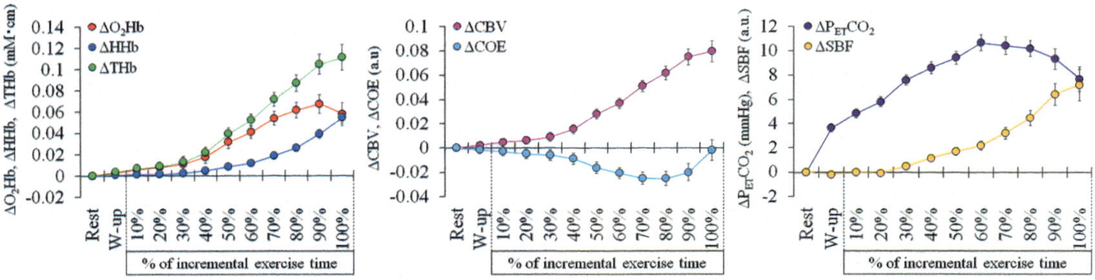

Fig. 19.2 Temporal change of each parameter. Red dots are oxyhemoglobin (O_2Hb), blue dots are deoxyhemoglobin (HHb), green dots are total hemoglobin (THb), pink dots are cerebral blood volume (CBV), light blue dots are cerebral oxygen exchange (COE), purple dots are partial pressure end-tidal carbon dioxide ($P_{ET}CO_2$), and yellow dots are skin blood flow (SBF). Values are presented as mean ± standard error of the mean (SEM)

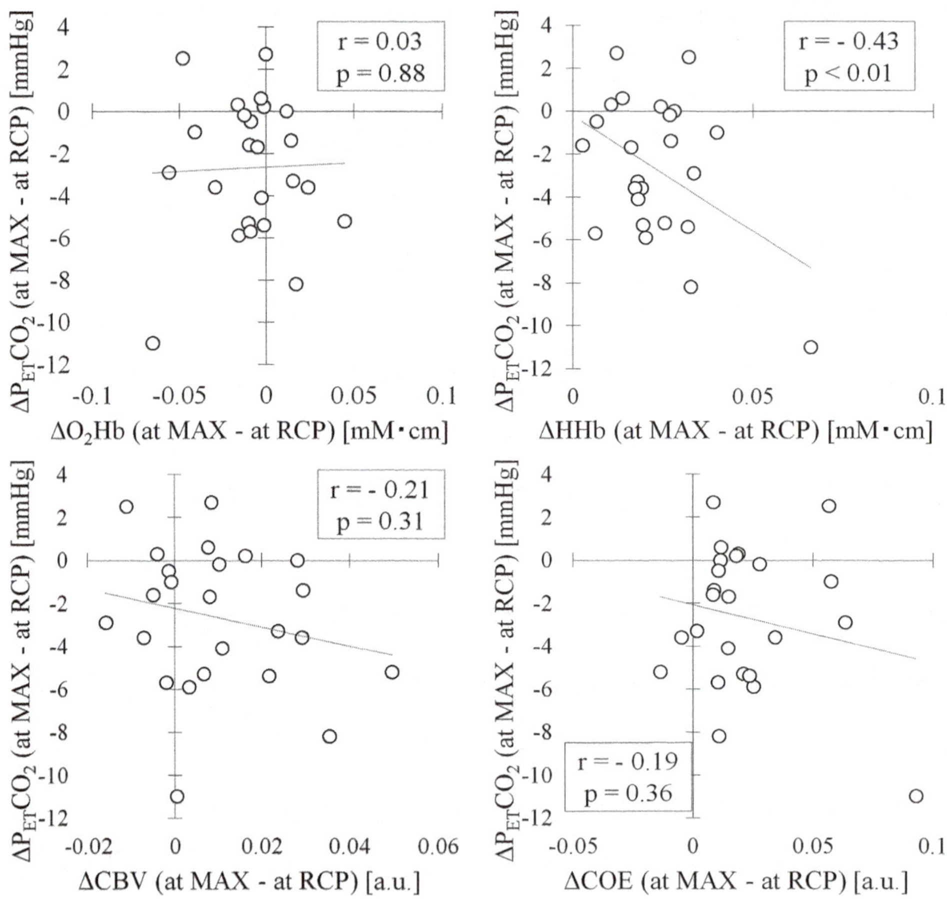

Fig. 19.3 Correlation between $P_{ET}CO_2$ and each parameter. O_2Hb,oxyhemoglobin; HHb deoxyhemoglobin, CBV cerebral blood volume, COE cerebral oxygen exchange, $P_{ET}CO_2$ partial pressure end-tidal carbon dioxide

19.4 Discussion

This study measured cortical O_2Hb, HHb, and THb in the PFC during incremental exercise using NIRS and estimated ΔCBV and ΔCOE from ratios of change in ΔO_2Hb and ΔHHb using NIRS vector analysis. In addition, we measured $P_{ET}CO_2$ and SBF. We focused on changes in each parameter from RCP to MAX.

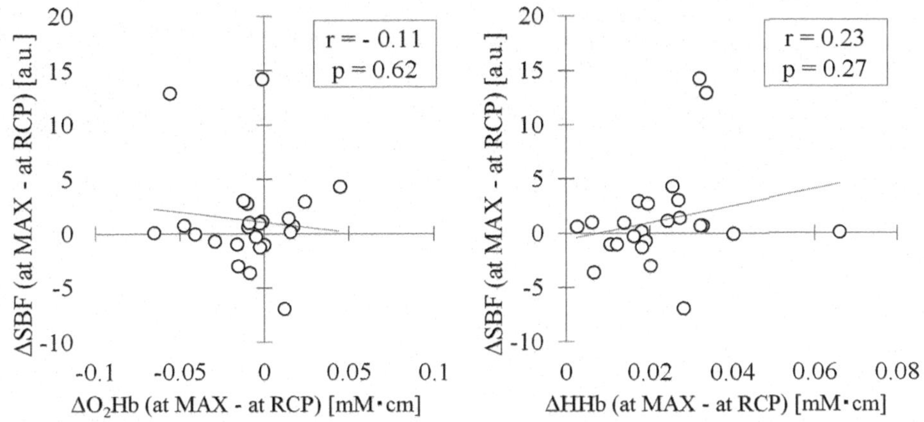

Fig. 19.4 Correlation between SBF and each parameter. O_2Hb oxyhemoglobin, HHb deoxyhemoglobin, CBV cerebral blood volume, COE cerebral oxygen exchange, SBF skin blood flow

The ΔO_2Hb moderately increased with an incremental load but decreased after 90%. The ΔSBF moderately continued to increase until 100%. A previous study reported that the changes in ΔO_2Hb significantly correlated with the changes in SBF [11]. However, changes in the SBF from RCP to MAX in this study did not correlate with the ΔO_2Hb and ΔHHb. Thus, we believed that the influence of SBF on O_2Hb and ΔHHb is small.

In this study, the main findings are that the $\Delta P_{ET}CO_2$ did not correlate with the ΔO_2Hb, ΔCBV, and ΔCOE. RCP correlated with the O_2Hb decrease point, and the $P_{ET}CO_2$ decreased by respiratory compensation after RCP [4, 10]. In addition, the $P_{ET}CO_2$ decrease correlated with the arterial partial pressure of carbon dioxide ($PaCO_2$) decrease [12], and the $PaCO_2$ decrease correlated with the decrease in CBF [5, 13]. Therefore, the previous study is thought to indicate that the O_2Hb decreases before maximal exercise during incremental exercise related to the $P_{ET}CO_2$ decrease after RCP [3–5]. However, this study did not show a significant correlation with the $\Delta P_{ET}CO_2$ with the ΔO_2Hb and ΔCBV. Another study reported that the $P_{ET}CO_2$ concentration did not affect the CBF [14]. Thus, we believe that it is challenging to explain the O_2Hb decrease by the $P_{ET}CO_2$ decrease.

The more the ΔCOE increases, the more the ΔO_2Hb decreases, and ΔHHb increases. A positive value for the ΔCOE shows hypoxic change from ΔCOE = 0, and a negative value for the ΔCOE shows a hyperoxic change [8, 9]. The ΔCOE increase from RCP to MAX shows hypoxic change, i.e., it is believed that it shows exchange from the O_2Hb to HHb by cerebral oxygen metabolism. Cerebral oxygen metabolism is invoked by promoting cortical neural activity [1, 15]. Therefore, we suggest that the O_2Hb decrease before maximal exercise during incremental exercise was related to cerebral oxygen metabolism by neural activity increase.

However, this study had the limitation that the ΔCBV and ΔCOE are estimated values and are not absolute values. The absolute value of the CBV and cerebral oxygen metabolism can be measured using positron emission tomography (PET), but measurements during whole-body exercise using PET is challenging. Transcranial Doppler ultrasonography (TCD) can measure the CBF of the middle cerebral artery during whole-body exercise. In the future, we need to measure using TCD and NIRS. In conclusion, change from RCP to MAX was not significantly correlated with $\Delta P_{ET}CO_2$, with the ΔO_2Hb and ΔCBV. In contrast, the ΔCOE increase is significantly correlated with the ΔO_2Hb decrease and ΔHHb increase. These results suggested that the O_2Hb decrease before maximal exercise during incremental exercise may be related to HHb increase via cerebral oxygen metabolism.

Acknowledgments This study was supported by a Grant-in-Aid for Scientific Research (C) from the Japan Society for the Promotion of Science (A. Tsubaki) and a Grant-in-Aid for Exploratory Research from Niigata University of Health and Welfare (A. Tsubaki).

Disclosure Statement The authors have no disclosures.

References

1. Lindauer U, Royl G, Leithner C et al (2001) No evidence for early decrease in blood oxygenation in rat whisker cortex in response to functional activation. NeuroImage 13:988–1001
2. Fox PT, Raichle ME (1986) Focal physiological uncoupling of cerebral blood flow and oxidative metabolism during somatosensory stimulation in human subjects. Proc Natl Acad Sci U S A 83:1140–1144
3. Rupp T, Perrey S (2008) Prefrontal cortex oxygenation and neuromuscular responses to exhaustive exercise. Eur J Appl Physiol 102(2):153–163
4. Oussaidene K, Prieur F, Tagougui S et al (2015) Aerobic fitness influences cerebral oxygenation response to maximal exercise in healthy subjects. Respir Physiol Neurobiol 205:53–60
5. Bhambhani Y, Malik R, Mookerjee S (2007) Cerebral oxygenation declines at exercise intensities above the respiratory compensation threshold. Respir Physiol Neurobiol 156(2):196–202
6. Kojima S, Morishita S, Qin W et al (2020) Cerebral oxygenation dynamics of the prefrontal cortex and motor-related area during cardiopulmonary exercise test: a near-infrared spectroscopy study. Adv Exp Med Biol 1232:231–237
7. Tempest GD, Eston RG, Parfitt G (2014) Prefrontal cortex haemodynamics and affective responses during exercise: a multi-channel near infrared spectroscopy study. PLoS One 9(5):e95924
8. Yoshino K, Kato T (2012) Vector-based phase classification of initial dips during word listening using near-infrared spectroscopy. Neuroreport 23(16):947–951
9. Kato T (2018) Vector-based approach for the detection of initial dips using functional near-infrared spectroscopy. In: Neuroimaging-structure, function and mind. IntechOpen. London, UK.
10. Wasserman K, Whipp BJ, Koyl SN et al (1973) Anaerobic threshold and respiratory gas exchange during exercise. J Appl Physiol 35:236–243
11. Miyazawa T, Horiuchi M, Komine H et al (2013) Skin blood flow influences cerebral oxygenation measured by near-infrared spectroscopy during dynamic exercise. Eur J Appl Physiol 113(11):2841–2848
12. Razi E, Moosavi GA, Omidi K (2012) Correlation of end-tidal carbon dioxide with arterial carbon dioxide in mechanically ventilated patients. Arch Trauma Res 1(2):58–62
13. von Kummer R (1984) Local vascular response to change in carbon dioxide tension. Long term observation in the cat's brain by means of the hydrogen clearance technique. Stroke 15(1):108–114
14. Vovk A, Cunningham DA, Kowalchuk JM et al (2002) Cerebral blood flow responses to changes in oxygen and carbon dioxide in humans. Can J Physiol Pharmacol 80(8):819–827
15. Lindauer U, Dirnagl U, Füchtemeier M et al (2010) Pathophysiological interference with neurovascular coupling – when imaging based on hemoglobin might go blind. Front Neuroenerg 2:25

Cerebral Oxygenation Dynamics During Incremental Exercise: Comparison of Arm Cranking and Leg Cycling

20

K. Hashimoto, K. Hotta, S. Morishita, R. Kanai, H. Takahashi, and A. Tsubaki

Abstract

This study aimed to compare cerebral oxyhemoglobin (O_2Hb) levels during incremental exercise by cycling vs. arm cranking in 12 healthy adult men aged 20.8 ± 0.2 years old. O_2Hb was measured by near-infrared spectroscopy. Regions of interest included the left and right prefrontal cortices (LtPFC and RtPFC, respectively), the left and right premotor cortices (LtPMC and RtPMC, respectively), and the supplementary motor area (SMA) bilaterally. After 4 min of rest, 4 min of warm-up was performed by using ergometer followed by incremental exercise (increasing work rate by 5 W/min for arm cranking and 20 W/min for cycling exercise). All values were averaged every tenth of the participant's exercise time period from beginning of incremental exercise to end point. At the middle exercise intensity (50% exercise time), the averaged O_2Hb values obtained at all regions of interest seemed to be higher during arm cranking exercise as compared to cycling; however, there were no significant differences between two types of exercise. At the end point of incremental exercise (100% exercise time), the O_2Hb obtained at all regions of interest was significantly higher during arm cranking exercise compared to cycling (LtPFC 0.081 ± 0.019 vs. –0.001 ± 0.013 mM·cm, RtPFC 0.076 ± 0.021 vs. 0.018 ± 0.015 mM·cm, SMA 0.012 ± 0.040 vs. 0.040 ± 0.016 mM·cm; arm cranking vs. cycling; $p < 0.05$, respectively). We conclude that exercise-induced cerebral oxygenation is greater with arm cranking than with leg cycling.

Keywords

Near-infrared spectroscopy · Incremental exercise · Prefrontal cortex · Premotor cortex · Supplementary motor area

20.1 Introduction

Near-infrared spectroscopy (NIRS) is widely used for monitoring real-time hemodynamic changes related to cortical neural activation during gross motor tasks. According to a systematic review of NIRS studies of cerebral oxygenation during incremental exercise, oxygenation of the prefrontal cortex (PFC) increases from rest to moderate intensity and decreases from high

K. Hashimoto · R. Kanai · H. Takahashi
Department of Physical Therapy, Niigata University of Health and Welfare, Niigata, Japan

K. Hotta (✉) · S. Morishita · A. Tsubaki
Institute for Human Movement and Medical Sciences, Niigata University of Health and Welfare, Niigata, Japan
e-mail: kazuki-hotta@nuhw.ac.jp

E. M. Nemoto et al. (eds.), *Oxygen Transport to Tissue XLII*, Advances in Experimental Medicine and Biology 1269, https://doi.org/10.1007/978-3-030-48238-1_20

intensity to exhaustion [1]. However, there has been no report on cerebral oxygenation during arm cranking.

Local cerebral blood flow (CBF) increase is associated with neural activation [2]. In past NIRS studies, enhanced premotor cortex (PMC) activation was associated with locomotor recovery in stroke patients [3]. Thus, NIRS is used to evaluate supplementary motor area (SMA) and PMC activation during exercise, and because of this, we anticipated that evaluating O_2Hb in healthy adult men during arm cranking would be clinically important. In addition, activation of the PFC during exercise is associated with improvement in cognitive function, executive function in particular [4]. It is important to clarify the changes in cerebral oxygenation occurring during arm cranking from low intensity to exhaustion to ensure appropriate clinical prescriptions for exercise for stroke patients. Furthermore, we considered that the characteristics of arm cranking can best be clarified by comparisons with cycling, which is the subject of many previous studies.

NIRS measures the concentrations of oxyhemoglobin (O_2Hb) in tissues, based on their differential absorptions at multiple wavelengths [5], and O_2Hb changes are the most sensitive indicators of changes in regional cerebral blood flow in NIRS measurements [6]. Our study aimed to compare the regional cerebral O_2Hb levels during incremental arm cranking exercise with that of cycling.

20.2 Methods

Twelve healthy adult men, 20.75 ± 0.17 years old, participated in the present study. The participants did not exhibit symptoms of any neurological, medical, or cardiovascular diseases and were not taking any medications. Each subject provided written consent after receiving information regarding the potential risk, study objectives, measurement techniques, and benefits associated with the study. This study was approved by the Ethics Committee of Niigata University of Health and Welfare (approval number 18133–190123). Participants performed arm cranking and cycling exercise tests. The participant was seated, the shoulder was at the height of the crank, and the pedals were driven by both arms. After a 4-min rest and a 4-min warm-up, incremental exercise began at work rate that gradually increased at 5 W/min for arm cranking and 20 W/min for cycling. The cycling and cranking rates were maintained at 50–55 r.p.m. Exhaustion was defined as previously described [7]. The two kinds of exercise were performed by each participant with a rest of 3 days or more between. During experiments, all items were measured continuously.

A multichannel NIRS imaging system (LABNIRS; Shimadzu Co., Kyoto, Japan) with multiple continuous wavelengths (780, 805, and 830 nm) was used to detect changes in O_2Hb at a sampling interval of 135 ms. NIRS optodes using eight light-sourcing and eight light-detecting optical fibers and providing simultaneous recordings from 24 channels (labeled Ch 1–24) were set in a 4 × 4 multichannel probe holder (Fig. 20.1). A 30-mm interoptode distance was employed to measure cortical tissue oxygenation. Regions of interest (ROI) included the left prefrontal cortex (Ch 1, 4, and 5; LtPFC), the right prefrontal cortex (Ch 3, 6, and 7; RtPFC), the left premotor area (Ch 8 and 11; LtPMA), the right premotor area (Ch 10 and 14; RtPMA), and the supplementary motor area bilaterally (Ch 12, 13, and 16; SMA). Cardiac output (CO) was measured using a noninvasive, impedance-type system (PhysioFlow Q-Link, Manatec Biomedical, Paris, France). Oxygen uptake (VO_2) and end-tidal carbon dioxide partial pressure ($P_{ET}CO_2$) were recorded with a respiratory gas analyzer (Aero Monitor AE300s, Minato Medical Science Co., Osaka, Japan). Skin blood flow (SBF) was measured at the forehead using a laser tissue-blood-flow oxygen monitor (OMEGAFLOW FLO-Cl, Omega Wave, Inc., Tokyo, Japan).

All ROIs O_2Hb were expressed as changes from the average of the rest. During rest and warm-up, all parameters were calculated mean value for 4 minutes. During incremental exercise, the time from start to end varied across groups and participants. Therefore, in the present study,

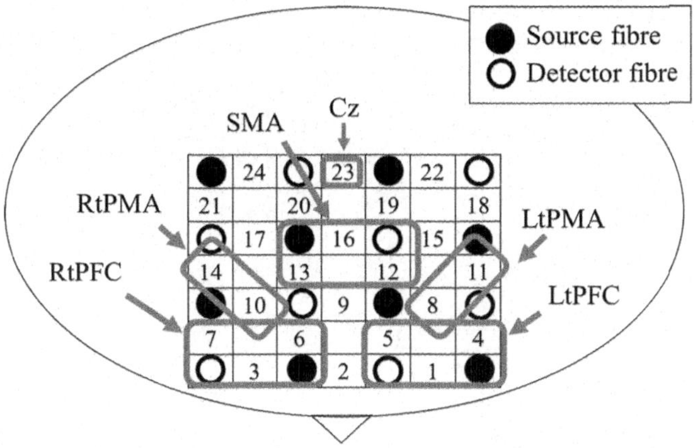

Fig. 20.1 Near-infrared spectroscopy optode placement and regions of interest. Cz the central position of the standard 10–20 electroencephalographic montage; LtPFC left prefrontal cortex, RtPFC right prefrontal cortex, LtPMC left premotor cortex, RtPMC right premotor cortex, SMA supplementary motor area; numerals, channel numbers

the time from the start of incremental exercise to the end was taken as 100%, and the value of each index was averaged at 50% and 100% peak work rate for each participant. Statistical processing was by two-factor, repeated-measures analysis of variance (two-way ANOVA) for a between-groups factor (arm cranking group, cycling group) and a time factor (pre-exercise, incremental exercise load) in all items. p less than 0.05 was taken to indicate significance. When a significant interaction or main effect was observed, paired t-tests were applied. In the present study, the same cortical area was compared between cranking and cycling. Values are presented as mean ± standard error of the mean.

20.3 Results

The incremental exercise time of arm cranking (787 ± 71 s) was significantly longer than cycling (523 ± 30 s) ($p < 0.05$).

Two-way ANOVA with O_2Hb showed group main effects in LtPMA ($p < 0.05$), and in all ROIs, time main effects and interaction were also observed ($p < 0.05$, respectively). During exercise intensity of 50%, in all ROIs, we found no significant differences from rest in the arm cranking and cycling (Fig. 20.2a). Furthermore, we found no significant differences comparing arm cranking with cycling (Fig. 20.2a). During exercise intensity of 100%, in all ROIs, we found significant differences from rest in the arm cranking ($p < 0.05$, respectively; Fig. 20.2b). Furthermore, we found significant differences comparing arm cranking with cycling (Fig. 20.2b; $p < 0.05$, respectively).

At rest, SBF, CO, $P_{ET}CO_2$, and VO_2 were not different between arm cranking and cycling groups (8.23 ± 0.79 a.u., 6.99 ± 0.37 L/min, 39.88 ± 2.86 mmHg, 3.72 ± 0.48 mL/kg/min in cranking and 7.78 ± 0.79 a.u., 6.26 ± 0.44 L/min, 39.3 ± 2.88 mmHg, 3.89 ± 0.49 mL/kg/min in cycling). Group main effects and time main effects and interactions were observed in CO, VO_2, and $P_{ET}CO_2$ (Fig. 20.3b–d; $p < 0.05$, respectively), but only time main effects were observed in SBF (Fig. 20.3a; $p < 0.05$). During exercise intensity of 50%, CO, VO_2, and $P_{ET}CO_2$ showed significantly higher values from rest in cranking and cycling. Comparing arm cranking with cycling at the exercise intensity of 50% peak work rate, arm cranking showed significantly lower values for $P_{ET}CO_2$ and VO_2 ($p < 0.05$, respectively). During exercise intensity of 100%, SBF, CO, $P_{ET}CO_2$, and VO_2 showed significantly higher values from rest in cranking and cycling. Comparing arm cranking with cycling at the exercise intensity of 100% peak work rate, arm cranking showed significantly lower values for $P_{ET}CO_2$ and VO_2 ($p < 0.05$, respectively).

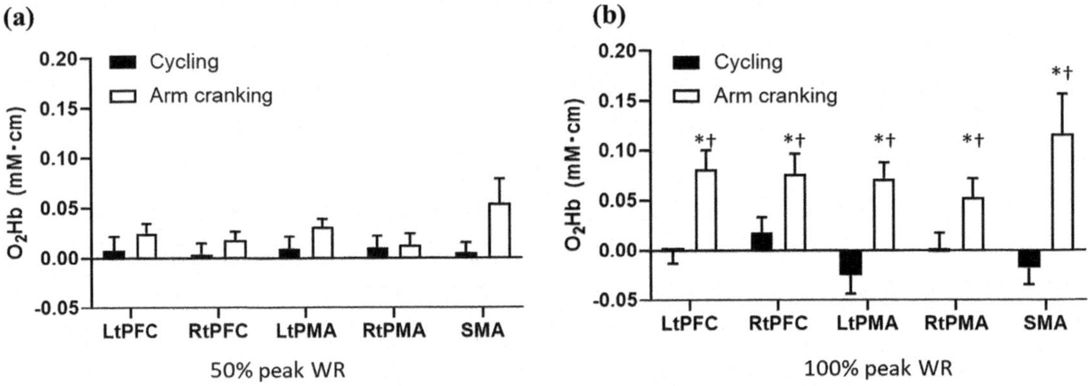

Fig. 20.2 Oxygenated hemoglobin during exercise at the intensity of 50% (**a**) and 100% peak work rate (**b**). LtPFC left prefrontal cortex, RtPFC right prefrontal cortex, LtPMA left premotor area, RtPMA right premotor area, SMA supplementary motor area. *$p < 0.05$ vs. cycling; +$p < 0.05$ vs. rest

20.4 Discussion

One of main findings of this study was that O_2Hb was greater during incremental exercise with arm cranking as compared to cycling in healthy volunteers. The difference in O_2Hb was observed at 100% peak work rate. The O_2Hb signals obtained by NIRS are known to be affected by various factors such as (1) SBF [8], (2) partial pressure of arterial carbon dioxide ($PaCO_2$), (3) blood pressure, and (4) neural activity. No differences in forehead SBF and CO during incremental exercise were observed between arm cranking and cycling, suggesting that increased O_2Hb levels could be independent of hemodynamic factors. Comparing $P_{ET}CO_2$ during cycling with that during arm cranking, arm cranking showed a significantly lower value at time points 50% and 100%. It has been reported that $P_{ET}CO_2$ is measured lower than $PaCO_2$ due to the effect of respiratory dead space at rest and that it decreases during exercise [9]. Hypocapnia reduces cerebral blood flow in healthy men [10]. Although the $P_{ET}CO_2$ during exercise was lower in arm cranking than cycling, O_2Hb was higher in arm cranking than cycling. Therefore, it is likely that hypocapnia may not be a cause of arm cranking exercise-induced higher O_2Hb. Neural activity increases local capillary blood flow. The VO_2 was significantly lower during arm cranking exercise than cycling. These results suggest that neural activity could be one of the causes of increased O_2Hb during arm cranking exercise in healthy male volunteers. These results also indicate that arm cranking exercise increased O_2Hb without excessive hemodynamic and metabolic stress.

Previous studies have reported that dorsolateral PFC and right ventrolateral PFC respond in a manner dependent on motor effort during right-arm cranking [11]. Our results showed O_2Hb increased in bilateral PFC during high-intensity arm cranking exercise, supporting the previous study [11]. The PMA has strong neural connections with the primary motor cortex (M1). The M1 somatotopy is larger in the upper limb than in the lower limb [12]. In general, arm cranking does not constitute the sort of refined movement that is thought to require the activation of M1. However, in the present study, it was necessary to grip the pedal during cranking, and M1 may have been activated in this way. The SMA helps to coordinate behavior during a bimanual task [13]. The change in SMA observed in the present study may have been due to a differential reliance on spinal central pattern generators (CPGs) between the two tasks. Previous studies have reported that the pattern of cutaneous reflex modulation in each arm during arm cranking is relatively independent of the activity of the contralateral limb [14]. Thus, it is considered that CPGs are less involved in arm cranking than in cycling, and the SMA was observed to be more activated by the arm cranking exercise.

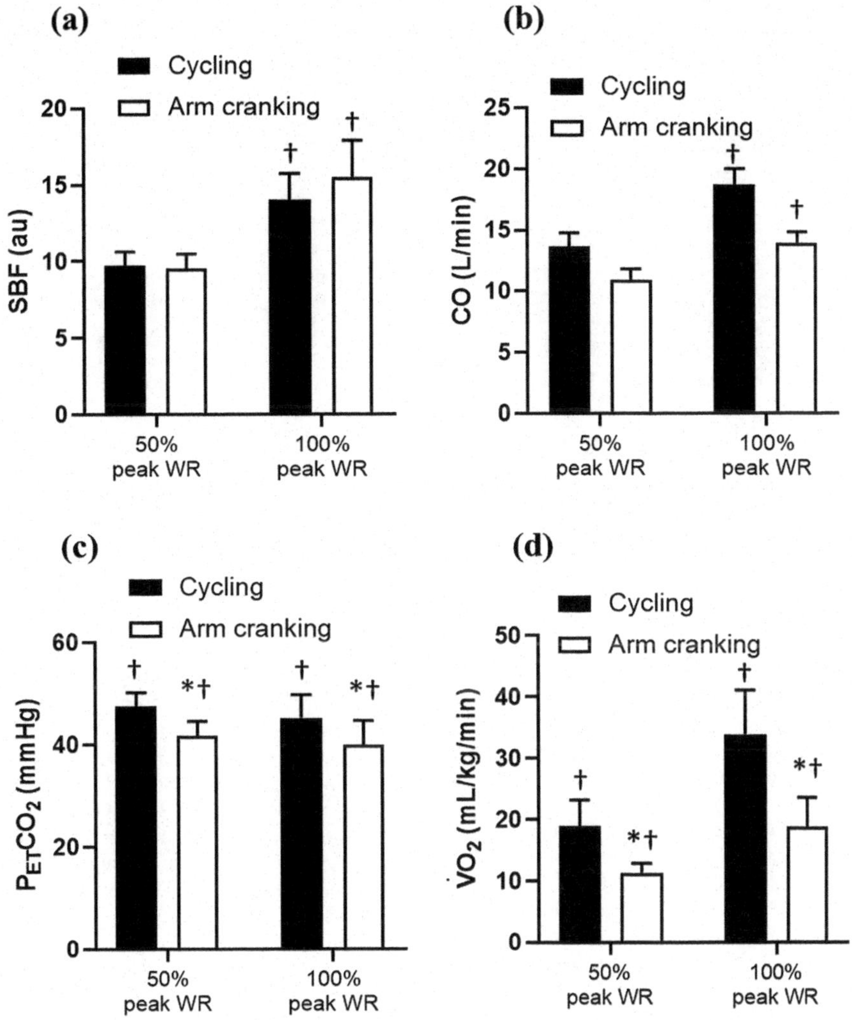

Fig. 20.3 Changes in skin blood flow (**a**), cardiac output (**b**), end-tidal partial pressure of CO_2 (**c**), and oxygen consumption (**d**) during exercise at the intensity of 50% and 100% peak work. SBF skin blood flow, CO cardiac output, $P_{ET}CO_2$ end-tidal partial pressure of CO_2, $\dot{V}O_2$, oxygen consumption. *$p < 0.05$ vs. cycling; +$p < 0.05$ vs. rest

This study has a few limitations. First, it has not been possible to determine possible effects of blood pressure and pH on O_2Hb. To measure the blood pressure response during arm cranking, it would have been necessary to place the cuff in a nonstandard and uncalibrated anatomical location such as the lower limbs. Blood pressure obtained at the relative intensity of exercise was similar for both arm cranking and cycling exercise [15]. In the present study, arm cranking and cycling were compared by relative exercise intensity. Therefore, it may have been unaffected by MAP. In addition, glucose, lactic acid, muscle mechanoreceptors, catecholamines, and oxygen partial pressure may be considered regulators of CBF [16], so it will be necessary to determine the contributions of all these factors in the future. Second, the exercise time was different between arm cranking and cycling. The reason that O_2Hb did not change during cycling may be because exercise time was short. Third, since the exercise intensity is high for stroke patients, it is necessary to devise measures such as high-intensity interval training in the future.

In conclusion, the present study found arm cranking increased O_2Hb levels with a higher efficiency than leg cycling.

References

1. Rooks CR, Thom NJ, McCully KK et al (2010) Effects of incremental exercise on cerebral oxygenation measured by near-infrared spectroscopy: a systematic review. Prog Neurobiol 92:134–150. https://doi.org/10.1016/j.pneurobio.2010.06.002
2. Perrey S (2013) Promoting motor function by exercising the brain. Brain Sci 3:101–122. https://doi.org/10.3390/brainsci3010101
3. Miyai I, Yagura H, Hatakenaka M et al (2003) Longitudinal optical imaging study for locomotor recovery after stroke. Stroke 34:2866–2870. https://doi.org/10.1161/01.STR.0000100166.81077.8A
4. Yanagisawa H, Dan I, Tsuzuki D et al (2010) Acute moderate exercise elicits increased dorsolateral prefrontal activation and improves cognitive performance with Stroop test. NeuroImage 50:1702–1710. https://doi.org/10.1016/j.neuroimage.2009.12.023
5. Boas DA, Gaudette T, Strangman G et al (2001) The accuracy of near infrared spectroscopy and imaging during focal changes in cerebral hemodynamics. NeuroImage 13:76–90. https://doi.org/10.1006/nimg.2000.0674
6. Hoshi Y (2007) Functional near-infrared spectroscopy: current status and future prospects. J Biomed Opt 12:62106. https://doi.org/10.1117/1.2804911
7. Riebe D (ed) (2018) ACSM's guidelines for exercise testing and prescription, 10th edn. Wolters Kluwer Health, Philadelphia. ISBN:9781496339072 149633907X
8. Miyazawa T, Horiuchi M, Komine H et al (2013) Skin blood flow influences cerebral oxygenation measured by near-infrared spectroscopy during dynamic exercise. Eur J Appl Physiol 113:2841–2848. https://doi.org/10.1007/s00421-013-2723-7
9. Wasserman K, Van Kessel AL, Burton GG (1967) Interaction of physiological mechanisms during exercise. J Appl Physiol 22:71–85. https://doi.org/10.1152/jappl.1967.22.1.71
10. Ito H, Kanno I, Ibaraki M, Hatazawa J, Miura S (2003) Changes in human cerebral blood flow and cerebral blood volume during hypercapnia and hypocapnia measured by positron emission tomography. J Cereb Blood Flow Metab 23(6):665–670
11. Ishii K, Liang N, Asahara R et al (2018) Feedforward- and motor effort-dependent increase in prefrontal oxygenation during voluntary one-armed cranking. J Physiol 596:5099–5118. https://doi.org/10.1113/JP276956
12. Penfield W, Boldrey E (1937) Somatic motor and sensory representation in the cerebral cortex of man as studied by electrical stimulation. Brain 60:389–443. https://doi.org/10.1093/brain/60.4.389
13. Brinkman C (1984) Supplementary motor area of the monkey's cerebral cortex: short- and long-term deficits after unilateral ablation and the effects of subsequent callosal section. J Neurosci 4:918–929. https://doi.org/10.1523/JNEUROSCI.04-04-00918.1984
14. Carroll TJ, Zehr EP, Collins DF (2005) Modulation of cutaneous reflexes in human upper limb muscles during arm cycling is independent of activity in the contralateral arm. Exp Brain Res 161:133–144. https://doi.org/10.1007/s00221-004-2050-7
15. Miles DS, Sawka MN, Glaser RM et al (1983) Plasma volume shifts during progressive arm and leg exercise. J Appl Physiol Respir Environ Exerc Physiol 54(2):491–495
16. Querido JS, Sheel AW (2007) Regulation of cerebral blood flow during exercise. Sports Med 37:765–782. https://doi.org/10.2165/00007256-200737090-

21

Localization of Deep Ischemia and Hemorrhage in Preterm Infants' Head with Near-Infrared Optical Tomography: A Numerical Case Study

Jingjing Jiang, Aldo Di Costanzo Mata, Scott Lindner, Martin Wolf, and Alexander Kalyanov

Abstract

Background and aim: Preterm infants have a high incidence of brain lesions that may lead to long-term disabilities. Early diagnosis of cerebral ischemia and hemorrhage may enable protection of the brain by prevention or neuroprotective treatment. Our recently developed time-domain near-infrared optical tomography (TD NIROT) system provides images to diagnose neonatal brain injury. Our aim is to study the image quality achievable from the TD NIROT signals perturbed by noise for two common cases: ischemia and hemorrhage. *Methods:* We implemented simulations on a spherical model of diameter 60 mm representing a typical neonatal head where the absorption $\mu_a = 0.08$ cm^{-1} and the reduced scattering $\mu'_s = 4.1$ cm^{-1}. Injury-mimicking spherical inclusions of various diameters (1 ~ 10 mm) were placed at depths of 10 ~ 20 mm in the ischemia case (2.5 × μ_a) and 14 ~ 30 mm for the hemorrhage case (50 × μ_a). TD data were generated from a large number of source-detector pairs, i.e., 208 detectors placed within a circle of diameter 40 mm on the surface surrounded by 18 sources. Up to 5% Gaussian noise was added in the simulations. 3D images were reconstructed with the modified Tikhonov minimization with the initial guess of a homogeneous phantom, and the images were evaluated by positional error and Dice similarity. *Results:* The inclusions were localized correctly with low positional errors (<1 mm), and the segmented images share a high Dice similarity with the ground truth for both the ischemia and the hemorrhage case, even for tiny inclusions of 1 mm in deep tissue. The hemorrhage case with a high contrast tolerates a substantial level of noise even though the performance drops with higher noise as expected. *Conclusions:* The large amount of data provided by our novel TD NIROT system provides rich enough information for correctly locating hemorrhage and ischemia in the neonatal brain.

Keywords

Near-infrared optical tomography · Brain imaging · Finite element methods

J. Jiang (✉) · A. Di Costanzo Mata · S. Lindner · M. Wolf · A. Kalyanov
Biomedical Optics Research Laboratory (BORL), Department of Neonatology, University Hospital Zürich and University of Zürich, Zurich, Switzerland
e-mail: Jingjing.Jiang@usz.ch

E. M. Nemoto et al. (eds.), *Oxygen Transport to Tissue XLII*, Advances in Experimental Medicine and Biology 1269, https://doi.org/10.1007/978-3-030-48238-1_21

21.1 Introduction

Early recognition of preterm infants at risk for brain injuries may make it possible to protect them from lifelong disabilities or even mortality [1, 2]. Near-infrared optical tomography (NIROT) is a promising technique to detect and locate the brain lesions without the need for the assumption of tissue homogeneity as in near-infrared spectroscopy (NIRS). It is intrinsically sensitive to oxyhemoglobin and deoxyhemoglobin which are two chromophores representing oxygenation that are directly related to absorption (μ_a) being the main absorbers in tissue [3]. A typical NIROT system consists of near-infrared light sources (e.g., laser or LED) and camera or fiber detectors placed on the surface of the target. Light intensity and possibly photon arrival times are measured for generating image reconstructions. Unfortunately, the inverse problem of recovering μ_a or μ'_s in three dimensions is usually ill-posed, and therefore recognition of small objects is challenging especially when they are located deep in tissue. To improve the performance in the application of diagnosis of neonatal brain lesions, we developed the time-resolved TD NIROT system Pioneer with a SPAD camera Piccolo and a picosecond pulsed laser described previously [4, 5]. The large volume of TD data provided by the large number of source-detector pairs is expected to substantially improve the resolution and sensitivity of NIROT. The aim of the study was to evaluate the performance of the TD NIROT system through a numerical study in two common cases of neonatal brain injuries: ischemia and hemorrhage.

21.2 Methods

21.2.1 Forward Model

Light propagation can be approximated as a diffusion process, because biological tissue is highly scattering in the near-infrared region. To solve the diffusion equations for a complex geometry, finite element methods (FEMs) are often used. We implemented the simulations in an open-source software NIRFAST, which provides numerical models based on FEM [6, 7]. We created a spherical tetrahedral mesh representing a typical neonatal head and placed 208 detectors for a circular field of view (FOV) of diameter 40 mm on the surface and 18 sources around the FOV (Fig. 21.1, Left). The optical properties of the head, specifically the absorption $\mu_a^B = 0.08\text{cm}^{-1}$ and scattering value $\mu'^B_s = 4.1\text{cm}^{-1}$ at 692 nm, were obtained from the literature for a preterm neonate at the gestational age of 32 weeks [2]. The hypoxia-ischemia usually shows more absorption at 692 nm and happens within the top 2 cm tissue, whereas bleeding occurs in deeper tissue and is highly absorbing due to the high concentration of blood.

Therefore, for the ischemia case, we placed spherical inclusions ($\mu_a^I = 2.5 \times \mu_a^B$) of various diameters 1 ~ 10 mm at depths of 10 ~ 20 mm and, for the hemorrhage case, inclusions of 1 ~ 7 mm in the diameters at 14 ~ 30 mm ($\mu_a^I = 50 \times \mu_a^B$) as illustrated in Fig. 21.1, Right. To evaluate the robustness, the TD data generated were perturbed by 1%, 2%, and 5% Gaussian noise.

21.2.2 Image Reconstruction

A discrete Fourier transform is taken on the TD data, and a set of amplitudes and phases is obtained for a discrete set of frequencies [3]. The Fourier domain data for the heterogeneous models were used for the image reconstruction. The target of the reconstruction is to recover the optical properties μ of all mesh nodes to make the calculated boundary values Φ^S agree with the measured forward results for the ground truth optical properties Φ^M. The Tikhonov regularization is applied to smooth the results:

$$\mu^* = \arg\min_{\mu}\left(\| \Phi^S - \Phi^M \|_2^2 + \lambda\Lambda(\mu)\right)$$

where λ is the Tikhonov regularization parameter and $\Lambda(\mu)$ is a quadratic Tikhonov regularization term. To better compare the results, we kept the λ = 10 for the first iteration and the initial guess as

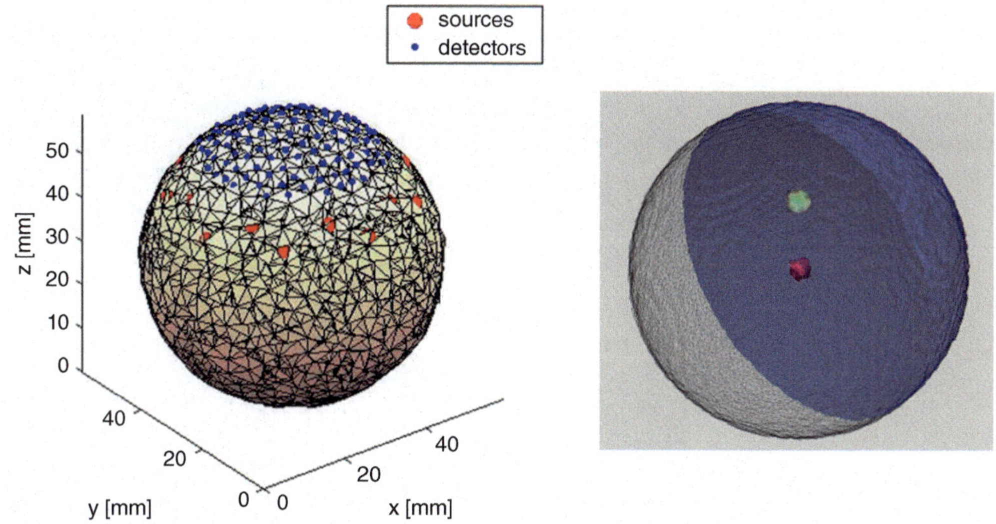

Fig. 21.1 Left: Geometry of neonatal head model; Right: 3D model of a simulated hemorrhage (pink) at the center of the brain and ischemia (green) at depth of 16 mm

a homogeneous model of the universal μ for reconstructions in all cases. A coarser mesh of 2208 nodes was generated from the fine mesh to simplify and speed up the inverse problem-solving. We set the maximum number of iterations to 20, and in addition the iteration stops when the performance of the optimization function stops improving the agreement.

21.2.3 Evaluation Parameters

The reconstructed images were segmented by intensity-based thresholding into the foregrounds representing brain injuries and the backgrounds representing normal tissue. The threshold values were set by averaging the maximum and the minimum of μ_a in the volume. Two parameters were utilized to evaluate the reconstruction performance: Dice similarity and positional error. The MATLAB function dice computed the Sørensen-Dice similarity coefficient between the reconstructed images and the ground truth defined by the following equation:

$$\text{dice}(A,B) = \frac{2|A \cap B|}{(|A| + |B|)}$$

where A and B are sets of binary values from the segmented 3D images of the reconstructed and initial meshes. The closer the Dice index is to 1, the more the volumes are overlapping. Positional errors were defined by the Euclidean displacement of the centroids of the reconstructed foregrounds from the ground truth.

21.3 Results and Discussion

In both scenarios, the Dice similarity generally decreases when the inclusion is smaller or embedded in deeper tissue as shown in the contour plots of Figs. 21.2 and 21.3. The exceptions are big inclusions located at shallow positions in the zero-noise cases where Dice indices are relatively low. The reason is that the reconstructed μ_a in the area of inclusion is peaked resulting in a smaller segmented area after thresholding than the ground truth. An example of such a case is illustrated in Fig. 21.4, Right, where the recovered lesion size is smaller than 10 mm, i.e., the original size. Nevertheless, the central position is recovered accurately with a positional error <1 mm. In the noise-free cases, the segmented images and the ground truth show a high Dice similarity for both scenarios. In the region with

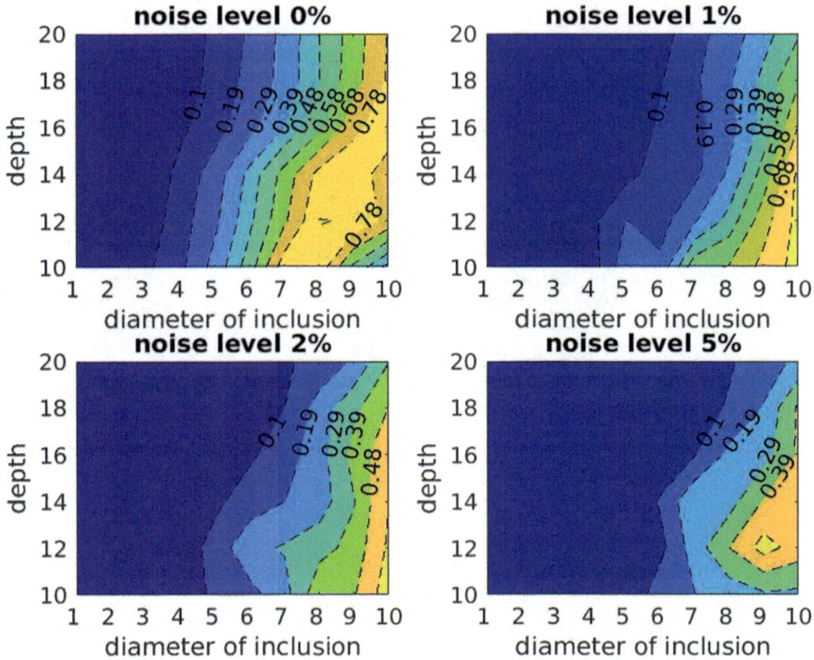

Fig. 21.2 Dice similarity for inclusions of different sizes (1 ~ 10 mm) at different depths (10 ~ 20 mm) for the ischemia case

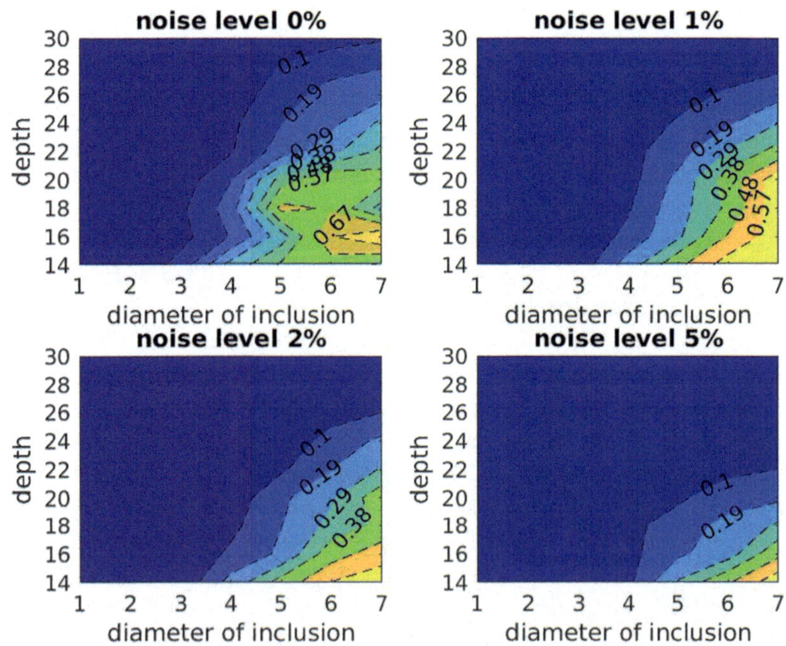

Fig. 21.3 Dice similarity for inclusions of different sizes (1 ~ 7 mm) at variant depths (14 ~ 30 mm) for the hemorrhage case

lower Dice similarity (upper left), the positional error is still small (<1 mm), even in the most challenging case of a tiny inclusion of 1 mm embedded deeply, as shown in Fig. 21.5, Right.

With added noises from 1% to 5% (Figs. 21.2 and 21.3), the similarity drops as expected. But the hemorrhage case with a high contrast is robust against a substantial level of noise.

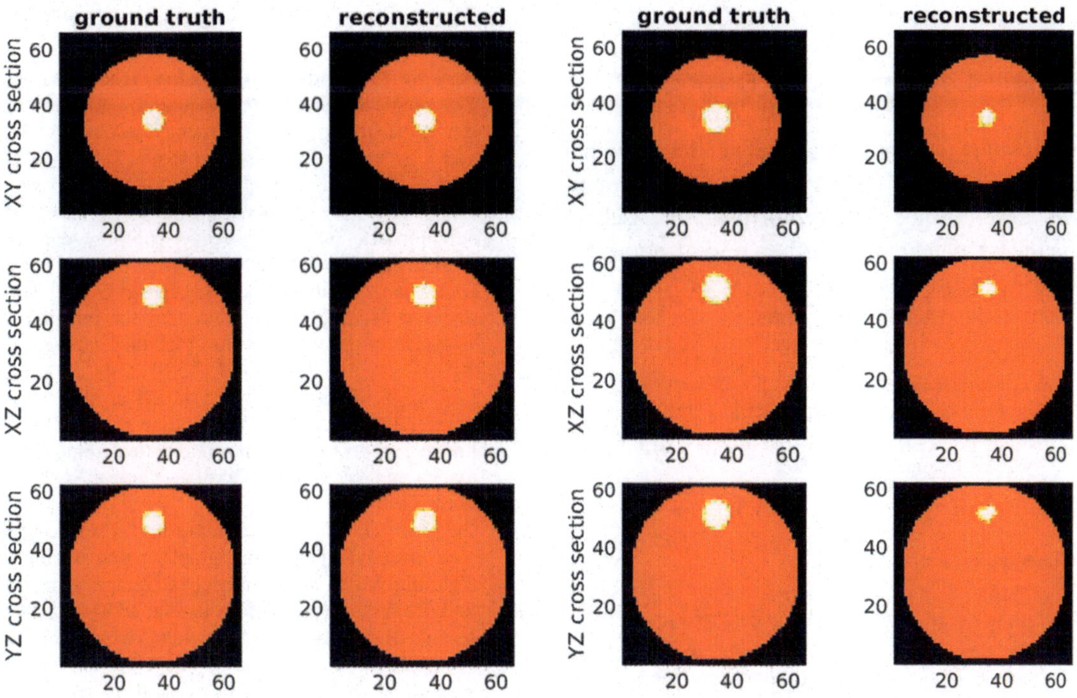

Fig. 21.4 Images of a simulated ischemia of size 8 mm at depth of 12 mm (Left) and size 10 mm at depth of 10 mm (Right) and their reconstructed results in the noiseless case. Compared with the left where the reconstructed area is approximately the same as the ground truth, the reconstructed area on the right is smaller than the ground truth which yields low similarity index. Nevertheless, the position of the ischemia is correctly reconstructed

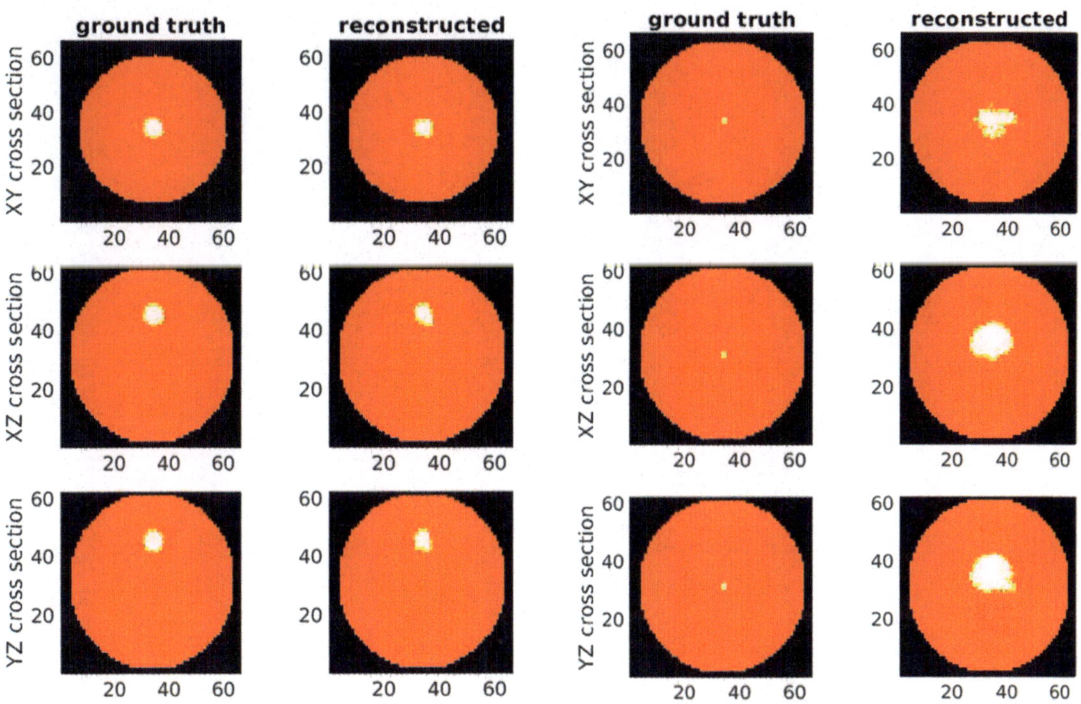

Fig. 21.5 Images of a target hemorrhage of size 7 mm at depth of 16 mm (Left) and size 1 mm at the center of the tissue (Right) and their reconstructed results in the noiseless case. The reconstruction algorithm used in this paper with the universal regularization L2 parameter tends to reconstruct a bigger area for tiny lesion in deep tissue as illustrated on the right. Even in this case of low contrast, the position is correct as the high-contrast case shown on the left where the reconstructed area is almost identical

21.4 Conclusion and Outlook

This study proves that the data generated with the Pioneer system contains rich enough information for correctly locating hemorrhage and ischemia in the neonatal brain. Further, optimization in the reconstruction algorithms will improve the accuracy in the area of the lesions.

Acknowledgments This research was supported by the Swiss Cancer Research grant KFS-3732-08-2015, the Swiss National Science Foundation project 159490, and CONACyT by the CVU-627802.

References

1. Wolf M, Bucher HU, Dietz V et al (1997) How to evaluate slow oxygenation changes to estimate absolute cerebral haemoglobin concentration by near infrared spectrophotometry in neonates. Adv Exp Med Biol 411(495–501):1997
2. Arri S, Muehlemann T, Biallas M et al (2011) Precision of cerebral oxygenation and hemoglobin concentration measurements inneonates measured by near-infrared spectroscopy. J Biomed Opt 16(4):047005
3. Jiang J, Wolf M, Sánchez Majos S (2017) Fast reconstruction of optical properties for complex segmentations in near infrared imaging. J Mod Opt 64(7):732
4. Di Costanzo-Mata A, Jiang J, Lindner S et al Time-resolved NIROT 'Pioneer' system for imaging the oxygenation of the preterm brain (accepted ISOTT 2018)
5. Lindner S, Zhang C, Antolovic IM et al (2018) A novel 32× 32, 224 Mevents/s time resolved SPAD image sensor for near-infrared optical tomography, Optics and the Brain, JTh5A. 6. Optical Society of America
6. Dehghani H, Eames ME, Yalavarthy PK et al (2009) Near infrared optical tomography using NIRFAST: algorithm for numerical model and image reconstruction. Commun Numer Methods Eng 25:711–732
7. Jermyn M, Ghadyani H, Mastanduno MA et al (2013) Fast segmentation and high-quality three-dimensional volume mesh creation from medical images for diffuse optical tomography. J Biomed Opt 18(8):086007

Discerning Membrane Steady-State Oxygen Flux by Monte Carlo Markov Chain Modeling

22

Gary Angles and Sally C. Pias

Abstract

Molecular oxygen (O_2) permeability coefficients for lipid bilayers have previously been estimated using both electron paramagnetic resonance (EPR) oximetry and molecular dynamics simulation data. Yet, neither technique captures the fluxes that exist physiologically. Here, the dynamic steady state is modeled using a stochastic approach built on atomic resolution molecular dynamics simulation data. A Monte Carlo Markov chain technique is used to examine membrane-level fluxes of oxygen in lipid-water systems. At steady state, the concentration of oxygen is found to be higher inside the model membranes than in surrounding water, consistent with the known favorable partitioning of O_2 toward the lipid phase. Pure phospholipid 1-palmitoyl,2-oleoyl-phosphatidylcholine (POPC) bilayers accrue ~40% more O_2 molecules at steady state than POPC/cholesterol bilayers (1:1 molecular ratio) mimicking the red blood cell membrane. Steady-state levels of oxygen were reached inside both bilayer types within the same timeframe, but depletion of oxygen from the bilayer interior occurred 17% faster for POPC than for POPC/cholesterol. Likewise, first-order rate constants estimated for accrual to steady state were the same for POPC and POPC/cholesterol, at 190 μs^{-1}, while first-order rate constants for depletion of the accrued O_2 from the bilayers differed, at 95 μs^{-1} for POPC and 81 μs^{-1} for POPC/cholesterol (lower by 15%). These results are consistent with prior experiments in red blood cells (RBCs) with varying membrane cholesterol content, in which additional cholesterol slowed oxygen uptake and release. Further work is needed to understand whether differences in RBC membrane cholesterol content would affect the delivery of oxygen to tissues.

Keywords

Molecular dynamics simulation · Hypoxia · Cholesterol · Stochastic model · Permeability

22.1 Introduction

Poor delivery of oxygen within tissues has been implicated as a possible cause of health anomalies associated with hypoxia, which may result from high tissue oxygen demand and/or low oxygen supply [1]. Oxygen transport depends on circulating red blood cells (RBCs), which take up

G. Angles · S. C. Pias (✉)
Department of Chemistry, New Mexico Institute of Mining and Technology (New Mexico Tech), Socorro, NM, USA
e-mail: sally.pias@nmt.edu

E. M. Nemoto et al. (eds.), *Oxygen Transport to Tissue XLII*, Advances in Experimental Medicine and Biology 1269, https://doi.org/10.1007/978-3-030-48238-1_22

oxygen in the alveolar capillaries through binding to hemoglobin. In tissues, O_2 release from hemoglobin generates a momentary oxygen gradient across the RBC membrane. This gradient drives O_2 transport across the membrane and involves a momentary steady state at the membrane level. Under normal physiological conditions, RBC membranes have a cholesterol-to-phospholipid molecular ratio of 1:1 or 50 mol% cholesterol [2]. Cholesterol at this level has been shown to slow the penetration of molecular oxygen [3, 4], but our previous work suggests that cholesterol-rich lipid bilayers should not be rate-limiting for oxygen diffusive transport [1].

Electron paramagnetic resonance (EPR) spin-label oximetry has provided valuable experimental data on membrane-level oxygen transport in 1-palmitoyl,2-oleoyl-phosphatidylcholine (POPC) and 1:1 POPC/cholesterol bilayers [2]. We have conducted prior molecular dynamics (MD) simulation studies of oxygen transport, which compare well with the EPR data and generate additional insight [1, 3]. In both the EPR and the MD techniques, observations are generated from systems at equilibrium, where the rate of oxygen diffusion in each direction is equal. Oxygen is neither consumed nor generated and, therefore, a steady state cannot be established. In contrast, biological oxygen transport occurs primarily under unidirectional, nonequilibrium steady-state conditions, where metabolic consumption of oxygen drives its transport.

The MD method does not readily support nonequilibrium simulations, as periodic boundary conditions are required to avoid boundary effects and to handle long-range electrostatic interactions. The use of periodic boundary conditions, where a molecule that leaves the simulation box on one side reenters on the opposite side, enables small-nanoscale systems (e.g., 30,000 atoms) to be treated as infinitely large, approximating the behavior of real macroscopic systems. While valuable for studying membrane permeation processes at atomic resolution, the MD technique alone does not provide a basis for studying steady-state flux. We have sought to overcome this limitation through stochastic modeling.

To probe unidirectional steady-state flux, we have developed a Monte Carlo Markov chain (MCMC) modeling technique [4] based on MD diffusional trajectories of O_2 molecules. The MCMC technique uses a Monte Carlo (random) simulator to propagate motion of oxygen molecules by way of a transition probability matrix built from MD simulations. The propagation of O_2 molecules across a lipid bilayer is treated as a Markov process, where the assumption is made that the probability for an O_2 molecule to transition to a new spatial position depends only on its current position. This MCMC technique enables approximation of unidirectional steady-state oxygen flux and overcomes the limitations of periodic boundary conditions while benefitting from the atomic resolution of unrestrained atomistic MD simulations.

Here, we use our MCMC technique to study the ebb and flow of oxygen at the level of a model lipid bilayer representing the RBC membrane as O_2 is taken up in the lungs or released in tissues. The MCMC technique enables generation of an oxygen gradient across a lipid bilayer, by holding the oxygen concentration on one side constant and by consuming oxygen on the other side. Due to its nonpolarity and small size, oxygen is at least three times more soluble in lipids than in water [5]. Therefore, at steady state, the oxygen content of the bilayer exceeds that of neighboring water.

We first study systems as they progress toward and then reach steady-state oxygen flux, as indicated by a constant number of O_2 molecules within the bilayer. Then, we study the depletion process for oxygen contained in a bilayer by ceasing to add O_2 molecules on the supply side and continuing to remove them on the consumption side. We compare these "accrual" and "depletion" processes for lipid bilayers composed of 1:1 POPC/cholesterol (RBC mimic) and POPC without cholesterol (control), to illuminate the role of cholesterol in RBC membrane-leveloxygen transport.

22.2 Methods

All-atom, unrestrained molecular dynamics simulations of hydrated POPC and POPC/cholesterol bilayers incorporating O_2 were used as the basis for constructing the Markov transition matrix. Conditions of the MD simulations were identical to those in our earlier work [1], with the following exceptions. First, the temperature was controlled using Langevin dynamics with a collision frequency of 1 ps^{-1}. Second, the O_2 model was adjusted to correct for overpartioning toward the lipid phase, by adopting the Lennard-Jones parameters for the ester carbonyl oxygen (oC) atom type in the Lipid14 force field; all other O_2 model parameters were maintained as in Ref. [1]. Finally, 15–45% higher O_2 levels were used, namely, 40 O_2 molecules in the POPC simulation system or 44 O_2 in the POPC/cholesterol system, along with 128 lipids and 4440 water molecules. The results of the current work are consistent with simulations done at the lower O_2 levels (data not shown).

For each bilayer system, a transition matrix for O_2 was constructed along the lipid bilayer normal (the axis of permeation, or z axis), using bins spaced at 1 Å intervals and a time step of 1 ps. For binning, only the depth of the oxygen molecules along this z axis was considered (ignoring the xy spatial distribution, which does not contribute directly to permeation). MD trajectories for 40 or 44 O_2 molecules over 156 ns with 1 ps sampling (6–7 million data points) were pooled to generate the matrix, which held the probabilities of O_2 molecule transition from every bin to every other bin along the z axis. Thus, the number of rows and columns of the matrix was equal and matched the number of 1 Å bins required to encompass the whole system, including the lipid bilayer and surrounding water layers.

After construction of the transition matrix, Monte Carlo moves were used to generate "runs" simulating O_2 transport at 1 ps and 1 Å (in z) intervals, with spatial transitions influenced by the probabilities held in the matrix. More specifically, the instantaneous O_2 molecule configuration along the z axis was held in a Markov chain vector, π_t. This vector was transformed by the transition probability matrix, P, resulting in a subsequent oxygen configuration, π_{t+1}. The configuration was iteratively transformed by the transition matrix to yield subsequent configurations, π_{t+2} and so on: $P\pi_t = \pi_{t+1}$, $P\pi_{t+1} = \pi_{t+2}$, etc. O_2 molecules were treated as whole particles, i.e., fractional occupation of a particular bin was disallowed. The code was developed using the Python programming language [6].

For the steady-state scheme, an oxygen concentration gradient was generated by holding the number of O_2 molecules constant on one side of the bilayer and consuming O_2 molecules on the other side. For POPC/cholesterol, the "supply" zone consisted of water layer bins 0–6 (Å), and the "consumption" zone consisted of water layer bins 88–94. For POPC, the supply zone spanned bins 0–6, and the consumption zone bins 68–73. (These zones are shaded in Fig. 22.1)

22.3 Results and Discussion

To study oxygen accrual within POPC/cholesterol and POPC lipid bilayers as each system progressed toward steady state, the total number of O_2 molecules in the system was initially set to zero. At each subsequent time step of an MCMC run, a threshold of 2 O_2 molecules was applied in the supply zone of the water region ("entry side" shaded areas in Fig. 22.1a, b), and one O_2 molecule was added at each time step if needed to meet the threshold. O_2 molecules were added in the supply zone, as needed to maintain at least two molecules in this zone at each time step. When the number of O_2 molecules accrued within the lipid bilayer reached a plateau, the system was considered to have reached steady state.

The steady-state accrual levels were 56 O_2 molecules for POPC (Fig. 22.1c) and 34 O_2 molecules for POPC/cholesterol (Fig. 22.1d). These levels reflect lower solubility of O_2 in cholesterol-rich bilayers [1]. Twenty 100 ns accrual runs (blue lines) were conducted for each bilayer system, and their running average is shown (black line). For both the POPC and the POPC/choles-

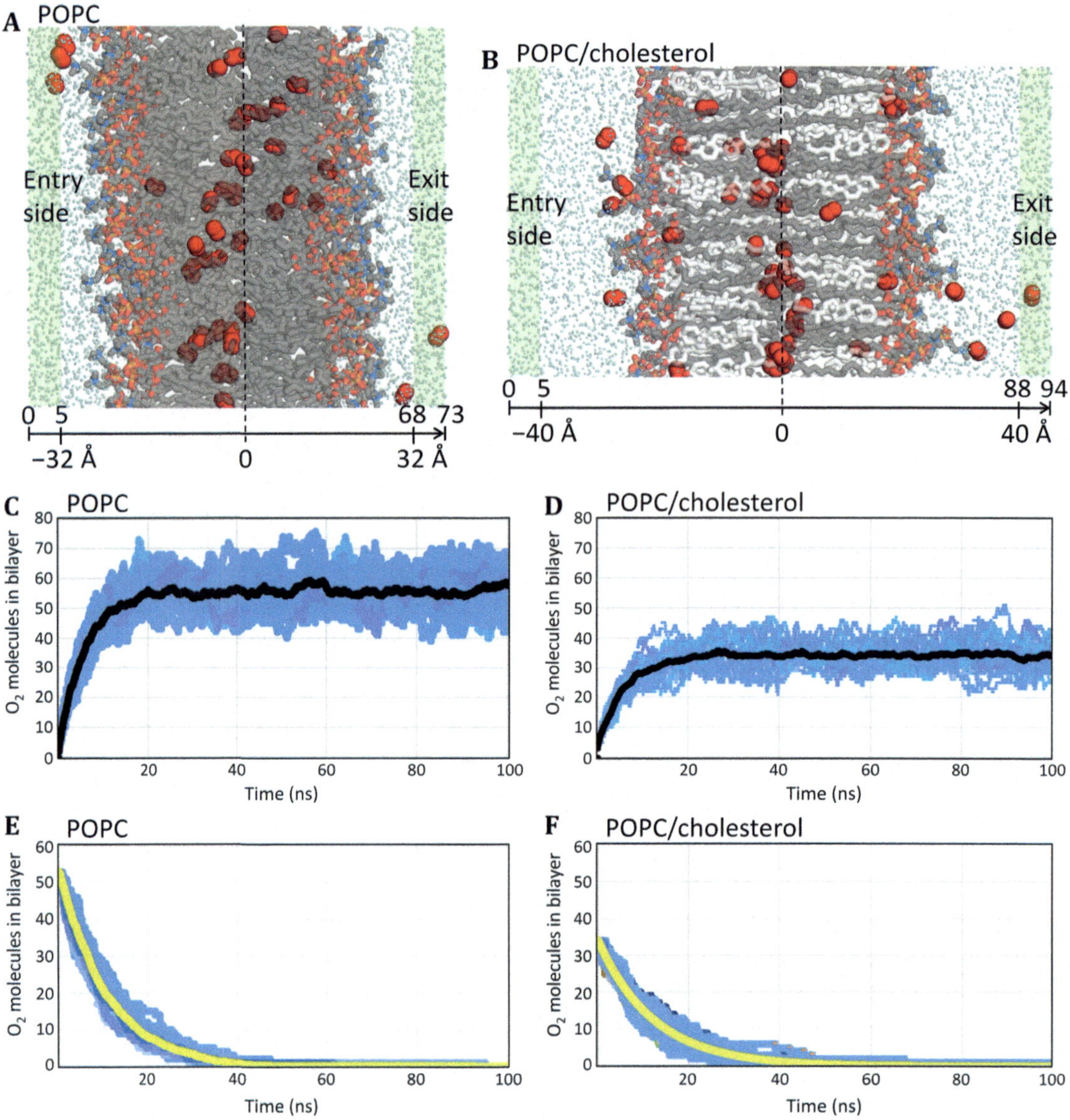

Fig.22.1 (**a**, **b**) Schematic representations of the MCMC steady-state models for the POPC and POPC/cholesterol bilayer systems. The bilayer images are MD simulation snapshots, with O_2 shown as red spheres, POPC as gray sticks with headgroups colored by element, cholesterol as white sticks, and surrounding water molecules as reduced-size dots. All H atoms hidden for clarity. (**c**, **d**) Accrual curves showing progression to steady state in POPC and POPC/cholesterol. Black curves are the average of 20 MCMC runs (blue lines). (**e**, **f**) Depletion curves for POPC and POPC/cholesterol. Yellow curves are the average of 20 runs (blue lines)

terol bilayer systems, steady state was reached within ~24 ns.

To study depletion of oxygen from the bilayers after reaching steady state, removal of O_2 molecules in the consumption zone was continued, while no further molecules were added in the supply zone. As before, 20 × 100 ns runs were conducted for each bilayer system (blue lines in Fig. 22.1e, f), and their running average is shown (yellow lines). As expected, the number of O_2 molecules within each lipid bilayer diminished, rapidly at first and then more slowly. Full depletion of O_2 occurred within ~48 ns for POPC and ~56 ns for POPC/cholesterol (17% longer).

Mathematical regression of the curves revealed the rates of accrual and depletion to be first order (dependent only on the O_2 concentration). The rate constants for accrual, k_{accr}, were calculated to be 190 μs^{-1} (or 1.9×10^8 s^{-1}) for both POPC and POPC/cholesterol. The rate constants for depletion, k_{depl}, reflect the differences in the depletion curves and are estimated to be 95 μs^{-1} (or 9.5×10^7 s^{-1}) for POPC and 81 μs^{-1} for POPC/cholesterol (lower by 15%). This difference is consistent with the ~10% reduction of 50 mol% POPC/cholesterol permeability relative to POPC estimated in our previous work, based on equilibrium MD simulations [1]. The kinetics observed here are also congruent with experimental work by Buchwald and colleagues, in which both the kinetics and the amount of O_2 uptake and release by RBCs were found to diminish with above-normal RBC membrane cholesterol content [7].

22.4 Conclusions and Expansion of the Model

The steady-state stochastic MCMC technique piloted here shows promise to generate valuable insights into physiological oxygen transport by RBCs. It also provides a basis for interpreting other experimental findings, such as magnified O_2 gradients across cholesterol-enriched Chinese hamster ovary (CHO) cell plasma membranes observed by Swartz and colleagues [8]. Moreover, the MCMC technique enables rapid simulation of model membrane systems on longer time and distance scales than are typically accessible at atomic resolution. Expansion of the spatial scale can be achieved through replication of the Markov transition matrix, to test whether oxygen diffusion over longer distances and multiple cell layers could be rate-limiting for oxygen delivery in some tissues. With the current bilayer systems, we have been able to reach simulation times of ~250 ns per hour, compared with 60–90 ns of MD simulation time per day on graphics processing unit (GPU) accelerators. The MCMC technique further enables modeling of intermittent variations, keeping in mind that RBCs are not continually at steady state.

The current results are intriguing, though further work is needed to determine their significance. The data indicate that membrane cholesterol diminishes the capacity of membranes to hold oxygen at steady state, with accompanying reduction in transmembrane oxygen flux. Additional study is required to evaluate whether hypercholesterolemia, and accompanying RBC membrane cholesterol elevation, would reduce RBC oxygen release to tissues. Such evaluation will require consideration of the effects of other potential barriers to oxygen diffusion. The structure of the vessel and target tissue presents many possible barriers, including the blood plasma, the endothelial cell membranes, and cytoplasm, as well as the interstitial fluid, membranes, and cytoplasm of the tissue. To a first approximation, the permeability of the aqueous layers immediately surrounding the RBC membrane should be considered: the RBC cytoplasm on one side and a layer of plasma on the other. Oxygen has relatively low solubility in water, compared with lipids, and is expected to have even lower solubility in aqueous fluids rich in proteins and other solutes [9, 10]. As such, the cytoplasm and plasma layers may pose diffusion barriers of comparable or greater magnitude than the RBC membrane barrier. Because permeability depends directly on thickness, close attention must be given to the thickness of the plasma layer surrounding the RBC. This layer may be especially thin in microcapillaries, where RBCs fit so snugly within the vessel that their shape is altered. In future work, we intend to pursue a formal comparison of the membrane barriers described here with aqueous barriers encountered upon O_2 transfer from RBCs to endothelial tissue.

Acknowledgments The authors thank James Kindt for reading the manuscript. This work has been supported by the National Institutes of Health under NIGMS grant P20GM103451 and by a gift from the Glendorn Foundation.

References

1. Dotson RJ, Smith CR, Bueche K, Angles G, Pias SC (2017) Influence of cholesterol on the oxygen permeability of membranes: insight from atomistic simulations. Biophys J 112:2336–2347. https://doi.org/10.1016/j.bpj.2017.04.046. PMCID: PMC5474842
2. Widomska J, Raguz M, Subczynski WK (2007) Oxygen permeability of the lipid bilayer membrane made of calf lens lipids. Biochim Biophys Acta 1768:2635–2645. https://doi.org/10.1016/j.bbamem.2007.06.018. S0005-2736(07)00233-7 [pii]
3. Angles G, Dotson R, Bueche K, Pias SC (2017) Predicted decrease in membrane oxygen permeability with addition of cholesterol. Adv Exp Med Biol 977:9–14. https://doi.org/10.1007/978-3-319-55231-6_2. PMCID: PMC5673249
4. Durrett R (2012) Essentials of stochastic processes. Springer New York, New York, NY
5. Möller MN, Denicola A (2018) Diffusion of nitric oxide and oxygen in lipoproteins and membranes studied by pyrene fluorescence quenching. Free Radic Biol Med 128:137–143. https://doi.org/10.1016/j.freeradbiomed.2018.04.553
6. Python Software Foundation. The Python Language Reference, version 2.6.11. Available at http://www.python.org
7. Menchaca HJ, Michalek VN, Rohde TD, O'Dea TJ, Buchwald H (1998) Decreased blood oxygen diffusion in hypercholesterolemia. Surgery 124:692–698. https://doi.org/10.1067/msy.1998.90944. S0039-6060(98)00298-0 [pii]
8. Khan N, Shen J, Chang TY, Chang CC, Fung PC, Grinberg O, Demidenko E, Swartz H (2003) Plasma membrane cholesterol: a possible barrier to intracellular oxygen in normal and mutant CHO cells defective in cholesterol metabolism. Biochemistry 42:23–29. https://doi.org/10.1021/bi026039t
9. Battino R, Rettich TR, Tominaga T (1983) The solubility of oxygen and ozone in liquids. J Phys Chem Ref Data 12:163–178
10. Skulachev VP (1990) Power transmission along biological membranes. J Membr Biol 114:97–112

Part III

Tumor Oxygenation and Modeling

23 The Role of MicroRNA Expression for Proliferation and Apoptosis of Tumor Cells: Impact of Hypoxia-Related Acidosis

L. Lange, T. Hüsing, M. Rauschner, Anne Riemann, and O. Thews

Abstract

The metabolic microenvironment in tumors is characterized by hypoxia and acidosis. Extracellular pH sometimes decreases to even below 6.0. Previous experiments showed that tissue pH has an impact on tumor cell proliferation and apoptosis. However, the mechanism of how cell cycle progression is affected by decreased pH is not fully understood yet. One possible mechanism includes changes in the expression of miRNAs. The aim of this study was to analyze the impact of pH-regulated miRNAs (miR-183 and miR-215) on proliferation, apoptosis, and necrosis of tumor cells. Therefore, AT1 prostate and Walker-256 mammary carcinoma cells were transfected with the miRNAs or with the respective antagomirs and incubated at pH 7.4 and 6.6 for 24 h. AT1 cells underwent a G0/G1 cell cycle arrest under acidic conditions and showed a marked reduction of the number of actively DNA-synthesizing cells. In Walker-256 cells, acidosis induced a reduction of apoptosis and additionally a significant increase in necrotic cell death. Transfection of tumor cells with miR-183 or miR-215, which were significantly downregulated under acidic conditions, had no impact on cell death of AT1 or Walker-256 cells. Overexpression of miR-183, which is also downregulated by acidosis, intensified G0/G1 cell cycle arrest in AT1 cells. Previous studies revealed that hypoxia-related tumor acidosis affects the expression of different small noncoding RNAs. However, not all of these acidosis-regulated miRNAs seem to have an impact on proliferation, apoptosis, and necrosis of tumor cells. While miR-215 had no influence, miR-183 seems to be an interesting candidate that could amplify the impact of extracellular acidosis on malignant behavior of tumor cells.

Keywords

Tumor acidosis · MicroRNA · Proliferation · Apoptosis · Necrosis

23.1 Introduction

Compared to normal organs, solid tumors exhibit an altered metabolic microenvironment which is characterized by hypoxia and acidosis. Insufficient angiogenesis leads to hypoxic areas within the rapidly growing tissue [1]. To fulfill energy requirements, cells increase glycolysis,

L. Lange · T. Hüsing · M. Rauschner · A. Riemann (✉) · O. Thews
Julius-Bernstein-Institute of Physiology, University of Halle, Halle (Saale), Germany
e-mail: anne.riemann@medizin.uni-halle.de

E. M. Nemoto et al. (eds.), *Oxygen Transport to Tissue XLII*, Advances in Experimental Medicine and Biology 1269, https://doi.org/10.1007/978-3-030-48238-1_23

but tumors also use glycolytic metabolism even with sufficient oxygen supply (Warburg effect), resulting in an increased lactic acid production and in an acidic extracellular pH even below 6.0 [2, 3]. Previous experiments showed that extracellular acidosis has an impact on metastasis and migration [4]. Small noncoding regulatory RNAs, so-called microRNAs, might be the link between metabolic microenvironment and malignant behavior. The single-stranded RNAs with an approximate length of around 22 nucleotides have a function in posttranscriptional RNA silencing [5, 6]. They can act as tumor suppressors and oncogenes [6] and can influence the metabolic microenvironment [6–8]. But the metabolic microenvironment (e.g., the extracellular tumor pH) can in turn also modulate the expression of microRNAs [9]. Four miRNAs (miR-7, miR-183, miR-203, miR-215) were identified to be pH regulated; miR-183 and miR-215 were downregulated under acidic conditions [9]. In this study, the impact of acidosis on proliferation, apoptosis, and necrosis in tumor cells was analyzed. Two different tumor cell lines (AT1 prostate and Walker-256 mammary carcinoma cells) were used in all experiments. Cells were transfected with the miRNAs (mimics) or with the respective antagomirs (inhibitors) and incubated at pH 7.4 (control conditions) or 6.6 (acidosis) for 24 h. Subsequently, the influence on proliferation, apoptosis, and necrotic cell death was measured. The effect on proliferation was examined with BrdU staining and cell cycle analysis, whereas apoptosis and necrosis were analyzed with caspase-3 activity and LDH release, respectively.

23.2 Methods

23.2.1 Cell Line

The subline AT1 of the rat Dunning R-3327 prostate carcinoma was grown in RPMI medium supplemented with 10% fetal calf serum (FCS). The rat mammary carcinoma cell line Walker-256 was grown in RPMI medium supplemented with 20 mM HEPES, 10 mM L-glutamine, 0.15% $NaHCO_3$, and 10% FCS. Cells were grown at 37 °C under humidified 5% CO_2 atmosphere and were split twice a week.

23.2.2 Experimental Settings

For the experiments, cells were transfected with 1.5 μl *Lipofectamine 2000* in 50 μl RPMI medium and 1 pmol miRNA mimic or 10 pmol miRNA inhibitor. After 24 h, cells were incubated in HEPES- and MES-buffered medium supplemented (BrdU assay) or lacking (caspase-3 activity, LDH release) with FCS at pH 7.4 (control) and 6.6 (acidosis) for 24 h (at 37 °C in a humidified atmosphere with 5% CO_2).

For BrdU staining, cells were kept at different pH conditions for 24 h after which they were incubated with 5 μM BrdU for 1 h. Cells were then fixed with 70% ethanol and stained with anti-BrdU antibody or isotype control (BD Biosciences, San Jose, CA, USA) and anti-mouse FITC antibody (1:100) (Rockland, Limerick, PA, USA). Additionally, cells were stained for 10 min with 50 μg/ml propidium iodide + RNase to measure cell cycle distribution. Apoptosis was examined with caspase-3 activity, and necrosis was measured with LDH release, as described in [10].

23.3 Results

In AT1 cells, an acidic extracellular pH (pH 6.6) leads to a decrease of the number of proliferating cells compared to the level of actively DNA-synthesizing cells under control conditions (pH 7.4), while in Walker-256 cells, only a trend of a decrease in proliferation could be seen (Fig. 23.1). Antagonizing the acidosis-induced downregulation of miR-215 by transfection with miR-215 mimic and incubation at pH 6.6 for 24 h, the number of proliferating cells (BrdU positive) was unaffected in both cell lines. However, antagonizing the acidosis-induced downregulation of miR-183 by transfection of miR-183 and incubation at low pH led to a decrease in the number of actively DNA-synthesizing AT1 cells from 23.8% to 16.3%

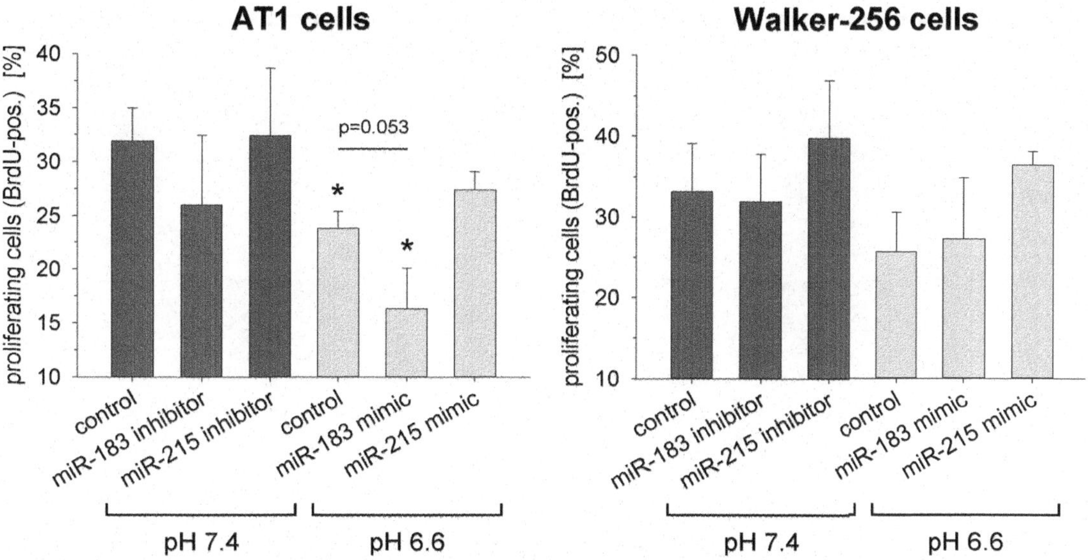

Fig. 23.1 Fraction of actively proliferating cells (BrdU positive) after transfection with microRNAs (mimics, antagomirs/inhibitors) and incubation at pH 7.4 and 6.6 for 24 h. Values are expressed as mean ± SEM, $n = 5–9$, (*) $p < 0.05$ vs. control pH 7.4

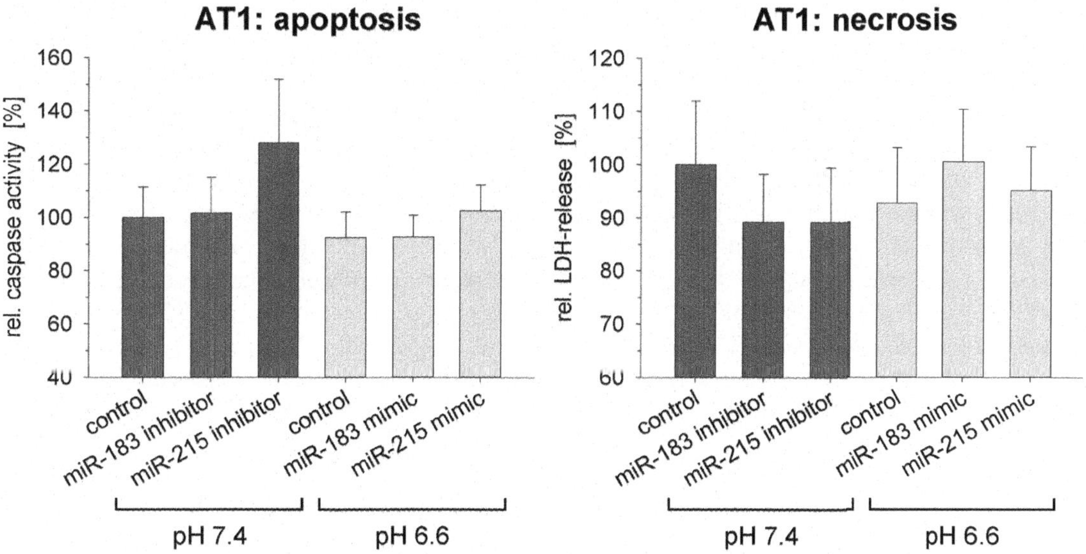

Fig. 23.2 Relative caspase-3 activity (apoptosis) and LDH release (necrosis) in AT1 cells after transfection with microRNAs (mimics, antagomirs/inhibitors) and incubation at pH 7.4 and 6.6 for 24 h. Values are expressed as mean ± SEM, $n = 5–9$, (*) $p < 0.05$ vs. control pH 7.4

($p = 0.053$), while Walker-256 cells were not affected by this artificial overexpression. Additionally, cell cycle analysis showed that AT1 cells underwent a significant G0/G1 cell cycle arrest under acidic conditions (fraction of G0/G1 cells: 62.0% at pH 7.4 vs. 73.3% at pH 7.4, $p < 0.02$). Overexpression of miR-183 at pH 6.6 intensified the G0/G1 arrest significantly (G0/G1 average value: 82.6% at pH 6.6, $p < 0.01$). In line with previous findings, extracellular acidification had no effect on cell cycle distribution of Walker-256 cells.

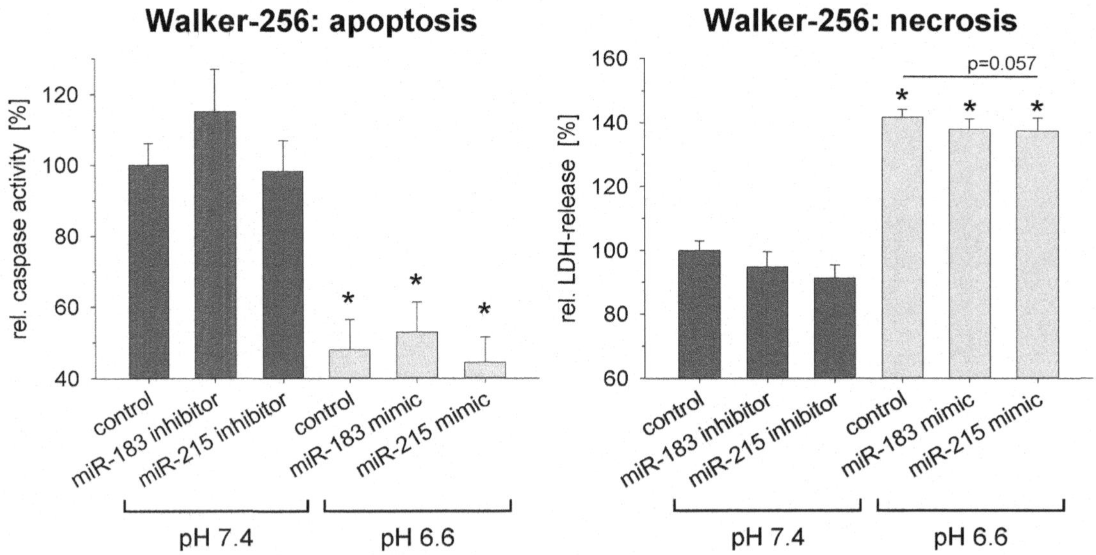

Fig. 23.3 Relative caspase-3 activity (apoptosis) and LDH release (necrosis) in Walker-256 cells after transfection with microRNAs (mimics, antagomirs/inhibitors) and incubation at pH 7.4 and 6.6 for 24 h. Values are expressed as mean ± SEM, $n = 5–9$, (*) $p < 0.05$ vs. control pH 7.4

Figure 23.2 shows the effect of acidosis on apoptosis and necrosis in AT1 cells. As standard error is quite high, only trends could be seen. Apoptosis and necrosis were not changed under acidic conditions. Overexpression of miR-183 (at pH 6.6) led to the trend of a slight increase of necrosis, while an inhibition of this miRNA at pH 7.4 shows the trend of a slight decrease of necrotic cell death by about 10% comparable with the level of necrosis at pH 6.6. In Walker-256 cells, acidosis led to a significant decrease of apoptosis of about 50% and a significant increase of necrotic cell death of approximately 40% (Fig. 23.3). Concerning the impact of microRNA expression, an altered microRNA expression level had no impact on apoptosis and necrosis of Walker-256 cells.

23.4 Conclusion

Hypoxia-related extracellular acidosis in tumors per se influences cell proliferation and cell death. Studies demonstrated that lactic acidosis not only markedly reduces apoptosis but also increases the resistance of tumor cells against stress-induced apoptosis [11, 12]. However, the results of the present study reveal that this effect is cell line-dependent. Whereas, in AT1 cells, proliferation (BrdU-positive cells, cell cycle arrest) is preferentially affected by low pH, Walker-256 cells are much more sensitive regarding cell death. The results also indicate that both mechanisms of cell death always have to be considered, since in Walker-256 cells low pH induced a marked reduction of apoptosis but in parallel a comparable increase in necrosis (Fig. 23.3) so that the net effect on overall cell survival is difficult to estimate in advance. But it becomes obvious that low extracellular pH influences the proliferation/cell death kinetics of tumors.

The mechanism by which acidosis modulates proliferation/cell death has been discussed controversially. Besides a direct impact on mitochondrial metabolism, G-protein-coupled signaling cascades have been discussed (for a review, see [13]). In the present study, we analyzed the hypothesis whether pH-dependent regulatory microRNAs can act as signaling mediators. Acidosis has been shown to influence the expression of different miRNAs (i.e., miR-183, miR-215) [9]. Modulating the microRNA expression by transfection with mimics or antagomirs/inhibitors revealed that only the level of miR-183 had a marginal impact on proliferation and/or cell death. However, just AT1 cells were influenced by this miRNA. In this cell line, transfection of miR-183 and incubation at low pH led to a further decrease in proliferation with only borderline significance ($p = 0.053$). Besides, this artificial overexpression intensified G0/G1 cell cycle arrest significantly. Concerning the impact on necrotic cell death, miR-183 increased LDH release at pH 6.6, while miR183 inhibition at pH 7.4 reduced necrosis. However, our data showed only slight tendencies because the standard error is quite high.

These results suggest that some effects of extracellular acidosis on proliferation and cell death could be mediated by acidosis-regulated miRNAs. While miR-215 seems to have no impact on cell cycle progression or cell death, miR-183 might amplify malignant potential of AT1 cells. Since the impact of microRNAs is clearly cell line-dependent, further studies are needed to analyze the impact of extracellular pH on different targets of the pH-sensitive microRNAs in both cell lines.

Acknowledgments The study was supported by the Deutsche Forschungsgemeinschaft (DFG) (grant TH482/6-1) and HaPKoM (PK24).

References

1. Vaupel P, Kallinowski F, Okunieff P (1989) Blood flow, oxygen and nutrient sup-ply, and metabolic microenvironment of human tumors: a review. Cancer Res 49(23):6449–6465
2. Vander Heiden MG, Cantley LC, Thompson CB (2009) Understanding the Warburg effect: the metabolic requirements of cell proliferation. Science 324(5930):1029–1033. https://doi.org/10.1126/science.1160809
3. Corbet C, Feron O (2017) Tumour acidosis: from the passenger to the driver's seat. Nat Rev Cancer 17(10):577–593. https://doi.org/10.1038/nrc.2017.77
4. Riemann A, Schneider B, Gündel D, Stock C, Thews O, Gekle M (2014) Acidic priming enhances metastatic potential of cancer cells. Pflugers Arch 466(11):2127–2138. https://doi.org/10.1007/s00424-014-1458-6
5. Ha M, Kim VN (2014) Regulation of microRNA biogenesis. Nat Rev Mol Cell Biol 15(8):509–524. https://doi.org/10.1038/nrm3838
6. Esquela-Kerscher A, Slack FJ (2006) Oncomirs – microRNAs with a role in cancer. Nat Rev Cancer 6(4):259–269. https://doi.org/10.1038/nrc1840
7. Jansson MD, Lund AH (2012) MicroRNA and cancer. Mol Oncol 6(6):590–610. https://doi.org/10.1016/j.molonc.2012.09.006
8. Lin S, Gregory RI (2015) MicroRNA biogenesis pathways in cancer. Nat Rev Cancer 15(6):321–333. https://doi.org/10.1038/nrc3932
9. Riemann A, Reime S, Thews O (2019) Acidic extracellular environment affects miRNA expression in tumors in vitro and in vivo. Int J Cancer 144(7):1609–1618. https://doi.org/10.1002/ijc.31790
10. Riemann A, Schneider B, Ihling A, Nowak M, Sauvant C, Thews O, Gekle M (2011) Acidic environment leads to ROS-induced MAPK signaling in cancer cells. PLoS One 6(7):e22445. https://doi.org/10.1371/journal.pone.0022445
11. Wu H, Ding Z, Hu D, Sun F, Dai C, Xie J, Hu X (2012) Central role of lactic acidosis in cancer cell resistance to glucose deprivation-induced cell death. J Pathol 227(2):189–199. https://doi.org/10.1002/path.3978
12. Hunter A, Hendrikse A, Renan M, Abratt R (2006) Does the tumor microenvironment influence radiation-induced apoptosis? Apoptosis 11(10):1727–1735. https://doi.org/10.1007/s10495-006-9789-1
13. Thews O, Riemann A (2019) Tumor pH and metastasis: a malignant process beyond hypoxia. Cancer Metastasis Rev 38(1–2):113–129. https://doi.org/10.1007/s10555-018-09777-y

Functional Impact of Acidosis-Regulated MicroRNAs on the Migration and Adhesion of Tumor Cells

24

T. Hüsing, L. Lange, M. Rauschner, Anne Riemann, and O. Thews

Abstract

Tumor tissue shows special features in metabolism in contrast to healthy tissue. Besides a distinctive oxygen deficiency, tumors often show a reduced extracellular pH (acidosis) resulting from an intensified glycolysis not only under hypoxic but also under normoxic conditions (Warburg effect). As shown in previous studies, cell migration is increased in AT1 prostate carcinoma cells after incubation at pH 6.6, and this leads to an increased number of lung metastases in vivo. However, the signaling pathway causing these functional changes is still unknown. Possible mediators could be acidosis-regulated microRNAs (miR-7, miR-183, miR-203, miR-215). The aim of the study was therefore to analyze whether a change in the expression of these microRNAs has an impact on the tumor cell migration and adhesion. Studies were performed with AT1 rat prostate cancer cells which were incubated for 24 h at pH 7.4 or 6.6. Keeping AT1 tumor cells at low pH increased the migratory capacity by about 100%. But also the decrease of miR-203 and miR-215 expression (at normal pH) led to an increase in migration velocity by 50%. In contrast, cell adhesion was increased by about 75% at low pH. However, an increase in miR-215 expression at pH 6.6 reduced the adhesion by trend. These results clearly indicated that the extracellular pH has an impact on migration and adhesion of tumor cells. In this mechanism, pH-regulated microRNAs could play a role since changes in the expression of these microRNAs (especially miR-203) are also able to modulate the migratory behavior.

Keywords

Tumor acidosis · MicroRNA · Migration · Adhesion · Metastasis

24.1 Introduction

Tumor tissue differs strongly from normal tissue due to its special features in metabolism. It is characterized by distinctive oxygen deficiency caused by insufficient vascularization combined with a high metabolic demand leading to intensified glycolytic metabolism. In addition, tumor cells employ glycolysis even if oxygen is available (Warburg effect) [1]. Glycolysis causes increased formation of protons and lactate, accumulating in the extracellular space leading to an

T. Hüsing · L. Lange · M. Rauschner · A. Riemann (✉) · O. Thews
Julius-Bernstein-Institute of Physiology, University of Halle-Wittenberg, Halle (Saale), Germany
e-mail: anne.riemann@medizin.uni-halle.de

E. M. Nemoto et al. (eds.), *Oxygen Transport to Tissue XLII*, Advances in Experimental Medicine and Biology 1269, https://doi.org/10.1007/978-3-030-48238-1_24

acidification (down to pH 6.0) [2]. Acidosis induces various changes at the cellular level such as alterations in cellular protein expression and changes of enzymatic activity [3]. However, functional properties of tumor cells are also affected by low pH. As shown in previous studies, extracellular acidosis (pH 6.6) leads to an enhanced cellular motility of tumor cells in vitro and an increased number of metastases in experimental tumors in vivo [4]. Furthermore, acidosis induced a reduced cell adhesion and the loss of the apical-basal polarity of the cells [5]. The signaling pathway mediating these effects is not completely understood. It is possible mechanisms include the actions of microRNAs. MicroRNAs are small noncoding RNAs (~20–22 bp) that regulate the gene expression at a post-transcriptional level and can function as tumor suppressors or oncogenes [6]. Therefore, an altered microRNA expression can cause tumor development, affect the chemosensitivity, or promote metastasis formation [5]. Previous studies identified four acidosis-regulated microRNAs: miR-7, miR-183, miR-203, and miR-215. MiR-7 was upregulated at low pH, whereas miR-183, miR-203, and miR-215 were downregulated by acidosis [7]. The aim of our study was to analyze whether changing the expression levels of miR-203 and miR-215 induces alterations of tumor cell migration and adhesion.

24.2 Methods

24.2.1 Cell Line

Prostate carcinoma cells (AT1, Dunning R-3327) were grown in RPMI medium supplemented with 10% fetal calf serum (FCS). The respective microRNAs (miR-203, miR-215) were modulated by transfecting the cells either with the microRNAs themselves (mimics, 10 μM) or with antagomirs (inhibitor, 40 μM) with Lipofectamine 2000. After 24 h, cells were incubated in HEPES- or MES-buffered RPMI medium at pH 7.4 (control) or 6.6 (acidosis) at 37 °C in a humidified atmosphere with 5% CO_2 for 24 h (migration experiments) or up to 40 h (adhesion measurements).

24.2.2 Experimental Settings

The migratory capacity of the cells was measured by time-lapse microscopy (Keyence, Osaka, Japan) over 100 min analyzing the migration velocity and the distance covered (meaning the Euclidian distance) of individual cells with ImageJ (Ibidi Chemotaxis and Migration Tool, Gräfelfing, Germany). Cell adhesion was measured by continuous impedance measurements of monolayer cells (xCELLigence DP; OLS OMNI Life Science, Bremen, Germany) in accordance with the manufacturer's instructions. After transfection and incubation, the cells were grown in special 16-well plates which contain gold biosensors embedded in the bottom of each well. The impedance between these sensors depends on the adherence of the cell and increases with stronger adhesion.

24.3 Results

Incubation of AT1 cells in an acidic medium for 24 h (pH 6.6) led to an increase of the migration velocity by about 50 to 60% compared to the cells at pH 7.4 (Figs. 24.1 and 24.2). The migration distance even increased by as much as 80 to 100% at low pH. In order to mimic the microRNA changes during acidosis, in which miR-203 and miR-215 expression was reduced, cells were kept at normal pH and simultaneously transfected with an inhibitor of the respective microRNA. With the miR-203 inhibitor, the migration speed increased from 0.6 to 0.9 μm/min which was, however, not statistically significant (Fig. 24.1). In contrast to the miR-203, the inhibition of miR-215 had an effect neither on the migratory speed nor on the covered distance of the cells (Figs. 24.2). To block the effect of acidosis, cells were kept at low pH and transfected with the respective microRNA mimic (Figs. 24.1 and 24.2). This procedure had no effect on the migratory capacity (velocity or distance).

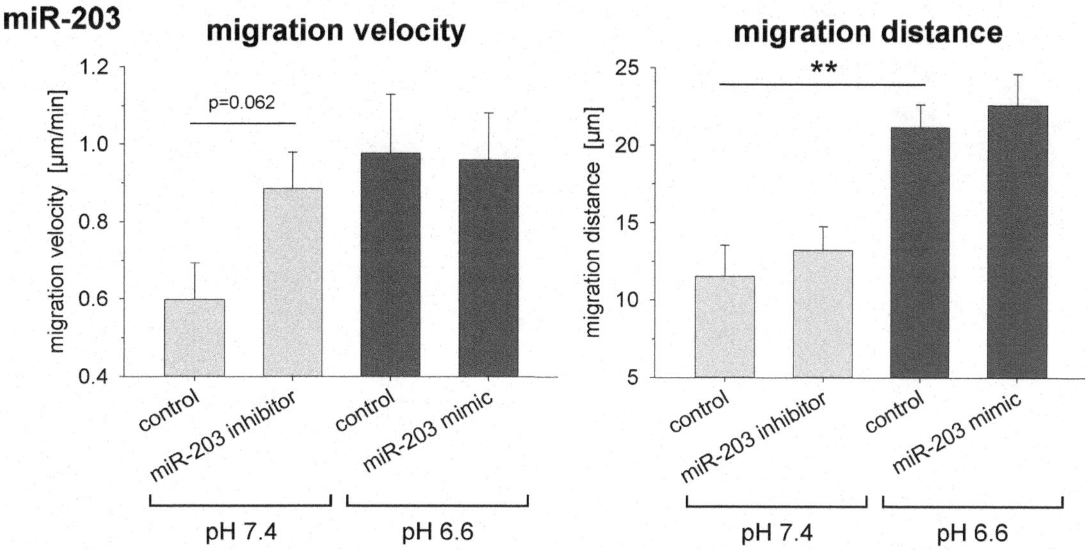

Fig. 24.1 Effect of extracellular acidosis and downregulation (inhibitor) or upregulation (mimic) of miR-203 on migration velocity and distance of AT1 cells. Cells were incubated during measurement in HEPES- or MES-buffered RPMI medium at pH 7.4 (control) or 6.6 (acidosis). Values as mean ± SEM, $n = 5–6$, $^{**}p < 0.01$

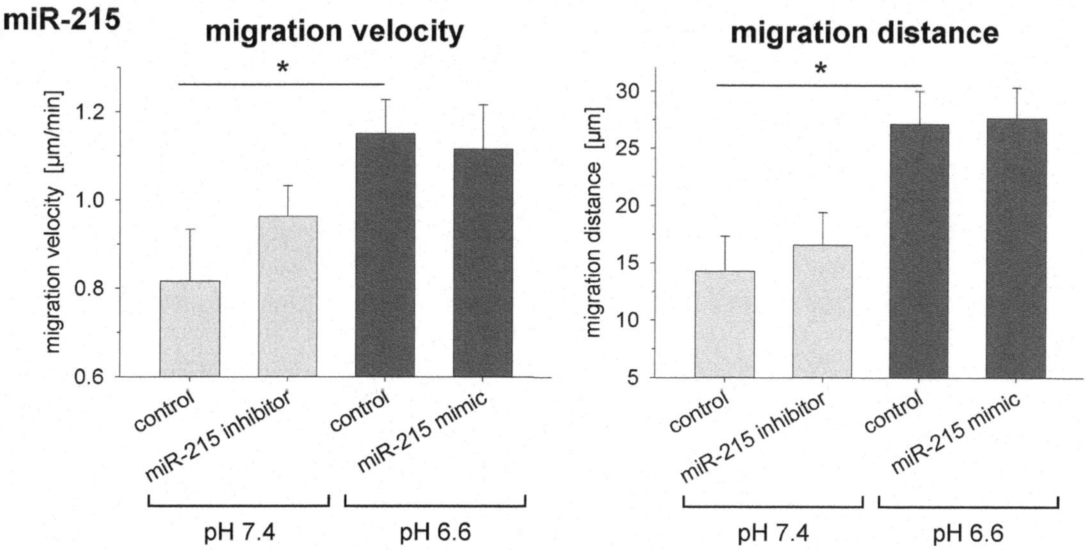

Fig. 24.2 Effect of extracellular acidosis and downregulation (inhibitor) or upregulation (mimic) of miR-203 on migration velocity and distance of AT1 cells. Cells were incubated during measurement in HEPES- or MES-buffered RPMI medium at pH 7.4 (control) or 6.6 (acidosis). Values as mean ± SEM, $n = 5–6$, $^{*}p < 0.05$

In order to analyze whether acidosis-regulated microRNAs influence cell adhesion, the adherence was determined by an impedance technique over a time period of 40 h. Cells were kept at pH 7.4 or 6.6 and additionally transfected with the respective microRNA inhibitor or mimic. Initially after plating (2 h), the adherence was reduced in all groups as compared to control cells at pH 7.4 (Fig. 24.3). Afterward, cells that were kept at low pH before (without microRNA transfection) showed a long-lasting increase in adhesion of about 70%, which was, however, due to the marked inter-

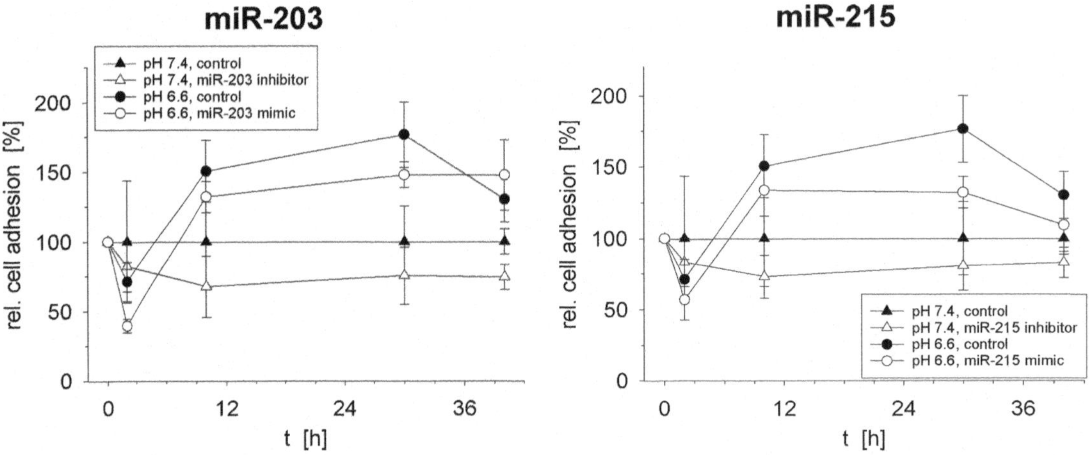

Fig. 24.3 Influence of acidosis and down- or upregulation of miR-203 and miR-215 on the adhesion of AT1 tumor cells in vitro. All measurements were normalized to control cells (sham transfection) at pH 7.4 at the respective time point. Values as mean ± SEM, $n = 4$–7

individual variability of the experiments, not statistically significant ($p = 0.07$ at $t = 30$ h). This increased adhesion was slightly reduced by trend by about 20% if the cells were transfected with miR-215 mimic (upregulation) (Fig. 24.3). No effect was seen when the cells were transfected with the inhibitors (downregulation) of both microRNAs at a controlled pH of 7.4 before. In summary, the inhibition of miR-203 at pH 7.4 might modulate the cell motility, whereas the overexpression of miR-215 at low pH seems to affect tumor cell adhesion.

24.4 Conclusion

Extracellular acidosis is found in many tumors and is caused by insufficient vascularization with functionally abnormal vessels, leading to hypoxia-induced glycolytic metabolism and accumulation of metabolic waste products [2, 8]. The signaling pathway for these alterations is still unknown, but since microRNAs have been shown to be regulated by low pH in previous experiments [7], the manuscript addresses the question whether low pH may modulate migration and adhesion via changes in microRNA expression. The present study clearly confirms the impact of extracellular acidosis on the migratory capacity of prostate carcinoma cells. Inhibition of miR-203 at normal pH increased the migratory speed and the distance covered by tumor cells. Since acidosis reduced the expression of this microRNA, the results may confirm the initial hypothesis of the study. The results are also in good accordance with the study of Tian et al. who described a significant promotion of cellular migration when suppressing miR-203 [9]. However, the hypothesis could not be completely confirmed, since the overexpression of miR-203 in acidic cells (which should counteract the acidosis-induced impact on migration) had no effect. The reason for the results in the overexpression experiments remains unclear at the moment; however, from the experiments at pH 7.4, it seems that acidosis-regulated microRNAs may increase tumor cell migration, and this may affect metastasis formation. The adhesion experiments showed that acidosis may promote the adherence of tumor cells to neighboring structures. Acidosis-regulated miR-215 might reduce this effect, although the changes were not statistically significant. Thus, it seems that the effect of the miRNAs could not overlay the effect driven by acidosis. Contradictory results were obtained in other (also clinical) studies, too [5]. For instance, miR-215 is characterized in several publications as a suppressor of proliferation and migration in different cancer types [10]. However, in clinical studies, a negative association of a reduced miR-215 expression level and lymphatic metastasis was shown [10]. The increase in adhesion, which seems not to fit to the increased migration, might be due to our experimental settings. Migration was analyzed directly in an acidic environment, while for the adhesion experiments, tumor cells were transfected and incubated at pH 6.6 before they were seeded. In conclusion, the present study clearly confirms that the extracellular pH has an impact on migration and adhesion of tumor cells. In this mechanism, pH-regulated microRNAs could possibly play a role, since changes in the expression of these microRNAs might also be able to modulate the migratory behavior (miR-203) and to a lesser extent adhesion (miR-215). However, further studies are needed to clearly demonstrate in which steps of metastasis microRNAs are relevant.

Acknowledgments The study was supported by the Dr. med. h.c. Erwin Braun Foundation, Basel, Switzerland, and the Deutsche Forschungsgemeinschaft (DFG) (grant TH482/6-1).

References

1. Warburg O (1925) Über den Stoffwechsel der Carcinomzelle. Klin Wschr 4:534–536
2. Vaupel P, Kallinowski F, Okunieff P (1989) Blood flow, oxygen and nutrient supply, and metabolic microenvironment of human tumors: a review. Cancer Res 49(23):6449–6465
3. Corbet C, Feron O (2017) Tumour acidosis: from the passenger to the driver's seat. Nat Rev Cancer 17(10):577–593. https://doi.org/10.1038/nrc.2017.77
4. Riemann A, Schneider B, Gündel D et al (2014) Acidic priming enhances metastatic potential of cancer cells. Pflugers Arch 466(11):2127–2138. https://doi.org/10.1007/s00424-014-1458-6
5. Thews O, Riemann A (2019) Tumor pH and metastasis: a malignant process beyond hypoxia. Cancer Metastasis Rev. https://doi.org/10.1007/s10555-018-09777-y
6. Ha M, Kim VN (2014) Regulation of microRNA biogenesis. Nat Rev Mol Cell Biol 15(8):509–524. https://doi.org/10.1038/nrm3838
7. Riemann A, Reime S, Thews O (2019) Acidic extracellular environment affects miRNA expression in tumors in vitro and in vivo. Int J Cancer 144(7):1609–1618. https://doi.org/10.1002/ijc.31790
8. Molls M, Vaupel P, Brown JM (2000) Blood perfusion and microenvironment of human tumors: implications for clinical radiooncology, 2nd edn. Medical radiology. Springer, Berlin, New York
9. Tian X, Tao F, Zhang B et al (2018) The miR-203/SNAI2 axis regulates prostate tumor growth, migration, angiogenesis and stemness potentially by modulating GSK-3β/β-CATENIN signal pathway. IUBMB Life 70(3):224–236. https://doi.org/10.1002/iub.1720
10. Yao Y, Shen H, Zhou Y et al (2018) MicroRNA-215 suppresses the proliferation, migration and invasion of non-small cell lung carcinoma cells through the downregulation of matrix metalloproteinase-16 expression. Exp Ther Med 15(4):3239–3246. https://doi.org/10.3892/etm.2018.5869

Impact of Acidosis-Regulated MicroRNAs on the Expression of Their Target Genes in Experimental Tumors In Vivo

25

Mandy Rauschner, A. Riemann, S. Reime, and O. Thews

Abstract

In comparison to normal tissue, solid tumors show an acidic extracellular pH, which results from hypoxia-induced glycolytic metabolism and the Warburg effect. Since acidosis modulates the expression of different microRNAs (e.g., miR-7, miR-183, miR-203, miR-215), microRNAs and their targets might be mediators between tumor acidosis and malignant behavior. The aim of this study was to investigate how modulation of these microRNAs affects the expression of their targets (Crem, cAMP-responsive element modulator; Gls2, glutaminase 2; Txnip, thioredoxin-interacting protein) in experimental tumors in vivo and whether these changes are acidosis dependent. The study was performed in two experimental tumor lines of the rat (AT-1 prostate carcinoma, Walker-256 mammary carcinoma). The results showed that all three targets were regulated by acidosis in vivo, Crem and Gls2 being downregulated and Txnip upregulated in both models. In AT-1 tumors at normal tumor pH, miR-203 overexpression increased Txnip expression by about 75%, whereas in Walker-256 tumors, miR-7 reduced protein expression. In more acidic tumors, no impact of microRNAs on Txnip expression was seen. On the other hand, Gls2 was significantly increased in acidic tumors by miR-183 or miR-7 overexpression (cell line dependent). As this increase was not present under control conditions, an acidosis-dependent effect can be assumed. These results indicate that tumor acidosis modulates the expression of targets of pH-sensitive microRNAs in experimental tumors. Especially the protein expression of Gls2 might be regulated via changes of microRNAs, which then affects the malignant progression of tumors.

Keywords

Acidosis · Experimental tumors · MicroRNAs · Crem · Gls2 · Txnip

25.1 Introduction

In comparison to normal tissue, solid tumors show an altered metabolic environment, which results from an insufficient vascular network, leading to hypoxia-induced glycolytic metabolism. These metabolic changes and the Warburg effect cause an acidification of extracellular tumor pH [1], which can affect, amongst others, metas-

M. Rauschner (✉) · A. Riemann · S. Reime · O. Thews
Julius-Bernstein-Institute of Physiology, University of Halle-Wittenberg, Halle (Saale), Germany
e-mail: mandy.rauschner@medizin.uni-halle.de

E. M. Nemoto et al. (eds.), *Oxygen Transport to Tissue XLII*, Advances in Experimental Medicine and Biology 1269, https://doi.org/10.1007/978-3-030-48238-1_25

tasis, invasiveness, and the expression of factors causing chemoresistance [2, 3]. MicroRNAs have been discussed for the signaling pathway from acidosis to gene expression. MicroRNAs are small noncoding RNAs, which regulate gene expression posttranscriptionally by 3′-UTR binding of target mRNAs, frequently leading to mRNA cleavage or translational repression [4]. Not only posttranscriptional silencing but also posttranscriptional stimulation is controlled by microRNAs [5], elucidating their function as important regulators in differentiation, cell proliferation, and metabolism. Recent studies showed that the expression of several microRNAs is acidosis regulated: miR-7, miR-183, miR-203, and miR-215 were uniformly regulated in different tumor lines [6]. Although the regulation of these microRNAs in cancer is discussed controversially, miR-7 is predominantly described as tumor suppressive in human breast cancer [7]. In human prostate cancer, miR-203 has antitumoral functions [8], whereas especially miR-183 is considered as prognostic biomarker [9].

The aim of this study was to evaluate whether those acidosis-regulated microRNAs are able to modulate the expression of their target genes in vivo, thereby mediating acidosis-induced functional effects. The cAMP-responsive element modulator (Crem), glutaminase 2 (Gls2), and the thioredoxin-interacting protein (Txnip), which are targets of the pH-sensitive microRNAs and which have been shown to be regulated by the extracellular pH, were therefore analyzed. All three proteins play a relevant role in oncology, and their expression is correlated with the malignant behavior of tumors [10–12].

25.2 Methods

25.2.1 Cell Culture and In Vivo Tumor Models

The subline AT-1 of the rat Dunning R-3327 prostate carcinoma was cultured in RPMI supplemented with 10% fetal calf serum (FCS), and the rat breast carcinoma cell line Walker-256 was grown with additional 10 mM L-glutamine, 20 mM HEPES, and 0.15% $NaHCO_3$. In order to increase the microRNA expression, tumor cells were transfected with microRNA mimics (miR-7, miR-183, miR-203, miR-215) and the corresponding mimic control using Lipofectamine 2000 reagent (Thermo Fisher Scientific, Waltham, MA, USA). Solid tumors were induced by subcutaneous implantation of tumor cells (6×10^6 cells within 0.5 mL isotonic saline) on the hind foot dorsum of male rats: Copenhagen or Wistar rats. Tumor volume was determined, and tumors were analyzed at a volume of 0.5–1.0 mL. To induce a more pronounced acidosis in vivo, animals were treated with a combination of respiratory hypoxia (8% O_2) and a single injection of meta-iodobenzylguanidine (MIBG). After 24 h, animals were sacrificed and tumors surgically removed. All experiments had previously been approved by the regional animal ethics committee and were conducted in accordance with the German law for animal protection and the UKCCCR Guidelines [13]. After excision, tumors were minced and lysed with cell lysis buffer (Cell Signaling Technology, Danvers, MA, USA) for protein isolation or RNA extracted using TRIzol Reagent (Thermo Fisher Scientific, Waltham, MA, USA).

25.2.2 Experimental Settings

The expression of Crem, Gls2, and Txnip was assessed after control or acidotic conditions by quantitative PCR. In brief, 1 μg RNA was subjected to reverse transcription with SuperScript II Reverse Transcriptase (Invitrogen, Carlsbad, CA, USA), and expression changes were studied by qPCR using the Platinum SYBR Green qPCR Supermix (Invitrogen, Carlsbad, CA, USA) with hypoxanthine-guanine phosphoribosyltransferase (HPRT) as housekeeping gene. Acidosis- and microRNA-induced regulation of Crem, Gls2, and Txnip on protein level was determined by western blot analysis. Protein lysates were separated by 12% SDS-PAGE and transferred to nitrocellulose membranes. Incubation was performed with the indicated primary antibodies for Crem, Gls2 (Thermo Fisher Scientific, Waltham,

MA, USA), Txnip, and β-actin (Cell Signaling Technology, Danvers, MA, USA) as housekeeping gene. Samples were detected by an Odyssey Imaging System (LI-COR Biosciences, Lincoln, NE, USA). All experiments were performed at least in triplicates, and results are presented as mean ± SEM.

25.3 Results

The model of intensified tumor acidosis by inspiratory hypoxia and MIBG application reduced the pH in both tumor lines by about 0.5 (AT-1: from 7.02 ± 0.04 to 6.48 ± 0.08, Walker-256: from 7.16 ± 0.03 to 6.65 ± 0.07). As shown in Fig. 25.1, intensified tumor acidosis led to a strong increase in Txnip expression (AT-1: 132.7 ± 40.4%, Walker-256: 53.1 ± 10.5%), whereas Gls2 expression was significantly diminished in both tumor models in vivo. Crem expression was downregulated in AT-1 tumors as well, although in Walker-256 tumors no distinct change was seen. To investigate whether microRNAs are involved in these acidosis-induced changes, the microRNA content was modulated with mimics of acidosis-regulated microRNAs. As the acidosis regulation of microRNAs was tumor-type specific in previous experiments in vivo, miR-7 was investigated in Walker-256 tumors, whereas miR-183, miR-203, and miR-215 were studied in AT-1 tumors.

Figure 25.2 shows that Crem expression is lowered by miR-215 combined with acidosis in AT-1 tumors (65.3 ± 4.5%) although no pH-independent effects were seen. MiR-183 mimic induced a significant increase in Gls2 expression under acidosis (170.8 ± 25.1%), even though miR-183 mimic alone at a normal pH had no effect. Unexpectedly, no distinct acidosis-induced downregulation of Gls2 was found, which is possibly due to transfection of the mimic control. Acidosis alone led to a higher Txnip expression (Fig. 25.1), but also overexpression of the miR-203 at normal pH increased the protein level by about 75%. If, however, the tumors had already been exposed to low pH, a further increase in Txnip expression by miR-203 overexpression was not possible.

In Walker-256 tumors (Fig. 25.3), miR-7 mimic significantly reduced Crem expression at normal pH, but under acidic conditions, there was only a trend of this effect. In contrast, miR-7 mimic alone did not lead to changes in Gls2 expression, whereas in combination with acidosis, a significant increase was seen (181.4 ± 24.5%). As described before, acidosis per se forced a strong upregulation of Txnip, but no remarkable change was found when miR-7 was overexpressed.

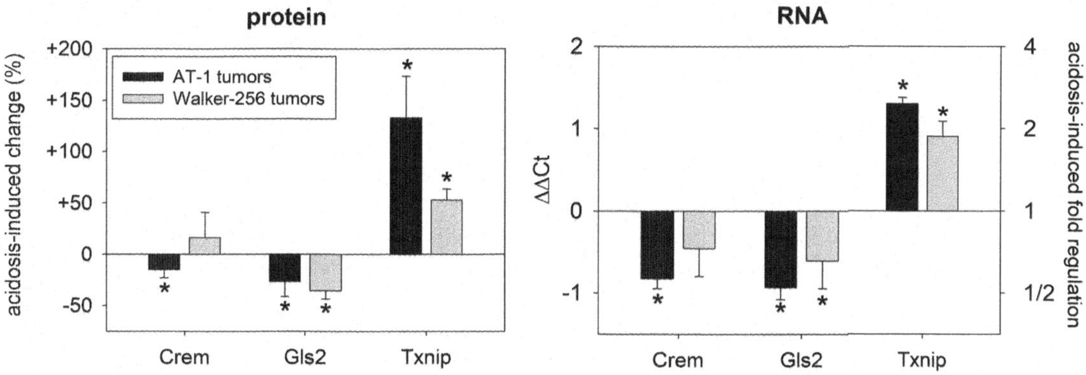

Fig. 25.1 Acidosis-induced change of the expression of Crem, Gls2, and Txnip in experimental tumors in vivo on RNA and protein level. Acidosis was induced by inspiratory hypoxia and MIBG injection. Values were normalized to control conditions during room air breathing. Values as mean ± SEM, $n = 4$–19. (*) $p < 0.05$

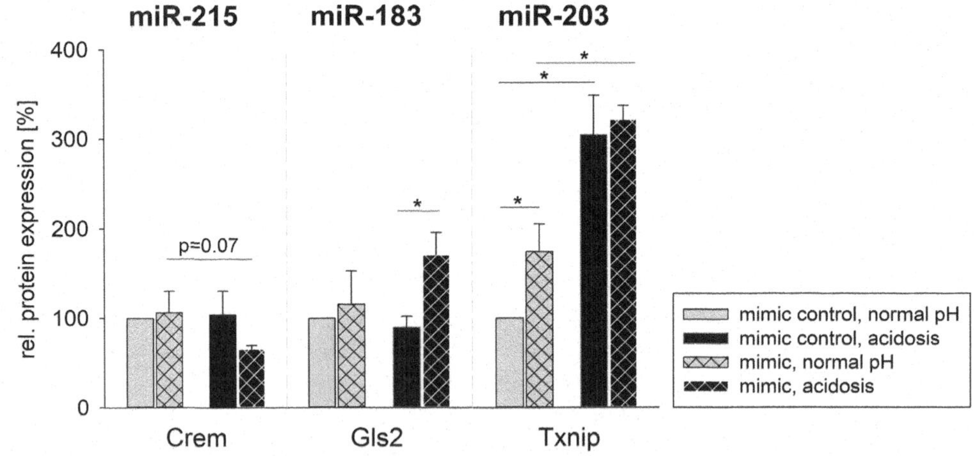

Fig. 25.2 Effect of microRNA overexpression on Crem, Gls2, and Txnip protein expression in AT-1 tumors at acidic and normal tumor pH for 24 h. Values were normalized to tumors at room air breathing and with unspecific transfection. Values as mean ± SEM, $n = 3–11$. (*) $p < 0.05$

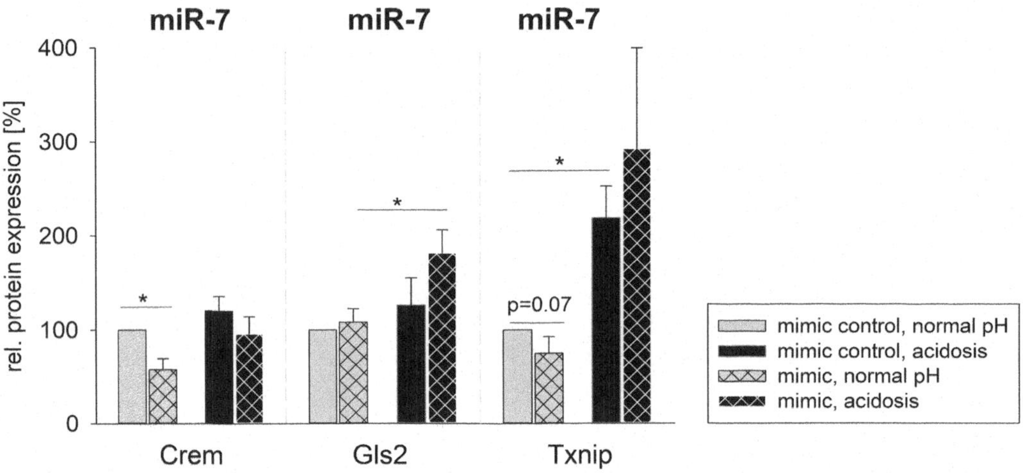

Fig. 25.3 Effect of miR-7 overexpression on Crem, Gls2, and Txnip protein expression in Walker-256 tumors at acidic and normal tumor pH for 24 h. Values were normalized to tumors at room air breathing and with unspecific transfection. Values as mean ± SEM, $n = 3–7$. (*) $p < 0.05$

25.4 Conclusion

Acidification of the extracellular space in experimental tumors affects mRNA and protein expression in both experimental tumor models studied. Txnip showed a strong upregulation at low pH (Fig. 25.1). This effect was also seen in cultured cells (data not shown). The role of Txnip in oncology has been discussed controversially. In human tumors, Txnip is often described as a tumor suppressor [14], whereas cellular stress like hypoxia and lactic acidosis induced an upregulation [15]. Hagen et al. showed that Txnip is regulated in a biphasic manner with an initial downregulation and an upregulation under prolonged hypoxia (18 h) [16], which is in line with our results under prolonged hypoxia-related tumor acidosis (24 h). Although Txnip expression was affected by miR-203 in AT-1 tumors (Fig. 25.2) and miR-7 in Walker-256 tumors (Fig. 25.3) at a normal pH, no additional mimic effect was observed under acidification, which might be explained by a predominant effect of acidosis on Txnip expression, which cannot be further increased by the microRNAs. Nevertheless, acidosis-independent modulation by microRNAs could be of importance and thus mediate metastasis in tumors [10].

Although no distinct acidosis-induced regulation of Crem in Walker-256 tumors was found, a significant downregulation in AT-1 tumors was determined. But also an overexpression of the miR-215 or miR-7 had similar effects, indicating that Crem might be an interesting target in the mediation of acidosis-induced malignant phenotypes, which is in accordance with in vitro results by others [12].

Since Gls2 has been shown to act as a tumor suppressor [11], our results of an acidosis-induced Gls2 downregulation could indicate a mechanism by which low pH forces tumor malignancy. Moreover, miR-183 mimic in AT-1 tumors (Fig. 25.2) and miR-7 mimic in Walker-256 tumors (Fig. 25.3) led to a significant increase in Gls2 expression under acidosis, which reverses the acidosis-induced decrease of Gls2 and goes in hand with the result that miR-183 and miR-7 are downregulated under acidosis.

In conclusion, this study indicates that a reduction of the extracellular pH affects the expression of proteins which are relevant for the malignant potential of tumors. But also changes in the expression of pH-sensitive microRNAs modulate the protein level. From these results, it appears possible that, at least partially, the effect of tumor acidosis is mediated by pH-sensitive microRNAs, which could also be of clinical importance due to their regulatory function in human breast and prostate carcinoma.

Acknowledgments The study was supported by the Deutsche Forschungsgemeinschaft (DFG) (grant TH482/6-1).

References

1. Justus CR, Dong L, Yang LV (2013) Acidic tumor microenvironment and pH-sensing G protein-coupled receptors. Front Physiol 4:354
2. Taylor S et al (2015) Microenvironment acidity as a major determinant of tumor chemoresistance: proton pump inhibitors (PPIs) as a novel therapeutic approach. Drug Resist Updat 23:69–78
3. Thews O, Riemann A (2019) Tumor pH and metastasis: a malignant process beyond hypoxia. Cancer Metastasis Rev 38(1–2):113–129
4. Eulalio A, Huntzinger E, Izaurralde E (2008) Getting to the root of miRNA-mediated gene silencing. Cell 132(1):9–14
5. Vasudevan S (2012) Posttranscriptional upregulation by microRNAs. Wiley Interdiscip Rev RNA 3(3):311–330
6. Riemann A, Reime S, Thews O (2019) Acidic extracellular environment affects miRNA expression in tumors in vitro and in vivo. Int J Cancer 144(7):1609–1618
7. Kong X et al (2012) MicroRNA-7 inhibits epithelial-to-mesenchymal transition and metastasis of breast cancer cells via targeting FAK expression. PLoS One 7(8):e41523
8. Viticchie G et al (2011) MiR-203 controls proliferation, migration and invasive potential of prostate cancer cell lines. Cell Cycle 10(7):1121–1131
9. Waseem M et al (2019) MicroRNA-183-5p: a new potential marker for prostate cancer. Indian J Clin Biochem 34(2):207–212
10. Chen D et al (2015) MiR-373 drives the epithelial-to-mesenchymal transition and metastasis via the miR-373-TXNIP-HIF1alpha-TWIST signaling axis in breast cancer. Oncotarget 6(32):32701–32712
11. Kuo TC et al (2016) Glutaminase 2 stabilizes Dicer to repress Snail and metastasis in hepatocellular carcinoma cells. Cancer Lett 383(2):282–294
12. Wang Y et al (2013) Low expression of cyclic AMP response element modulator-1 can increase the migration and invasion of esophageal squamous cell carcinoma. Tumour Biol 34(6):3649–3657
13. Workman P et al (2010) Guidelines for the welfare and use of animals in cancer research. Br J Cancer 102(11):1555–1577
14. Nishizawa K et al (2011) Thioredoxin-interacting protein suppresses bladder carcinogenesis. Carcinogenesis 32(10):1459–1466
15. Chen JL et al (2010) Lactic acidosis triggers starvation response with paradoxical induction of TXNIP through MondoA. PLoS Genet 6(9):e1001093
16. Wong RW, Hagen T (2013) Mechanistic target of rapamycin (mTOR) dependent regulation of thioredoxin interacting protein (TXNIP) transcription in hypoxia. Biochem Biophys Res Commun 433(1):40–46

An Observation on Enhanced Extracellular Acidification and Lactate Production Induced by Inhibition of Lactate Dehydrogenase A

26

Jinxia Jiang, Jeffrey Roman, He N. Xu, and Lin Z. Li

Abstract

The Warburg effect, representing enhanced glycolysis and lactate production in adequately oxygenated cancer cells, has been widely regarded to cause increased extracellular acidification. Converting pyruvate to lactate by lactate dehydrogenase A (LDHA) is the last step of glycolysis. Here, we report an interesting counterintuitive observation that inhibition of LDHA resulted in enhanced glycolysis in MDA-MB-231 breast cancer cells. The cells were treated with FX11 (7-benzyl-2,3-dihydroxy-6-methyl-4-propylnaphthalene-1-carboxylic acid), a specific LDHA inhibitor. Seahorse assay reported dose-dependent increases in both oxygen consumption rate (OCR) and extracellular acidification rate (ECAR). Independent biochemical measurements also confirmed the increase of lactate production under FX11 treatment. The reasons and mechanism of these observations of elevated ECAR and lactate production in the MDA-MB-231 breast cancer cells under FX11 treatment remain to be investigated.

J. Jiang · J. Roman · H. N. Xu · L. Z. Li (✉)
Department of Radiology, Perelman School of Medicine, University of Pennsylvania, Philadelphia, PA, USA
e-mail: linli@pennmedicine.upenn.edu

Keywords

Lactate dehydrogenase A · FX11 · OCR · ECAR · Lactate production · Triple-negative breast cancer

26.1 Introduction

Cancers are a large family of diseases that involve the abnormal growth of cells and the potential to invade and spread to other parts of the body. To understand the underlying mechanisms involved in cancer, many studies on cancer metabolism have been performed. One of the first such observations, as described by Otto Warburg, shows that the metabolic activities in cancer cells rely heavily on glycolysis, even in the presence of oxygen [1]. Although it was hypothesized that the glycolytic phenotype in cancer is due to a permanent impairment of cancer mitochondrial oxidative phosphorylation (OXPHOS), many studies have challenged this view to show that cancer cells have normal mitochondrial OXPHOS [2]. The Warburg effect or enhanced glycolysis under aerobic condition has been demonstrated in many types of cancers, including breast cancer [3].

The very last step of glycolysis is catalyzed by lactate dehydrogenase A (LDHA), which converts pyruvate to lactate coupled by NADH and NAD^+. Although various LDH isoforms

E. M. Nemoto et al. (eds.), *Oxygen Transport to Tissue XLII*, Advances in Experimental Medicine and Biology 1269, https://doi.org/10.1007/978-3-030-48238-1_26

have been detected in breast cancer cells [4], studies have shown that LDHA is critical to cancer cells exhibiting the highly glycolytic Warburg phenotype and is overexpressed in many cancer types including breast cancer [5–7], indicating LDHA as a promising target for cancer prevention and treatment. In the current study, we explore the bioenergetics and metabolic effects of LDHA inhibition by FX11, which competes with NADH for LDHA binding, on the triple-negative breast cancer (TNBC) cell line, MDA-MB-231. We hypothesized that FX11-treated cells will show a decrease in lactate efflux to extracellular space as pyruvate cannot be converted to lactate effectively. Furthermore, we expected cells treated with FX11 to show higher reliance on OXPHOS and suppressed aerobic glycolysis since more pyruvate may be diverted to mitochondrial metabolism. However, counterintuitively, we observed that enhanced glycolysis and lactate generation were induced by FX11 treatment.

26.2 Methods

MDA-MB-231 cells were cultured in phenol-red-containing RPMI 1640 (Invitrogen, Cat no. 11875-085) supplemented with 10% fetal bovine serum (FBS). Cells were maintained at 37 °C with 5% CO_2 and passaged at approximately 80% confluency using 0.25% trypsin-EDTA.

The Seahorse XFe96 Extracellular Flux Analyzer was used to perform the metabolic analysis. Briefly, MDA-MB-231 cells were seeded on a microplate at 20,000 cells per well and incubated at 37 °C with 5% CO_2 overnight. The following day, the culture medium was replaced with Seahorse XF RPMI Medium (Agilent, Cat no. 103576-100) supplemented with 11 mM glucose and 2 mM L-glutamine. The plate was placed in a non-CO_2 incubator about 1 hour before the start of the assay. For treatment, chemical agents at various concentrations were preloaded into the injection ports. After instrument calibration, three basal oxygen consumption rate (OCR) and extracellular acidification rate (ECAR) measurements (3-0-3, mix-wait-measure cycle) were performed, followed by control and FX11 injections (blank control with Seahorse medium; 0.1% DMSO; 1 μM, 3 μM, 5 μM, and 10 μM FX11). FX11 concentrations were prepared using serial dilutions, with 10 μM FX11 having the highest percentage of DMSO (0.1%). The effect of FX11 was monitored for a total of 15 cycles, approximately 100 minutes. There were seven wells as technical replicates for each concentration of FX11 and six biological replicates in total.

The amount of protein in each well was determined using the bicinchoninic acid (BCA) assay (Pierce Biotechnology, Cat no. G7570). Briefly, medium was removed from the wells, which were then rinsed with PBS with Ca^{2+} and Mg^{2+}. Albumin concentrations (0, 0.125, 0.25, 0.5, and 1 mg/mL) were loaded into cell-free wells as standards. Cells were lysed using RIPA buffer with 0.5% PMSF protease inhibitor. Working reagent was added into all wells, and the plate was wrapped in aluminum foil and incubated for 30 minutes at 37 °C. Absorbance at 562 nm was measured using a plate reader (Enspire Multimode Plate Reader, model: 2300, Perkin Elmer). A linear regression of the reference standard absorbance and their concentrations was performed, and the results were used to quantify the protein concentrations in wells with cells.

The Seahorse metabolic flux assay data was exported from Wave software (v.2.6.0, Agilent Technologies) and analyzed using Microsoft Excel. Data from each well were first normalized to its protein amount. To combine all biological replicates, OCR and ECAR measurements were normalized to the third basal measurement to account for minor differences in basal OCR and ECAR across replicates. Data values greater than 1.5 times the interquartile ranges below the first quartile or above the third quartile were classified as outliers and removed from the analysis. The OCR and ECAR of individual wells were averaged across technical replicates first and then biological replicates.

Extracellular lactate and glucose concentrations were measured as with follows: MDA-MB-231 cells were seeded in a six-well plate at 0.5 million cells per well with 2 mL culture medium. After cells had attached overnight, the medium was removed, and the wells were rinsed with PBS with Ca^{2+} and Mg^{2+}, followed by the addition of 1 mL FBS-free RPMI with phenol red. Treatments (0.1% DMSO and 5 μM FX11) were added to wells, and the plate was then incubated at 37 °C and 5% CO_2. Cells treated with FX11 had equal amounts of DMSO as in the control. Samples of the medium (30 μL) were collected at 2, 6, and 24 hours post treatment and measured for extracellular glucose and lactate concentrations using the YSI 2300 STAT Plus Glucose and Lactate Analyzer (YSI Inc.) calibrated with YSI 2747 dual standards. Glucose and lactate measurements were also analyzed using Microsoft Excel.

To assess statistical significance, unpaired heteroscedastic two-tailed t-tests were performed. A modified alpha = 0.005 was used to mitigate type 1 error (Bonferroni correction). All p-values below this alpha indicate statistical significance and are reported as significant results.

26.3 Results

FX11 induced metabolic responses in the TNBC cell line, MDA-MB-231. After the initial baseline measurements and FX11 injection, we observed a dose-dependent increase in OCR (Fig. 26.1a). In particular, we observed a significant difference ($p < 0.005$) between DMSO and 3 μM FX11 at the first and last time points and a significant difference between DMSO and 5 μM at the first time point after FX11 injection (Fig. 26.1c). These results were in line with our hypothesis, where LDHA inhibition by FX11 leads to an increase in OCR, an indicator of increased OXPHOS.

For the ECAR, we also observed a concentration-dependent increase induced by FX11 (Fig. 26.1b). In particular, we observed significant differences between DMSO and 3 μM and 5 μM at their first and last time points and between DMSO and 10 μM at the first time point after FX11 injection (Fig. 26.1d). These observations were not as expected, as we had hypothesized that inhibition of the last step of glycolysis by FX11 would decrease glycolysis and ECAR due to ineffective pyruvate to lactate conversion.

In both the OCR and ECAR responses, the 10 μM FX11 treatment showed a decrease over time. In fact, its OCR 2 hour post treatment was lower than its initial baseline measurement. This might reflect cytotoxic effects of high FX11 concentrations.

To further validate our ECAR observations, we performed extracellular lactate and glucose measurements on cells treated with DMSO and 5 μM FX11. Our results showed significantly higher extracellular lactate levels in extracellular media at 2, 6, and 24 hours post 5 μM FX11 treatment compared to that of the DMSO-treated group (Fig. 26.2a). Two additional independent experiments performed with differing seeding densities and medium volumes also showed significantly higher extracellular lactate levels in the medium of cells treated with 5 μM FX11 compared to that of the DMSO control (data not shown). This lactate enhancement phenomenon was further confirmed by an experiment using newly purchase MDA-MB-231 cells from ATCC. Extracellular glucose measurements showed lower levels of glucose in the medium of the 5 μM FX11-treated group at all treatment times but with the 24-hour treatment group being significantly different from the DMSO control (Fig. 26.2b), indicating an increased glucose consumption associated with increased ECAR and lactate production.

26.4 Discussion and Conclusion

Our results showed that FX11 increased the oxygen consumption rate in MDA-MB-231, as expected by our hypothesis, because reduced LDHA activity would favor the entry of pyruvate into the mitochondria for OXPHOS. This observation has also been reported in another human B-cell lymphoma cell line P493, where Le et al. observed increased oxygen consumption with the reduction of LDHA by siRNA and FX11 treatment [8]. With the halt in the conversion between pyruvate and lactate, we could assume that the aerobic glycolysis activity would

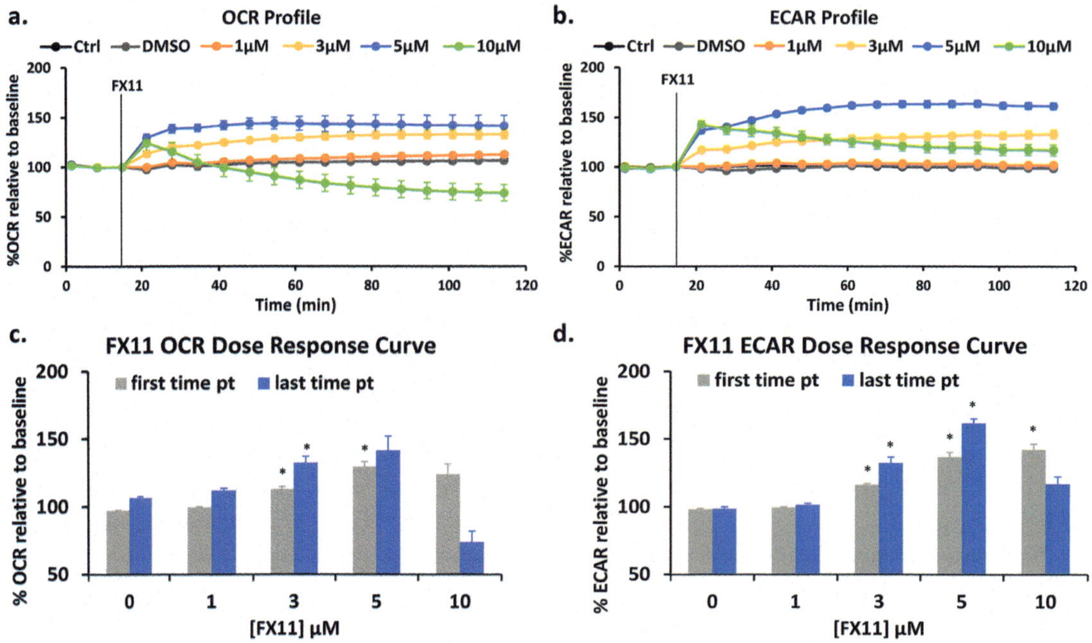

Fig. 26.1 Effect of FX11 on the oxygen consumption rate (OCR) and extracellular acidification rate (ECAR) in MDA-MB-231 cells. (**a**) OCR profile and (**b**) ECAR profile for control (Ctrl and DMSO) and FX11 treatments at various concentrations. Ctrl indicates blank control with medium. Results are reported as %OCR or %ECAR relative to the third time point (pt) baseline measurement ± SEM. The FX11 dose-dependent response was also plotted for (**c**) OCR and (**d**) ECAR based on first and last time points during the treatment period. Zero μM FX11 indicates DMSO control. The first time point indicates approximately 6 minutes post treatment, and the last time point indicates approximately 100 minutes post treatment. $n = 6$, $*p < 0.005$ with DMSO control

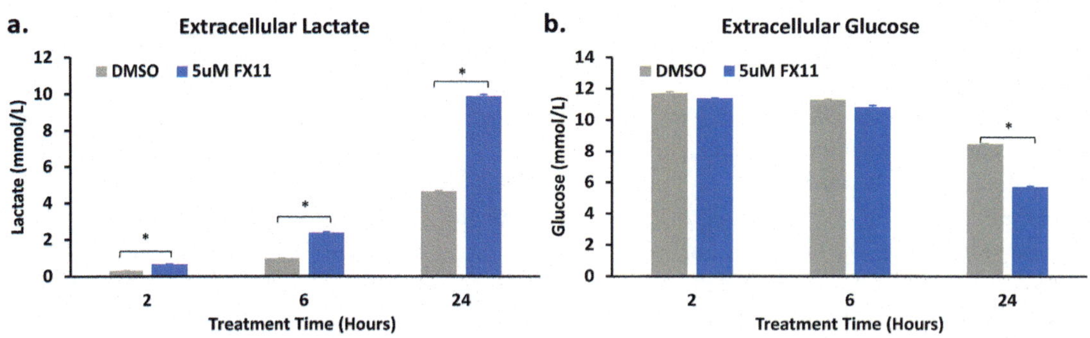

Fig. 26.2 Effect of FX11 on extracellular lactate and glucose levels. (**a**) Lactate and (**b**) glucose concentration in the extracellular medium at 2, 6, and 24 hours post treatment. Lactate and glucose levels are reported as mean + SEM. $n = 3$, $*p < 0.005$

decrease, which has been demonstrated in neuroblastoma cells treated with FX11 showing a decrease in lactate production [9] and in osteosarcoma cells also showing a decrease in lactate production and ECAR by genetic knockdown of LDHA [10].

Contrary to these observations and our hypothesis, our results showed an increased extracellular acidification rate, lactate production, and glucose consumption in breast cancer MDA-MB-231 cells, indicating an enhanced glycolytic activity. One possible explanation for this observation is to consider the role of the other major lactate dehydrogenase isoforms such as LDHB. It has been reported that neither LDHA nor LDHB genetic knockouts strongly reduced lactate efflux and that double disruption of LDHA and LDHB was required to ablate the lactate production in tumor cells [11]. It has also been reported that highly glycolytic TNBC cells exhibited high LDHB expression [4, 12] and that LDHB was used as a metabolic marker for neoadjuvant chemotherapy response in breast cancers [13]. These reports suggest that LDHB also likely plays an important role in regulating breast cancer metabolism. For future studies, we can investigate LDHB activity and whether LDHB contributes to the enhancement of ECAR and lactate production in MDA-MB-231 cells as observed here. We can also investigate whether FX11 may cause other effects on MDA-MB-231 cell metabolism, e.g., changing intracellular pH and extracellular glucose uptake rate. Although the glucose level used in cell culture is much higher than the extracellular glucose level in solid tumors [14, 15] and thus the results may not be applicable to clinical tumors, this study presents an interesting phenomenon worthy of further investigation.

Acknowledgments This work was supported by US NIH Grant R01CA191207 (L. Z. Li). We thank David Nelson for his assistance in the operation of the YSI instrument.

References

1. Hsu PP, Sabatini DM (2008) Cancer cell metabolism: Warburg and beyond. Cell 134:703–707
2. Zheng J (2012) Energy metabolism of cancer: glycolysis versus oxidative phosphorylation (review). Oncol Lett 4:1151–1157
3. Robey IF, Lien AD, Welsh SJ et al (2005) Hypoxia-inducible factor-1alpha and the glycolytic phenotype in tumors. Neoplasia 7:324–330
4. Hussien R, Brooks GA (2011) Mitochondrial and plasma membrane lactate transporter and lactate dehydrogenase isoform expression in breast cancer cell lines. Physiol Genomics 43:255–264
5. Goldman RD, Kaplan NO, Hall TC (1964) Lactic dehydrogenase in human neoplastic tissues. Cancer Res 24:389–399
6. Koukourakis MI, Kontomanolis E, Giatromanolaki A et al (2009) Serum and tissue LDH levels in patients with breast/gynaecological cancer and benign diseases. Gynecol Obstet Investig 67:162–168
7. Huang X, Li X, Xie X et al (2016) High expressions of LDHA and AMPK as prognostic biomarkers for breast cancer. Breast 30:39–46
8. Le A, Cooper CR, Gouw AM et al (2010) Inhibition of lactate dehydrogenase A induces oxidative stress and inhibits tumor progression. Proc Natl Acad Sci U S A 107:2037–2042
9. Rellinger EJ, Craig BT, Alvarez AL et al (2017) FX11 inhibits aerobic glycolysis and growth of neuroblastoma cells. Surgery 161:747–752
10. Gao S, Tu DN, Li H et al (2016) Pharmacological or genetic inhibition of LDHA reverses tumor progression of pediatric osteosarcoma. Biomed Pharmacother 81:388–393
11. Zdralevic M, Brand A, Di Ianni L et al (2018) Double genetic disruption of lactate dehydrogenases A and B is required to ablate the "Warburg effect" restricting tumor growth to oxidative metabolism. J Biol Chem 293:15947–15961
12. McCleland ML, Adler AS, Shang Y et al (2012) An integrated genomic screen identifies LDHB as an essential gene for triple-negative breast cancer. Cancer Res 72:5812–5823
13. Dennison JB, Molina JR, Mitra S et al (2013) Lactate dehydrogenase B: a metabolic marker of response to neoadjuvant chemotherapy in breast cancer. Clin Cancer Res 19:3703–3713
14. Gullino PM, Clark SH, Grantham FH (1964) The interstitial fluid of solid tumors. Cancer Res 24:780–794
15. Vaupel P (2004) Tumor microenvironmental physiology and its implications for radiation oncology. Semin Radiat Oncol 14:198–206

The Warburg Effect: Historical Dogma Versus Current Rationale

27

Peter Vaupel and Gabriele Multhoff

Abstract

Contrary to Warburg's original thesis, accelerated aerobic glycolysis is not a primary and permanent consequence of dysfunctional mitochondria compensating for a poor ATP yield per mole glucose. Instead, the Warburg effect is an essential part of a "selfish" metabolic reprogramming, which results from the interplay between (normoxic or hypoxic) HIF-1 overexpression, oncogene activation (cMyc, Ras), loss of function of tumor suppressors (mutant p53, mutant PTEN, microRNAs and sirtuins with suppressor functions), activated (PI3K/Akt/mTORC1, Ras/Raf/Mek/Erk/c-Myc) or deactivated (AMPK) signaling pathways, components of the tumor microenvironment, and HIF-1 cooperations with epigenetic mechanisms. Molecular and functional processes of the Warburg effect include (a) considerably accelerated glycolytic fluxes; (b) adequate ATP generation per unit time to maintain energy homeostasis; (c) backup and diversion of glycolytic intermediates facilitating the biosynthesis of nucleotides, nonessential amino acids, lipids, and hexosamines; (d) inhibition of pyruvate entry into mitochondria; (e) excessive formation and accumulation of lactate which stimulates tumor growth and suppression of antitumor immunity (in addition, lactate can serve as an energy source for normoxic cancer cells, contributes to extracellular acidosis, and thus drives malignant progression and resistances to conventional therapies); (f) maintenance of the cellular redox homeostasis and low ROS formation; and (g) HIF-1 overexpression, mutant p53, and mutant PTEN which inhibit mitochondrial biogenesis and functions, thus negatively impacting cellular respiration rate. The glycolytic switch is an early event in oncogenesis and primarily supports cell survival. All in all, the Warburg effect, i.e., aerobic glycolysis in the presence of oxygen and – in principle – functioning mitochondria, constitutes a major driver of the cancer progression machinery, resistance to conventional therapies, and – finally – poor patient outcome.

Keywords

Aerobic glycolysis · Warburg effect · Metabolic reprogramming · Glycolytic phenotype · Glycolytic switch · Tumor glucose metabolism · Biosynthesis of

P. Vaupel (✉)
Department of Radiation Oncology, Tumor Pathophysiology Group, University Medical Center, Mainz, Germany
e-mail: vaupel@uni-mainz.de

G. Multhoff
Center for Translational Cancer Research, Klinikum rechts der Isar, Technical University Munich, Munich, Germany

E. M. Nemoto et al. (eds.), *Oxygen Transport to Tissue XLII*, Advances in Experimental Medicine and Biology 1269, https://doi.org/10.1007/978-3-030-48238-1_27

macromolecules · ATP generation · Energy homeostasis · Lactate accumulation · Tumor acidosis · Tumor mitochondria · Oncogenesis · Redox homeostasis

27.1 Introduction

In the early 1920s, Warburg published experimental data on the enhanced, accelerated conversion of glucose to pyruvate (followed by lactate formation) even in the presence of abundant oxygen (aerobic glycolysis, Warburg effect) [1, 2]. He attributed this metabolic trait to a (primary) "respiratory injury" [3] (Fig. 27.1) and considered this a universal metabolic alteration in carcinogenesis [7]. This interpretation of the data has been questioned since the early 1950s by Chance et al. [8–11], Weinhouse [12, 13], and Aisenberg [14] showing that cytochromes of tumor cells were intact and functional, which clearly argues against a general mitochondrial dysfunction. Additional arguments speaking against Warburg's initial "respiration injury theory" include a methodological problem, i.e., tumor tissue sections used in Warburg's experiments were definitely thicker than critical O_2 diffusion distances and, thus, tissue slices were at least partially hypoxic [4]. Furthermore, there is clear indication that the O_2 uptake rates of most malignant tumors in vivo are determined by O_2 availabilities, not by sequelae to damaged mitochondria [15, 16].

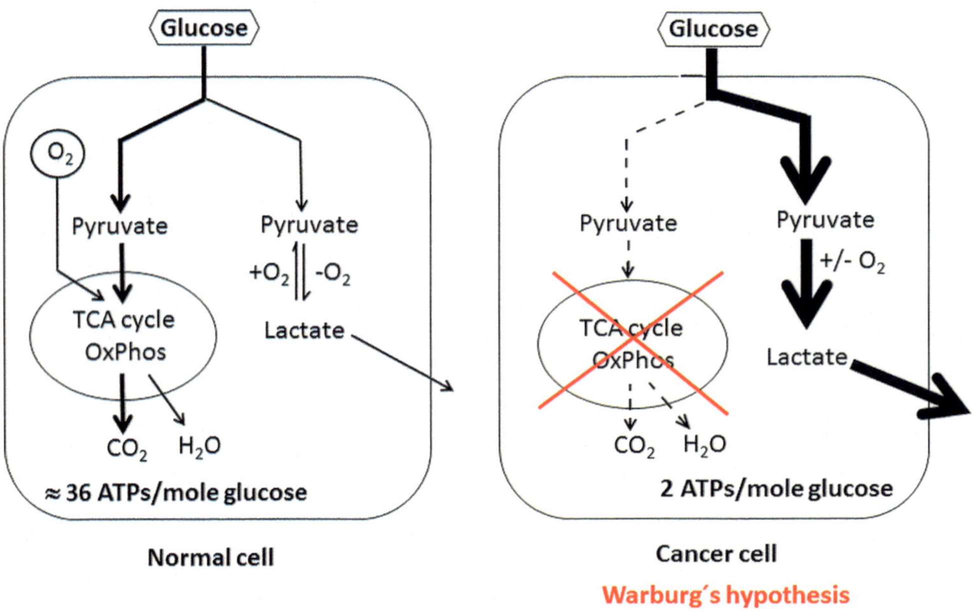

Fig. 27.1 Warburg's historical postulate. Cancer cells – as a sequela to (primarily) damaged mitochondria – have a 10–40-fold higher glucose uptake rate and a lactate production which is 10–100 times faster than the complete oxidation of glucose in mitochondria ("facilitated glycolytic flux") in order to maintain energy homeostasis. Lactate is accumulated in the tumor extracellular space upon export from cancer cells (right panel). In normal cells, lactate is produced only under hypoxic/anoxic conditions (anaerobic or hypoxic glycolysis, e.g., during strenuously exercising muscle, left panel). ATP adenosine triphosphate, TCA tricarboxylic acid, OxPhos oxidative phosphorylation. Lactate formation not only is restricted to hypoxic tumor areas (at a certain distance away from tumor microvessels) but also occurs in normoxic ("aerobic") tumor tissue volumes. *Note*: The absolute values of O_2 radial diffusion distances in tumor tissues decrease from the arterial to the venous end of the tumor microvessels and depend on the vessel arrangement and blood flow directions (e.g., centripetal diffusion from vessels surrounding tumors cords (Hill-model) vs. centrifugal diffusion from a central vessel within a cord (Krogh-model) vs. irregular vascular networks and existence of concurrent vs. countercurrent flow in neighboring vessels) and vary between different tumor types with different blood flow and respiration rates [4–6]

Considering contributions by modern genomic and mass spectrometry-based proteomic analyses, realistic causative mechanisms and consequences of the Warburg effect were described only during the past 15 years and are summarized in this chapter.

27.2 The Warburg Effect: Essential Part of Metabolic Reprogramming and Favoring Biosynthesis Pathways

Conversion of glucose to lactate (lactic acid) in the presence of oxygen and functioning mitochondria (aerobic glycolysis, Warburg effect) is certainly more than a simple adaptation to hypoxia [17]. It is instead a crucial component of the malignant phenotype and a central feature of the "selfish" metabolic reprogramming of cancer cells, which is considered a "hallmark of cancer" (updated list, [18]). The switch to aerobic glycolysis is acquired very early in carcinogenesis (oncogenesis), even before tumor cells are exposed to hypoxic conditions [19]. The Warburg phenotype constitutes a metabolic signature of 70–80% of human cancers, which results from the interplay between the normoxic/hypoxic activation of the hypoxia-inducible transcription factor-1 (HIF-1), oncogene activation, loss of function of tumor suppressors, altered signaling pathways, and interaction with components of the tumor microenvironment (TME), sometimes working in concert with epigenetic mechanisms. The Warburg effect reflects a metabolic program of cancer cells driving sustained proliferation and accelerates malignant progression [4].

27.2.1 Major Biochemical Steps of Aerobic Glycolysis

The glycolytic pathway involves the catabolism of glucose to pyruvate in 9–10 biochemical steps, which are schematically shown in Fig. 27.2. Key transcriptional activations include the glucose transporter GLUT1 and lactate exporter monocarboxylate transporter 4 (MCT4) and key ("crucial") glycolytic enzymes: hexokinase 2 (HK2), phosphofructokinase 1 (PFK1), enolase 1 (ENO1), the low-activity pyruvate kinase M2 (PKM2), and the strongly overexpressed lactate dehydrogenase A (LDHA). Transcriptional activation also includes the mitochondrial pyruvate dehydrogenase kinase 1 (PDK1), which inactivates the "bottleneck" or "gatekeeper" enzyme pyruvate dehydrogenase (PDH) and thus impedes the intramitochondrial conversion of pyruvate to acetyl-CoA. As a result, pyruvate is shunted from the mitochondria and is converted to lactate within the cytosol. Lactate is exported into the extracellular space, where it accumulates (up to 40 mM).

The overexpression of the poorly active/nearly inactive pyruvate kinase M2, another "gatekeeper" enzyme, limits the phosphoenolpyruvate to pyruvate conversion (i.e., the final step of glycolysis) and thus leads to a backup of upstream glycolytic intermediates ("glucose carbons") which are shuttled into biosynthesis pathways allowing for sustained proliferation and unlimited growth.

These pathways can satisfy the anabolic demands of the macromolecular biosynthesis of nucleotides, lipids, proteins, and hexosamines. For nucleotide synthesis (and NADPH production), glucose-6-phosphate (G-6-P) is diverted via the pentose phosphate pathway (PPP). For biosynthesis of cell membrane components, phospholipids and triglycerols, glyceraldehyde-3-phosphate (GA-3-P), and dihydroxyacetone phosphate (DHA-P) are precursors. Nonessential amino acids emanate from GA-3-P (serine, glycine) and pyruvate (alanine). Fructose-6-phosphate is the glycolytic intermediate for the hexosamine pathway.

Of note Normoxic cancer cells can utilize lactate produced by – and exported from – hypoxic cancer cells as an energy source for OxPhos following MCT1-mediated import from the tumor microenvironment ("metabolic symbiosis" between hypoxic and normoxic cancer cells [20, 21]). In addition, normoxic cancer cells can utilize lactate produced by stressed stromal cells of the TME (e.g., cancer-associated fibroblasts, CAFs). This phenomenon is called the "reverse Warburg effect" [22, 23].

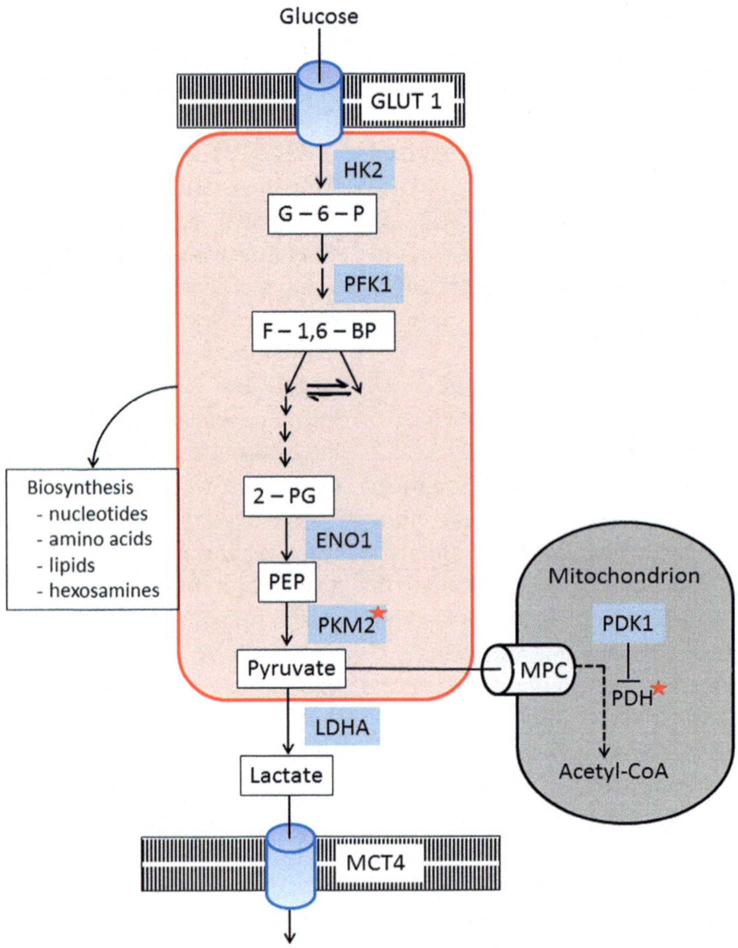

Fig. 27.2 Schematic illustration of biochemical steps of the Warburg phenotype. Upon enhanced import through overexpressed GLUT1 transporters, glucose is converted into two pyruvate molecules, the end product of aerobic glycolysis. In a following step, pyruvate is converted into lactate, which is exported via upregulated MCT4 transporters into the extracellular space, where it contributes to acidification (pH < 6.8). "Gatekeeper" enzymes (marked with a red star) lead (a) to an accumulation of upstream glycolytic intermediates (PKM2*) utilized for the biosynthesis of nucleic acids, nonessential amino acids, lipids, and hexosamines and (b) to a diversion of pyruvate away from the mitochondria (TCA cycle, OxPhos) by encoding PDK1, which in turn activates the "gatekeeper" enzyme PDH*. G-6-P: glucose-6-phosphate, F-1,6-BP: fructose-1,6-bisphosphate, 2-PG: 2-phosphoglycerate, PEP: phosphoenolpyruvate, acetyl-CoA: acetyl-coenzyme A, MPC: mitochondrial pyruvate carrier. Red box: 9(−10) biochemical steps of aerobic glycolysis in the cytosol

27.2.2 The Warburg Effect and Energy Homeostasis

In order to maintain energy homeostasis, cancer cells must consume large amounts of glucose (and glutamine, the second principal growth-supporting substrate). This can lead to glucose deprivation in the extracellular space, as illustrated in Fig. 27.3 (upper panel). Low-glucose conditions in the TEM in turn can cause a loss of stromal caveolin-1, yielding an oxidative stress which mimics hypoxia ("pseudohypoxia") through activation of HIF-1 and NFκB (see "reverse Warburg effect," Subchapter 27.2.1).

Aerobic glycolysis has been described as an inefficient means of energy metabolism, since the net production is only 2 moles of ATP per glucose molecule, whereas the total yield is approxi-

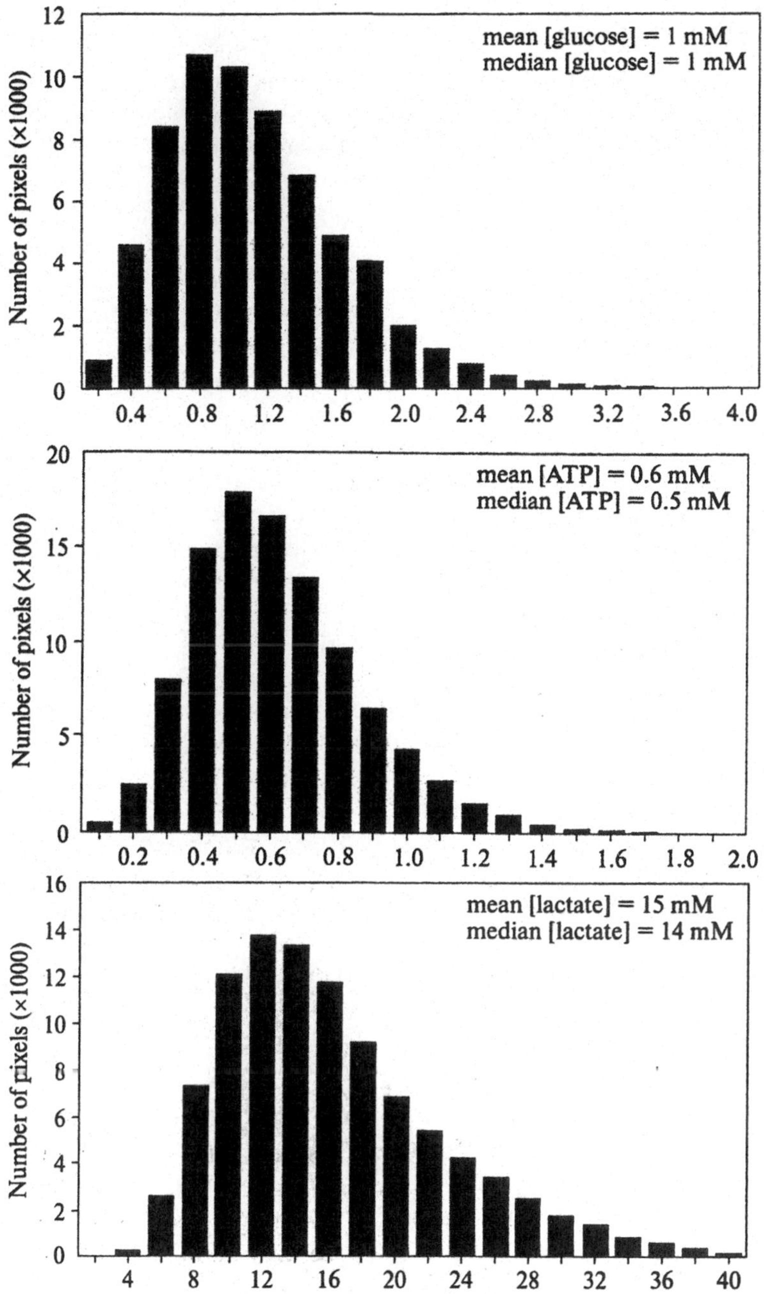

Fig. 27.3 Histograms of glucose (upper panel), ATP (central panel), and lactate concentrations (lower panel) in cancers of the uterine cervix. Abscissae: Concentration units: mM [24]

mately 36 (−38) ATPs from the complete oxidation of one glucose molecule. However, the speed of the cytosolic ATP generation is approx. 100 times faster (range: 20–300 times) than in mitochondria ("low yield but high-speed ATP production"). ATP provision *per unit time* is higher than in oxidative glucose metabolism as long as an adequate glucose supply is maintained in the extracellular compartment [4]. In cases of greatly increased ATP demand by cancer cells, aerobic glycolysis can rapidly increase, while OxPhos remains quite constant due to the much faster ATP production through the Warburg effect. Representative ATP levels in cancer tissue are depicted in Fig. 27.3 (central panel).

27.2.3 The Warburg Effect Ensures Redox Homeostasis and Reduces ROS Production

The Warburg effect provides reducing equivalents benefitting cancer cell proliferation: (a) during aerobic glycolysis, two NADHs per mole glucose are generated, and (b) the activated pentose phosphate pathway provides NADPH, which maintains the antioxidative power of glutathione (GSH), thus increasing the radioresistance of cancer cells, and can act as a directly operating antioxidant in the mitochondrial compartment [4, 25]. Furthermore, glycolysis can minimize the production of reactive oxygen species, which, at lower concentrations, can promote increased survival of cancer cells.

27.3 Regulatory Network of the Warburg Effect

As schematically illustrated in Fig. 27.4, major mechanisms acting independently or in cooperation to sustain aerobic glycolysis in cancer cells are (a) hypoxic/normoxic activation of HIF-1 ("master regulator," which can also work in concert with epigenetic mechanisms), (b) activation (gain of function) of oncogenes (e.g., cMyc, mTORC1, Akt, K-ras), (c) inactivation (loss of function) of tumor suppressors (e.g., mutant p53, mutant PTEN), (d) activation of e.g. RTK-PI3K/Akt/mTORC1 signaling pathway, (e) inactivation of AMPK signaling pathway, (f) downregulation/loss of function of several microRNAs (miRs) and sirtuins (SIRTs), (g) allosteric regulation by glycolytic intermediates, (h) interactions with the hostile TME and cancer-associated stromal cells, and (i) maintenance of the pH_i/pH_e gradient [26–35].

As mentioned above, downregulation or loss of several miRs and SIRTs with tumor suppressor functions can create a tumor-permissive phenotype via activation of the Warburg effect (not shown in Fig. 27.4) [36, 37]. These include miR-29, miR-143, and miR-144. Loss of these miRs and the tumor suppressors SIRT3 and SIRT6 can – inter alia – activate HIF-1, cMyc, Akt (= "Warburg kinase"), and key glycolytic enzymes; expedite PI3K/Akt/mTOR and Ras/Raf/MEK/ERK pathways; and activate GLUT1 and MCT4 transporters or inactivate the MPC carrier.

Mitochondrial contributions may also drive maintenance of aerobic glycolysis. These include (a) inhibition of OxPhos by mutant p53 (through regulators TIGAR and SOC2), (b) inhibition of mitochondrial biogenesis (by deactivated AMPK pathway and HIF-1), (c) miR-210-triggered inhibition of the electron transport chain, (d) BNIP3 (= B-cell lymphoma 2-interacting protein 3)-induced mitochondrial autophagy (mitophagy), and (e) mitochondrial DNA mutations.

27.4 Warburg Effect: The Role of Lactate Accumulation and Extracellular Acidosis

High lactate levels in the TME (up to 40 mM) primarily result from the upregulation of aerobic glycolysis. In addition, enhanced glutaminolysis, to a certain extent, contributes to lactate accumulation.

Lactate (lactate anion) probably is the only *oncometabolite* involved and necessary in nearly all main sequelae for malignant progression. A series of these pathophysiological conditions result after binding of the ligand lactate to the GPR81 receptor and activation of the PI3K/Akt/mTOR pathway and HIF-1 stabilization. Major sequelae driving malignant progression have been described in detail recently [e.g., 4, 29, 3840]. The use of lactate to fuel oxidative phosphorylation (OxPhos) in normoxic cancer cells has been described in Chap. 27.2.1.

Extracellular acidosis ($pH_e < 6.8$) is another detrimental trait arising from aerobic glycolysis. Its key role in driving malignant progression has

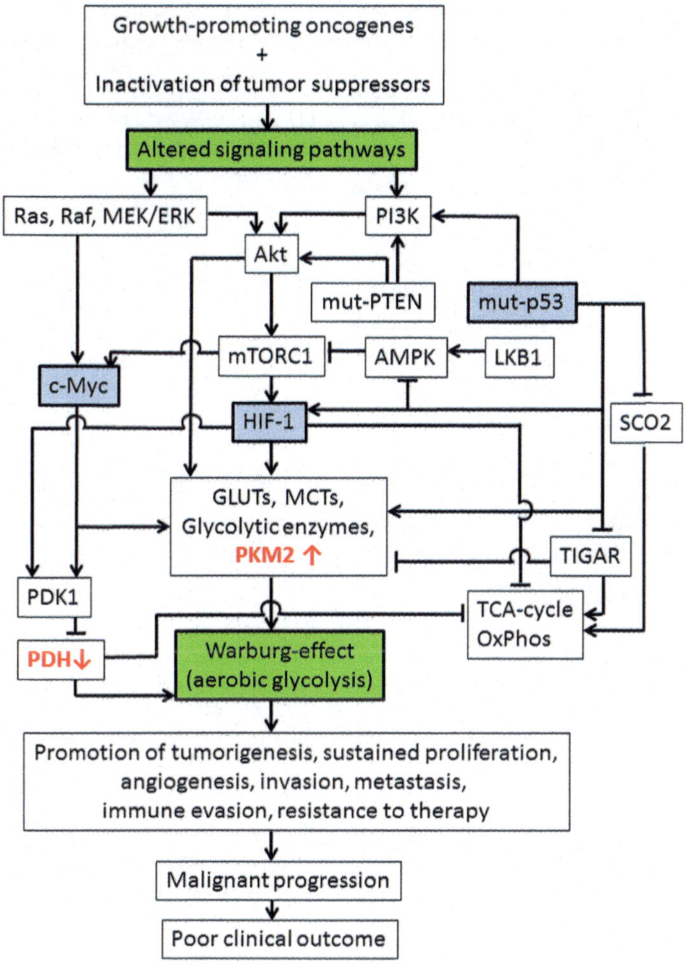

Fig. 27.4 Regulatory network of the Warburg effect, mitochondrial contributions to sustained glycolysis, and major mechanisms leading to cancer progression. Green boxes: "landmarks," grey boxes: key regulators, enzymes in red: gatekeeper/bottleneck enzymes (upregulated low-activity PKM2, downregulated PDH complex). Arrows represent positive impacts/activations; T-bars represent negative impacts/inhibitions. MEK/ERK: MAPK/ERK kinase, ERK: extracellular signal-regulated kinase, PI3K: phosphatidylinositol-3-kinase, Akt: protein kinase A ("Warburg kinase"), mut-p53: mutant p53, mut-PTEN: mutant PTEN (PTEN phosphatase and tensin homologue), mTOR: mechanistic ("mammalian") target of rapamycin, AMPK: AMP-activated protein kinase, cMyc: cellular Myc oncogene, LKB1: liver kinase B1 (tumor suppressor), SCO2: synthesis of cytochrome oxidase factor 2, PDH: pyruvate dehydrogenase (complex), TIGAR: tp53-inducible glycolysis and apoptosis regulator. (Jak/Stat3 signaling pathway not shown in Fig. 27.4)

been comprehensively reviewed recently [e.g., 3943]. There is ample information that lactate anions, H^+ (acidosis), and hypoxia are independent parameters (i.e., they can act independently) promoting malignant phenotypes in many instances but may also interact in regulatory systems (e.g., hypoxia-inducible pH regulation).

Footnote Diagnostic aspects of the Warburg effect (e.g., ^{18}F-FDG-PET, ^{13}C-MRS, ^{13}C-MRI, use of PKM2 and LDHA as biomarkers) and metabolic targeting in cancer therapy (e.g., inhibition or activation of key elements of the Warburg effect) are intentionally not discussed in this chapter.

27.5 Conclusions

Genetic instability, mutagenesis, aberrant gene expression, and altered signaling pathways cause a glycolytic switch in 70–80% of human cancers leading to aerobic glycolysis (Warburg effect). The glycolytic phenotype constitutes an essential component of the metabolic reprogramming of cancer cells and occurs early in oncogenesis, i.e., before tissue hypoxia develops. A series of molecular intricacies allow cancer cells to escape from typical regulatory constraints ensuring sustained, uncontrolled growth, invasion, and metastasis. Survival advantages and malignant progression, resistance to radio-/chemotherapy and other conventional cancer therapies, and escape from antitumor immune responses ultimately lead to poor patient outcome.

Acknowledgments The authors want to thank Anett Lange for her help in preparation of the manuscript.

References

1. Warburg O (1923) Versuche an überlebendem Carcinomgewebe. Biochem Zschr 142:317–333
2. Warburg O, Posener K, Negelein E (1924) Über den Stoffwechsel der Carcinomzelle. Biochem Zschr 152:319–344
3. Warburg O (1956) On the respiratory impairment in cancer cells. Science 124:269–270
4. Vaupel P, Schmidberger H, Mayer A (2019) The Warburg effect: essential part of metabolic reprogramming and central contributor to cancer progression. Int J Radiat Biol 95:912–919
5. Vaupel P (1990) Oxygenation of human tumors. Strahlenther Onkol 166:377–386
6. Vaupel P (2004) Tumor microenvironmental physiology and its implication for radiation oncology. Semin Radiat Oncol 14:198–206
7. Warburg O (1956) On the origin of cancer cells. Science 123:309–314
8. Chance B (1953) Dynamics of respiratory pigments of ascites tumor cells. Trans N Y Acad Sci 16:74–75
9. Chance B, Castor NL (1952) Some patterns of the respiratory pigments of ascites tumors of mice. Science 116:200–202
10. Chance B, Hess B (1956) On the control of metabolism in ascites tumor cell suspensions. Ann N Y Acad Sci 63:1008–1016
11. Chance B, Hess B (1959) Metabolic control mechanisms. III. Kinetics of oxygen utilization in ascites tumor cells. J Biol Chem 234:2416–2427
12. Weinhouse S (1956) On respiratory impairment in cancer cells. Science 124:267–269
13. Weinhouse S (1976) The Warburg hypothesis fifty years later. Cancer Res Clin Oncol 87:115–126
14. Aisenberg AC (1961) The glycolysis and respiration of tumors. Academic Press, New York
15. Vaupel P (1974) Atemgaswechsel und Glucosestoffwechsel von Implantationstumoren (DS-Carcinosarkom) in vivo. Funktionsanalyse Biolog Systeme 1:1–138
16. Vaupel P, Mayer A (2012) Availability, not respiratory capacity governs oxygen consumption in solid tumors. Int J Biochem Cell Biol 44:1477–1481
17. Gatenby RA, Gillies RJ (2004) Why do cancers have high aerobic glycolysis? Nat Rev Cancer 4:891–899
18. Hanahan D, Weinberg RA (2011) Hallmarks of cancer: the next generation. Cell 144:646–674
19. Vander Heiden MG, Cantley LC, Thompson CB (2009) Understanding the Warburg effect: the metabolic requirements of cell proliferation. Science 324:1029–1033
20. Semenza GL (2008) Tumor metabolism: cancer cells give and take lactate. J Clin Invest 118:3835–3837
21. Sonveaux P, Vegran F, Schroeder T et al (2008) Targeting lactate-fueled respiration selectively kills hypoxic tumor cells in mice. J Clin Invest 118:3930–3942
22. Fu Y, Liu S, Yin S et al (2017) The reverse Warburg effect is likely to be an Achilles heel of cancer that can be exploited for cancer therapy. Oncotarget 8:57813–57825
23. Pavlides S, Whitaker-Menezes D, Castello-Cros R et al (2009) The reverse Warburg effect: aerobic glycolysis in cancer associated fibroblasts and the tumor stroma. Cell Cycle 8:3984–4001
24. Vaupel P (1992) Physiological properties of malignant tumours. NMR Biomed 5:220–225
25. Kirsch M, De Groot H (2001) NAD(P)H, a directly operating antioxidant? FASEB J 15:1569–1574
26. Tameemi WA, Dale TP, Al-Jumaily RMK et al (2019) Hypoxia-modified cancer cell metabolism. Front Cell Dev Biol 7:4
27. Semenza GL (2010) HIF-1: upstream and downstream of cancer metabolism. Curr Opin Genet Dev 20:51–56
28. Nagao A, Kobayashi M, Koyasu S et al (2019) HIF-1 dependent reprogramming of glucose metabolic pathway of cancer cells and its therapeutic significance. Int J Mol Sci 20:238
29. Kato Y, Maeda T, Suzuki A et al (2018) Cancer metabolism: new insights into classic characteristics. Jpn Dent Sci Rev 54:8–21
30. Lu J, Tan M, Cai Q (2015) The Warburg effect in tumor progression: mitochondrial oxidative metabolism as an anti-metastasis mechanism. Cancer Lett 356:156–164
31. Ganapathy-Kanniappan S (2019) Molecular intricacies of aerobic glycolysis in cancer: current insights into the classic metabolic phenotype. Crit Rev Biochem Mol Biol 53:667–682

32. Cantor JR, Sabatini DM (2012) Cancer cell metabolism: one hallmark, many faces. Cancer Discov 2:881–898
33. He X, Li C, Ke R et al (2017) Down-regulation of adenosine monophosphate-activated protein kinase activity: a driver of cancer. Tumor Biol. https://doi.org/10.1177/1010428317697576
34. Tran Q, Lee H, Park J (2016) Targeting cancer metabolism-revisiting the Warburg effect. Toxicol Res 32:177–193
35. Counihan JL, Grossman EA, Nomura DK (2018) Cancer metabolism: current understanding and therapies. Chem Rev 118:6893–6923
36. Yu L, Chen X, Sun X et al (2017) The glycolytic switch in tumors: how many players are involved? J Cancer 8:3430–3440
37. Martinez-Pastor B, Mostolavsky R (2012) Sirtuins, metabolism, and cancer. Front Pharmacol 3:22
38. San-Millan I, Brooks GA (2017) Reexamining cancer metabolism: lactate production for carcinogenesis could be the purpose and explanation of the Warburg effect. Carcinogenesis 38:119–133
39. Mayer A, Vaupel P (2013) Hypoxia, lactate accumulation and acidosis: siblings or accomplices driving tumor progression and resistance to therapy. Adv Exp Med Biol 789:203–209
40. Vaupel P, Multhoff G (2018) Hypoxia-/HIF-1α-driven factors of the tumor microenvironment impeding antitumor immune responses and promoting malignant progression. Adv Exp Med Biol 1072:171–176
41. Thews O, Riemann A (2019) Tumor pH and metastasis: a malignant process beyond hypoxia. Cancer Metastasis Rev 38:113–129
42. Corbet C, Feron O (2017) Tumour acidosis: from the passenger to the driver's seat. Nat Rev Cancer 17:577–593
43. Riemann A, Schneider B, Gündel D et al (2016) Acidosis promotes metastasis formation by enhancing tumor cell motility. Adv Exp Med Biol 876:215–220

28 The Acidic Tumor Microenvironment Affects Epithelial-Mesenchymal Transition Markers as Well as Adhesion of NCI-H358 Lung Cancer Cells

Anne Riemann, M. Rauschner, M. Gießelmann, S. Reime, and O. Thews

Abstract

Epithelial-mesenchymal transition (EMT), which is involved in metastasis formation, requires reprogramming of gene expression mediated by key EMT transcription factors. However, signals from the cellular microenvironment, including hypoxia, can also modulate the process of EMT. Hypoxia is often associated with a reduction in the extracellular pH of the tumor microenvironment (acidosis). Whether acidosis alone has an impact on the expression of the EMT markers E-cadherin, N-cadherin, and vimentin was studied in NCI-H358 lung cancer cells. Reducing extracellular pH decreased E-cadherin mRNA, while vimentin and N-cadherin mRNA were doubled. However, at the protein level, E-cadherin and N-cadherin were both reduced, and only vimentin was upregulated. E-cadherin and N-cadherin expression at the cell surface, which is the relevant parameter for cell-cell and cell-matrix interaction, decreased too. The reduction of cell surface proteins was due to diminished protein expression and not changes in cellular localization, since localization of EMT markers in general was not affected by acidosis. Acidosis also affected NCI-H358 cells functionally. Adhesion was decreased when the cells were primed in an acidic medium before measuring cell adherence, which is in line with the reduced expression of cadherins at the cell surface. Additionally, migration was decreased after acidic priming. A possible mechanism for the regulation of EMT markers involves the action of microRNA-203a (miR-203a). In NCI-H358 lung cancer cells, miR-203a expression was repressed by acidosis. Since a decrease in the level of miR-203a has been shown to induce EMT, it might be involved in the modulation of EMT marker expression, adhesion, and migration by the acidic tumor microenvironment in NCI-H358 lung cancer cells.

Keywords

Acidosis · EMT · Adhesion · Migration · MiR-203a

A. Riemann (✉) · M. Rauschner · M. Gießelmann · S. Reime · O. Thews
Julius Bernstein Institute of Physiology, University of Halle-Wittenberg, Halle (Saale), Germany
e-mail: anne.riemann@medizin.uni-halle.de

E. M. Nemoto et al. (eds.), *Oxygen Transport to Tissue XLII*, Advances in Experimental Medicine and Biology 1269, https://doi.org/10.1007/978-3-030-48238-1_28

28.1 Introduction

Epithelial-mesenchymal transition (EMT) is a critical step in metastasis formation, which is still the leading cause of cancer-associated death worldwide [1]. During EMT, tumor cells lose their epithelial properties and gain mesenchymal features. This involves a reprogramming of gene expression that is mediated by key transcription factors including SNAIL and ZEB [2]. Additionally, signals from the cellular microenvironment, including hypoxia, can modulate the process of EMT [1, 3]. Hypoxia is often associated with a reduction of extracellular pH of the tumor microenvironment (acidosis) in the range of 6.0–7.0. Furthermore, metabolic reprogramming independent of hypoxia (Warburg effect) can induce acidosis. Acidosis has been shown to affect tumor aggressiveness through modulating metastasis and chemoresistance [4, 5]. Thus, the aim of this study was to analyze whether acidosis alone has an impact on EMT, both at the level of EMT marker expression (E-cadherin, N-cadherin, and vimentin) and concerning cellular function, including adhesion and migration of NCI-H358 lung cancer cells.

28.2 Methods

28.2.1 Cell Line

NCI-H358 human bronchioalveolar carcinoma cell line (ATCC CRL-5807) was grown in RPMI medium supplemented with 10% fetal calf serum (FCS). Cells are weakly differentiated with glandular features and are frequently used as an EMT model in the literature [6]. To study the changes in expression, cells were incubated in FCS-lacking medium pH 7.4 or 6.6 with 10 mM HEPES/10 mM MES for either 24 (RNA/microRNA) or 48 h (protein). For adhesion and migration experiments, cells were preincubated for 24 h at pH 7.4 or 6.6 as described above and subsequently transferred to RPMI medium with FCS for adhesion or lacking FCS to minimize proliferation to study migration.

28.2.2 Experimental Settings

qPCR was performed using SuperScript II Reverse Transcriptase and Platinum SYBR Green qPCR Supermix (Thermo Fisher Scientific, Waltham, USA) according to the manufacturer's instructions. Data was normalized to Rn 18S. Taqman qPCR for microRNA expression (Thermo Fisher Scientific) was performed according to the manufacturer's protocols with U6 snRNA for normalization. Western blot, flow cytometry, and immunofluorescence were performed according to standard protocols using the Molecular Imager ChemiDoc XRS system (Bio-Rad, Munich, Germany), LSRFortessa flow cytometer (BD Bioscience, Franklin NJ, USA), and inverse microscope BZ-8100E (Keyence, Osaka, Japan) for data acquisition, respectively. Antibodies were obtained from Cell Signaling (Danvers, USA) or BD Biosciences. Adhesion was studied either by a standard adhesion assay, rinsing the cells twice with 1× PBS 2 h after seeding, and counting of adherent cells with the CASY cell counter (Innovatis, Reutlingen, Germany) or by continuous impedance measurements (xCELLigence DP, OLS OMNI Life Science, Bremen, Germany) according to the manufacturer's instructions. After incubation at pH 7.4/6.6, cells were mechanically detached and transferred to 6-well cell culture plates before rinsing or 16-well plates containing gold biosensors to measure impedance. Migration was analyzed by a wound closure assay with the IncuCyte S3 Live-Cell Analysis System and Software (Sartorius, Göttingen, Germany). All experiments were performed with at least three passages, and results are presented as mean ± SEM. Differences between groups were assessed by unpaired Student's t-test, and the significance level was set at $\alpha = 5\%$.

28.3 Results

Acidosis led to a decrease in E-cadherin by a factor of 2 and a doubling of N-cadherin and vimentin mRNA (Fig. 28.1a). However, when looking at the protein level, only E-cadherin and vimentin

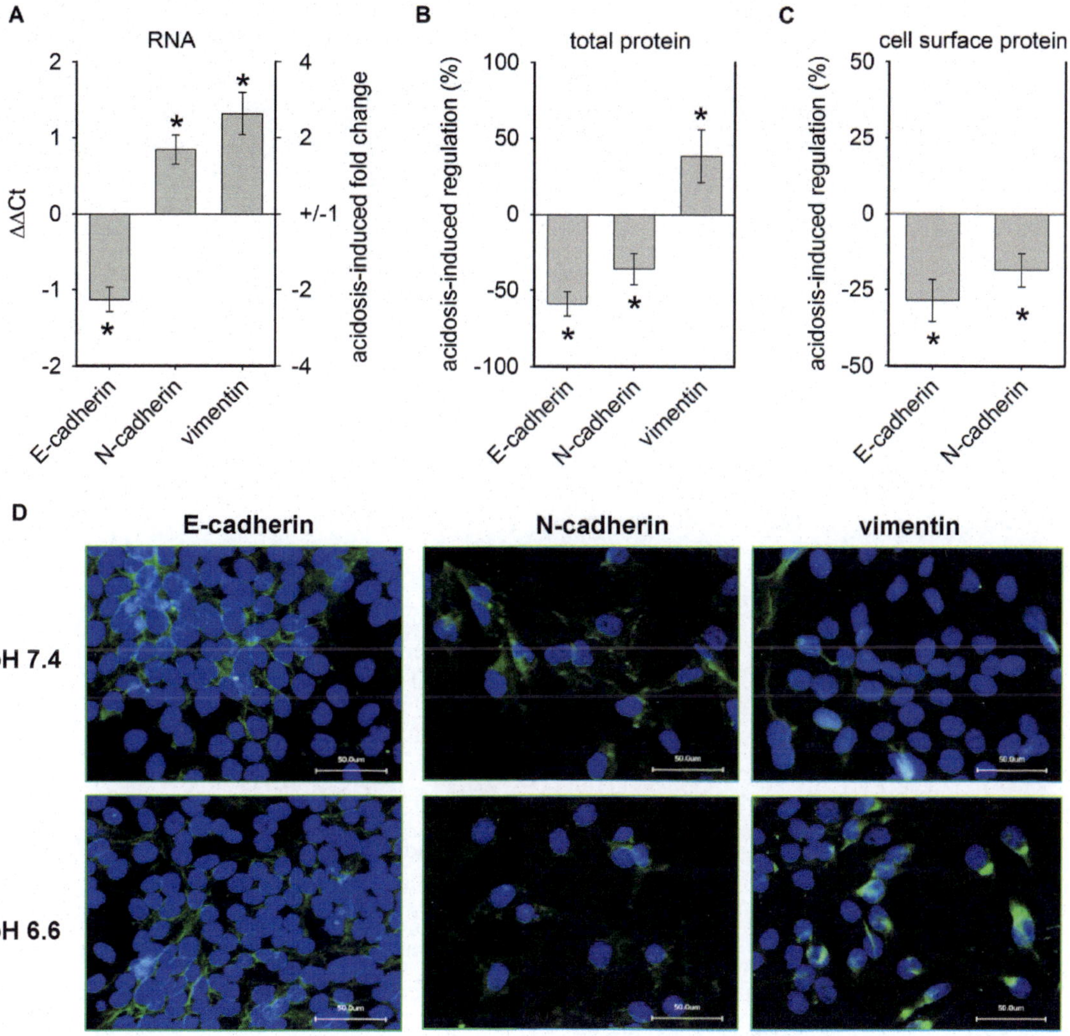

Fig. 28.1 Impact of extracellular acidosis on EMT marker expression and localization in NCI-H358 cells. Relative acidosis-induced modulation of EMT markers at (**a**) mRNA ($n = 6–8$), (**b**) total protein ($n = 7–11$), and (**c**) cell surface protein level ($n = 8–9$). The values are normalized to control conditions at pH 7.4, $^{*}p < 0.05$. (**d**) Representative immunofluorescence images of E-cadherin, N-cadherin, and vimentin (in green) after 48 h at pH 7.4 or 6.6, merged with staining of cell nuclei with DAPI (in blue), bar = 50 μm

had comparable results, while N-cadherin protein was decreased by acidosis (Fig. 28.1b). E- and N-cadherin at the cell surface were decreased by about 25% as analyzed by flow cytometry (Fig. 28.1c). Immunofluorescence images after 48 h of pH 7.4 or 6.6 showed that this decrease was not due to changes in cellular localization (Fig. 28.1d). Adhesion of NCI-H358 cells to a surface was measured by standard cell adhesion assays. Acidic pre-treatment for 24 h reduced adhesion by about 25% (Fig. 28.2a). The results were validated by continuous impedance measurements using the xCELLigence RTCA DP system. Cell index resembles adhesion to a plastic surface as well as cell-cell contact. After 6 h, the difference between pre-treatment at pH 6.6 and control (pH 7.4) was statistically significant, and it increased further over time (Fig. 28.2b). These results are in line with the reduced expression of cadherins at the cell surface. Migration was analyzed by a wound closure assay. To minimize the impact of proliferation on gap closure,

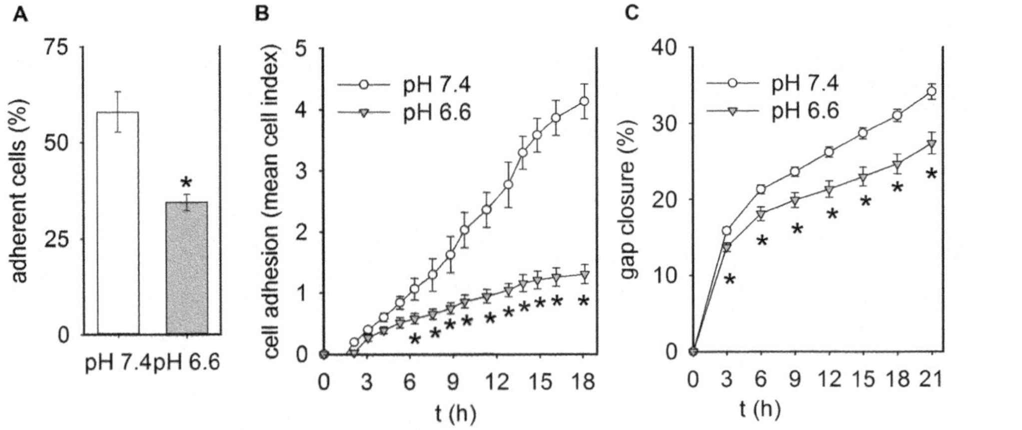

Fig. 28.2 Reduction in adhesion and migration by acidic preincubation of NCI-H358 cells. (**a**) Adherent cells after washing (n = 12–15), (**b**) changes in cell adhesion over time analyzed by impedance measurements (n = 3), and (**c**) wound closure assay to determine cell migration (n = 32–35). *$p < 0.05$

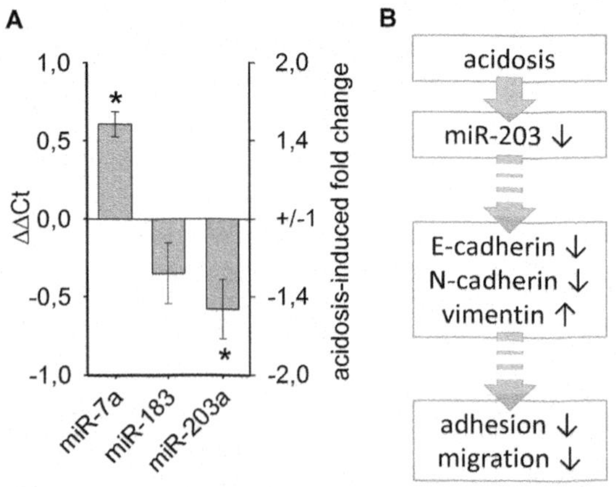

Fig. 28.3 Acidosis-induced regulation of microRNAs and its possible impact. (**a**) MicroRNA expression after 24 h at pH 6.6 compared to control (pH 7.4), n = 4–5, *$p < 0.05$. (**b**) A possible mechanism for acidosis-induced changes in EMT marker expression comprises the repression of miR-203. Reduced E-cadherin expression in turn might be involved in the decrease in cell adhesion in an acidic tumor microenvironment

the cells were kept in medium lacking FCS after their pre-treatment at pH 7.4/6.6. Gap closure was impeded when cells were primed at an acidic pH (Fig. 28.2c). Thus, acidosis led to a decrease in migration in NCI-H358 cells. A possible mechanism comprises microRNAs, which are often deregulated in cancer and are involved in EMT and metastasis formation [7, 8]. We recently identified miR-7a, mir-183, and miR-203a as regulated by acidosis in prostate and breast carcinoma cells [9]. Thus, their expression was analyzed in NCI-H358 lung cancer cells. Acidosis increased the expression of miR-7a and reduced the level of miR-203a (Fig. 28.3a).

28.4 Conclusions

An acidic microenvironment modulates processes involved in EMT, such as the expression of EMT markers E-cadherin, N-cadherin, and vimentin, cellular adhesion, and migration. However, the regulation by acidosis was not always concordant with the expected regulation during EMT. The epithelial marker E-cadherin was downregulated as was cell adhesion, while the mesenchymal-related protein vimentin was increased, which is in line with EMT induction [10]. In contrast, mesenchymal marker N-cadherin was downregulated as was the migratory behavior of NCI-H358 lung cancer cells. In line with this, it has been shown in the literature that upregulation of N-cadherin can be linked to fostered migration [10]. The diminished surface expression of both E- and N-cadherin might be mechanistically linked to reduced adhesion. A decrease in E-cadherin, for instance, is linked to a destabilization of adherens junctions [11]. As well as the reduced level of N-cadherin at the cell surface, acidosis can also weaken N-cadherin binding activity [12]. Mechanistically, the reduction of miR-203a in NCI-H358 cells by acidosis might be involved. MicroRNAs repress their targets posttranscriptionally and are linked to EMT and metastasis formation [7]. They often affect EMT marker expression by regulation of the critical EMT master transcription factors but are sometimes even able to regulate cadherin expression directly [11]. MiR-203a is said in the literature to repress EMT, including EMT marker expression, adhesion, and migration, as well as subsequently metastases [13–16]. In lung adenocarcinoma cells, it has been shown that the molecular mechanism comprises miR-203 repression which in consequence increases EMT transcription factors SNAI1 and SNAI2 [13]. Thus, acidosis does not induce a classical EMT in NCI-H358 cancer cells, but affects EMT marker expression and reduces adhesion and migration possibly via downregulation of miR-203a (Fig. 28.3b) and subsequent upregulation of SNAI1 and SNAI2.

Acknowledgments This study was supported by the Deutsche Forschungsgemeinschaft (DFG) (grant TH482/6-1).

References

1. Redfern AD, Spalding LJ, Thompson EW (2018) The Kraken Wakes: induced EMT as a driver of tumour aggression and poor outcome. Clin Exp Metastasis 35:285–308
2. Tania M, Khan MA, Fu J (2014) Epithelial to mesenchymal transition inducing transcription factors and metastatic cancer. Tumour Biol 35:7335–7342
3. Yeo CD, Kang N, Choi SY et al (2017) The role of hypoxia on the acquisition of epithelial-mesenchymal transition and cancer stemness: a possible link to epigenetic regulation. Korean J Intern Med 32:589–599
4. Thews O, Riemann A (2019) Tumor pH and metastasis: a malignant process beyond hypoxia. Cancer Metastasis Rev 38:113–129
5. Taylor S, Spugnini EP, Assaraf YG et al (2015) Microenvironment acidity as a major determinant of tumor chemoresistance: proton pump inhibitors (PPIs) as a novel therapeutic approach. Drug Resist Updat 23:69–78
6. Wang D, Haley JD, Thompson P (2017) Comparative gene co-expression network analysis of epithelial to mesenchymal transition reveals lung cancer progression stages. BMC Cancer 17:830
7. Díaz-López A, Moreno-Bueno G, Cano A (2014) Role of microRNA in epithelial to mesenchymal transition and metastasis and clinical perspectives. Cancer Manag Res 6:205–216
8. Kim J, Yao F, Xiao Z et al (2018) MicroRNAs and metastasis: small RNAs play big roles. Cancer Metastasis Rev 37:5–15
9. Riemann A, Reime S, Thews O (2019) Acidic extracellular environment affects miRNA expression in tumors in vitro and in vivo. Int J Cancer 144:1609–1618
10. Le Bras GF, Taubenslag KJ, Andl CD (2012) The regulation of cell-cell adhesion during epithelial-mesenchymal transition, motility and tumor progression. Cell Adhes Migr 6:365–373
11. Lamouille S, Xu J, Derynck R (2014) Molecular mechanisms of epithelial-mesenchymal transition. Nat Rev Mol Cell Biol 15:178–196
12. Baumgartner W, Osmanagic A, Gebhard M et al (2013) Different pH-dependencies of the two synaptic adhesion molecules N-cadherin and cadherin-11 and the possible functional implication for long-term potentiation. Synapse 67:705–715
13. Ge X, Li G-Y, Jiang L et al (2019) Long noncoding RNA CAR10 promotes lung adenocarcinoma metastasis via miR-203/30/SNAI axis. Oncogene 38:3061–3076
14. Ge XJ, Zheng LM, Feng ZX et al (2018) H19 contributes to poor clinical features in NSCLC patients and leads to enhanced invasion in A549 cells through regulating miRNA-203-mediated epithelial-mesenchymal transition. Oncol Lett 16:4480–4488
15. Gao P, Wang S, Jing F et al (2017) MicroRNA-203 suppresses invasion of gastric cancer cells by targeting ERK1/2/Slug/ E-cadherin signaling. Cancer Biomark 19:11–20
16. Tian X, Tao F, Zhang B et al (2018) The miR-203/SNAI2 axis regulates prostate tumor growth, migration, angiogenesis and stemness potentially by modulating GSK-3β/β-CATENIN signal pathway. IUBMB Life 70:224–236

29

Assessment of the Probability of Tumour Control for Prescribed Doses Based on Imaging of Oxygen Partial Pressure

Ana Ureba, Emely Kjellsson Lindblom, Iuliana Toma-Dasu, Alexandru Dasu, and Marta Lazzeroni

Abstract

In radiotherapy, hypoxia is a known negative factor, occurring especially in solid malignant tumours. Nitroimidazole-based positron emission tomography (PET) tracers, due to their selective binding to hypoxic cells, could be used as surrogates to image and quantify the underlying oxygen distributions in tissues. The spatial resolution of a clinical PET image, however, is much larger than the cellular spatial scale where hypoxia occurs. A question therefore arises regarding the possibility of quantifying different hypoxia levels based on PET images, and the aim of the present study is the prescription of corresponding therapeutic doses and its exploration.

A tumour oxygenation model was created consisting of two concentric spheres with different oxygen partial pressure (pO_2) distributions. In order to mimic a PET image of the simulated tumour, given the relation between uptake and pO_2, fundamental effects that limit spatial resolution in a PET imaging system were considered: the uptake distribution was processed with a Gaussian 3D filter, and a re-binning to reach a typical PET image voxel size was performed. Prescription doses to overcome tumour hypoxia and predicted tumour control probability (TCP) were calculated based on the processed images for several fractionation schemes. Knowing the underlying oxygenation at microscopic scale, the actual TCP expected after the delivery of the calculated prescription doses was evaluated. Results are presented for three different dose painting strategies: by numbers, by contours and by using a voxel grouping-based approach.

The differences between predicted TCP and evaluated TCP indicate that careful consideration must be taken on the dose prescription strategy and the selection of the number of fractions, depending on the severity of hypoxia.

A. Ureba (✉)
The Skandion Clinic, Uppsala, Sweden

Karolinska Institutet, Medical Radiation Physics, Department of Oncology-Pathology, Stockholm, Sweden
e-mail: ana.ureba@ki.se

E. Kjellsson Lindblom · I. Toma-Dasu · M. Lazzeroni
Karolinska Institutet, Medical Radiation Physics, Department of Oncology-Pathology, Stockholm, Sweden

Stockholm University, Medical Radiation Physics, Department of Physics, Stockholm, Sweden

A. Dasu
The Skandion Clinic, Uppsala, Sweden

E. M. Nemoto et al. (eds.), *Oxygen Transport to Tissue XLII*, Advances in Experimental Medicine and Biology 1269, https://doi.org/10.1007/978-3-030-48238-1_29

Keywords

Dose painting · Hypoxia · Mathematical modelling · TCP · PET

29.1 Introduction

In radiation therapy, decreased oxygen in tissues entails an increased radioresistance. Hypoxia in solid tumours results from malformed vasculature lacking hierarchical vessel arrangement [1]. The possibility of identifying hypoxia in vivo, before or during the treatment, with a minimally invasive protocol, may be of great value, especially using techniques which are routinely available in the clinic, such as positron emission tomography (PET) or magnetic resonance (MR). In particular, for PET imaging, a broad range of radiotracers, such as nitroimidazole-based tracers, able to identify hypoxia expression in tumours are available [1, 2].

PET has improved the ability to delineate biological targets aiming to boost radiation-resistant regions. However, while PET imaging is routinely used for delineation purposes, there is still lack of general consensus in handling this information for dose prescription (dose painting, DP) [3]. DP approaches could be tested in a theoretical framework by parameterising the main features relevant for the effects of radiation, such as the role of the oxygen concentration in tissues [4], while studies of clinical outcomes bring the ultimate validation.

The PET macroscopic information provides an insight on the metabolic pathways of dedicated radiotracers, such as tracers whose bindings are correlated to hypoxic microenvironments [2, 5]. Nevertheless, the PET ability to distinguish between different characteristics of a heterogeneous tissue is highly limited by the PET camera resolution, the reconstruction algorithm and the image acquisition time [6, 7]. While the reconstruction algorithm is known and the image acquisition time is unavoidable, the spatial resolution of the PET camera strongly limits the ability to represent the biological tumour heterogeneity.

A few theoretical studies aiming at quantifying tumour hypoxia by PET imaging, at evaluating the practical limitations of imaging-based DP [3, 8] or at estimating the expected cellular heterogeneity [9], are available. However, studies considering the impact of the hypoxia spatial scale and its change in time on the treatment outcome using several DP strategies are still scarce [3].

This study aims at assessing the tumour control probability (TCP) for different dose prescription strategies based on PET imaging of oxygen partial pressure (pO_2) taking the resolution of the image explicitly into account.

29.2 Methods

An in silico 3D tumour model consisting of two concentric regions (rim and core) with heterogeneous oxygenation was simulated. The model accounts for the impact of different blood inter-vessel distance distributions simulated by a Monte Carlo-based algorithm (Fig. 29.1a) [8]. Three different hypoxia levels are considered for the core (low, medium and high) corresponding to those resulting from three different mean blood inter-vessel distances (120, 140 and 160 μm, respectively). The average pO_2 and hypoxic fraction (HF) corresponding to the rim were 19 mmHg and 15%, respectively. The average pO_2 and HF for the three hypoxia levels were 12, 10 and 8 mmHg and 46, 61 and 69%, respectively. Fast reoxygenation after every fraction was simulated by resampling the oxygenation for each fraction, so the temporal variation in oxygenation was taken into account. The same overall hypoxic level was assumed at every fraction.

A previously proposed model by Toma-Dasu et al. [4], which describes the relationship between ^{18}F-fluoromisonidazole (FMISO) radiotracer uptake and oxygen partial pressure distribution based on the inhibition of a chemical reaction ($\digamma$), was used (Fig. 29.1b).

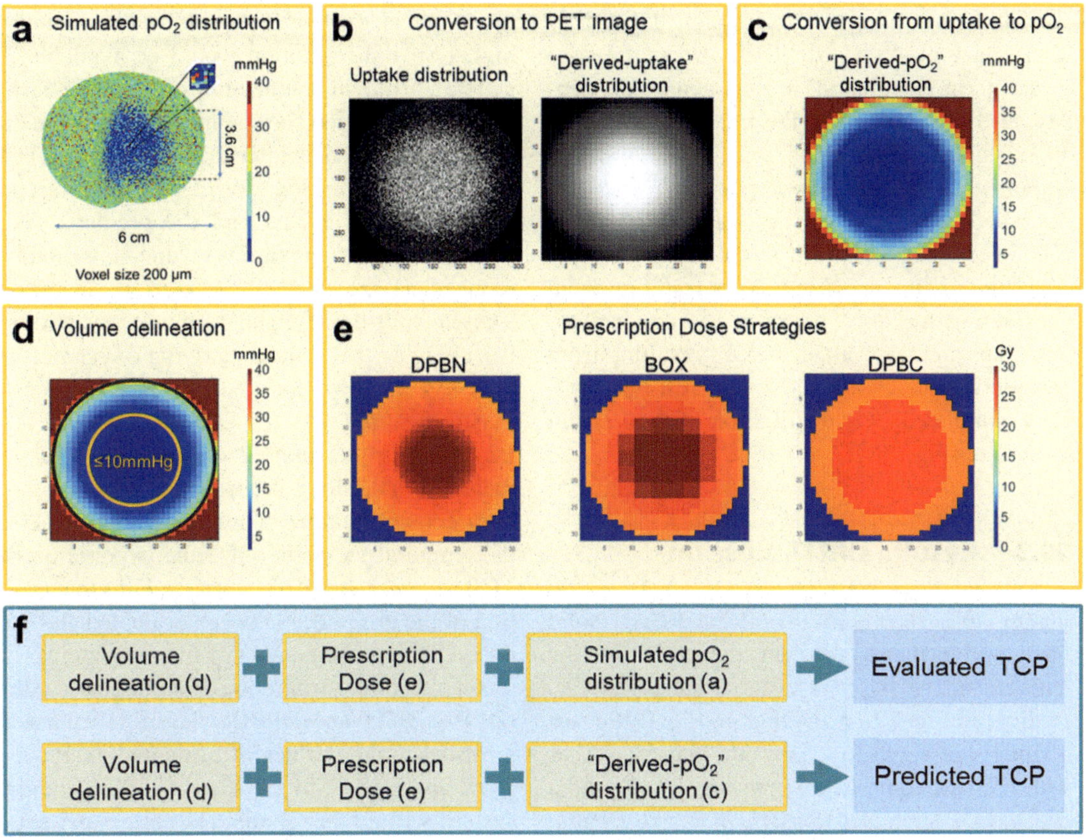

Fig. 29.1 Schematic illustration of the workflow of the study: (**a**) simulated in silico 3D model of a tumour with heterogeneous oxygenation; (**b**) left: corresponding uptake distribution at microscopic scale, right: derived-uptake distribution mimicking the spatial resolution and reconstructed voxel size of a positron emission tomography (PET) imaging system; (**c**) derived-pO_2 distribution obtained from derived-uptake map; (**d**) hypoxic region delineation (threshold equal to 10 mmHg); (**e**) dose prescription distribution with three dose painting strategies: by numbers (DPBN), by contours (DPBC) and by a voxel grouping-based approach (BOX); (**f**) input data used for the calculation of the evaluated and predicted tumour control probabilities (TCPs)

Fundamental effects that limit the spatial resolution in a PET imaging system were mimicked by processing the uptake maps (derived-uptake distribution) [4]. The derived-uptake distribution was convolved with a Gaussian 3D filter (full width at half maximum, FWHM, of 0.5, 6.1 and 12.2 mm) and re-binned to increase the initial voxel size from 0.2 to 2 and 4 mm, respectively (Fig. 29.1b).

A new derived-pO_2 distribution from the derived-uptake distribution was then calculated using the inverse of the function previously described (F^{-1}) to convert uptake into pO_2 values (Fig. 29.1c). A hypoxic region was contoured on the obtained image by considering as threshold for hypoxia a pO_2 value equal to 10 mmHg (Fig. 29.1d).

Prescription doses needed to overcome tumour radioresistance for different fractionation schedules (1–30 fractions) were calculated by assuming that the only factor that affects radioresistance is the hypoxia level [4, 10].

Three different DP strategies were adopted, mimicking a DP strategy with different 'brush' sizes (Fig. 29.1e): (a) prescription dose assigned at voxel level aiming at 95% of TCP (DPBN), (b) prescription dose to groups of voxels of 3 × 3 × 3 (BOX) assigning the maximum dose within each group and (c) prescription dose assigned uniformly within each contoured region (i.e. hypoxic core and rim) using the expression derived by Toma-Dasu et al. [4, 10] (DPBC). For the dose prescription calculation, a clonogenic cell density, at the beginning of the treatment, equal to 10^6 cells/cm^3 was assumed.

For each of the dose painting strategies described above, the corresponding TCPs were calculated using the two different underlying pO_2 distributions: the predicted TCPs resulting from considering the dose prescriptions on derived-pO_2 maps and the evaluated TCPs resulting from considering the dose prescriptions on the originally simulated pO_2 distribution with 0.2 mm voxel size (Fig. 29.1f).

29.3 Results and Discussion

Figure 29.2 shows results of predicted (solid lines) and evaluated (dashed lines) TCP for the three considered hypoxia levels (low in Fig. 29.2a, medium in Fig. 29.2b and high in Fig. 29.2c) for a voxel size equal to 2 mm and Gaussian filter with FWHM equal to 6.1 mm and for the three adopted DP strategies (DPBN, BOX and DPBC) as a function of the number of fractions in which the treatment is delivered.

For each DP strategy, for each number of fractions and for each hypoxic level, a prescription dose distribution was calculated. The dose required for achieving a TCP higher than 90% for the simulated tumour with a higher hypoxic level corresponding to the lower PET spatial resolution (Fig. 29.2c), for example, is 58 Gy to the rim and 69 Gy to the hypoxic core, for the DPBC strategy when the treatment is delivered in 30 fractions, while the mean and standard deviation of the dose distribution for the BOX are 59.0 ± 1.2 Gy to the rim and 71 ± 5 Gy to the core and for the DPBN are 57.7 ± 1.3 Gy to the rim and 68 ± 5 Gy to the core for the same number of fractions. The selection of the presented combination of FWHM and voxel size is intended to mimic the typical spatial resolution of clinically available PET imaging system [7]. In Fig. 29.2d, calculations are also presented for an increased spatial resolution (FWHM equal to 0.5 mm) of the PET image and voxel size equal to the initially simulated pO_2 map (i.e. 0.2 mm, Fig. 29.1a) for the high hypoxia case, in order to study the hypothetical case where a PET camera with a higher spatial resolution would be available. In general, different combinations of hypoxia levels and PET resolution show similar trends in the differences between predicted and evaluated TCP. As illustrated in Fig. 29.2a–c, the difference between the evaluated and the predicted TCP increases with hypoxia level, and it is notably reduced as the number of fractions increases. These results therefore confirm previous findings [9], showing that if the underlying oxygen distribution is unknown, the predicted TCP is overestimated. Regardless of the DP strategy used, TCP increases as the number of fraction increases, meaning that, along the treatment course, for a high enough number of fractions, the impact of the temporal variability of acute hypoxia on the TCP becomes lower. This fact explains the reduction of the difference between evaluated and predicted TCP as the number of fractions increases.

Of the three different DP strategies studied (DPBN, BOX and DPBC), the more robust, in terms of higher values of evaluated TCP, were BOX and DPBC. In the case of a PET imaging system with higher spatial resolution and small reconstructed voxel size (Fig. 29.2d), the DPBC strategy appears to be the most robust one (Fig. 29.2). However, it should be noted that, in this scenario, the edge of the grouped BOX is only 0.6 mm, which is unrealistic to be delivered by conventional radiotherapy. Further studies focused on optimising the size of the grouping matrix for the BOX DP strategy accounting both for feasibility in delivery of the treatment and for increased TCP values are ongoing. Furthermore, the simulation of the results from a PET imaging system with high resolution also showed the lowest difference between predicted and evaluated TCP for the DPBC strategy in the high hypoxic scenario (Fig. 29.2d). This indicates that a more precise knowledge of the underlying radiosensitivities allows for a better prescription dose, even using the biggest 'brush' size, DPBC. The results also showed that DPBN strategy is the least robust among all the studied strategies (Fig. 29.2) since it implies highly heterogeneous dose distributions that are prone to mismatching the underlying radiosensitivity when hypoxia fluctuates over time.

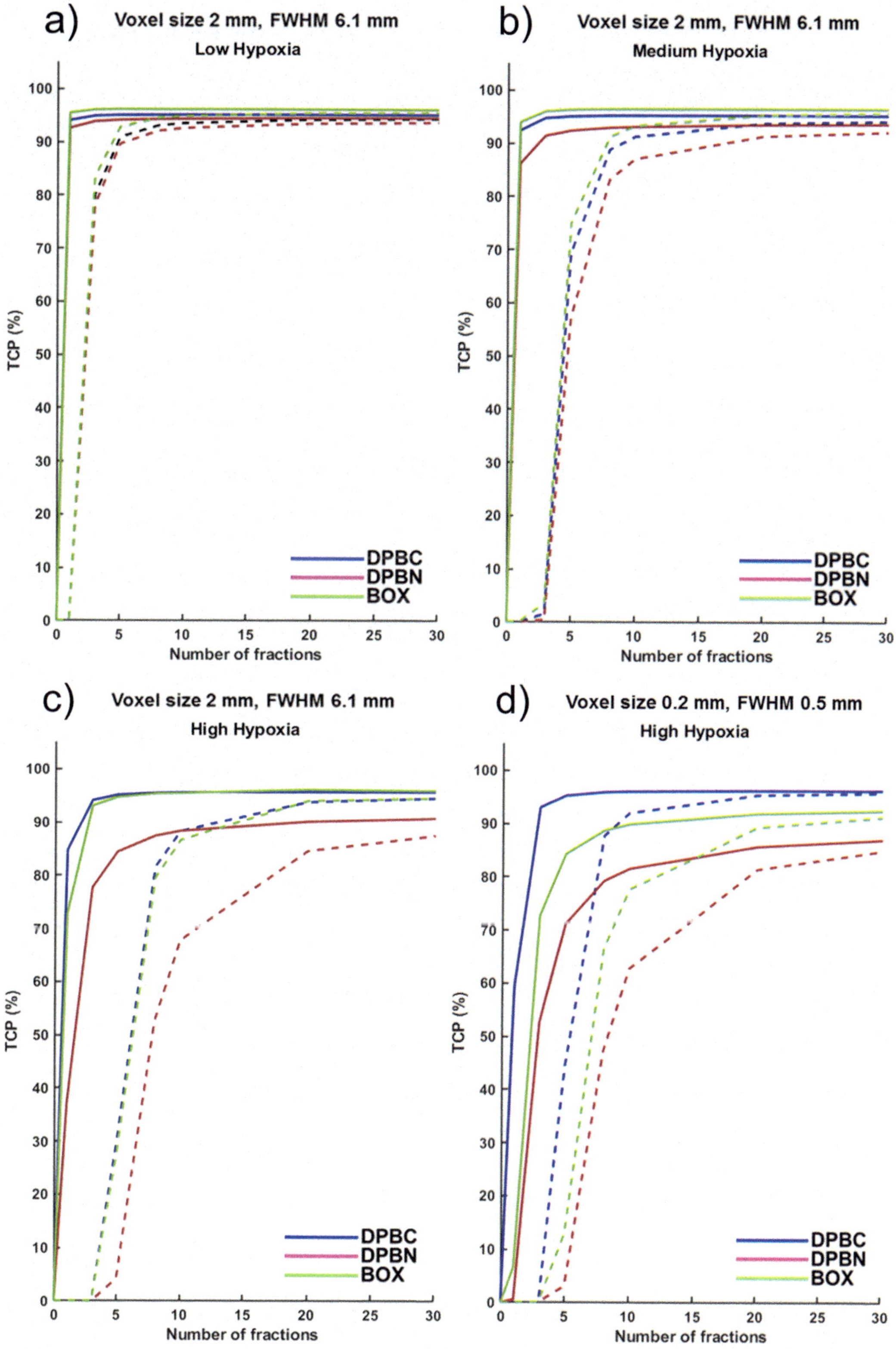

Fig. 29.2 Predicted (solid lines) and evaluated (dashed lines) tumour control probabilities (TCP) as a function of the number of fractions for two positron emission tomography resolutions: full width at half maximum (FWHM) equal to 6.1 mm (**a**–**c**) and FWHM equal to 0.5 mm (**d**). Results are shown for three different dose painting strategies: by numbers (DPBN), by contours (DPBC) and by using a voxel grouping-based approach (BOX)

29.4 Conclusions

Differences between predicted and evaluated TCP values indicate that careful consideration must be taken of the dose prescription strategy. An increasing number of fractions, depending on the severity of hypoxia, helps to compensate hypoxia radioresistance. DP strategies, such as DPBC or BOX, mimicking dose painting with a larger 'brush', offer a more robust DP solution.

Acknowledgements This project has received funding from the European Union's Horizon 2020 research and innovation programme under grant agreement no. 730983 and from the Swedish Cancer Research Funds of Radiumhemmet (RaHFo).

References

1. Harada H (2011) How can we overcome tumor hypoxia in radiation therapy? J Radiat Res 52(5):545–556
2. Zhu A, Shim H (2011) Current molecular imaging positron emitting radiotracers in oncology. Nucl Med Mol Imaging 45(1):1–14
3. Tanderup K, Olsen DR, Grau C (2006) Dose painting: art or science? Radiother Oncol 79(3):245–248
4. Toma-Dasu I, Uhrdin J, Antonovic L et al (2012) Dose prescription and treatment planning based on FMISO-PET hypoxia. Acta Oncol 51(2):222–230
5. Thorwarth D (2015) Functional imaging for radiotherapy treatment planning: current status and future directions—a review. Br J Radiol 88(1051):20150056
6. Grimes DR, Warren DR, Warren S (2017) Hypoxia imaging and radiotherapy: bridging the resolution gap. Br J Radiol 90:20160939
7. Moses WW (2011) Fundamental limits of spatial resolution in PET. Nucl Instrum Methods Phys Res A 648:S236–S240
8. Dasu A, Toma-Dasu I (2013) Dose painting by numbers-do the practical limitations of the technique decrease or increase the probability of controlling tumours? IFMBE Proc 39:1731–1734
9. Petit SF, Dekker AL, Seigneuric R et al (2009) Intravoxel heterogeneity influences the dose prescription for dose-painting with radiotherapy: a modelling study. Phys Med Biol 54(7):2179–2196
10. Toma-Dasu I, Dasu A, Brahme A (2009) Dose prescription and optimisation based on tumour hypoxia. Acta Oncol 48:1181–1192

On the Feasibility of Skin Water Content Imaging Adjuvant to Tissue Oximetry

30

Guennadi Saiko

Abstract

Oxygen supply to tissues can be seriously impacted during wound healing. In particular, edema can increase the distance between capillaries, thus decreasing oxygen supply to cells. Thus, the detection of edema, preferably at the preclinical stage, is of great importance. However, there is no reference standard for a cross-sectional, objective measurement of edema. Multispectral imaging can be such adjuvant technology to elucidate the impact of edema on oxygen transport to tissues. The purpose of the current study is to assess the feasibility of multispectral imaging for visualization of water content in surface tissues. *Methods*: The skin (hand and forearm) of healthy volunteers was imaged using the Multi-Spectral Imaging Device (MSID). MSID is a multispectral imaging system for visualization of tissue chromophores in surface tissues. It uses a 12-bit scientific-grade NIR-enhanced monochrome camera and ten wavelength light source (600–1000 nm range) to visualize the distribution of oxy- and deoxy-hemoglobins, methemoglobin, water, and melanin. The imaging distance is 30 cm and the field of view: 7 × 7 cm. *Results*: Water content was extracted using various subsets of two and three wavelengths. To mimic the use of a consumer-grade camera, four least significant bits for each pixel value of a 12-bit image were discarded during preprocessing. Eight-bit results were compared with 12-bit results. *Conclusions*: Rough numerical calculations and initial experiments show feasibility of water content imaging in the skin using 970 nm band illumination and 12- and 8-bit cameras.

Keywords

Wound healing · Edema · Tissue imaging · Tissue water content imaging

30.1 Introduction

Edema (accumulation of fluids in interstitial space) is a common clinical sign in a wide variety of conditions. Being a nonspecific finding, it often poses a challenge for the clinician. While, in many cases, it has a benign origin, in other instances, it can be a sign of life-threatening conditions. Because the interstitium can easily accommodate several liters of fluid, a patient's weight may increase nearly 10% before pitting edema is evident. Thus, early detection of edema (preferably preclinical) is of great importance,

G. Saiko (✉)
Swift Medical Inc., Toronto, ON, Canada
e-mail: gennadi.saiko@swiftmedical.com

E. M. Nemoto et al. (eds.), *Oxygen Transport to Tissue XLII*, Advances in Experimental Medicine and Biology 1269, https://doi.org/10.1007/978-3-030-48238-1_30

especially for patients with compromised health (diabetes, kidney or heart conditions, etc.).

Edema can seriously impact wound healing by restricting oxygen supply to tissues. For example, edema can increase the distance between capillaries, thus decreasing oxygen supply to cells, or it may compress small vessels to shut off the local blood supply at all, thus creating ischemic tissue. On another side, it is known that oxygen diffusivity (oxygen diffusion constant) increases with increasing tissue water content [1].

There is no gold standard for an objective measurement of edema. In particular, for peripheral edema, the most widely used technique is a subjective clinical assessment where an examiner applies pressure with an index finger to a patient's ankle [2] to capture pit depth and the time needed for the skin to return to its original state (recovery time). Despite common use, this method has not been proven to be a sufficiently objective, reliable, or sensitive assessment of edema. Several quantitative methods to measure peripheral edema have been proposed [3], but they are mostly used in physical therapy and sports medicine.

Several quantitative technologies have been used to assess edema or the hydration of skin noninvasively. They include skin impedance methods, ultrasound, and magnetic resonance imaging and spectroscopy.

The major part of existing methods of measuring of edema suffers from various shortcomings, namely, subjectivity [4], inability to detect on early stages [5], and impossibility to be applied in certain clinical or field settings (e.g., water displacement for postoperative patients, MRI, and ultrasound in field settings).

Thus, it would be useful to have a more widely accessible way to investigate edema and ideally visualize it in various clinical and field settings.

Optical spectroscopy, along with the skin impedance [6], is a promising modality for the noninvasive diagnosis and monitoring of skin water content in various care settings, including point of care and home care. Multispectral/hyperspectral imaging is one of the emerging imaging modalities to visualize and quantify blood supply in surface tissues such as skin or mucosa. It extends the utility of spectroscopy to a large field of view. If this technology was capable of visualizing skin water content alongside with the oxygenation, it would be a useful clinical tool adjuvant to diagnostics of peripheral vascular disease and pressure injuries.

Our group works on multispectral imaging modalities adjuvant to tissue oximetry, which can be used to elucidate various factors affecting the blood supply to tissues. In our previous works, we have demonstrated the feasibility of multispectral methemoglobin visualization in the tissue [7] and the impact of methemoglobin presence on oximetry results [8]. The scope of the current study is to assess the feasibility of multispectral imaging of water content in the skin.

30.2 Methods

The feasibility of water content imaging in the skin using a 970 nm band was assessed through numerical calculations and multispectral imaging.

30.2.1 Imaging

The Multi-Spectral Imaging Device (MSID) (Swift Medical Inc., Toronto) is a multispectral imaging system for visualization of the distribution of oxy- and deoxyhemoglobins, methemoglobin, water, and melanin in the skin. The MSID consists of an illumination unit (a ten wavelength light source (630, 660, 690, 735, 810, 830, 850, 880, 940, and 970 nm)), a scientific-grade camera (a 12-bit NIR-enhanced monochrome camera acA1300-60gmNIR (Basler, Germany)), and a processing unit, which coordinates them. The illumination unit produces a sequence of light flashes, each flash at a particular wavelength, while the camera captures a series of images, each with illumination at a particular wavelength. The acquired images are arranged into a 3D hypercube (λ, i, j) for further processing. The imaging distance is 30 cm and the field of view 7×7 cm.

The skin (hand and forearm) of healthy volunteers was imaged using the MSID. In order to have a contrast of water content distribution, the skin segments with large superficial veins were imaged. In this case, one can expect that the area above the vein will have larger water content than nearby areas.

30.2.2 Processing

During each measurement, the MSID device captures 11 images: 10 with illumination at a particular wavelength and 1 without additional illumination (ambient light only). The processing consists of the following consequential steps: (a) calculate diff images (subtract the image without additional illumination from the image with illumination at a particular wavelength), (b) obtain reflectance images by dividing the diff image by the diff image of the reference object, (c) extract index of absorption μ_a from reflectance using tissue light transport model (e.g., Beer-Lambert), and (d) extract tissue chromophore concentrations using least square fitting.

To emulate a compact device scenario, various subsets of captured images (two or three of them) were used to extract water content. The MSID device uses the 12-bit scientific-grade camera. To emulate the use of a consumer-grade camera (8-bit), four least significant bits for each pixel value of a 12-bit image were discarded. False-color maps were used to visualize water content.

30.3 Results

In lean individuals, water accounts for 60% of total body weight. Total body water is divided between the intracellular and extracellular spaces; the latter further comprises the intravascular plasma volume and the extravascular interstitial volume [9]. Different tissues have different water content, an extracellular fluid fraction (ECF) of total water [10], and interstitial fluid volume (IFV).

Calculations based on a model presented in [11] show that we can expect approximately −0.4% change in reflectance for every 1% increase in the absorption coefficient at 970 nm. Given that the water is the primary absorber in this range, we can expect that it will be possible to detect even preclinical peripheral edema with an expected increase in water content. In particular, if we assume 50% increase in IFV, then the final water content (WC_f) can be found using initial water content (WC_i) and extracellular fluid fraction (ECF) using the following formula:

$$WC_f = \frac{1.5 * WC_i * ECF + WC_i * (1 - ECF)}{1.5 * WC_i * ECF + (1 - WC_i * ECF)} \quad (30.1)$$

Based on Eq. (30.1), we can expect 5–6% increase in total water content in the skin, adipose tissue, and connective tissue (see Table 30.1), which will translate into 2–2.4% change in tissue reflectance. This difference can be detected even by consumer-grade 8-bit cameras.

To validate these high-level estimations, we have processed the multispectral images of the skin. On the first step to establishing a benchmark, we extracted water content using all ten illumination channels.

Then, the subsets of images were used to extract water content per pixel using the normal equation [12] to solve the least squares fitting problem. In particular, two and three wavelength subsets were used. To limit the number of possible permutations, only subsets containing 970 nm were considered. In Fig. 30.1, one can see water content reconstruction using two (630 and 970 nm) and three (630, 660, and 970 nm) wavelengths (panels a and c, respectively). Cross sections at 600th (orange line) and 800th (blue line) columns using two and three wavelengths are depicted in panels b and d, respectively.

Table 30.1 Initial and expected water content for 50% increase in IFV for different tissue types

Tissue	WC_i, % [10]	ECF, % [10]	WC_f, %
Skin	72	95	79.1
Skeletal muscle	76	16	77.4
Adipose tissue	14	80 (85)	18.5 (18.8)
Connective tissue	80	100	85.7

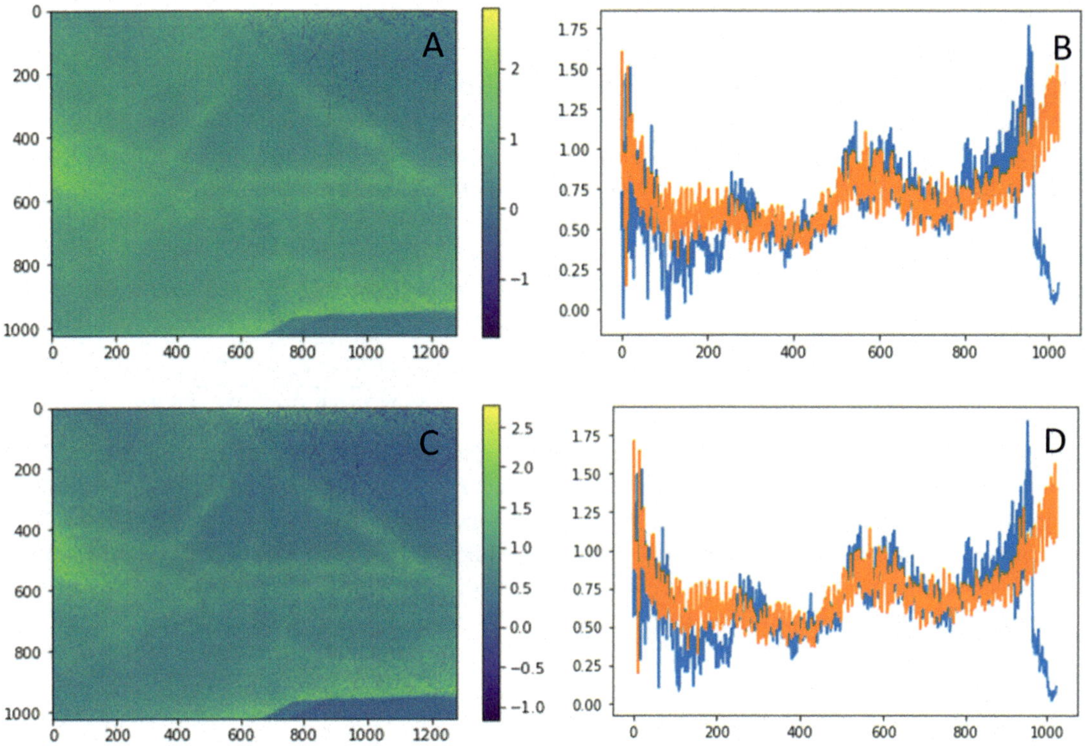

Fig. 30.1 Water content reconstruction maps using two and three wavelengths (panels **a** and **c**, respectively) and cross sections at 600th (orange line) and 800th (blue line) columns using two and three wavelengths (panels **b** and **d**, respectively). Water content (color bar on panels **a** and **c** and *y*-axis on panels **b** and **d**) is displayed in arbitrary units

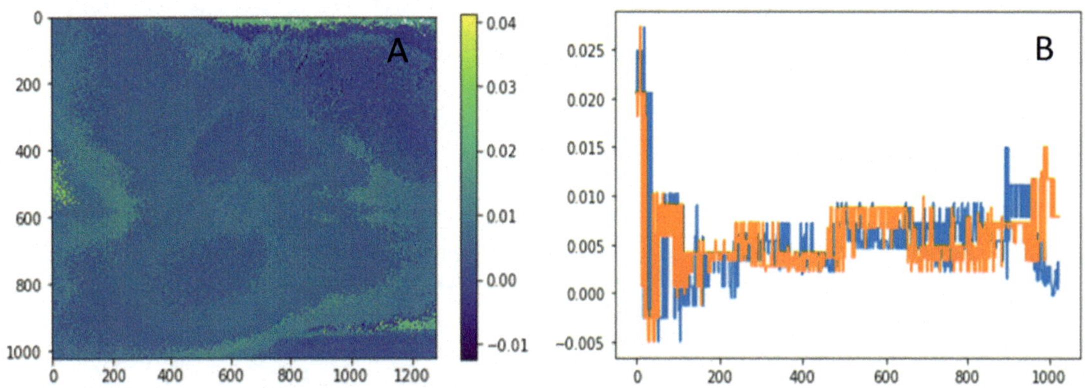

Fig. 30.2 Water content reconstruction map (panel **a**) and cross sections (panel **b**) at 600th (orange line) and 800th (blue line) columns using 8-bit images. Water content (color bar on panel **a** and *y*-axis on panel **b**) is displayed in arbitrary units

Finally, to emulate the use of an 8-bit camera, we discarded four least significant bits and applied the processing algorithm to two and three wavelength subsets. In Fig. 30.2, one can see water content reconstruction using 8-bit images (Fig. 30.2, panel a) for a two wavelength subset (630, 970 nm) similar to 12-bit reconstruction (Fig. 30.1, panel a). Cross sections at 600th (orange line) and 800th (blue line) columns using 8-bit images are depicted in panel b.

30.4 Conclusions

Our rough calculations and initial experiments show the feasibility of water content imaging in the skin.

Two and three wavelengths (including 970 nm) are sufficient to extract water content. There is no noticeable improvement in water content reconstruction with three wavelengths (panels c and d, Fig. 30.1) over the two wavelength case (panels a and b, Fig. 30.1). Even the use of a single band at 970 nm (results not presented in this article) allows seeing the contrast, which may be sufficient for qualitative purposes. However, several (at least two) wavelengths are required for quantitative measurements and to improve the robustness of the algorithm.

The difference between water content reconstruction using 12-bit (panels a and b, Fig. 30.1) and 8-bit (panels a and b, Fig. 30.2) images is more noticeable; however, even 8-bit image reconstruction retains all major features.

The current study was designed to prove the concept. Due to the complexity to control or even measure water content in the skin, there is a great need for realistic lab models with well-controlled parameters. The focus of future work will be to create such water-responsive skin models. In future work, we also plan to conduct more rigorous validations on volunteers.

In summary, rough numerical calculations and initial experiments show the feasibility of water content imaging in the skin using a 970 nm band.

References

1. Vaupel P (1976) Effect of percentual water content in tissue and liquids on the diffusion coefficient of O2, CO2, N2, and H2. Pflügers Arch 361:201–204
2. Seidel HM, Ball JW, Dains JE et al (1995) Heart and blood vessels. In: Schrefer S (ed) Mosby's guide to physical examination, 3rd edn. Mosby, St. Louis, p 419
3. Perrin M, Guex JJ (2000) Edema and leg volume: methods of assessment. Angiology 51(1):9–12
4. Brodovicz KG, McNaughton K, Uemura N et al (2009) Reliability and feasibility of methods to quantitatively assess peripheral edema. Clin Med Res 7(1–2):21–31
5. Hedlund LW, Putman CE (1985) Methods for detecting pulmonary edema. Toxicol Ind Health 1(2):59–68
6. Mayrovitz HN (2007) Assessing local tissue edema in postmastectomy lymphedema. Lymphology 40:87–94
7. Saiko G, Zheng X, Betlen A et al (2018) Visualization of methemoglobin distribution in tissues: phantom validation. Adv Exp Med Biol 1072:387–390
8. Saiko G, Zheng X, Betlen A et al (2020) Fabrication and optical characterization of gelatin-based phantoms for tissue oximetry. Adv Exp Med Biol 1232:369–374
9. Braunwald E (1994) Edema. In: Isselbacher KJ, Braunwald E, Wilson JD et al (eds) Harrison's principles of internal medicine, 13th edn. McGraw-Hill, New York, pp 183–187
10. Bhave G, Neilson EG (2011) Body fluid dynamics: back to the future. J Am Soc Nephrol 22(12):2166–2181
11. Saiko G, Betlen A (2020) Optimization of band selection in multispectral and narrow-band imaging: an analytical approach. Adv Exp Med Biol 1232:361–367
12. Dodge Y (2008) Normal equations. In: The concise encyclopedia of statistics. Springer, New York

Mechanisms of Sound-Induced Opening of the Blood-Brain Barrier

31

O. Semyachkina-Glushkovskaya, D. Bragin, O. Bragina, Y. Yang, A. Abdurashitov, A. Esmat, A. Khorovodov, A. Terskov, M. Klimova, I. Agranovich, I. Blokhina, A. Shirokov, N. Navolokin, V. Tuchin, and J. Kurths

Abstract

The blood-brain barrier (BBB) poses a significant challenge for drug delivery to the brain. The limitations of our knowledge about the nature of BBB explain the slow progress in the therapy of brain diseases and absence of methods for drug delivery to the brain in clinical practice. Here, we show that the BBB opens for high-molecular-weight compounds after exposure to loud sound (100 dB 370 Hz) in rats. The role of stress induced by loud sound and the systemic and molecular mechanisms behind it are discussed in the framework of the BBB. This opens an informative platform for novel fundamental knowledge about the nature of BBB and for the development of a noninvasive brain drug delivery technology.

Keywords

Loud sound · Blood-brain barrier · Mechanisms · Cerebral blood oxygen saturation · Meningeal lymphatic clearance

31.1 Introduction

The blood-brain barrier (BBB) is a highly selective barrier, which controls the penetration of blood-borne agents into the brain or the release of metabolites and ions from the brain tissue to blood. Therefore, the BBB plays a vital role in central nervous system (CNS) health protecting

O. Semyachkina-Glushkovskaya (✉) · A. Abdurashitov · A. Esmat · A. Khorovodov · A. Terskov · M. Klimova · I. Agranovich · I. Blokhina · V. Tuchin
Saratov State University, Saratov, Russia

D. Bragin
Lovelace Biomedical Research Institute, Albuquerque, NM, USA

University of New Mexico School of Medicine, Departments of Neurology and Neurosurgery, Albuquerque, NM, USA

O. Bragina
Lovelace Biomedical Research Institute, Albuquerque, NM, USA

Y. Yang
University of New Mexico, College of Pharmacy, Albuquerque, NM, USA

A. Shirokov
Institute of Biochemistry and Physiology of Plants and Microorganisms, Russian Academy of Sciences, Saratov, Russia

N. Navolokin
Saratov State Medical University, Saratov, Russia

J. Kurths
Saratov State University, Saratov, Russia

Humboldt University, Physics Department, Berlin, Germany

Potsdam Institute for Climate Impact Research, Potsdam, Germany

E. M. Nemoto et al. (eds.), *Oxygen Transport to Tissue XLII*, Advances in Experimental Medicine and Biology 1269, https://doi.org/10.1007/978-3-030-48238-1_31

the brain against pathogens and toxins. Although this protective mechanism is essential for normal functioning of CNS, it also creates a hindrance to the entry of drugs into the brain. In this context, it is not surprising that CNS diseases account for 28% of the total burden of all diseases [1]. This is the reason why approaches for reversible overcoming of the BBB have received significant attention in the last four decades. Currently, over 70 different methods are suggested for overcoming the BBB [2, 3]. Nevertheless, these methods are not widely applied in daily clinical practice for many reasons including invasiveness (e.g., photodynamic opening of the BBB that requires trepanation) [4], challenges in performing (intra-arterial injection of mannitol that usually only a few specialists in clinics can do) [5], limitation of drug concentration (intranasal drug delivery) [6], or small area of treatment (only 1–3 mm at usage of focused ultrasound that opens the BBB with additional use of microbubbles) [7]. All these methods require further studies to improve the reproducibility and technological robustness.

In this study on rats, we demonstrate that a factor such as loud sound, which we can meet in daily life when listening to MP3/MP4 players or at a rock concerts, reversibly opens the BBB to low- and high-molecular-weight molecules. We also discuss mechanisms underlying the sound-related opening of BBB.

31.2 Methods

The experiments were done on four groups: (1) no sound – the control group; 2, 3, and 4–1, 4, and 24 h after sound exposure in freely moving mongrel male rats (250–280 g), respectively; $n = 10$ in each group in all experiments.

To produce loud sound (100 dB, 370 Hz), we used a sound speaker (7A, 12 V, Auto VAZ PJSC, Tolyatti, Russia). The sound exposure was performed using the sequence of 60 s, sound on, and then 60 s – sound off over 2 h.

For quantitative assessment of the BBB permeability, we used (1) fluorescent microscopy for in vivo visualization of extravasation of albumin complex of Evans Blue dye (EBAC, 68.5 kDa, 2 mg/body weight, 1% solution in saline, iv, Sigma-Aldrich) via an optically cleared skull window in anaesthetized rats (2% isoflurane at 1 L/min N_2O/O_2–70:30) [8], (2) a spectrofluorometric assay for ex vivo analysis of EBAC leakage [9], and (3) confocal imaging of extravasation of fluorescein isothiocyanate (FITC)-dextran 70 kDa (FITCD, 1 mg/body weight, 0.5% solution in saline, iv, Sigma-Aldrich).

A custom-made laser speckle contrast imaging (LSCI) system was used to monitor relative cerebral blood flow (rCBF) in the cerebral microvessels and in the sagittal sinus [8, 10]. The blood oxygen saturation (SpO2) in the brain was monitored using a pulse oximeter (model CMS60D, Contec Medical Systems Co., Ltd., Qinhuangdao, China). Oxyhemoglobin saturation is presented as a percentage of HbO2 vs. the total Hb in the blood. LSCI and SpO2 were monitored in the same rats before and at 1h/4h after sound exposure via an optically cleared skull window in anaesthetized rats (2% isoflurane at 1 L/min N_2O/O_2–70:30).

The plasma epinephrine level (ng/ml) was determined using ELISA kits (Abnova, Taiwan) at normal state (before sound), during sound stress (at the last minute (120 min) of sound stress), and in the post-stress period (1h and 4h after sound exposure) in rats ($n = 10$ in each group).

Expression of tight junction (TJ) proteins such as claudin-5 (CLND-5), occludin (Occ), zonula occludens-1 (ZO-1), junctional adhesion molecule (JAM), pericyte marker (NG_2), and lymphatic endothelium (LYVE-1) was evaluated using the standard method of simultaneously combined staining (Abcam protocol) using antibodies for indicated proteins (1:500; Santa Cruz Biotechnology, Santa Cruz, USA) with further confocal microscopy of the rat cerebral cortex or the dura mater (Olympus, Japan).

31.3 Results

31.3.1 Blood-Brain Barrier Opening to High-Molecular-Weight Molecules

In the first step, we demonstrated effects of loud sound on the BBB permeability to EBAC and FITCD in in vivo and ex vivo experiments. Using

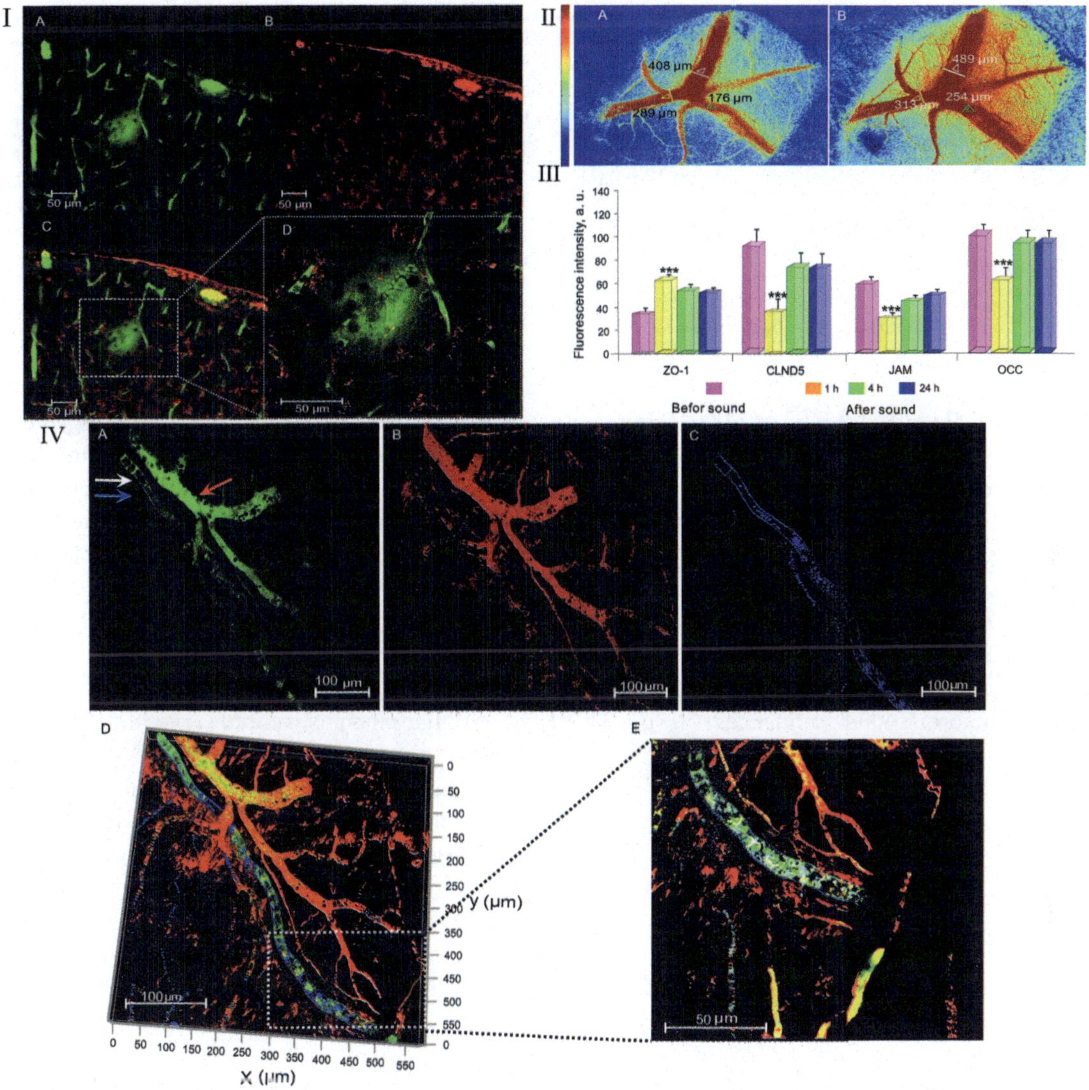

Fig. 31.1 Mechanisms of the sound-induced BBB opening: I – Fluorescent microscopy of EBAC leakage before (A) and 1h after (B) sound exposure. II – Confocal microscopy of the BBB permeability to FITCD before (A–C) and 1h after sound exposure (D–G): A: FITCD is inside of the cerebral vessels (green color), B: the cerebral vessels labelled by pericyte marker NG2 (red color), C: the merged image from A and B, D: FITCD leakage presented as green fluorescence around the cerebral vessel, E: the cerebral vessels labelled by pericyte marker NG2 (red color), F: the merged image from D and E showing FITCD leakage, and G: FITCD leakage at higher magnification from F. III – LSCI of rCBF before (A) and 1h after (B) sound exposure (the time of opening of the BBB). IV – The expression of TJ proteins in the control group (before sound exposure) and 1/4/24 h after sound impact ($n = 10$ for each group): $^{***}p < 0.001$ vs. the control group (before sound). V – The clearance of FITCD from the brain via MLVs after its crossing of the opened BBB: A: the fluorescent signal from FITDC in both anatomical positions of MLV (white arrow) and the cerebral vein (red arrow); B: the cerebral vessels (red color) labelled by NG_2 (pericyte marker); C: MLV (blue color) labelled by LYVE-1 (marker of lymphatic endothelium); D: the merged image from A, B, and C; and E: the same area at higher magnification from D

an in vivo method of real-time fluorescent microscopy, we observed significant EBAC leakage 1h after sound exposure (Fig. 31.1I (A, B)). Afterward, the brains of the same rats were collected for spectrofluorimetric assay and quantitative analysis of the BBB integrity. The results of ex vivo data showed the level of EBAC in the brain tissues was increased 23.1-fold vs. the control group in all rats

Table 31.1 The sound-induced changes in the level of serum epinephrine, rCBF, and SpO_2

	Before sound	After sound			
		0h	1h	4h	24h
rCBF, a.u. (in the sagittal sinus)	0.91 ± 0.05	2.10 ± 0.09 ***	1.84 ± 0.07 **	1.12 ± 0.02	0.97 ± 0.02
rCBF, a.u. (in the cerebral microvessels)	0.37 ± 0.02	0.89 ± 0.04 ***	0.61 ± 0.01 **	0.42 ± 0.03	0. 40 ± 0.01
SpO_2, %	97 ± 3	127 ± 5 *	114 ± 2 *	99 ± 2	97 ± 5
Epinephrine level, ng/ml	5.1 ± 1.9	31.4 ± 5.0 ***	17.0 ± 6.2 **	5.7 ± 2.3	4.9 ± 1.8

***$p < 0.001$; **$p < 0.01$; *$p < 0.05$ vs. the control group (before sound)

(2.61 ± 0.07 vs. 0.11 ± 0.03, $p < 0001$). For qualitative assessment of the BBB permeability, we used confocal imaging of FITCD leakage. Figure 31.1II (D–G) clearly illustrates FITCD extravasation from the cerebral capillaries to the brain tissues 1h after sound exposure. It is important to notice that we did not find an increased BBB permeability to FITCD and EBAC 4h and 24h after sound exposure as well as at the normal state (before sound influences) (Fig. 31.1II (A–C)).

31.3.2 Systemic and Metabolic Responses Induced by Loud Sound

Since loud sound is a stress, we analyzed the general systemic and metabolic stress responses such as changes in the plasma level of epinephrine, rCBF, and SpO_2. The results showed that sound exposure was accompanied by significant increase in epinephrine level vs. the basal value (Table 31.1). The sound stress off was associated with slow normalization of hormone level. One hour after sound exposure, when the BBB was opened, the epinephrine level was decreased but continued to be higher compared with the normal state (Table 31.1). When the BBB closed (4h after sound exposure), the level of epinephrine was over the normal value, and it was not changed to the next day.

LSCI data of rCBF demonstrated an increase in rCBF in both venous and microcirculatory levels immediately after sound stress off (Table 31.1). The BBB opening (1h after sound exposure) was associated with a tendency to normalization of rCBF; however, the level of rCBF was significantly elevated compared to the normal state. Figure 31.1III (A, B) illustrates an increase in rCBF in the time of BBB opening (1h after sound exposure) compared with the control group (before sound). The complete normalization of rCBF was observed at the time of BBB closing (4h after sound exposure) and preserved at the normal level in the next day (Table 31.1).

Similar changes were observed in SpO_2. The sound stress was characterized by a significant increase in SpO_2 that then gradually decreased but continued to be higher at the time of BBB opening (1h after sound exposure) and had returned to the normal values by the time of BBB closing (4 h after sound exposure). In the next day after sound effects on the BBB permeability, we did not observe any changes in SpO_2.

31.3.3 Sound-Induced Changes in TJ Machinery

In the next step, we aimed to study the brain expression of TJ such as CLDN-5, Occ, JAM, and ZO-1 at the time of opening of the BBB (1h after sound) and its recovery (4h and 24h after sound) compared with the control group (before sound exposure). Figure 31.1IV shows that the BBB opening was accompanied by a decrease in expression of CLDN-5, Occ, and JAM and by an increase in expression of ZO suggesting the disorganization of TJ assembly with fast restoration of expression of TJ proteins 4h after sound exposure and without any further changes in the BBB integrity.

31.3.4 Sound-Induced BBB Opening Is Associated with Activation of Lymphatic Clearance of Molecules Crossing the Opened BBB

The important question is how the brain recovers after the sound-induced opening of BBB. To answer this question, we studied clearance of FITCD from the brain after its crossing of the opened BBB via the meningeal lymphatic vessels (MLVs), which play a crucial role in the brain recovery and clearance [11]. With this aim, FITCD was injected intravenously at the time of full opening of the BBB (1h after sound) and circulated for 5 min. Afterward, the brains were removed, and the meninges were collected for confocal microscopy analysis. The results presented in Fig. 31.1V clearly show the presence of FITCD in MLVs suggesting rapid clearance of FITCD from the brain after its crossing of the opened BBB via MLVs.

31.4 Conclusions

We show that loud sound reversibly opens the BBB via stress-mediated TJ machinery disorganization that is accompanied by elevation of serum epinephrine level, rCBF, and SpO_2, as well as by meningeal lymphatic clearance of molecules crossing the BBB. Our data are consistent with the hypothesis suggesting an important role of stress in the BBB opening via mechanisms underlying epinephrine-induced enhancement of the BBB permeability including (1) vasodilation of cerebral vessels and widening of TJs, (2) changes of ultrastructure of endothelial cells and astroglial endfeet, and (3) an increase in transport and the pinocytotic activity of endothelial cells [12–17]. This method has a high potential for clinical applications as an easily used, noninvasive, low-cost, labeling-free perspective and completely new approach for the treatment of brain diseases. The fact that loud sound, which we can meet in daily life, opens the BBB is socially important and should be considered in daily life.

Acknowledgments This work was supported by grants from the Russian Science Foundation (20-15-00090): Visualization of the meningeal lymphatics; RFBR 20-015-00308a: SpO2 recording; grant from the RF Governmental grant 075-15-2019-1885: Methods for the BBB opening. DB was supported by NIH R01 NS112808.

References

1. Silberberg D, Anand N, Michels K et al (2015) Brain and other nervous system disorders across the lifespan – global challenges and opportunities. Nature 527(7578):S151–S154
2. Mitragotri S (2013) Devices for overcoming biological barriers: the use of physical forces to disrupt the barriers. Adv Drug Deliv Rev 65:100–103
3. Pandey P, Sharma A, Gupta U et al (2016) Blood brain barrier: an overview on strategies in drug delivery, realistic in vitro modeling and in vivo live tracking. Tissue Barriers 4(1):e1129476
4. Semyachkina-Glushkovskaya O, Kurths J, Borisova E et al (2017) Photodynamic opening of blood-brain barrier. Biomed Opt Express 8(11):5040–5048
5. Kiviniemi V, Korhonen V, Kortelainen J et al (2017) Real-time monitoring of human blood-brain barrier disruption. PLoS One 12(3):e0174072
6. Wu S, Li K, Yan Y et al (2013) Intranasal delivery of neural stem cells: a CNS-specific, non-invasive cell-based therapy for experimental autoimmune encephalomyelitis. J Clin Cell Immunol 4(3). https://doi.org/10.4172/2155-9899.1000142
7. Chu P-C, Chai W-Y, Tsai C-H et al (2016) Focused ultrasound-induced blood-brain barrier opening: association with mechanical index and cavitation index analyzed by dynamic contrast-enhanced magnetic-resonance imaging. Sci Rep 6:33264. https://doi.org/10.1038/srep33264
8. Yisong Q, Yu T, Jianyi X et al (2019) FDISCO: advanced solvent-based clearing method for imaging whole organs. Sci Adv 5(1). https://doi.org/10.1126/sciadv.aau8355
9. Wang H-L, Lai TW (2014) Optimization of Evans blue quantitation in limited rat tissue samples. Sci Rep 4:6588. https://doi.org/10.1038/srep06588
10. Abdurashitov A, Lychagov V, Sindeeva O et al (2015) Histogram analysis of laser speckle contrast image for cerebral blood flow monitoring. Front Optoelectron 8(2):187–194
11. Semyachkina-Glushkovskaya O, Postnov D, Kurths J (2018) Blood–brain barrier, lymphatic clearance, and recovery: Ariadne's thread in labyrinths of hypotheses. Int J Mol Sci 19:3818

12. Johansson B, Martinsson L (1980) The blood-brain barrier in adrenaline-induced hypertension: circadian variations and modification by beta-adrenoreceptor antagonists. Acta Nellrol Scand 62:96–102
13. Murphy V, Johanson C (1985) Adrenergic-induced enhancement of brain barrier system permeability to small nonelectrolytes: choroid plexus versus cerebral capillaries. JCBFM 5:01–12
14. Sarmento A, Borges N, Azevedo I (1991) Adrenergic influences on the control of blood-brain barrier permeability. Naunyn Schmiedeberg's Arch Pharmacol 343(6):633–637
15. Chi O, Wang G, Chang Q, Weisss H (1998) Effects of isoproterenol on blood-brain barrier permeability in rats. Neurol Res 20(3):259–264
16. Akihiko U, Grubb J, Babks W, Sly W (2007) Epinephrine enhances lysosomal enzyme delivery across the blood-brain barrier by up-regulation of the mannose 6-phosphate receptor. PNAS 104(31):12873–12878
17. Santha P, Veszelka S, Hoyk Z, Meszaros M et al (2016) Restrain stress-induced morphological changes at the blood-brain barrier in adult rats. Front Mo Neurosci 8:88. https://doi.org/10.3389/fnmol.2015.00088

Multimodal Measurements of Brain Tissue Metabolism and Perfusion in a Neonatal Model of Hypoxic-Ischaemic Injury

32

Gemma Bale, Ajay Rajaram, Matthew Kewin, Laura Morrison, Alan Bainbridge, Linshan Liu, Udunna Anazodo, Mamadou Diop, Keith St Lawrence, and Ilias Tachtsidis

Abstract

This is the first multimodal study of cerebral tissue metabolism and perfusion post-hypoxic-ischaemic (HI) brain injury using broadband near-infrared spectroscopy (bNIRS), diffuse correlation spectroscopy (DCS), positron emission tomography (PET) and magnetic resonance spectroscopy (MRS). In seven piglet preclinical models of neonatal HI, we measured cerebral tissue saturation (StO_2), cerebral blood flow (CBF), cerebral oxygen metabolism ($CMRO_2$), changes in the mitochondrial oxidation state of cytochrome c oxidase (oxCCO), cerebral glucose metabolism (CMRglc) and tissue biochemistry (Lac+Thr/tNAA). At baseline, the parameters measured in the piglets that experience HI (not controls) were 64 ± 6% StO_2, 35 ± 11 ml/100 g/min CBF and 2.0 ± 0.4 μmol/100 g/min CMRO2. After HI, the parameters measured were 68 ± 6% StO_2, 35 ± 6 ml/100 g/min CBF, 1.3 ± 0.1 μmol/100 g/min $CMRO_2$, 0.4 ± 0.2 Lac+Thr/tNAA and 9.5 ± 2.0 CMRglc. This study demonstrates the capacity of a multimodal set-up to interrogate the pathophysiology of HIE using a combination of optical methods, MRS, and PET.

Keywords

Near-infrared spectroscopy · Diffuse correlation spectroscopy · Metabolism · Hypoxic ischaemic encephalopathy

32.1 Introduction

Hypoxic-ischaemic encephalopathy (HIE) is responsible for a quarter of neonatal deaths globally and is one of the largest causes of preventable childhood disabilities such as cerebral palsy [1]. The injury evolves throughout treatment, so a continuous monitoring of brain tissue health deployed at the cotside is highly desirable. The progression of the brain health during HIE can be

G. Bale (✉) · I. Tachtsidis
Biomedical Optics Research Laboratory, University College London, London, UK
e-mail: g.bale@ucl.ac.u

A. Rajaram · M. Kewin · L. Morrison · L. Liu · U. Anazodo · M. Diop · K. S. Lawrence
Medical Biophysics, Western University, and Lawson Health Research Institute, London, ON, Canada

A. Bainbridge
Medical Physics, University College London Hospital, London, UK

E. M. Nemoto et al. (eds.), *Oxygen Transport to Tissue XLII*, Advances in Experimental Medicine and Biology 1269, https://doi.org/10.1007/978-3-030-48238-1_32

characterised in terms of the metabolism, progressing from a 'latent phase' where metabolism recovers, to normal levels, to 'secondary energy failure' which may cause further injury. The metabolic state after HIE can be measured using proton (^1H) magnetic resonance spectroscopy (MRS) [2]. The ^1H MRS-derived thalamic Lac/NAA peak area ratio is a robust predictor of neurodevelopmental outcome in babies with HIE and has been used as a surrogate outcome measure in clinical neuroprotection studies of HIE. This metabolic information is vital for prognostication but only gives a snapshot of the cerebral injury at a particular time point, usually after treatment has been completed. Glucose consumption, measured by FDG PET, is valuable but is also non-continuous and requires injection of radioisotopes so is not ideal for neonatal care [3].

Diffuse optics provides a continuous measurement of brain metabolism. Broadband near-infrared spectroscopy (bNIRS) yields information about cerebral haemodynamics (via oxy- and deoxyhaemoglobin: HbO_2 and HHb, respectively), tissue oxygenation (StO_2) and metabolism from cytochrome c oxidase (CCO). CCO is the terminal electron acceptor in the electron transport chain (ETC): the final stage of oxidative metabolism [4]. We have recently shown that the signal is associated with the level of HI injury [5]. Another optical technique, diffuse correlation spectroscopy (DCS), measures an index of cerebral blood flow, which, combined with oxygenation from NIRS and pulse oximetry, measures cerebral metabolic rate of oxygen ($CMRO_2$) [6]. We have recently shown that it is possible to simultaneously measure CBF and CCO [7]; the aim of this study is to demonstrate how through a combination of optics (bNIRS, DCS), FDG PET and MR measurements we can obtain a full description of the haemodynamic, oxygenation and metabolism status of the brain following HI.

32.2 Methods

32.2.1 Animal Model of HI

This study was approved by the Animal Use Subcommittee of the Canadian Council on Animal Care at Western University (London, Ontario). Piglets were anesthetised under 3% isoflurane during preparatory surgery (2% post surgery), tracheotomised and mechanically ventilated on an oxygen-medical air mixture. Incisions were made lateral to the trachea, and vascular occluders were placed around the carotid arteries posterior to the clavicle (In Vivo Metric, CA). Catheters were inserted into an ear vein for injections and into a femoral artery to monitor vitals (SurgiVet, Smiths Medical, MN), as well as to collect arterial blood samples for gas and glucose analyses. SaO_2 was measured via a pulse oximeter attached to the piglet's right forelimb. The bNIRS and DCS emission/detection fibres were secured to the piglet's left brain, avoiding the sagittal sinus, using an in-house 3D-printed probe holder.

The HI insult was induced by first inflating the occluders around the carotid arteries, followed by reducing the inspired oxygen from 21% to 8%. bNIRS and DCS data were acquired continuously throughout the insult, starting 5 minutes prior to carotid clamping to acquire baseline measurements. The real-time DCS flow index was used to confirm successful clamping, i.e. an immediate drop in CBF. Following this confirmation, inspired oxygen concentration was reduced, and the HI insult was maintained for a minimum duration of 10 minutes once the blood flow index reached its nadir. At the end of the HI insult, recovery was initiated by deflating the carotid occluders and returning oxygen supply to baseline levels.

Data were recorded from seven newborn piglets (four female, aged 10–40 hours): severe HI injury was induced in five piglets and there were two controls.

32.2.2 Measurements of Cerebral Metabolism

Cerebral metabolism was assessed by different modalities: bNIRS and DCS continuously before, during and after the HI and MRS and PET after HI.

The optical device has been fully described previously [7] and is described here briefly. Essentially, it is a bNIRS device and a DCS device which were run synchronously with a system of shutters to avoid crosstalk between them. The bNIRS device consists of a halogen bulb (Ocean Optics HL-2000-HP) and a custom-made spectrometer (iDus Andor camera, Oxford Instruments; P&P Optica, ON, Canada). For the DCS system, the light source was a long coherence length, continuous-wave laser emitting at 785 nm (DL785–100 s, CrystaLaser, NV) and the detector a single-photon counting module (SPCM-AQR4C, Excelitas, QC, Canada). The output of the SPCM was fed into a correlator board (Flex033LQ-1, Correlator.com, NJ) to generate normalised intensity autocorrelation functions.

The continuous recording of bNIRS and DCS data was set on a 14 s cycle, acquiring 12 bNIRS spectra over 3 s, followed by two DCS measurements over the following 10s, with a 0.5 s delay. These measurements were collected continuously before, during and after HI. Ninety min post HI, the DCS data was calibrated by measuring absolute CBF by DCE-NIRS [8]. The DCE-NIRS protocol consisted of a bolus injection of indocyanine green (ICG, 0.1 mg/kg) into a cannulated vein. The CBF was measured by monitoring the cerebral ICG concentration with bNIRS and the time-varying arterial ICG concentration by a dye densitometer attached to a front paw (DDG 2001, Nihon Kohden, Japan).

Magnetic resonance imaging and spectroscopy and FDG PET were performed after the optical monitoring on a 3 T Biograph mMR scanner (Siemens Healthcare). MR scans included measurements of (lactate + threonine)/(NAA + NAAG) (Lac+Thr/tNAA) from the left hemisphere cortex (ant) and thalamus (bas) with proton (^{1}H) MRS (PRESS: TR = 2 s; TE = 135 or 288 ms) (Fig. 32.1).

32.2.3 Data Analysis

bNIRS: The changes in chromophore concentrations (oxCCO, HbO_2 and HHb) were calculated from the measured changes in broadband near-infrared light attenuation using the modified Beer-Lambert law as applied with the UCLn algorithm [4] across 136 wavelengths (771–906 nm) with a fixed differential path length factor of 4.39 (preterm head) and 3 cm optode separation. To measure absolute StO_2, the spectral data were analysed using the solution to the diffusion approximation for a semi-infinite medium [9]. The absorption coefficient was defined as the sum of the three largest chromophores: HHb, HbO_2 and water. Chromophore concentrations and the scattering terms were determined in a series of steps involving fitting the numerical derivatives of the theoretical model (i.e. the analytical solution to the diffusion approximation) to the derivative spectra.

An algorithm was developed to quantify the recovery of Δ[HbT], Δ[HbDiff], Δ[oxCCO], StO_2 and CBF 1 hour after HI. Data at baseline and recovery were averaged over a 1 min window to calculate the recovery fraction of each signal relative to baseline. All the measurements were normalised against the nadir point:

$$\text{Recovery Fraction}\left(\text{RF}\right)=\frac{\text{Recovery}-\text{Nadir}}{\text{Baseline}-\text{Nadir}}\times 100\%$$

MRS data were analysed using Tarquin [10]. The fitted amplitudes of Lac and Thr were combined because they are not resolvable in in vivo spectra [11].

32.3 Results

Measured attenuation spectra and autocorrelation curves from this data set have been previously presented [7]. Figure 32.2 presents an example of the optical signals obtained and the resulting recovery fractions. The full results with all final absolute metabolic variables are shown in Table 32.1. At baseline, the parameters measured in the piglets that experienced HI (not controls) were 64 ± 6% StO_2, 35 ± 11 ml/100 g/min CBF and 2.0 ± 0.4 μmol/100 g/min $CMRO_2$. After HI, the parameters measured were 68 ± 6% StO_2, 35 ± 6 ml/100 g/min CBF, 1.3 ± 0.1 μmol/100 g/min $CMRO_2$, 0.4 ± 0.2 Lac+Thr/tNAA and 9.5 ± 2.0 CMRglc.

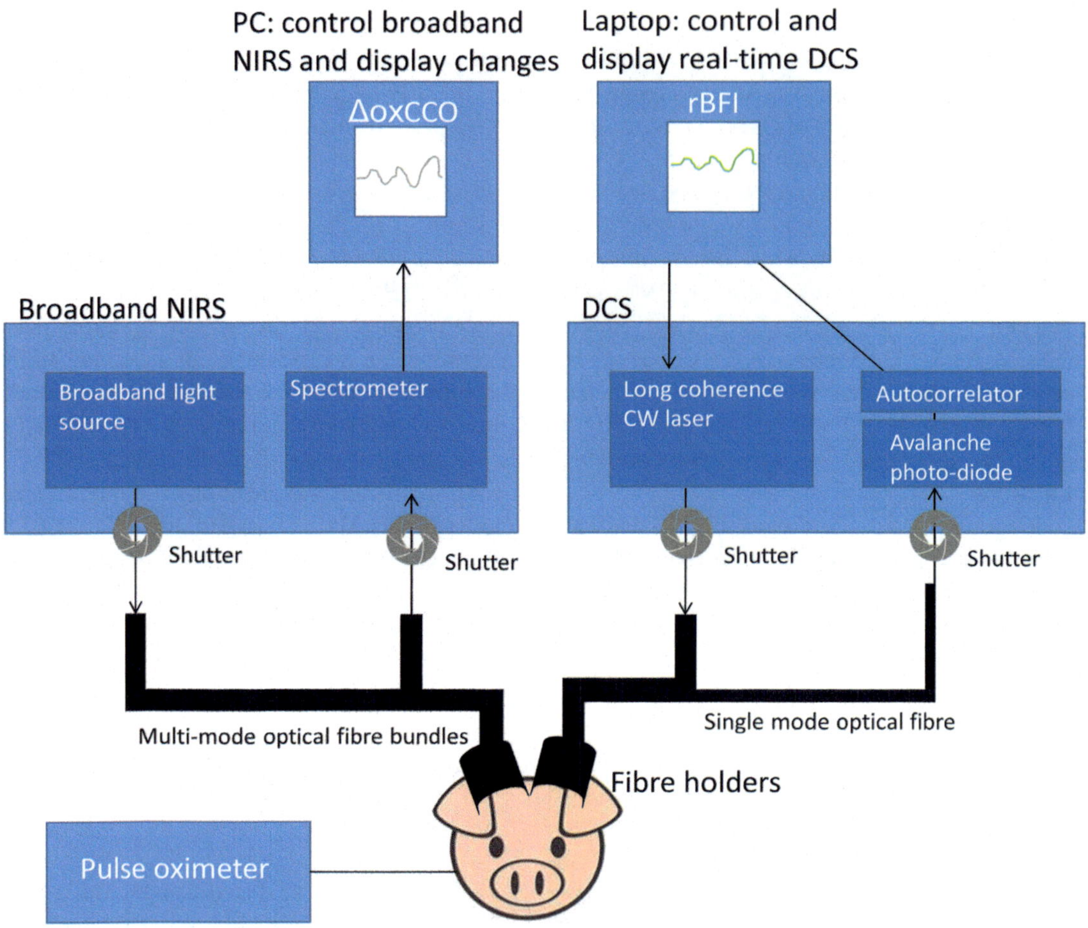

Fig. 32.1 Optical instrumentation for continuous broadband NIRS and DCS measurements

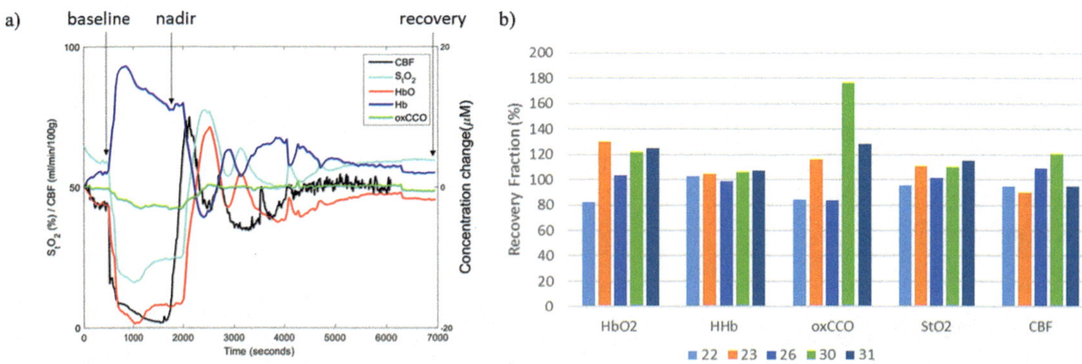

Fig. 32.2 (**a**) Example of optical signals used to calculate recovery fraction (from piglet 26). (**b**) Recovery fractions 1 hour after HI for all optical signals for all HI piglets

Table 32.1 Piglet details and final cerebral measurements. Units: CBF ml/100 g/min, $CMRO_2$ μmol/100 g/min, MRS is Lac+Thr/total NAA and CMRglc μmol/100 g/min. MRS data is missing in some anatomical locations for some animals due to low SNR

Pig	Age (hours)	Weight (kg)	Sex	HI (mins)	StO_2 (%)	CBF	$CMRO_2$	MRS Ant	MRS Bas	CMRglc
20	12	1.4	F	0	65.2	33.6	1.2		0.04	8.44
22	23	1.2	F	10	70.4	35.7	1.2		0.11	8.58
23	10	1.6	M	20	71.7	39.2	1.4		0.57	7.04
26	24	1.5	M	20	64.1	42.0	1.2	0.24	0.35	13.20
28	28	1.9	F	0	45.2	45.5	3.9	0.20	0.29	13.72
30	20	1.8	M	20	75.4	30.8	1.4	0.37	0.39	9.58
31	40	1.7	F	20	59.0	26.6	1.3	0.45		9.10

32.4 Discussion

In this work, we have demonstrated the ability of optical monitoring (bNIRS and DCS) to obtain metabolic information aligned with ^{1}H MRS and FDG PET in a piglet model of HIE. Further, due to the non-invasive, cotside nature of the optical devices, we highlight the potential for continuous measurements of metabolism. The measured parameters are aligned with those obtained by another device working alone; Kaynezhad et al. observed similar changes in HbO_2, HHb and oxCCO during a piglet model of HI [12], and the BFI changes are comparable to those obtained by Rajaram et al. [7].

The recovery fractions obtained with bNIRS and DCS showed that all signals recovered to around 100%, showing that the brain was able to recover to normal levels of oxygenation and metabolism after the insult suggesting that the injury was mild [13]. These optical measures agree with the results from the MR-PET which shown little difference in the recovered metabolic parameters between the control animals and the animals who experienced HI. This may be due to the measurements (both optical and MR-PET) being obtained within the first few hours post HI when the piglets are likely to be in the 'latent phase' of HIE.

This is one of the limitations of this study. Other limitations include the low number of animals involved due to technical issues with the multimodal monitoring which restricts our ability to perform statistical analysis at this stage. Future work includes increasing the number of animals studied and increasing the time between insult and final measurement to capture the metabolic decline during secondary energy failure.

Acknowledgements This research was funded by the Wellcome Trust, grant 104580/Z/14/Z, and an operating grant from the Canadian Institutes of Health Research (St Lawrence).

References

1. Chalak LF, Tian F, Tarumi T, Zhang R (2016) Cerebral hemodynamics in asphyxiated newborns undergoing hypothermia therapy: pilot findings using a multiple-time-scale analysis. Pediatr Neurol 55:30–36
2. Mitra S et al (2019) Proton magnetic resonance spectroscopy lactate/N-acetylaspartate within 2 weeks of birth accurately predicts 2-year motor, cognitive and language outcomes in neonatal encephalopathy after therapeutic hypothermia. Arch Dis Child Fetal Neonatal Ed 104(4):F424–F432
3. Thorngren-Jerneck K et al (2001) Cerebral glucose metabolism measured by positron emission tomography in term newborn infants with hypoxic ischemic encephalopathy. Pediatr Res 49(4):495–501
4. Bale G, Elwell CE, Tachtsidis I (2016) From Jöbsis to the present day: a review of clinical near-infrared spectroscopy measurements of cerebral cytochrome-c-oxidase. J Biomed Opt 21(9):091307
5. Bale G et al (2019) Oxygen dependency of mitochondrial metabolism indicates outcome of newborn brain injury. J Cereb Blood Flow Metab 39(10):2035–2047
6. Durduran T, Choe R, Baker WB, Yodh AG (2010) Diffuse optics for tissue monitoring and tomography. Reports Prog Phys 73(7):076701
7. Rajaram A et al (2018) Simultaneous monitoring of cerebral perfusion and cytochrome c oxidase by combining broadband near-infrared spectroscopy and diffuse correlation spectroscopy. Biomed Opt Express 9(6):2588–2603

8. Cooper JA et al (2011) Continuous monitoring of absolute cerebral blood flow by near-infrared spectroscopy during global and focal temporary vessel occlusion. J Appl Physiol 110(6):1691–1698
9. Yeganeh HZ, Toronov V, Elliott JT, Diop M, Lee T-Y, Lawrence KS (2012) Broadband continuous-wave technique to measure baseline values and changes in the tissue chromophore concentrations. Biomed Opt Express 3(11):2761–2770
10. Wilson M, Reynolds G, Kauppinen RA, Arvanitis TN, Peet AC (2011) A constrained least-squares approach to the automated quantitation of in vivo (1)H magnetic resonance spectroscopy data. Magn Reson Med 65(1):1–12
11. Kreis R, Hofmann L, Kuhlmann B, Boesch C, Bossi E, Hüppi PS (2002) Brain metabolite composition during early human brain development as measured by quantitative in vivo 1H magnetic resonance spectroscopy. Magn Reson Med 48(6):949–958
12. Kaynezhad P et al (2019) Quantification of the severity of hypoxic-ischemic brain injury in a neonatal preclinical model using measurements of cytochrome-c-oxidase from a miniature broadband-near-infrared spectroscopy system. Neurophotonics 6(04):1

Cerebral Spreading Depression Transient Disruption of Cross-Frequency Coupling in the Rat Brain: Preliminary Observations

33

Tongsheng Zhang and Edwin M. Nemoto

Abstract

Normal brain function requires an integrated, simultaneous communication between brain regions in a coordinated manner. In our studies on cortical spreading depolarization (CSD) induced electrically in the rat brain while recording electrocorticography (ECoG) and delta wave activity, we found for the first time that CSD suppressed delta wave activity, which began even before the CSD was fully developed. We pursued this observation to determine whether repeated CSD suppressed delta wave activity in rats. CSD was produced by electrical stimulation of the neocortex while recording the development of CSD and changes in the coupling of low-frequency band cross coupling to four typical physiological neuronal activity frequency bands, i.e., 5–7 Hz, 8–12 Hz, 13–30 Hz, and 30–80 Hz. Band-pass filters were applied to achieve the corresponding physiological band signals. Besides the cross-frequency coupling (CFC) analysis, the distribution of delta wave density in time domain was analyzed. We calculated the delta wave density per 30 seconds but represent the density as frequency per minute. A Generalized Linear Models (GLM) was used to carry out the CFC analysis in Matlab. Because delta waves dominated the ECoG recorded, we modeled the higher-frequency amplitude envelope as a function of low-frequency phase using a spline basis. Besides the CFC analysis, we also characterized the distribution of the delta wave density in time domain. Four CFC, Theta, Alpha, Beta, and Gamma were at very small values after CSD, and after about 8 minutes, the CFC recovered to the pre-CSD level. CFC were seen to decrease *before* a CSD occurred at the higher-frequency bands and tended to decrease quickly. Whether the attenuated CFC by CSD has long-term consequences remains to be determined. Future studies will explore the impact of cortical CSD on CFC with deeper brain structures, including the thalamus and the caudate putamen.

Keywords

Brain · Cortical spreading depression · Cross-frequency coupling · Delta waves · Electroencephalogram

T. Zhang · E. M. Nemoto (✉)
Department of Neurosurgery, University of New Mexico, Albuquerque, NM, USA
e-mail: enemoto@salud.unm.edu

E. M. Nemoto et al. (eds.), *Oxygen Transport to Tissue XLII*, Advances in Experimental Medicine and Biology 1269, https://doi.org/10.1007/978-3-030-48238-1_33

33.1 Introduction

Normal brain function requires coordinated communication between different brain regions on a short time scale in as simple a task as reading novel that is pleasurable or frightening. It requires the activation of the visual cortex, word recognition, memory recall of words, and memory recall of personal experiences and emotional content pleasurable or not in the amygdala and the medial-lateral temporal lobe. The concept of this organization of the brain was brought to fore by Raichle et al. [1–3]. Along this line of the integration of brain function also requires the functional coordination of the brain in very short if not an instantaneous time frame, which brings us to the existence of electrical cross-frequency coupling (CFC) which has also been a topic of intense interest as it relates to the functional organization of the brain combined with the role of functional MRI elucidating the resting state [4, 5] and its alteration in altered brain function [6, 7].

Since Leao [8] first demonstrated the occurrence of suppression of the electroencephalogram (EEG), the role of cortical spreading depolarizations (CSDs) and its role in increasing the severity of brain damage sustained after traumatic brain injury or cerebrovascular accidents have been well recognized and presented clinically over the past 20 years [9, 10] primarily through the persistent effort of Dr. Strong through the COSBID group [10]. It was in this environment that we came upon studying the effect of repetitive CSD on the injury to the brain and the observation for the first time that CSD suppressed cortical CFC coupling suppression of the delta frequency in CFC.

CFC supports the resting state neuronal network where lower-frequency activities engage larger brain areas that modulate spatially localized fast oscillations, known as cross-frequency coupling (CFC). CFC plays a fundamental role in connecting different regions of a brain to work as a whole [4]. CSD suppresses the underlying neurons temporarily losing connections to the rest of the brain. After the CSD, the affected neurons are gradually reconnected back to default network at rest in the brain. Thus, CSD interrupts the default network. Our interest is to explore how the affected neurons are connected back to the brain default network at rest after the connection is interrupted by the CSD and the function of cross-frequency coupling.

33.2 Material and Methods

33.2.1 Animal Model

Twelve male Sprague Dawley rats weighing 350–400 grams body weight were anesthetized with urethane 1.5 g/kg, i.p. The animal under anesthesia corresponds to stage N3 slow-wave sleep, with delta waves accounting for 20% or more of the EEG recording. The rats were intubated, and their lungs mechanically ventilated with 30% oxygen and 70% nitrogen with arterial blood gases and pH controlled within normal limits. Blood electrolytes and glucose and lactate were measured on a GEM4000 (Instrumentation Labs, Bedford, MA). Femoral artery and vein catheters were inserted for blood pressure monitoring, blood sampling, and fluid replacement with Lactated Ringers, 1.0 ml/hr. The rats were fixed in stereotaxic frame, and Ag/AgCl ball electrodes were inserted over the parietal cortex covering the somatosensory cortex. The electrodes were made from silver wire (125 micrometer in diameter with 25 micrometer of Teflon coating) by shaping the ball at the tip in flame of a lab lamp.

33.2.2 Recording System and Electrodes

Ag/AgCl ball bipolar electrodes were inserted over the parietal cortex covering the somatosensory cortex. The cortical recording electrodes were connected to high input impedance bioamplifiers (BIOPAC, Goleta, CA). The sampling frequency was set as high as 10 KHz and the data saved every hour. The reference electrode was attached to the left ear with conductive gel to ensure good contact. Before the application of any cortical electrical stimulation, background brain activities were recorded to establish baseline CFC.

33.2.3 Data Analysis

The data were preprocessed by removal of power line noise and transient interference and down sampled to 1 KHz to reduce the memory usage. We used the Generalized Linear Models (GLMs) in Matlab for CFC analysis [11]. Delta waves dominated the ECoG recorded during sleep stage N3; therefore, we modeled the higher-frequency amplitude envelope as a function of the low-frequency phase using a spline basis. Briefly, this modeling frame first finds a null model, representing the null hypothesis of no CFC. Then, a spline model is employed to fit a smooth function for the expected amplitude as a function of the phase slow waves. The amplitudes over different phases evenly spanned over 2π phase space were estimated based on those two models, and a ratio r of the amplitudes from the above two models was then derived. The maximum r is selected to describe the coupling intensity between low-frequency phase to higher-frequency amplitude, which will be denoted later. Visual inspection of the data indicates that the ECoG contains strong delta and slow waves, and we then select lower delta waves at 0.1–2 Hz and employ its phase as a predictor in GLM procedure. The phases are wrapped to $-\pi$ to π. We then study the phase of this low-frequency band cross coupling to four typical physiological neuronal activity frequency bands, i.e., ϑ (5–7 Hz), α (8–12 Hz), β (13–30 Hz), and γ (30–80 Hz). FIR band-pass filter was applied to achieve the corresponding physiological band signals.

We also characterized the distribution of the delta wave density in time domain. We first established a delta wave pattern and then used a pattern-matching approach to find all delta waves in the recording. In order to illustrate its changes with time more clearly, we calculate the delta wave density per 30 seconds but represent the density as frequency per minute. All the analysis programs were implemented in Matlab.

After preprocessing the data, each CFC analysis is carried out over 2 minutes of dataset. The procedure is continuously applied to the data before and after a CSD. The CFC analysis did not include CSD duration due to a lack of spontaneous activities. A typical CFC result (slow-wave phase to Gamma band amplitude) provides a coupling intensity index r that is defined in the equation below. The maximum of the amplitude Amax provided by the spline model is found. The coupling intensity r is then defined as follows:

$$r = \mathrm{abs}\left(1 - \frac{\mathrm{Amax}}{\mathrm{Ao}}\right)$$

where Ao is the amplitude from Null Model.

33.3 Results

Spontaneous CSD and CFC changes are shown in Fig. 33.1. For these spontaneous CSD, CFCs always decrease just before a CSD. Right after the CSD, the CFCs are smaller than normal at baseline. With repetitive CSD, the CFC at low-frequency bands, i.e., ϑ, tend to recover; however, the higher-frequency bands, i.e., β and γ, tend to decrease rapidly.

We mass averaged 4 CFCs over 12 animals over all the CSD. During 10 minutes recovery after a CSD, the CFCs gradually return to normal (Fig. 33.2). A mass average of the uncoupling and restoration of coupling after repetitive CSD is shown in Fig. 33.3.

The changes in delta wave density for evoked repetitive CSD and suppression of delta wave activity occurs in electrically, KCl, and spontaneous CSD (Fig. 33.4). Generally speaking, the delta wave density gradually recovers after a CSD, but the trend with repetitive CSD gradually decreased, indicating potential damage to the underlying neurons (Fig. 33.5).

33.4 Discussion and Conclusions

In this paper, we describe how CSD temporarily interrupts the default neuronal connections in resting brain and how those affected neurons

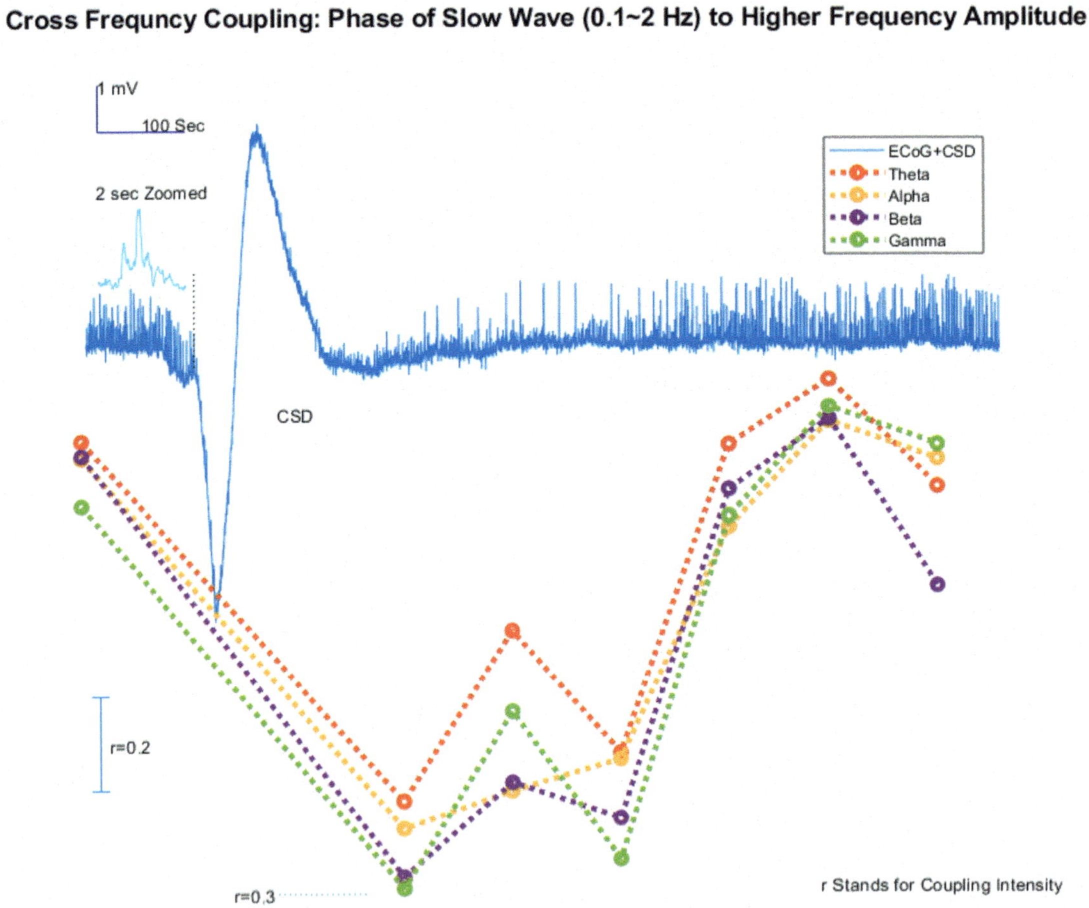

Fig. 33.1 CSD and CFC uncoupling of higher frequencies, i.e., Alpha, Beta, Theta, and Gamma bands. A zoomed 2 second recording right before CSD comes up is shown in the insert at the upper left of the figure, in order to illustrate the typical CFC activities that the higher frequency (referring to the spikes in the wavelet) spikes are clearly visible on top of a slow wave. The coupling strength is quantitatively described by the r value that is diminished during and right after a CSD

reconnect back to the default network in the mechanism of CFC. CSD caused a reduction in spontaneous synaptic and action potential (AP) firing that lasted over an hour. CSD alters both excitatory and inhibitory input, through both pre- and postsynaptic mechanisms, for at least an hour after passage of the wave [12]. Harmony [13] reviewed the role of delta waves in cognitive tasks and proposed that the sustained delta oscillations inhibit the external inferences that may affect the performance of the mental tasks. This role is possibly implemented by modulating the activity of those networks that should be inactive to accomplish the task.

The role of delta waves during mental tasks has been postulated to be associated with cortical deafferentation or with the inhibition of the sensory afferents that interfere with internal concentration [14].The rats were anesthetized and comparable to slow-wave sleep, which consists of rich delta wave activity. We postulate that in the sleep stage, the ubiquitous delta

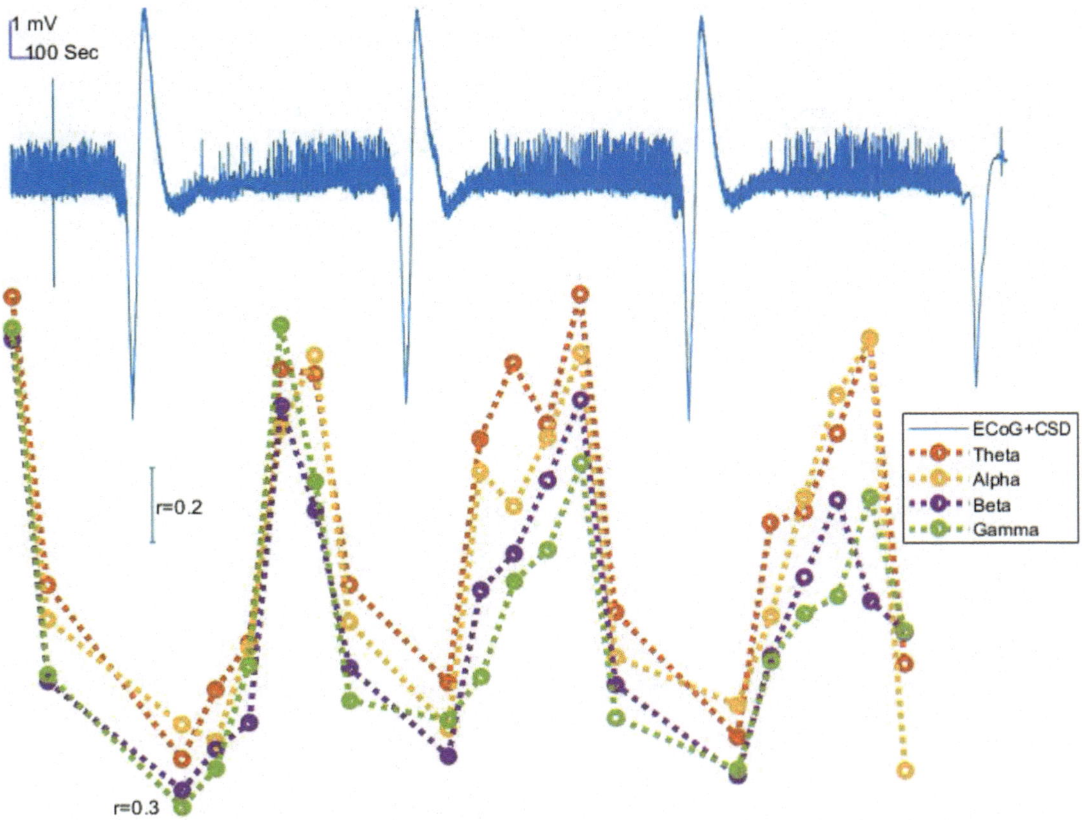

Fig. 33.2 CFC changes with repetitive CSDs. The CFC for higher frequencies, such as Beta and Gamma bands, is attenuated with repetitive CSDs obviously, while, in contrast, Theta and Alpha bands CFC seem to recover faster

waves play a role as suggested by Harmony [13] that the delta waves serve to isolate external stimuli from the default neuronal networks in the brain. In fact, in both human and mammals, there is enhanced delta wave activity after sleep deprivation, suggesting that they desperately attempt to isolate the external inference to achieve sleep [15].

The phase to amplitude CFC is calculated in the typical four physiological frequency bands, i.e., Theta (4–7 Hz), Alpha (7–13 Hz), Beta (13–30 Hz), and Gamma (12–80 Hz). The delta waves modulate CFC recovery during 10 minutes after disruption by a CSD; however, a repetitive CSD train may cause a permanent reduction of the CFC, in particular, at higher-frequency band like Gamma wave. Delta wave-Gamma Amplitude CFC is most affected by CSD. We found that CFC falls to very low values (about $r = 0.3$) after a CSD from about $r > 1$ before CSD using the GLM approach, which we suspect is due to CSD suppression of underlying neurons.

We also observed that CFC was decreasing before the arrival of the CSD. However, we do not know if this is accurate since the data were analyzed every 2 minutes. Shortening this dataset may reveal more details of this interesting change before CSD. Interestingly, before the CSD, the ECoG is unchanged, indicating that the local neurons were not yet affected, but the CFC was

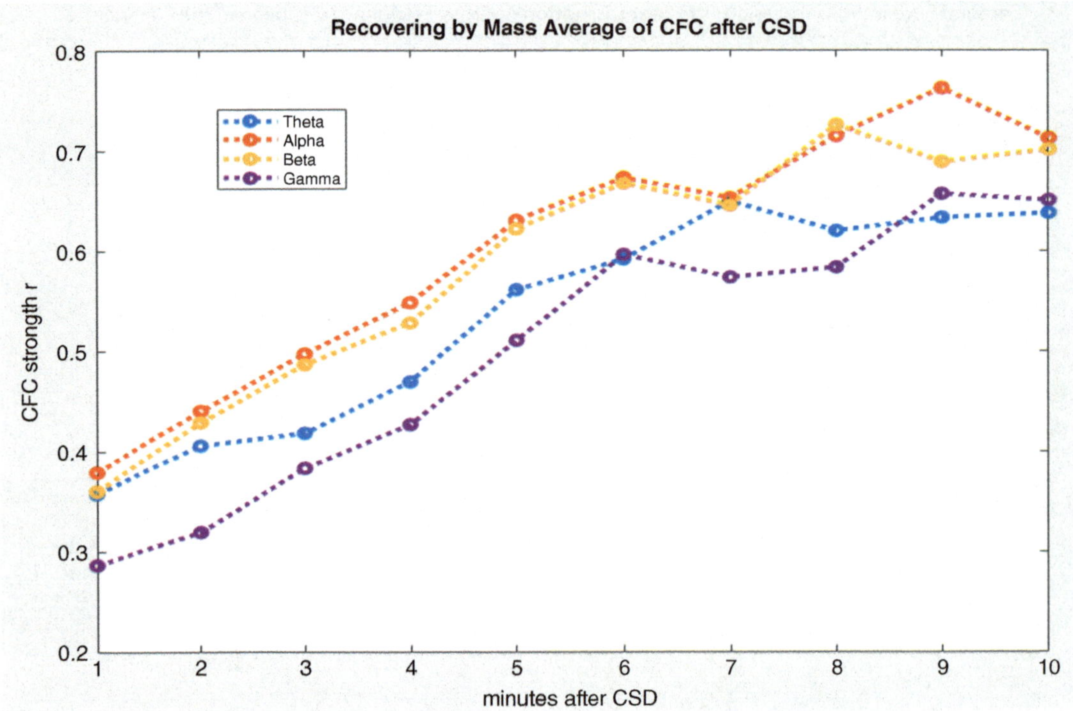

Fig. 33.3 Mass average of CFC after CSD during recovery. The CFC recoveries of the slow wave to four typical physiological frequency bands were similar. Interestingly, the Theta band CFC presents a smaller value for this mass average. Note that mass average of CFC was carried out over many data points from a single CSD

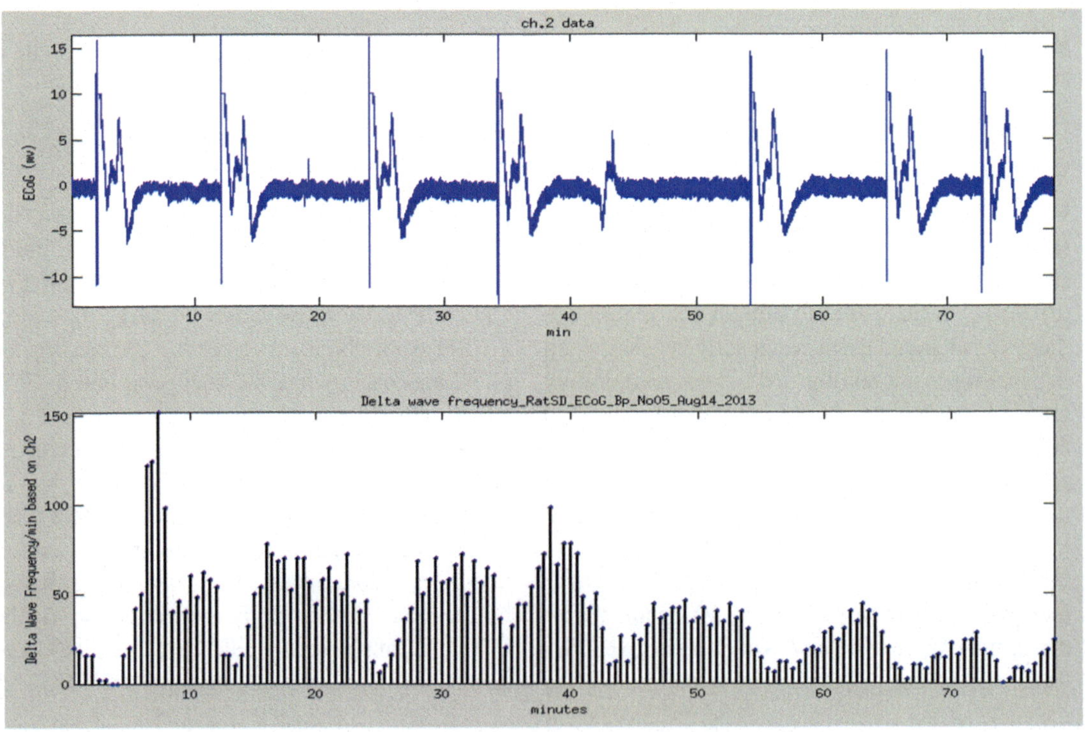

Fig. 33.4 Evoked CSD vs delta waves. The delta waves were found by pattern-matching approach (see text for details). With the repeated evoked CSDs, the delta wave density also diminished, indicating a smaller and smaller partial recovery of the neuronal networks in the neocortex

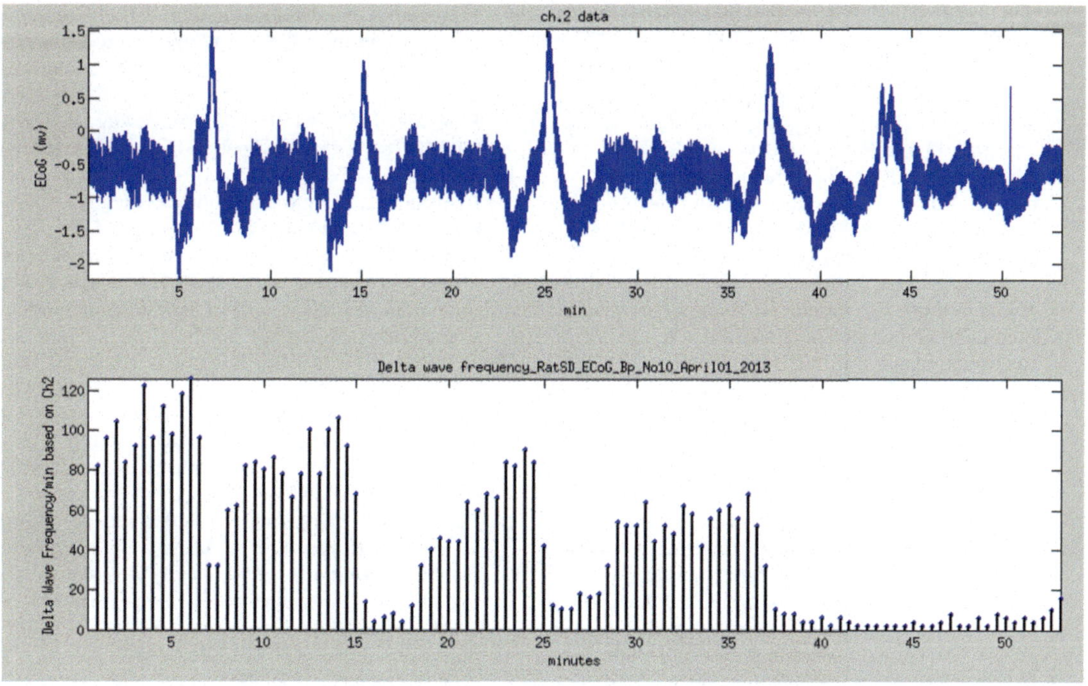

Fig. 33.5 Complex spontaneous CSD vs delta waves. For these spontaneous CSD, the delta wave density with the repeated CSD shows a similar pattern as the evoked CSD (see Fig. 33.4), indicating that both CSDs, no matter evoked or spontaneous, similarly affect the underlying neurons

already decreasing, which may be a problem of spatial resolution.

An interesting question in our data is that why do the delta waves return first after the CSD has passed followed by the higher frequencies. Harmony [13] proposed that delta activity is actually a characteristic of a state in which interneurons and thalamocortical inputs are inacvtive and inhibited. We hypothesize that the delta waves play the same role during sleep, i.e., to block external unwanted information for a proper internal sleep environment.

After CSD, presynaptic activities are inhibited [12], which gives rise to inhibition of all neurons underlying CSD. However, the sleep state establishes the mechanism that tries to block the external interference, which is characterized by delta activities as mentioned above. While all underlying neuronal networks affected by a CSD are inhibited, delta waves tend to come back first after a CSD. Higher-frequency activities, represented by the CFC of all the normal physiological frequency bands, gradually come back after recovery of the affected neurons.

References

1. Raichle ME, MacLeod AM, Snyder AZ, Powers WJ, Gusnard DA, Shulman GL (2001, 98) A default mode of brain function. Proc Natl Acad Sci U S A (2):676–682. PMID: 11209064
2. Raichle ME (2015) The restless brain: how intrinsic activity organizes brain function. Philos Trans R Soc Lond Ser B Biol Sci 370(1668):pii: 20140172. https://doi.org/10.1098/rstb.2014.0172. Review. PMID: 25823869
3. Goyal MS, Blazey TM, Su Y, Couture LE, Durbin TJ, Bateman RJ, Benzinger TL, Morris JC, Raichle ME, Vlassenko AG (2019) Persistent metabolic youth in the aging female brain. Proc Natl Acad Sci U S A 116(8):3251–3255. https://doi.org/10.1073/pnas.1815917116. Epub 2019 Feb 4. Erratum in: Proc

Natl Acad Sci U S A. 2019;116(11):5198. PMID: 30718410
4. Canolty RT, Knight RT (2010) The functional role of cross-frequency coupling. Trends Cogn Sci 14(11):506–515. https://doi.org/10.1016/j.tics.2010.09.001. Review. PMID: 20932795
5. Klimesch W (2018) The frequency architecture of brain and brain body oscillations: an analysis. Eur J Neurosci 48(7):2431–2453. https://doi.org/10.1111/ejn.14192. Review: PMID: 30281858
6. Antonakakis M, Dimitriadis SI, Zervakis M, Micheloyannis S, Rezaie R, Babajani-Feremi A, Zouridakis G, Papanicolaou AC (2016) Altered cross-frequency coupling in resting-state MEG after mild traumatic brain injury. Int J Psychophysiol 102:1–11. https://doi.org/10.1016/j.ijpsycho.2016.02.002. Epub 2016 Feb 22. PMID: 26910049
7. Wang J, Fang Y, Wang X, Yang H, Yu X, Wang H (2017) Enhanced gamma activity and cross-frequency interaction of resting-state electroencephalographic oscillations in patients with Alzheimer's disease. Front Aging Neurosci 9:243. https://doi.org/10.3389/fnagi.2017.00243. eCollection 2017.PMID:28798683
8. Leao AA (1944) Spreading depression of activity in the cerebral cortex. J Neurophysiol 7:359–390
9. Lauritzen M, Strong AJ (2017) Spreading depression of Leão' and its emerging relevance to acute brain injury in humans. J Cereb Blood Flow Metab 37(5):1553–1570. https://doi.org/10.1177/0271678X16657092. Epub 2016 Jan 1. Review
10. Hartings JA, the COSBID group (2017) Recording, analysis, and interpretation of spreading depolarizations in neurointensive care: review and recommendations of the COSBID research group. J Cereb Blood Flow Metab 37(5):1595–1625. https://doi.org/10.1177/0271678X16654496. Epub 2016 Jan 1. Review
11. Kramer MA, Eden UT (2013) Assessment of cross-frequency coupling with confidence using generalized linear models. J Neurosci Methods 220:64–74
12. Sawant-Pokam PM, Suryavanshi P, Mendez JM, Dudek FE, Brennan KC (2017) Mechanisms of neuronal silencing after cortical spreading depression. Cereb Cortex 27(2):1311–1325
13. Harmony T, Fernández T, Silva J, Bernal J, Díaz-Comas L, Reyes A et al (1996) EEG delta activity: an indicator of attention to internal processing during the performance of mental tasks. Int J Psychophysiol 24:161–171. https://doi.org/10.1016/s0167-8760(96)00053-0
14. Fernández T, Harmony T, Rodríguez M, Bernal J, Silva J, Reyes A et al (1995) EEG activation patterns during the performance of tasks involving different components of mental calculation. Electroencephalogr Clin Neurophysiol 94:175–182. https://doi.org/10.1016/0013-4694(94)00262-j
15. Kim Y, Laposky AD, Bergmann BM, Turek FW (2007) Repeated sleep restriction in rats leads to homeostatic and allostatic responses during recovery sleep. Proc Natl Acad Sci U S A 104:10,679–10,702

Long-Term Blue Light Exposure Changes Frontal and Occipital Cerebral Hemodynamics: Not All Subjects React the Same

34

Hamoon Zohdi, Felix Scholkmann, and Ursula Wolf

Abstract

Background: In modern society, we are increasingly exposed to numerous sources of blue light, including screens (e.g., TVs, computers, laptops, smartphones, tablets) and light from fluorescent and LED lamps. Due to this wide range of applications, the effects of blue light exposure (BLE) on the human physiology need to be thoroughly studied. Aim: To investigate the impact of long-term BLE on frontal and occipital human cerebral hemodynamics and oxygenation using functional near-infrared spectroscopy (fNIRS) neuroimaging. Materials and Methods: 32 healthy right-handed subjects (20 females, 12 males; age: 23.8 ± 2.2 years) were exposed to blue LED light for 15 minutes. Before (baseline, 8 min) and after (recovery, 10 min) the BLE, subjects were in darkness. We measured the concentration changes of oxyhemoglobin ([O_2Hb]) and deoxyhemoglobin ([HHb]) at the prefrontal cortex (PFC) and visual cortex (VC) by fNIRS during the experiment. Subjects were then classified into different groups based on their hemodynamic response pattern of [O_2Hb] at the PFC and VC during BLE. Results: On the group level (32 subjects), we found an increase in [O_2Hb] and a decrease in [HHb] at both cortices during BLE. Evoked changes of [O_2Hb] were higher at the VC compared to the PFC. Eight different hemodynamic response patterns were detected in the subgroup analysis, while an increase of [O_2Hb] in both cortices was the most common pattern (8 out of 32 cases, 25%) during BLE. Discussion and Conclusion: Our study showed that the hemodynamic and oxygenation changes at the PFC and VC during BLE (i) were generally higher in the VC compared to the PFC, (ii) showed an intersubject variability with respect to their magnitudes and shapes, and (iii) can be classified into eight groups. We conclude that blue light affects humans differently. It is essential to consider this when assessing the impact of the BLE on society.

Keywords

Blue light exposure · Functional near-infrared spectroscopy · Different hemodynamic response patterns · Prefrontal cortex · Visual cortex

H. Zohdi (✉) · U. Wolf
University of Bern, Institute of Complementary and Integrative Medicine, Bern, Switzerland
e-mail: hamoon.zohdi@ikim.unibe.ch

F. Scholkmann
University of Bern, Institute of Complementary and Integrative Medicine, Bern, Switzerland

University Hospital Zurich, University of Zurich, Department of Neonatology, Biomedical Optics Research Laboratory, Zurich, Switzerland

E. M. Nemoto et al. (eds.), *Oxygen Transport to Tissue XLII*, Advances in Experimental Medicine and Biology 1269, https://doi.org/10.1007/978-3-030-48238-1_34

34.1 Introduction

Blue light is increasingly prevalent in our modern society due to modern light sources such as light-emitting diodes (LEDs) and fluorescent lamps and the omnipresence of screens (e.g., TVs, computers). The adverse effect of blue light exposure (BLE) on human physiology is increasingly recognized [1–3]. But BLE can also be beneficial, for example, treating circadian and sleep dysfunction and seasonal affective disorder, as well as boosting alertness, helping cognitive function, and elevating mood [4, 5].

Functional near-infrared spectroscopy (fNIRS) is a technology for cost-effective and noninvasive neuroimaging in research and clinical practice. This technique measures cerebral blood oxygenation and perfusion [6, 7]. Absolute quantitation of the concentration of oxyhemoglobin ([O_2Hb]) and deoxyhemoglobin ([HHb]) is possible by applying the frequency-domain near-infrared spectroscopy (FD-NIRS) technique [8].

The effects of BLE on the visual and nonvisual pathway can be distinguished by the measurement of the visual cortex (VC) and prefrontal cortex (PFC). We measured both cortices in parallel in order to investigate the effects of BLE in the visual and nonvisual pathways associated with the processing of visual information. Moreover, it is known that colors may affect the emotional status and mood, and thus, we expected modulation of PFC activation by BLE.

In this study, we aimed to investigate the impact of long-term wide-angle BLE on frontal and occipital human cerebral hemodynamics using fNIRS. The results of the current study are expected to facilitate a better understanding of the beneficial and detrimental effects of BLE on society.

34.2 Material and Methods

Thirty-two healthy right-handed subjects (20 females, 12 males; age: 23.8 ± 2.2 years, range: 20–28 years) were assessed in this study. They were asked to sit upright in a comfortable chair while their feet were on the ground and a white wall was in front of them (distance eyes-wall: 160 ± 5 cm). The blue LED light (six LED PAR headlights: each has 12 × 35 mm RGBW LEDs; peak wavelength: 450 nm; illuminance: 120 lux at eye level) was continuously exposed to the white wall (width: 2.5 m, height: 3 m) for 15 minutes. Before (baseline, 8 min) and after (recovery, 10 min) the BLE, subjects were in darkness.

The focus of this study was on the intersubject variability of the hemodynamic responses.

The concentration changes of [O_2Hb] and [HHb] were measured bilaterally over the PFC and VC by FD-NIRS (Imagent, ISS Inc., Champaign, IL, USA). The PFC optodes were placed over the left (Fp_1) and right (Fp_2) PFC and over the right (O_2) and left (O_1) VC, respectively, according to the international 10–20 system. The source-detector separations of the optodes were 2.0, 2.5, 3.5, and 4.0 cm over the PFC and 2.0, 2.5, 3.0, and 3.5 cm over the VC. Movement artifacts in [O_2Hb] and [HHb] signals were detected and removed by the movement artifact reduction algorithm (MARA) [9]. To further remove high-frequency noise, signals were low pass filtered using a robust second-degree polynomial moving average (RLOESS) filter with a span of 4 min. Signals from the left and right PFC and VC were subsequently averaged to obtain signals for the whole PFC and VC, respectively. The signals were then normalized to the last 5 minutes of the baseline period to analyze the changes of [O_2Hb] and [HHb] for each subject. To compare the changes of [O_2Hb] and [HHb] between PFC and VC at the group level, the BLE phase was segmented into 60 parts, and the median of [O_2Hb] and [HHb] values for each segment was calculated for each subject. Then, the median value of each segment among all subjects was calculated. Finally, the median values obtained for all segments were averaged.

Subjects were finally classified into different groups based on their hemodynamic response pattern of [O_2Hb] at the PFC and VC during BLE. The BLE phase of normalized [O_2Hb] signal was segmented into 60 parts, and the median value for each segment was calculated. Then, the One-Sample Wilcoxon Signed Rank Test was applied to all median values of segments. Inconclusive (−) pattern indicates a failure to reject the null hypothesis (median is zero) at the 5% significant level ($p > 0.05$), while increase (↑) and decrease (↓) patterns indicate a rejection of the null hypothesis ($p < 0.05$).

34.3 Results

Group-Level Analysis The group-averaged long-term changes of [O_2Hb] and [HHb] at the PFC and VC are depicted in Fig. 34.1. We found an increase in [O_2Hb] and a decrease in [HHb] at both cortices during BLE. Evoked changes of [O_2Hb] were higher at the VC compared to the PFC ($p < 0.001$; effect size (Cohen's d): $d = 1.03$), while [HHb] changes at the PFC were more prominent than that of the VC ($p < 0.001$; $d = 1.15$). This change was observed, especially after light exposure in the recovery period.

Subgroup Analysis We observed a large inter-subject variability of the hemodynamic responses. Nevertheless, the hemodynamic responses were assigned to eight groups according to the changes of [O_2Hb] at the VC and PFC, i.e., eight different response pattern could be defined. Figure 34.2 and Table 34.1 show the classification of stimulus-evoked hemodynamic responses based on [O_2Hb] pattern at the PFC and VC during BLE. The most common fNIRS response pattern during BLE was an increase of [O_2Hb] associated with a decrease of [HHb] in both cortices (8 out of 32 cases, 25%). An increase and a decrease in [O_2Hb] at the PFC and VC, respectively, were the second most common pattern (6 out of 32 cases, 19%). In contrast to the latter pattern, we found a decrease in [O_2Hb] at the PFC and an increase in [O_2Hb] at the VC as the third pattern (5 out of 32 cases, 16%). Although the number of males investigated in this study was lower than females (20 females, 12 males), the frequency of the third most common pattern in the male group was considerably higher compared to female group (Group 3: 1 female, 4 males).

34.4 Discussion and Conclusions

Neuronal activation generally leads to an increase in [O_2Hb] with a concurrent decrease in [HHb] due to changes in cerebral hemodynamics and metabolism. At the group level, we observed in our study the typical hemodynamic changes in the PFC and VC during BLE. The mean increases in [O_2Hb] during BLE were less pronounced in the PFC than that in the VC. That the BLE also led to a change in the PFC is indicative for an activity increase of higher cognitive processes related to increase in activity of the PFC [10]. The reasons for the continued increase in the recovery phase are not yet clarified. Our hypothesis is that the BLE leads to long-lasting effects. Nevertheless, it is a valuable observation because it may have implications on the applications of blue light.

In spite of the typical hemodynamic response pattern observed at the group-level analysis, this pattern ([O_2Hb] increase in both cortices) was found in only 8 out of 32 cases. Different patterns

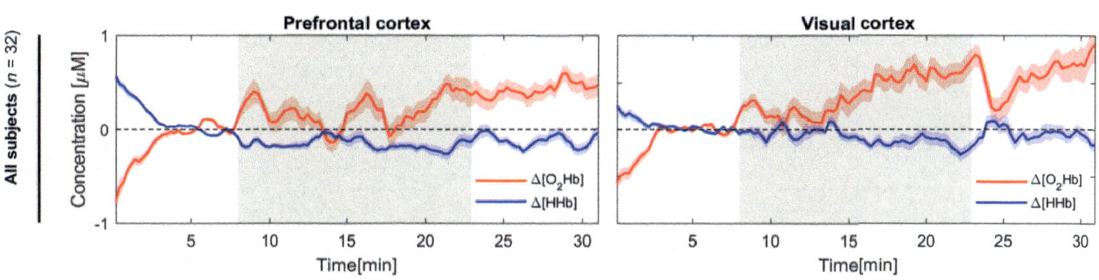

Fig. 34.1 Group-averaged changes in hemodynamic response ([O_2Hb] and [HHb]) of the PFC and VC. The gray-shaded areas represent the BLE. Median ± standard error of median (SEM) is shown

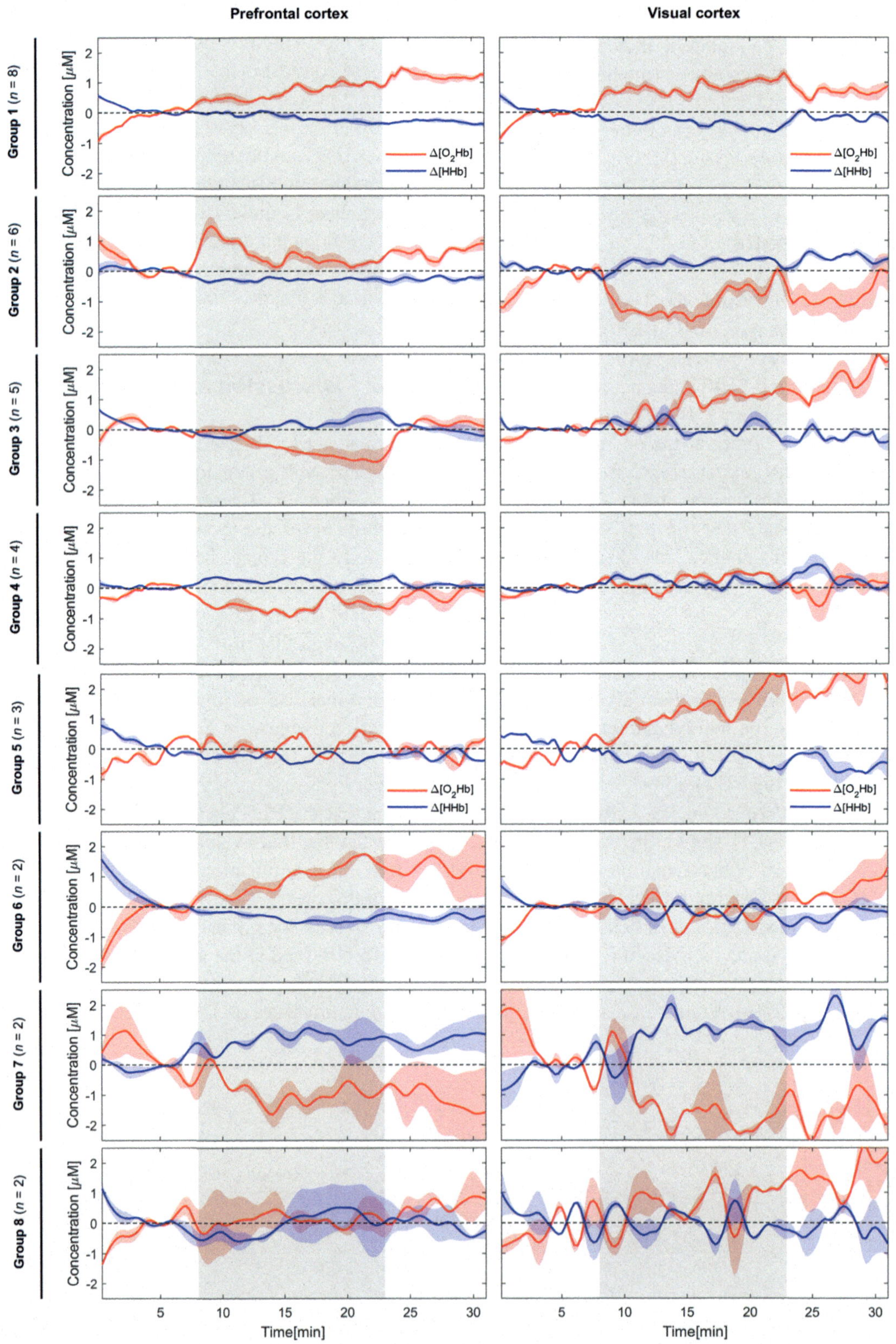

Fig. 34.2 Subgroup analysis (eight classes) of stimulus-evoked hemodynamic responses at the PFC and VC. The gray-shaded areas represent the BLE. Median ± SEM is shown

Table 34.1 Classification of hemodynamic response of [O_2Hb] patterns

	PFC	VC	Number of subjects within the group
Group 1	↑	↑	8 (5 females, 3 males); 63% female, 37% male
Group 2	↑	↓	6 (4 females, 2 males); 67% female, 33% male
Group 3	↓	↑	5 (1 female, 4 males); 20% female, 80% male
Group 4	↓	–	4 (4 females); 100% female
Group 5	–	↑	3 (1 female, 2 males); 33% female, 67% male
Group 6	↑	–	2 (2 females); 100% female
Group 7	↓	↓	2 (2 females); 100% female
Group 8	–	–	2 (1 female, 1 male); 50% female, 50% male

Decrease ↓, increase ↑, and inconclusive – at the PFC and VC during BLE

of cortical activation (characterized by the lack of [O_2Hb] increased or even decreased [O_2Hb]) were observed in the remaining subjects. In total, eight different hemodynamic response patterns were detected. Atypical changes in fNIRS signals can be triggered by systemic physiological noise, partial volume effects, or the presence of specific pathophysiological changes [11, 12]. Negative responses may also be explained by the interaction between neural activity, CBF, and cerebral metabolic rate of oxygen ($CMRO_2$). The decrease in [O_2Hb] may result from a further increase in oxygen consumption ($CMRO_2$) with a consequent mismatch between CBF and $CMRO_2$ increase, this time in favor of $CMRO_2$ [13]. Another possible reason for atypical patterns could be attributed to individual anatomical variability (e.g., diverse neuroanatomy) [12, 13]. Additionally, variations in CBF or arterial blood oxygenation, changes in intracranial pressure, hyper- or hypocapnia, and decreases of systemic blood pressure may alter the relationship between neuronal activity and fNIRS signals [14].

In conclusion, we found that blue light affects individual humans differently. Although a typical cortical activation pattern (an increase of [O_2Hb] associated with a decrease of [HHb]) was found for group-level analysis, such a pattern was observed in only eight subjects. However, we discovered eight different hemodynamic response patterns, which, in particular, should be taken into consideration when assessing the impact of BLE on society. We assume that the underlying reasons for the different patterns lie in individual changes in systemic physiology.

References

1. Hatori M, Gronfier C, Van Gelder RN et al (2017) Global rise of potential health hazards caused by blue light-induced circadian disruption in modern aging societies. NPJ Aging Mech Dis 3:9
2. O'Hagan JB, Khazova M, Price LLA (2016) Low-energy light bulbs, computers, tablets and the blue light hazard. Eye 30:230–233
3. Tosini G, Ferguson I, Tsubota K (2016) Effects of blue light on the circadian system and eye physiology Gianluca. Mol Vis 22:61–72
4. Vandewalle G, Maquet P, Dijk D-J (2009) Light as a modulator of cognitive brain function. Trends Cogn Sci 13:429–438
5. Viola AU, James LM, Schlangen LJM, Dijk D (2008) Blue-enriched white light in the workplace improves self-reported alertness, performance and sleep quality. Scand J Work Environ Health 34:297–306
6. Scholkmann F, Kleiser S, Metz AJ et al (2014) A review on continuous wave functional near-infrared spectroscopy and imaging instrumentation and methodology. NeuroImage 85:6–27
7. Zohdi H, Scholkmann F, Nasseri N, Wolf U (2018) Long-term changes in optical properties (μa, μ′s, μeff and DPF) of human head tissue during functional neuroimaging experiments. Adv Exp Med Biol 1072:331–337
8. Fantini S, Franceschini MA (2002) Frequency-domain techniques for tissue spectroscopy and imaging. Handb Opt Biomed Diag 7:405–453
9. Scholkmann F, Spichtig S, Muehlemann T, Wolf M (2010) How to detect and reduce movement artifacts in near-infrared imaging using moving standard deviation and spline interpolation. Physiol Meas 31:649–662
10. Scholkmann F, Hafner T, Metz AJ et al (2017) Effect of short-term colored-light exposure on cerebral hemodynamics and oxygenation, and systemic physiological activity. Neurophotonics 4:045005
11. Herold F, Wiegel P, Scholkmann F, Müller N (2018) Applications of functional near-infrared spectroscopy (fNIRS) neuroimaging in exercise–cognition science: a systematic, methodology-focused review. J Clin Med 7:466
12. Holper L, Shalóm DE, Wolf M, Sigman M (2011) Understanding inverse oxygenation responses during

motor imagery: a functional near-infrared spectroscopy study. Eur J Neurosci 33:2318–2328
13. Quaresima V, Ferrari M, Torricelli A et al (2005) Bilateral prefrontal cortex oxygenation responses to a verbal fluency task: a multichannel time-resolved near-infrared topography study. J Biomed Opt 10:011012
14. Lindauer U, Dirnagl U, Füchtemeier M et al (2010) Pathophysiological interference with neurovascular coupling – when imaging based on hemoglobin might go blind. Front Neuroenerg 2:25

Changes in Prefrontal Cortex Asymmetry Due to Standing Load in Stroke Patients Measured by NIRS

35

Masamichi Moriya and Kaoru Sakatani

Abstract

Autonomic disorders such as orthostatic hypotension often become a problem during the early mobilization of poststroke patients. We reported that the prefrontal cortex (PFC) oxyhemoglobin changes at rest are often on the right, and a positive correlation was observed between the left and right activity balance and the change in oxy-Hb. In this study, we focused on the asymmetrical changes associated with the standing load from rest. We assessed the left-right asymmetry of the PFC oxyhemoglobin changes at rest and standing load by calculating the Laterality Index at Rest (LIR) and laterality index during activity (LIA); positive values indicate the right-dominant activity, while negative values indicate left-dominant activity. As for left-right asymmetry LIA, the active dominant PFC was reversed in five patients. It should be noted that in almost all of the 13 cases, the active PFC and the lesion side matched. The detailed mechanism of overactivity up to the prefrontal cortex on the lesion side is unknown, but it may be a recovery mechanism that elicits plasticity in the brain network.

Keywords

Stroke · NIRS · Rehabilitation · Laterality · Mobilization

35.1 Introduction

In the acute phase of stroke, the autoregulation of cerebral blood flow (CBF) is often impaired, and CBF changes with systemic blood pressure. In addition, it has been reported that the autonomic nervous system (ANS) is also impaired during the acute phase of stroke, resulting in abnormal systemic blood flow [1]. However, the central mechanism of the dysfunction of the ANS in the acute phase of stroke is not yet clear.

Recently, employing near-infrared spectroscopy (NIRS), we evaluated the relationship between the prefrontal cortex (PFC) hemodynamic changes and the ANS function in poststroke patients who suffered consciousness disorder [2]. We assessed left-right asymmetry of the PFC hemodynamic changes at rest and compared it with the ANS function. We found that the right PFC dominant case showed an

M. Moriya (✉)
Department of Physical Therapy, Faculty of Health Care and Medical Sports, Teikyo Heisei University, Chiba, Japan

K. Sakatani
Universal Sport Health Science Laboratory, Department of Human and Engineered Environmental Studies, Graduate School of Frontier Sciences, The University of Tokyo, Chiba, Japan

E. M. Nemoto et al. (eds.), *Oxygen Transport to Tissue XLII*, Advances in Experimental Medicine and Biology 1269, https://doi.org/10.1007/978-3-030-48238-1_35

increase in oxy-Hb during standing loads, while the left PFC dominant case showed a decrease in oxy-Hb. In the present study, we focused on the asymmetrical changes associated with the standing load; we evaluated left-right asymmetry during standing loads and compared it with the ANS function.

35.2 Methods

35.2.1 Subjects

We studied 13 poststroke patients (six males, seven females, 73.5 ± 12.2 years; mean ± SD age). The diagnosis of the subject (affected side: Lt/Rt) was two (1/1) cases of a cerebral hemorrhage, five (2/3) cases of cerebral infarction, two cases of pontine hemorrhage, and four (1/3) cases of subarachnoid hemorrhage. All patients suffered consciousness disorders; mean Glasgow Coma Scale score was 9.5 ± 2.0. All patients were admitted to the ICU at the University Hospital of Nihon University (Tokyo, Japan). We performed the present study within 2 weeks after the onset of stroke. The data was measured after the informed consent and rehabilitation prescription from the doctor to the patient. Ethical approval was obtained from the Nihon University Itabashi Hospital (150210–2).

We studied the patients who showed the following physiological condition: (1) systolic blood pressure (SBP) 120–220 mmHg, (2) heart rate (HR) 40–100 bpm, (3) oxygen saturation >92%, and (4) temperature <38.5 °C. When the following physiological changes were observed during experiments, we immediately stopped the study: (1) mean blood pressure <70 or >120 mmHg; (2) HR <40 or >130 bpm; (3) respiratory rate <5 or >40 bpm; (4) oxygen saturation <88%; (5) if intracranial pressure (ICP) was monitored, ICP >15 mmHg; and (6) sudden changes of neurologic symptom or level of consciousness. This is based on the criteria of the Japanese Society of Critical Care Medicine [3].

35.2.2 NIRS Measurements

We used two-channel NIRS (Pocket NIRS Duo, Dyna Sense, Hamamatsu, Japan) for measurements of cerebral blood oxygenation (CBO) in the bilateral PFC. The NIRS probes were set symmetrically on the forehead with a flexible fixation pad so that the midpoint between the emission and detection probes was 3 cm above the centers of the upper edges of the bilateral orbital sockets; the distance between the emitter and detector was set at 3 cm. This positioning is similar to positions Fp1 (left) and Fp2 (right) of the international electroencephalographic 10–20 system.

In all subjects, the study was performed in the rehabilitation room of the Hospital of Nihon University. In order to evaluate orthostatic hypotension, we applied gradual standing loads on the participants using a tilt table. One trial consisted of the following steps: first, each subject remained on the tilt table in the supine position for 10 min. Second, the standing load was increased to 30°, 45°, and 60° at 5 min intervals. Finally, the table was returned to 0° and remained in this position for 5–10 min.

We diagnosed the subject as having orthostatic hypotension when the subject exhibited the following criteria [4]: (1) systolic blood pressure fell by over 20 mmHg within 3 minutes after the posture change, (2) the systolic blood pressure dropped to less than 90 mmHg, and (3) the diastolic blood pressure decreased by over 10 mmHg.

35.2.3 Data Analysis

Initially, we evaluated the left/right asymmetry of the PFC oxyhemoglobin changes at rest. Then, we evaluated the relation between the left-right asymmetry and the NIRS-measured CBO changes induced by standing loads.

We evaluated the left/right asymmetry of the PFC hemodynamic changes at rest by calculating the laterality index at rest (LIR) as follows:

$$\text{LIR} = \frac{\Sigma t\{(\text{oxyRt} - \text{oxyRmin}) - (\text{oxyLt} - \text{oxyLmin})\}}{\Sigma t\{(\text{oxyRt} - \text{oxyRmin}) + (\text{oxyLt} - \text{oxyLmin})\}}$$

LIR >0 indicates the right-dominant activity, while LIR <0 indicates the left-dominant activity. Previous studies demonstrated that LIR >0 is associated with sympathetic activity, while LIR <0 is associated with parasympathetic activity [5].

In a similar manner, laterality index during activity (LIA) was calculated.

Then, we evaluated the relation between the LIR and the oxy-Hb change in the PFC during standing loads 30° → 45° → 60°. We calculated the average changes of oxy-Hb: (Δoxy-Hb at 30° + Δoxy-Hb at 45° + Δoxy-Hb at 60°) ÷ 3.

Employing Spearman's rank correlation coefficient analysis, we investigated the correlation between the LIR and the oxy-Hb change in the PFC.

35.3 Results

Nine out of the 13 patients showed right-dominated PFC oxyhemoglobin changes at rest (LIR >0), while four cases showed a left-dominant activity (LIR <0). During standing loads, eight out of 13 patients showed right-dominant PFC oxyhemoglobin changes (LIA >0), while five patients showed left-dominant PFC activity (LIA <0). Five patients had LIR and LIA reversed (Table 35.1). Interestingly, the standing load increased oxy-Hb in the PFC on the lesion side during standing loads in ten out of 13; two cases had pontine hemorrhage.

The standing load increased oxy-Hb in the PFC in seven out of 13 poststroke patients. There was a significant positive correlation between the LIR and the oxy-Hb changes induced by the standing load ($r = 0.6$, $p < 0.05$) (Fig. 35.1).

The standing load decreased systemic blood pressure from 134.5 ± 21.5 mmHg to 114.4 ± 24.9 mmHg, while heart rate increased from 89.8 ± 16.1 bpm to 99.0 ± 17.8 bpm. We observed orthostatic hypotension in six poststroke patients. It should be noted that all six patients with orthostatic hypotension showed positive LIR (i.e., right-dominant PFC oxyhemoglobin changes at rest), but patients with negative LIR did not suffer orthostatic hypotension. The other three patients showed positive LIR but did not suffer orthostatic hypotension.

35.4 Discussion

The present study demonstrated a positive correlation between LIR and oxy-Hb changes during standing loads in poststroke patients. This finding is consistent with our previous study [2]. In the previous study, we hypothesized that the standing load might act on poststroke patients as a stressor, which caused an increase of PFC hemodynamic changes; NIRS studies on healthy adults demonstrated that mental stress could cause an increase of PFC *hemodynamic changes*, leading to an increase of oxy-Hb [6, 7]. The significant positive correlation between LIR and oxy-Hb changes during the standing load supports this hypothesis, since right-dominant PFC oxyhemoglobin changes at rest (i.e., high LIR score) are associated with high anxiety levels [5]. In addition, this hypothesis may be supported by the fact that the patient with left-dominant activity at rest did not show increased oxy-Hb in the PFC during the standing load, since left-dominant PFC hemodynamic changes at rest are associated with low anxiety levels [5].

Interestingly, seven out of 13 cases showed paradoxical increases of oxy-Hb in the PFC on the lesion side during standing loads; two cases had pontine hemorrhage. The physiological mechanism of the paradoxical increase of oxy-Hb is not yet clear since oxy-Hb should reduce on the lesion side where autoregulation was impaired. However, the following mechanism should be considered: it has been reported that the cerebral cortex including the lesion side is widely activated during the recovery process after stroke [8]. Such activation of the brain may be involved in the paradoxical increase of oxy-Hb. Further study is necessary to evaluate the mechanism of the paradoxical increase of oxy-Hb on the lesion side during standing loads.

Table 35.1 PFC hemodynamic changes dominant at rest and standing

	Rest			Standing			
Case	Lt	Rt		Lt	Rt		Laterality, diagnosis
1		■		■			**Lt** cerebral infarction
2		■		■			**Lt** cerebral infarction
3		■			■		Pontine hemorrhage
4	■				■		**Rt** caudate nucleus hemorrhage
5	■			■			Lt putamen hemorrhage
6		■			■		Rt subarachnoid hemorrhage
7		■			■		Pontine hemorrhage
8		■			■		Rt subarachnoid hemorrhage
9	■			■			Rt subarachnoid hemorrhage
10		■			■		Rt subarachnoid hemorrhage
11	■				■		**Rt** cerebral infarction
12		■			■		Rt cerebral infarction
13		■		■			**Lt** cerebral infarction

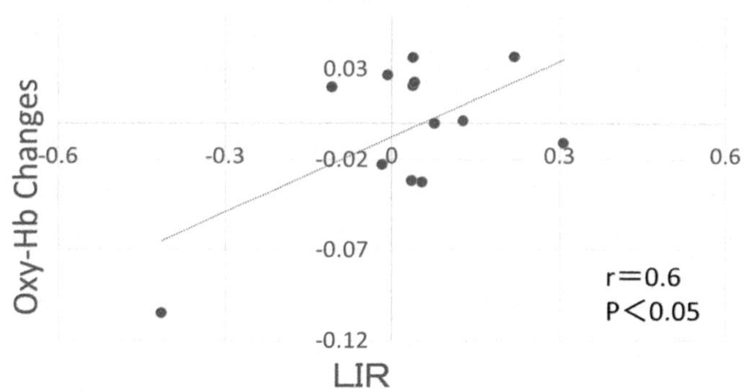

Fig. 35.1 Relation between LIR and oxy-Hb changes induced by standing loads

Finally, it should be noted that orthostatic hypotension was observed only in right-dominated cases as in previous studies. It is known that there is a functional left-right bias in the autonomic nerve itself, and the vagus and sympathetic nerves affect the right rather than the left. Resting LIR suggests the possibility of predicting orthostatic hypotension during rehabilitation. We have also estimated the LI for the deoxy-Hb response (results not shown) and found not significant correlation with the LI of the oxy-Hb.

35.5 Conclusions

The present study demonstrated that the PFC plays an important role in the ANS of poststroke patients. It may be useful for the prediction of orthostatic hypotension to evaluate left/right asymmetry of PFC oxyhemoglobin changes at rest; right dominant may predict orthostatic hypotension.

Acknowledgments This part of the present study was supported by Xebio Cooperation in Japan.

References

1. Phillips AM, Jardine DL, Parkin PJ et al (2001) Brain stem stroke causing baroreflex failure and paroxysmal hypertension. Stroke 31:1997–2001
2. Moriya M, Sakatani K (2018) Relation between asymmetry of prefrontal activity and autonomic nervous system in post-stroke patients with a disorder of consciousness. Adv Exp Med Biol 1072:53–58
3. Ad Hoc Committee for Early Rehabilitation, The Japanese Society of Intensive Care Medicine (2017) The Japanese Society of Intensive Care Medicine: evidence based expert consensus for early rehabilitation in the intensive care unit. J JPN Soc Intensive Care Med 24:255–3036
4. Brignole M, Moya A, de Lange FJ et al (2018) 2018 ESC Guidelines for the diagnosis and management of syncope. Eur Heart J 39:1883–19487
5. Ishikawa W, Sato M, Fukuda Y et al (2013) New method of analyzing NIRS data from prefrontal cortex at rest. Adv Exp Med Biol 789:391–397
6. Tanida M, Sakatani K, Takano R et al (2004) Relation between asymmetry of prefrontal cortex activities and the autonomic nervous system during a mental arithmetic task: near infrared spectroscopy study. Neurosci Lett 369:69–74
7. Kamiyama Y, Fujita Y, Fuchigami T et al (2014) Asymmetrical changes in cerebral blood oxygenation induced by an active standing test in children with postural tachycardia syndrome. Adv Exp Med Biol 812:271–278
8. Cramer SC, Nelles G, Benson RR et al (1997) A functional MRI study of subjects recovered from hemiparetic stroke. Stroke 28:2518–2527

Parasympathetic Nervous Activity Associated with Discoordination Between Physical Acceleration and Heart Rate Variability in Patients with Sleep Apnea

36

Kentaro Taniguchi, Akito Shimouchi, Naoya Jinno, Naoya Okumura, and Akitoshi Seiyama

Abstract

Sleep apnea syndrome (SAS) often accompanies alterations in heart rate variability (HRV). The severity of SAS is sometimes evaluated using the oxygen desaturation index (ODI). We hypothesized that effects of the autonomic nervous system could be involved in the coordination between HRV and physical acceleration during free movement in patients with SAS. Among 33 women aged 60 years or older, 19 had a high ODI (>5). Their HRV and physical acceleration were simultaneously obtained every minute for 24 hours. The low frequency/high frequency (LF/HF) ratio and the high frequency in normalized units (HFnu) were used as HRV indices. Low levels of %Lag0, defined as the percentage of the lag = 0 min in 1 h, indicated coordination between physical acceleration and HRV. Nineteen participants were divided into group A (high %Lag0 before sleep [$n = 9$]) or group B (low %Lag0 [$n = 10$]). In group B participants with a high ODI and low %Lag0 in the hour after waking, HFnu was significantly increased compared to that in group A participants with high ODI and high %Lag0 in the hour after waking ($p < 0.05$). These results suggest that close associations between high ODI and discoordination between HRV and physical acceleration may be due to higher parasympathetic nervous system activity after waking.

Keywords

Oxygen desaturation index · Heart rate variability · Physical acceleration · Older women · Parasympathetic nervous activity

K. Taniguchi
Human Health Sciences, Graduate School of Medicine, Kyoto University, Kyoto, Japan

Department of Bioscience, Nagahama Institute of Bio-Science and Technology, Nagahama, Japan

National Cerebral and Cardiovascular Research Center, Osaka, Japan

A. Shimouchi (✉)
College of Life and Health Science, Chubu University, Kasugai, Japan

National Cerebral and Cardiovascular Research Center, Osaka, Japan
e-mail: ashimouc@isc.chubu.ac.jp

N. Jinno · N. Okumura
College of Life and Health Science, Chubu University, Kasugai, Japan

A. Seiyama
Human Health Sciences, Graduate School of Medicine, Kyoto University, Kyoto, Japan

E. M. Nemoto et al. (eds.), *Oxygen Transport to Tissue XLII*, Advances in Experimental Medicine and Biology 1269, https://doi.org/10.1007/978-3-030-48238-1_36

36.1 Introduction

Sleep apnea syndrome (SAS) is one of several major diseases that cause general hypoxemia and are linked to oxidative stress [1], and the prevalence of obstructive sleep apnea is reportedly 26% among adults in the USA [2]. SAS is usually diagnosed using polysomnography, which is expensive and not suitable for screening. Pulse oximetry, on the other hand, is a convenient technique used to measure oxygen saturation (SpO_2). Using a pulse oximeter to measure the oxygen desaturation index (ODI), the number of times blood oxygen levels drop 3% or more during 1 h of night sleep, is a simple and easy method to screen for SAS [2].

Monitoring an individual's heart rate variability (HRV) and any variations in the beat-to-beat intervals (R-R intervals) and autonomic nervous system is a noninvasive way to obtain health information [3]. Normalized spectral indices such as the ratio of low frequency/high frequency (LF/HF) and the high frequency in normalized units (HFnu) are regarded as markers of the parasympathetic nervous system [4]. The LF/HF ratio may indicate a shift toward sympathetic predominance or reduced vagal activity [5]. It is generally acknowledged that sleep-wake stages are associated with dramatic changes in the autonomic nervous system [6]. During sleep, the heart rate and LF/HF ratio decline, while the HFnu increases. After waking, the heart rate and LF/HF ratio increase, while the HFnu decreases [7].

In addition to an increase in heart rate, an increase in sympathetic activity and a decrease in vagal discharge are observed during exercise with increasing physical acceleration [8]. In healthy conditions, physical acceleration causes an immediate HRV response; in impaired conditions, however, the response may be altered. Therefore, we considered the lag between physical acceleration and HRV to reflect the coordination between physical acceleration and the autonomic nervous system. Based on a cross-correlation analysis of the relationship between HRV and physical acceleration, we observed that the lag increases with age in the daily lives of free-moving adults [9]. We found that 1 h before night sleep was the most appropriate time to detect impairments in coordination between HRV and physical acceleration.

Although the prevalence and severity of SAS is lower in women than in men, the consequences of the disease may be worse [10]. Habitual activity and HRV have both been reported to differ between men and women [11], but data is lacking on SAS in aged women without the effects of menopausal and menstruation cycles, which may alter autonomic control [12].

In this study, we examined whether SAS in older women is accompanied by impaired coordination between physical acceleration and HRV and observed any autonomic alteration differences among sleep and awake stages.

36.2 Methods

36.2.1 Subjects

Forty-two women (aged 60 years or older) volunteered to participate in this study. We excluded from the analysis two subjects who consumed alcohol on the day of the experiment, six subjects with severe arrhythmia, three subjects for whom there was excessive electrical noise in the devices, and one subject taking a beta-blocker. These numbers overlap; in total, nine subjects were excluded based on their responses during medical interviews, physical findings, blood and breath test results, and electrocardiography (ECG) findings. We identified arrhythmia based on the assessment of a 12-lead ECG and electrocardiographic complexes derived from Lorenz plots. Finally, 33 subjects were included in the analysis.

36.2.2 Protocols

Subjects arrived at the laboratory at approximately 13:00 and promptly underwent venous blood sampling and ECG. Each wore a portable monitor (Active Tracer AC301; GMS Inc., Tokyo) to record physical acceleration and R-R intervals over a period of 24 h. During monitoring, subjects were instructed to avoid bathing but to otherwise continue with their daily routines. They donned a portable pulse oximeter (Pulsleep LS-100 Fukuda. co. Ltd) before night sleep at home. After the completion of the 24-h monitoring, subjects returned to the laboratory. Experimental protocols were described further in our previous study [9].

36.2.3 Oxygen Desaturation Index

The pulse oximeter recorded SpO_2. SpO_2 data was obtained every second. ODI was calculated as the average number of desaturation episodes, which dropped 3% or more during 1 h of night sleep. We defined high ODI (>5) based on the American Academy of Sleep Medicine criteria [13].

36.2.4 Questionnaire

We used the General Health Questionnaire 28, which has four subscales (A: somatic symptoms, B: anxiety and insomnia, C: social impairments, and D: severe depression), the Self-Depression Scale, and the Cornell Medical Index, which determines neurosis tendency.

36.2.5 Physical Acceleration

For physical acceleration measurement, an activity tracer equipped with a triaxial accelerometer (72 g in weight) [14] was positioned on the frontal midline of the waist above the navel to allow free movement. The resolution of acceleration was specified as 2 mG, and the sensitivity ranged between 0 and 4.0 G. The absolute values of the resultant vector, which was calculated from the signals of triaxial acceleration, were averaged for every 1 min.

36.2.6 Analysis

Spectral analysis of HRV was performed at 1-min intervals using the maximal entropy combined with the method of least squares (MEMCalc System; Suwa Trust Co., Ltd., Tokyo), and then, the data was separated into HF and LF ranges for a power analysis [3]. We estimated the times at which subjects fell asleep and woke based on the changes in body positions revealed by the activity tracer.

Lag was determined as the time difference indicated by the maximum correlation coefficient obtained from an analysis of the cross-correlation between the HRV components and the physical acceleration. Cross-correlation coefficients were calculated for 10-min windows of moving time over consecutive 60-min periods. We identified impairments of coordination between HRV and physical acceleration when the lag time was 1 min or longer; lag analysis is discussed in greater detail in our previous study [9]. We defined %Lag0 as the percentage of the lag = 0 min in 1 h and considered it an index of coordination between HRV and physical acceleration. Low levels of %Lag0 would indicate discoordination between physical acceleration and HRV.

36.2.7 Statistics and Ethics

Data are expressed as the mean ± standard deviation. Statistical analyses were performed using analysis of variance and Tukey's range test. *P*-values <0.05 were considered statistically significant. This study was approved by the ethical committees at the National Cerebral and Cardiovascular Research Center (M18–19-2, M26–158), Chubu University (280031), and Kyoto University (R1758). All subjects gave written informed consent prior to participation in this study.

36.3 Results

Of the 33 participants, 14 had a low ODI (<5) and were categorized into the control group. Nineteen had a high ODI (>5) and were divided into two groups; nine with a high %Lag0 (>33) 1 h before night sleep were categorized into group A, and ten with low %Lag0 (<33) were categorized into group B.

Subjects in the control group had significantly longer sleeping hours than those of groups A and B. However, no other significant differences were observed (Table 36.1).

In the hour after waking, group B had significantly higher HFnu than group A. In the other ranges (the hour before sleep, during sleep, 2 hours after waking, or 3 hours after waking), HFnu did not differ significantly among the three groups (Fig. 36.1). On the other hand, there were no significant differences among the changes in LF/HF levels before sleep, during night sleep, or every hour for 3 hours after waking (data not shown).

36.4 Discussion

Among older women with a high ODI, we found that those with low %Lag0 in the hour before night sleep had high HFnu in the hour after waking. This indicates that the coordination between HRV and physical acceleration before sleep may not only affect sleep but also the autonomic nervous system after waking in older women with SAS.

To our knowledge, this is the first study to report that HFnu in the hour after waking in the morning was significantly increased in patients with SAS and that %Lag0 levels indicated impaired coordination between physical acceleration and HRV.

HRV analysis has been proposed as a simple screening test for the detection of SAS [15]. The autonomic nervous system (in the brain stem) is anatomically close to the hindbrain, which houses the sleep-wake regulating system. Moreover, the parasympathetic center is directly regulated by the solitary tract nucleus (within the hindbrain sleep center) [16].

Table 36.1 Characteristics of each group

		Control group	Group A	Group B
n		14	9	10
Age		71.6 ± 4.0	71.1 ± 7.5	73.7 ± 4.3
Body mass index		22.8 ± 3.7	21.6 ± 1.6	24.2 ± 4.5
Sleeping hours		476 ± 74*	424 ± 51	422 ± 91
Frequency of nocturnal awakening		1.1 ± 1.0	1.2 ± 1.0	1.0 ± 0.8
General Health Questionnaire A		2.3 ± 1.9	2.4 ± 1.9	2.4 ± 1.9
General Health Questionnaire B		3.6 ± 2.6	3.0 ± 2.5	2.9 ± 2.5
General Health Questionnaire C		1.0 ± 1.5	2.1 ± 1.7	1.4 ± 1.3
General Health Questionnaire D		1.6 ± 2.4	0.3 ± 1.0	1.7 ± 2.8
General Health Questionnaire sum		8.6 ± 7.0	7.9 ± 5.7	8.4 ± 6.1
Self-Depression Scale		42.8 ± 10.9	38.2 ± 9.5	39.8 ± 7.0
CMI neurosis tendency		2.6 ± 1.3	2.3 ± 1.0	2.3 ± 0.9
Diseases	Hypertension	3	1	3
	Hepatic dysfunction	2	1	0
	Hyperlipidemia	7	6	4
Physical acceleration during last hour before sleep		38.6 ± 13.6	37.9 ± 12.3	42.4 ± 12.8
Physical acceleration during first hour after waking		51.5 ± 25.0	53.4 ± 27.9	44.2 ± 16.7

Control: low 3% oxygen desaturation index (ODI) <5
Group A: high 3% ODI (>5) and high %Lag0 during 1 h before night sleep (>33)
Group B: high 3% ODI (>5) and low %Lag0 during 1 h before night sleep (<33)
*$p < 0.05$ control vs group A or group B

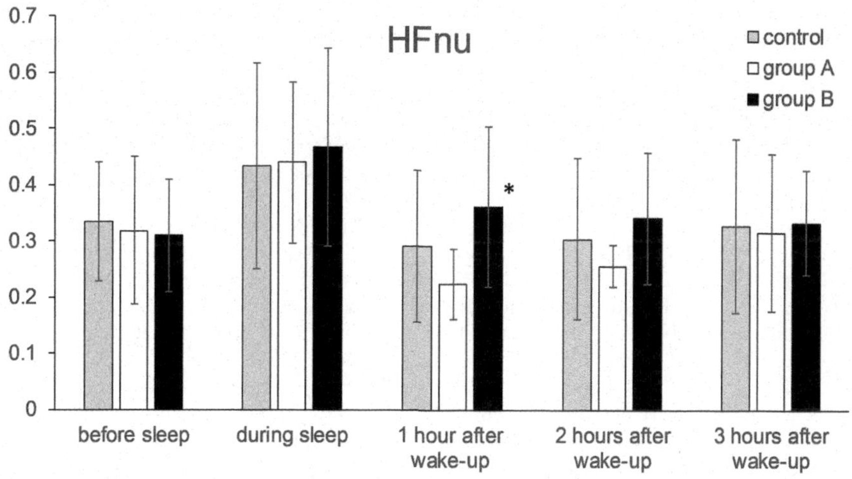

Fig. 36.1 Changes in the high frequency in normalized units (HFnu) before and during night sleep and every hour after waking for 3 hours. Control: low 3% ODI (<5); Group A: high 3% ODI (>5) and high %Lag0 during the hour before night sleep (>33); Group B: high 3% ODI (>5) and low %Lag0 during the hour before night sleep (<33) *$p < 0.05$ Group A vs. Group B

SAS causes systemic hypertension during waking and is associated with increased incidences of stroke, heart failure, atrial fibrillation, and coronary heart disease [1]. Generally, cardiovascular events are more likely to occur in the morning [17]. Thus, we consider that our new findings may be associated with impairments caused by SAS.

It is acknowledged that physical acceleration is linked with the autonomic nervous system [18]. Therefore, impairments to the coordination between HRV and physical acceleration may be derived from compromised links among the involved systems. Generally, HFnu was higher during sleep than after waking. The subjects with high ODI and low %Lag0 before sleep had high HFnu in the hour after waking. We considered that not only SAS but also low %Lag0 between HRV and physical acceleration before sleep may affect sleep quality and the autonomic nervous system during night sleep, which may, in turn, cause poor suppression of the parasympathetic nervous system in older women with SAS. Future studies are needed to clarify impairments to the mechanism responsible for the sleep-wake transition.

References

1. Javaheri S, Barbe F, Campos-Rodriguez F et al (2017) Sleep apnea: types, mechanisms, and clinical cardio-vascular consequences. J Am Coll Cardiol 69:841–858
2. Peppard PE, Young T, Barnet JH et al (2013) Increased prevalence of sleep-disordered breath- ing in adults. Am J Epidemiol 177:1006–1014
3. Task Force of the European Society of Cardiology and the North American Society of Pacing and Electrophysiology (1996) Heart rate variability: standards of measurement, physiological interpretation, and clinical use. Eur Heart J 93:1043–1065
4. Stein C, Dal Lago P, Ferreira JB et al (2011) Transcutaneous electrical nerve stimulation at different frequencies on heart rate variability in healthy subjects. Auton Neurosci 165:205–208
5. Malliani A, Montano N (2002) Heart rate variability as a clinical tool. Ital Heart J 3:439–445
6. Zemaityte D, Varoneckas G, Sokolov E (1984) Heart rhythm control during sleep. Psycho Physiol 21:279–289
7. Huikuri HV, Niemelä MJ, Ojala S et al (1994) Circadian rhythms of frequency domain measures of heart rate variability in healthy subjects and patients with coronary artery disease. Effects of arousal and upright posture. Circulation 90:121–126
8. Proper KI, Staal BJ, Hildebrandt VH et al (2002) Effectiveness of physical activity programs at worksites with respect to work-related outcomes. Scand J Work Environ Health 28(2):75–84

9. Taniguchi K, Shimouchi A, Seki J et al (2015) Factors affecting coordination between heart rate variability and physical acceleration in daily lives of free-moving adults. Adv Biomed Eng 4:35–41
10. Senaratna CV, Perret JL, Lodge CJ et al (2017) Prevalence of obstructive sleep apnea in the general population: a systematic review. Sleep Med Rev 34:70–81
11. Koenig J, Thayer JF (2016) Sex differences in healthy human heart rate variability: a meta-analysis. Neurosci Biobehav Rev 64:288–310
12. Brockbank CL, Chatterjee F, Bruce SA et al (2000) Heart rate and its variability change after the menopause. Exp Physiol 5:327–330
13. Kapur VK, Auckley DH, Chowdhuri S et al (2017) Clinical practice guideline for diagnostic testing for adult obstructive sleep apnea: an American academy of sleep medicine clinical practice guideline. J Clin Sleep Med 13(3):479–504
14. Iwashita S, Takeno Y, Okazaki K et al (2003) Triaxial accelerometry to evaluate walking ef- ficiency in older subjects. Med Sci Sports Exerc 35:1766–1772
15. Guilleminault C, Connolly S, Winkle R (1984) Cyclical variation of the heart rate in sleep apnoea syndrome. Mechanisms, and usefulness of 24 h electrocardiography as a screening technique. Lancet 1:126–131
16. Sakai K, Crochet S (2003) A neural mechanism of sleep and wakefulness. Sleep Biol Rhythm 1:29–42
17. Arntz HR, Willich SN, Oeff M et al (1993) Circadian variation of sudden cardiac death re- flects age-related variability in ventricular fibrillation. Circulation 88:2284–2289
18. Mueller PJ (2007) Exercise training and sympathetic nervous system activity: evidence for physical activity dependent neural plasticity. Clin Exp Pharmacol Physiol 34:377–384

The Changes in Brain Oxygenation During Transcranial Alternating Current Stimulation as Consequences of Traumatic Brain Injury: A Near-Infrared Spectroscopy Study

37

Alex O. Trofimov, Arthem A. Kopylov, Dmitry S. Martynov, Anna V. Zorkova, Ksenia Trofimova, Peter N. Cheremuhin, and Denis E. Bragin

Abstract

The aim was to evaluate the changes in brain tissue oxygenation, assessed by near-infrared spectroscopy (NIRS), during transcranial alternating current stimulation (tACS) in patients with mild and moderate traumatic brain injury (TBI). Nineteen patients with diffuse, blunt, non-severe TBI (mean age 32.7 ± 11.4 years; 4 women and 15 men; Glasgow Coma Score before tACS 14.1 ± 0.5) were treated by 10 Hz in-phase tACS applied for 30 minutes to the left and right lateral prefrontal cortex at 21 days after TBI. Regional cerebral tissue oxygen saturation ($SctO_2$) in the frontal lobes was measured simultaneously by the cerebral oximeter. Significance was preset to $P < 0.05$. The $SctO_2$ values before tACS were not different between hemispheres ~65%. After 15 minutes of tACS, a significant ($p < 0.05$) decrease in regional $SctO_2$ was observed with the minimum at the eighth minute of 53.4 ± 3.2% and 53.4 ± 3.2% in the left and right hemispheres, respectively. At the end of the stimulation (30 minutes), the hemispheric differences in cerebral oxygen saturation became statistically insignificant again ($p > 0.05$). Therefore, tACS causes a significant decrease in $SctO_2$, probably, due to neuronal activation. Our data indicate that tACS may need to be supplemented with oxygen therapy. Further research is required.

A. O. Trofimov (✉)
Department of Neurosurgery, Privolzhsky Research Medical University, Nizhny Novgorod, Russia

Department of Neurosurgery, Regional Hospital named after Semashko, Nizhny Novgorod, Russia

A. A. Kopylov · A. V. Zorkova · K. Trofimova
Department of Neurosurgery, Privolzhsky Research Medical University, Nizhny Novgorod, Russia

D. S. Martynov
Nizhny Novgorod State Technical University named after R.E. Alekseev, Nizhny Novgorod, Russia

P. N. Cheremuhin
Department of Neurosurgery, Regional Hospital named after Semashko, Nizhny Novgorod, Russia

D. E. Bragin
Lovelace Biomedical Research Institute, Albuquerque, NM, USA

University of New Mexico School of Medicine, Departments of Neurology and Neurosurgery, Albuquerque, NM, USA

E. M. Nemoto et al. (eds.), *Oxygen Transport to Tissue XLII*, Advances in Experimental Medicine and Biology 1269, https://doi.org/10.1007/978-3-030-48238-1_37

Keywords

Alternating current stimulation · Brain injury

37.1 Introduction

Traumatic brain injury (TBI) triggers an array of delayed pathological responses, making TBI a risk factor for neurodegenerative and other conditions such as posttraumatic encephalopathy. Transcranial alternating current stimulation (tACS) is a method of brain stimulation where a sinusoidal oscillating low-voltage electric current, adjusted to one's maximal endogenous frequency [1, 2], is applied to the scalp. Unlike transcranial direct current stimulation (tDCS), tACS has no visible motor effects [3]. The tACS leads to a shift in the oscillations of the membrane potential from its resting potential to slightly more depolarized but not hyperpolarized states. Thus, in a state of depolarization, neurons are triggered with greater frequency in response to other neurons (the so-called stochastic resonance) [4]. As a result, tACS has a modulating (but not imposing) effect on the neurovascular unit.

Oscillations within the alpha band range (8–12 Hz) have various correlations with brain states [5]. Several studies have proven to be effective in increasing alpha power using 10 Hz tACS. Previous studies have shown a reduction in saturation during tDCS [6, 7]. However, the dynamics of cerebral oxygenation during and after tACS in patients with TBI remains unknown.

We hypothesized that despite tACS being potentially different from tDCS, it causes a decrease in the oxygen saturation in the damaged brain. Thus, this work aimed to evaluate the changes in brain oxygenation, assessed by near-infrared spectroscopy (NIRS), during tACS in patients with TBI.

37.2 Methods

This is a prospective non-randomized single-center study that complies with the Declaration of Helsinki, and the protocol was approved by the local ethics committee. All the patients gave informed consent to participate in the study.

TACS was used as part of the rehabilitation treatment of patients with mild and moderate TBI.

We included patients who had the following: mild and moderate TBI within 21 days after a head injury with a GCS more than 12 and Marshall grade I.

The exclusion criteria were as follows: (1) younger than 16 years, (2) Glasgow Coma Score less than 12, (3) any intracranial volume injury with Marshall grades II–VI (intracranial hematoma, traumatic parenchymal lesions, etc.) and cardiovascular injury, and (4) before tACS were not taking neurotropic medications.

In total, 19 patients with diffuse, blunt, non-severe TBI admitted to the Nizhny Novgorod Regional Hospital were studied. The mean age was 32.7 ± 11.4 years (range 19–45 years). There were 4 women and 15 men. The level of wakefulness according to the Glasgow Coma Score before tACS was 14.1 ± 0.5 (range 12–15).

37.2.1 tACS

Each of the patients received in-phase tACS applied to the left frontal cortex and right lateral prefrontal cortex with a pair of gel-soaked surface sponge electrodes (Ambu, USA) as common in tDCS. According to previous studies [8], the applied current was always sinusoidal with a 2.0 mA amplitude and a 10 Hz frequency. The sinusoidal current waveform did not result in measurable higher harmonics. The voltage of the stimulator was always less than 20 V. The tACS device was designed and manufactured at Nizhny Novgorod State Technical University (Nizhny Novgorod, Russia). No complications caused by tACS were identified.

37.2.2 Cerebral Oximetry

The cerebral oximetry was simultaneously performed by a two-channel, space-resolved spectroscopy monitor Fore-Sight 2030 (CAS Medical Systems Inc., Branford, CT, USA). The NIRS probe was set symmetrically on the forehead: the positioning is similar to midpoint between electrode position Fp1–Fp3 (left) and Fp2–Fp4 (right) of the international 10–20 system) [9]. Received data were collected using a multimodality monitoring system providing half minute-by-half minute average values. Manual assessments of NIRS data were performed to avoid errors due to the patient's movements. The $SctO_2$ values were compared before stimulation, by the 15th minute and at the end of the tACS.

37.2.3 Statistical Analysis

Statistical analysis of all results was performed using T-criterion Wilcoxon. The level of significance was preset at $p < 0.05$. Data are shown as a mean ± standard deviation.

37.3 Results

Before the stimulation, $SctO_2$ value varied between 51% and 89%, with a mean of 64.9 ± 8.2% on the left side and 65.8 ± 6.9% on the right side. $SctO_2$ values were not significantly different between hemispheres of the brain (T-criterion Wilcoxon = 35; Z-score = 1.41; $p = 0.15$).

The tACS led to a significant decrease in the cerebral oxygen saturation in the frontal lobe (T-criterion Wilcoxon = 2; Z-score = 3.29; $p = 0.009$). $SctO_2$ value reached a minimum by the eighth minute of the stimulation and varied between 47% and 67% (mean $SctO_2$ = 53.4 ± 3.2% on the left side and 51.3 ± 3.9% on the right side).

The average duration of the "decline plateau" was 8 minutes. After that, the $SctO_2$ values gradually increased and reached the baseline levels by the end of the stimulation (T-criterion Wilcoxon = 23; Z-score = 1.57; $p = 0.115$), with a mean $SctO_2$ being 64.8 ± 5.5% on the left side and 63.6 ± 6.2% on the right side (Fig. 37.1).

37.4 Discussion

In the present study, we measured cerebral oxygenation in frontal cortex areas before, during, and after tACS. $SctO_2$ decreased during the procedure and then increased again after the stimulation was terminated o the initial values. A previous study showed that motor learning was improved by applying 10 Hz tACS [10]. In addition, alpha band tACS (7–12 Hz) decreased corticomuscular coherence over 30 min after the procedure [10].

As is known, near-infrared spectroscopy can be used to measure changes in the cerebral hemodynamic response and metabolic shifts, thus allowing for the use even of single-channel NIRS recording for functional optical imaging of the human brain activity during stimulation [11]. Although many studies have reported the changes of cerebral oxygenation levels during tDCS [11–13] or constant work rate [14, 15] and exercise, the effects of tACS on cerebral oxygenation at TBI were unknown. This study clarifies the effects of an alternating current on cerebral oxygenation and thus provides some fundamental data regarding neural plasticity induced by electrostimulation of the frontal lobe of the brain.

One of the main findings of this study is that tACS results in a significantly lower $SctO_2$ level throughout the frontal cortex. Another important finding is that the $SctO_2$ values during the stimulation are significantly lower than the values in the rest condition (before the procedure) and at the end of the stimulation. Regarding the decrease in $SctO_2$ in the entire frontal area, a similar change was observed in a study by Polania et al. [6] who reported that electric current changed the functional connections between different parts of the human brain; therefore, cerebral blood flow might be redistributed to the region of the stimulation. This suggests the possibility that $SctO_2$ decreased in the region where the connection was not strengthened. The strengthening of neuronal structures, which constitute the oscillatory network of the brain, by tACS may facilitate the spiking of neurons (and probably glial cells), which in turn may lead to further spiking by adjacent neurons [4].

According to Del Felice [2], brain intrinsic dynamic networks are highly non-entropic systems, which tend to spontaneously return to the point of equilibrium or into the physiological oscillatory range. We think that, probably, this mechanism, based on neurovascular coupling,

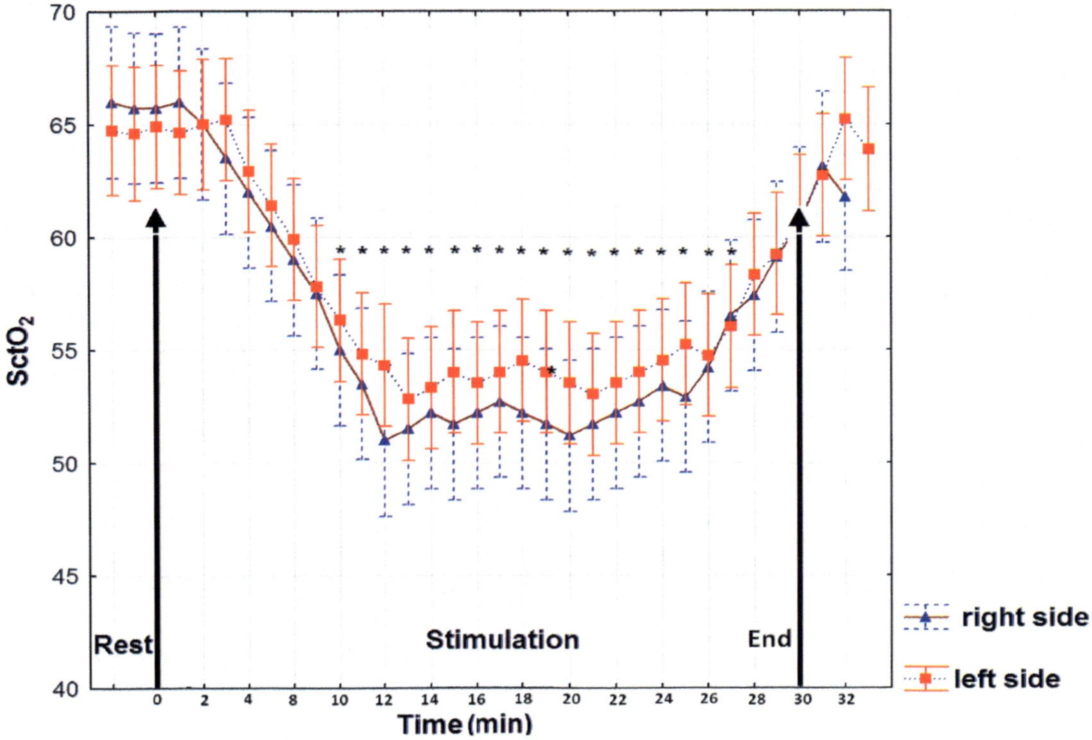

Fig. 37.1 Temporal changes in cerebral tissue oxygenation ($SctO_2$, red boxes – left frontal lobes, blue triangles – right frontal lobes) values before tACS (rest zone) and during procedures (stimulation zone). Values are presented as mean ± standard deviation of the mean. *Significant difference ($p < 0.05$)

led to the restoration of cerebral oxygenation in the frontal lobes at the end of the stimulation, which was demonstrated by our data. At the same time, a decrease in cerebral oxygenation during tACS indicates damage to the coupling between it and cerebral blood flow even at non-severe TBI, as confirmed by previous studies [8, 16].

However, our study had some limitations. First, we measured oxygenation only in the frontal lobes of the brain, and this study did not consider the distribution of cerebral oxygenation in other areas of the cortex during and after tACS. Second, the measurement sites were slightly different for stimulation probes and NIRS optodes, which could somewhat reduce the accuracy of the measurements. The creation of sensors combining both a stimulator and an oximeter could correct this drawback. Third, to clarify the mechanisms of the mismatch between neuronal activity and oxygenation, it is necessary to assess the state of cerebral autoregulation. All these issues require further study.

37.5 Conclusion

Transcranial alternating current stimulation causes a significant ($p < 0.05$) decrease in regional $SctO_2$, probably, due to a tissue reaction to neuronal activation. Our data indicate that tACS may need to be supplemented with oxygen therapy. Further research is required.

Acknowledgments The reported study was funded by RFBR, project number 20-015-00110; DB was supported by NIH R01 NS112808.

References

1. Helfrich RF, Knepper H, Nolte G (2014) Selective modulation of interhemispheric functional connectivity by HD-tACS shapes perception. PLoS Biol 12(12):e1002031
2. Del Felice A, Magalini A, Masiero S (2015) Slow-oscillatory transcranial direct current stimulation modulates memory in temporal lobe epilepsy by altering sleep spindle generators: a possible rehabilitation tool. Brain Stimul 8(3):567–573
3. Elsner B, Kwakkel G, Kugler J et al (2017) Transcranial direct current stimulation (tDCS) for improving capacity in activities and arm function after stroke: a network meta-analysis of randomised controlled trials. J Neuroeng Rehabil 14(1):95
4. McDonnell M, Abbott D (2009) What is stochastic resonance? Definitions, misconceptions, debates, and its relevance to biology. PLoS Comput Biol 5(5):e1000348
5. De Koninck BP, Guay S, Proulx-Begin L et al (2019) Optimized tACS parameters for modulation of alpha oscillation. Brain Stimul 12(2):507
6. Polanıa R, Paulus W, Antal A et al (2011) Introducing graph theory to track for neuroplastic alterations in the resting human brain: a transcranial direct current stimulation study. NeuroImage 54(3):2287–2296
7. Nitsche MA, Paulus W (2000) Excitability changes induced in the human motor cortex by weak transcranial direct current stimulation. J Physiol 527(3):633–639
8. Bikson M, Esmaeilpour Z, Adair D et al (2019) Transcranial electrical stimulation nomenclature. Brain Stimul 12(6):1349–1366
9. Tavakoli A, Yun K (2017) Transcranial alternating current stimulation (tACS) mechanisms and protocols. Front Cell Neurosci 11:1–10
10. Moriya M, Aoki C, Sakatani K (2016) Effects of physical exercise on working memory and prefrontal cortex function in post-stroke patients. Adv Exp Med Biol 923:203–208
11. Tamura M, Hoshi Y, Okada F (1997) Localized near-infrared spectroscopy and functional optical imaging of brain activity. Philos Trans R Soc Lond Ser B Biol Sci 352:737–742
12. Bhambhani Y, Malik R, Mookerjee S (2007) Cerebral oxygenation declines at exercise intensities above the respiratory compensation threshold. Respir Physiol Neurobiol 156:196–202
13. Rupp T, Perrey S (2008) Prefrontal cortex oxygenation and neuromuscular responses to exhaustive exercise. Eur J Appl Physiol 102:153–163
14. Peltonen JE, Paterson DH, Shoemaker JK et al (2009) Cerebral and muscle deoxygenation, hypoxic ventilatory chemosensitivity and cerebrovascular responsiveness during incremental exercise. Respir Physiol Neurobiol 169:24–35
15. Tsubaki A, Takai H, Kojima S et al (2016) Changes in cortical oxyhaemoglobin signal during low-intensity cycle ergometer activity: a near-infrared spectroscopy study. Adv Exp Med Biol 876:79–85
16. Zhao M, Ma H et al (2014) Neurovascular coupling methods. Springer New York Heidelberg Dordrecht London, p 335

Error Evaluation for Automated Diameter Measurements of Cerebral Capillaries Captured with Two-Photon Laser Scanning Fluorescence Microscopy

38

Hiroki Suzuki, Takuma Sugashi, Hiroshi Takeda,
Hiroyuki Takuwa, Iwao Kanno,
and Kazuto Masamoto

Abstract

Cerebral capillaries respond to changes in neural activity to maintain regional balances between energy demand and supply. However, the quantitative aspects of the capillary diameter responses and their contribution to oxygen supply to tissue remain incompletely understood. The purpose of the present study is to check if the diameters measured from large-scale angiographic image data of two-photon laser scanning fluorescent microscopy (2PLSM) are correctly determined with a custom-written MATLAB software and to investigate how the measurement errors can be reduced, such as at the junction areas of capillaries. As a result, nearly 17% of the measured locations appeared to be outliers of the automated diameter measurements, in particular arising from the junction areas where three capillary segments merged. We observed that about two-thirds of the outliers originated from the measured locations within 6 μm from the branching point. The results indicate that the capillary locations in the junction areas cause non-negligible errors in the automated diameter measurements. Considering the common site of the outliers, the present study identified that the areas within 6 μm from the branch point could be separately measured from the diameter analysis, and careful manual inspection with reference to the original images for these transition areas around the branch point is further recommended.

Keywords

Brain microcirculation · Optical imaging · 3D image analysis · Animal experiments · Neurovascular coupling

H. Suzuki (✉) · T. Sugashi · H. Takeda
Graduate School of Informatics and Engineering,
University of Electro-Communications, Tokyo, Japan
e-mail: suzuki@nvu.mi.uec.ac.jp

H. Takuwa · I. Kanno
Department of Functional Brain Imaging Research,
National Institute of Radiological Sciences,
Chiba, Japan

K. Masamoto
Department of Functional Brain Imaging Research,
National Institute of Radiological Sciences,
Chiba, Japan

Center for Neuroscience and Biomedical Engineering, University of Electro-Communications, Tokyo, Japan
e-mail: masamoto@mce.uec.ac.jp

E. M. Nemoto et al. (eds.), *Oxygen Transport to Tissue XLII*, Advances in Experimental Medicine and Biology 1269, https://doi.org/10.1007/978-3-030-48238-1_38

38.1 Introduction

Cerebral capillaries respond to changes in neural activity to maintain regional energy demand and supply. To better understand the quantitative relationship between oxygen supply from the capillaries and oxygen demand in tissue, precise structure and functional data on brain microvasculature are prerequisites.

Two-photon laser scanning fluorescent microscopy (2PLSM) allows us to capture a three-dimensional complex network of the cerebral microvessels in vivo by fluorescently imaging labeled blood plasma with a sequential scan (i.e., XYZ scanning) from the cortical surface to a depth of about 0.8 mm in the rodent cortex [1]. By extracting a centerline of the vessels and measuring the minimum distance from the vessel center to the boundary of the labeled blood plasma on each slice images, a vessel diameter (i.e., an intra-lumen diameter) can be automatically measured with the aid of MATLAB-based software [2]. However, it should be considered that the automated diameter measurements may produce false measurements around junction areas where three capillary segments merge at the single point.

The purpose of the present study is therefore to check if the diameters in the junction areas are correctly determined with the MATLAB software that automatically determines the vascular diameters along the centerline of the vessels on the 2PLSM angiographic images and to investigate how measurement errors can be reduced, such as in the junction areas of capillary networks.

38.2 Methods

The experimental protocol was approved by the institutional animal ethics committee of the National Institute of Radiological Sciences and the University of Electro-Communications. Two male and four female adult C57BL/6 mice (25–33 g) were used for the imaging experiments, in accordance with previously published studies [2–5]. Briefly, the cortical microvascular networks were visualized with two-photon microscopy (TCS-SP5MP, Leica Microsystems) excited at 910 nm by fluorescently labeling blood plasma with an intraperitoneal injection of sulforhodamine 101 (through a band-pass filter for 610/75 nm) [3]. The head of the animal was fixed under isoflurane anesthesia, and the skull was opened. The animals were then allowed to recover from anesthesia. Under fully recovered awake conditions, the whiskers of the animals were mechanically stimulated for 20–30 sec with a time interval of 30–180 sec [4, 5], while vascular responses were repeatedly measured with XYZ scanning (256 by 256 pixels with an in-plane resolution of 1.0 μm/pixel and a step size of 1.58 μm) over depths of 100–300 μm in the activated somatosensory cortex. It took about 30 sec to acquire a single volume image, and a total of 20 XYZ images were acquired for each stimulation and resting conditions. Additionally, high-resolution XYZ scanning (1024 by 1024 pixels with an in-plane resolution of 0.25 μm/pixel and a step size of 0.79 μm) was conducted to determine the fine structure of the measured microvessels before or after the functional experiments.

All images acquired with 2PLSM were analyzed with custom-written MATLAB software. First, a measured vessel region was defined using the high-resolution (i.e., 0.25 μm/pixel) anatomical image. The image was roughly binarized to extract the vessel regions, and 3D thinning was applied to determine a centerline of the vessels with manual corrections. Then, individual trial images were binarized according to a signal-to-noise ratio (i.e., at a full-width half-maximum point with a linear correction to the signal-to-noise ratio in each pixel location; see also Sugashi et al. in this book) over the cross section of the vessel, and its diameter was measured along the centerlines of the segment. The diameter was the minimum width of the cross section of the vessel, determined by measuring the widths of the cross section around the center point with 1 degree increments from 0 to 180 degrees in each trial image.

38.3 Results

A total of 4559–7096 pixel locations were obtained in each animal for 3D reconstruction over depths of 100–300 μm with 2PLSM in the awake mouse cortex. The custom-written MATLAB software successfully analyzed 2997–5813 pixel locations for automated diameter measurements, excluding large vessels in diameter more than 10 μm. A representative image is shown in Fig. 38.1 (n = 3187 capillary locations in N = 1 animal). The average diameter and length of the measured segments whose end points at both sides were identified as the branch points were 5.6 ± 1.2 μm and 68 ± 54 μm, respectively, over 78 segments in this representative animal. A mean segment diameter was slightly larger than those of the grand average diameter (5.2 ± 1.4 μm), which is due to a relatively larger contribution of large diameter segments which had shorter length (a small number of pixels per segment).

Next, the average diameter was compared in axial directions of the vessel segment. All segments were divided at the center of the segment and averaged at each pixel location from the branch point. Figure 38.2 represents axial distribution of the mean capillary diameter, showing that relatively large diameters and variations exist near the branch points. In these locations, most of the measured diameters had outliers (i.e., more or less than two standard deviations in all measured diameters over 3187 locations), indicating that the diameters around the branch points were inaccurately measured by the software. According to a histogram of the outlier locations along the capillary segment (Fig. 38.2, right), about two-thirds of the outliers originated from the junction areas within 6 μm from the branch point.

Those locations of the outliers were displayed in three-dimensionally reconstructed microvascular networks, and those junction areas (less than 6 μm from the branch point) were also highlighted (Fig. 38.3). Accordingly, 210 out of 337 outliers were observed to be overlapped in the junction areas. Considering the localization of the outliers in the junction areas, capillary diameters were re-averaged for other pixel locations (2642 points) excluding the junction areas (545 points), which resulted in 5.0 ± 1.2 μm. The mean segment diameters and lengths over 69 segments are 5.2 ± 1.1 μm and 75 ± 53 μm, respectively.

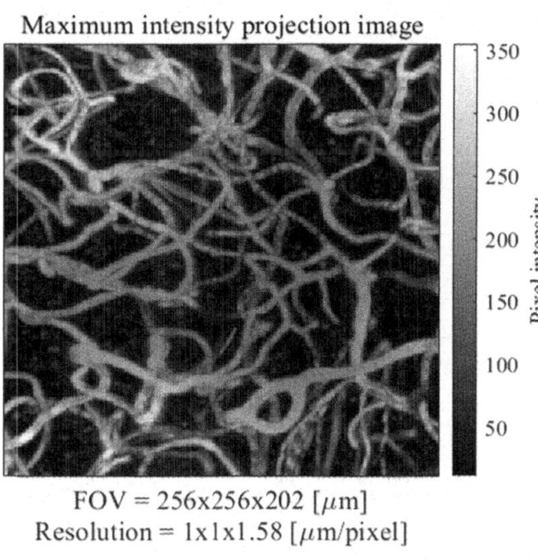

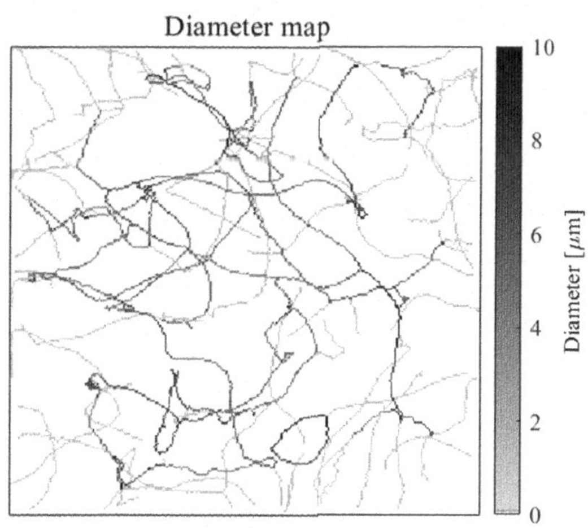

Fig. 38.1 A representative image of cortical microvasculature in the mouse cortex in vivo captured with 2PLSM. (Left) The image shows the maximum intensity projection over depths of 100–300 μm in the somatosensory cortex. (Right) A mean diameter map measured over 20 trials for resting states at the location shown in Left. The gray scale indicated to the right of the diameter map corresponds to the diameter measured at the pixel location on the left, and the line is a centerline of the extracted capillary segments. The capillary segment was defined as the capillary whose both ends are the branch point (connecting to other capillaries) within the field of view (FOV)

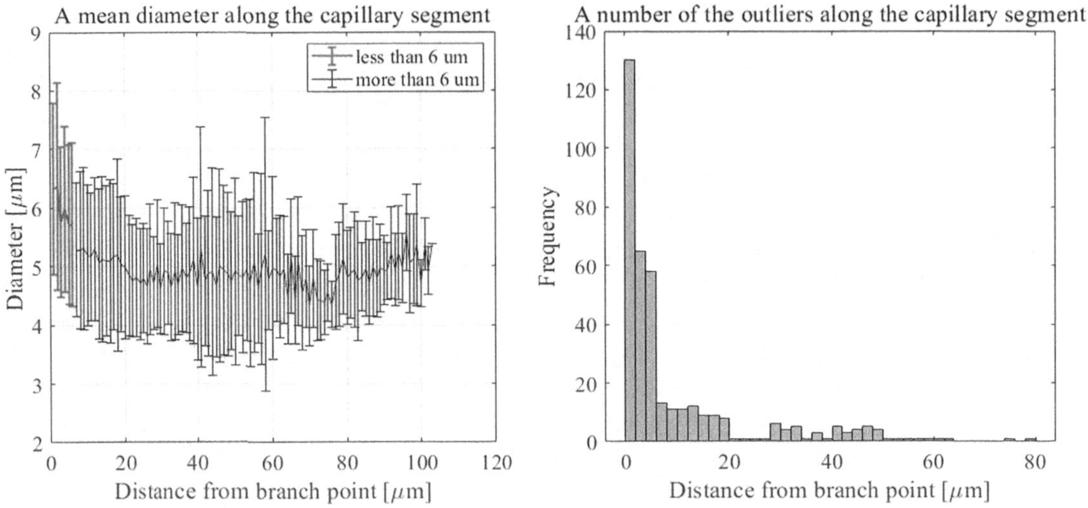

Fig. 38.2 A comparison for distribution of the measured diameters and outliers along the single capillary segments. (Left) A comparison of mean diameters over the segments in axial direction of the segment. Due to variable segment lengths, a single segment was divided in two at the center of the segment and includes both segments for this specific calculation. A total of 156 half segments (i.e., 78 capillary full segments) were used. Average diameters and standard deviation (an error bar) are noticeably larger around the branching points. (Right) A histogram of the outlier distribution, measured from all 3187 capillary locations. Two-thirds of the outliers (210 out of 337) were observed to be present within less than 6 μm from the branch point

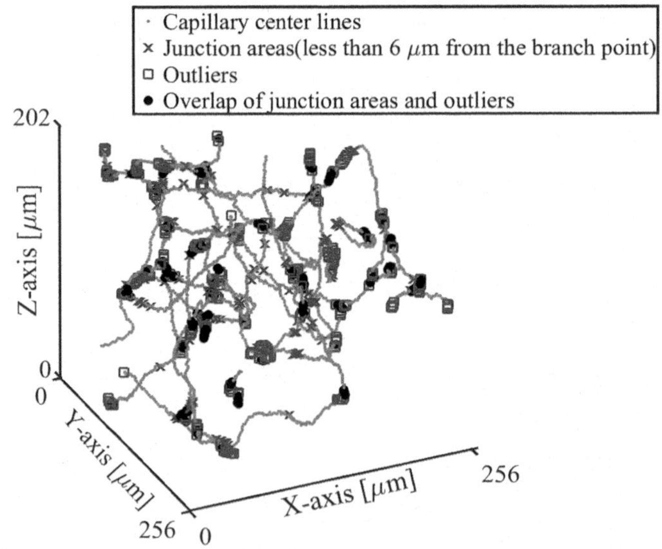

Fig. 38.3 Three-dimensionally (3D) reconstructed image of the capillary center point (n = 3187 points, shown as a gray dot). A total of 64 branch points were identified in this representative image shown in Fig. 38.1. Junction areas (within a distance of 6 μm from the branch point) were represented as dark gray lines, and outliers (more or less than two standard deviation of the measured dimeters over all locations) were displayed as a thick dark gray dot. The figure represents that 210 out of 337 outliers were produced in the junction areas (overlap, as shown as black dots)

38.4 Discussion

A total of 3187 capillary locations in single XYZ images of 2PLSM were analyzed with the custom-written software for the automated diameter measurements (Fig. 38.1). The software allows us to quantitatively measure large-scale 2PLSM image data, which has advantages in saving time and increasing statistical power. However, nearly 17% of the measured locations appeared to be producing outliers, and two-thirds of the outliers are localized in the junction areas where three capillary segments meet at a single point. Excluding those outliers within the junction areas, the mean capillary diameters measured over all measured locations and over segments were both slightly reduced. This is because the measured errors arising from the junction areas caused an overestimation due to the absence of the clear boundary on the cross section. According to a common site that preferentially produced the outliers (Fig. 38.2), the present study tentatively cuts off 6 μm from the branch point for the capillary segment measurements. This threshold is slightly larger than the mean capillary diameter, suggesting the potential exclusion of the important locations. Namely, the capillary segment which is applicable for the automated diameter measurements is limited to the capillaries whose length is larger than 12 μm. However, this condition satisfies most of the segments we analyzed in the present study (69/78 segments). In addition, this elimination is more effective for segmental analysis because of a larger reduction of mean segment diameter relative to the grand average. Nevertheless, it is likely missing important measurements near the branch points, such as for pericyte regulation and functional sphincters [6]. Therefore, careful consideration and further manual inspection with reference to the raw images are warranted.

Another technical viewpoint for the automated diameter measurements is that analytical consideration of transitions from the branch point to the capillary segment is needed for quantification of the blood volume responses in the 2PLSM images. One of the advantages in using the automated data analysis with the software relative to manual measurements is availability of the large-scale quantitative data from the reconstructed volume images. However, the present methods lack accuracy for the measurements around the junction areas. This shortcoming should be overcome in future studies, because our estimation showed that those junction areas account for 20.3% of the measured capillary locations, which is not negligible for quantification of entire vascular volumes.

In conclusion, the capillary locations in the junction areas cause non-negligible errors in the automated diameter measurements of the capillary segments. Based on the results of the common site of the outlier pixels, the present study identified that the areas within 6 μm from the branch point could be separately measured from the segment analysis, and further manual inspection with reference to the raw images (anatomical and/or functional images) specific to these transition areas is recommended.

Acknowledgments This study was partly supported by JSPS KAKENHI (JP201710551 to TS and 19K07795 to KM).

References

1. Yoshihara K, Takuwa H, Kanno et al (2013) 3D analysis of intracortical microvasculature during chronic hypoxia in mouse brains. Adv Exp Med Biol 765:357–363
2. Sekiguchi Y, Masamoto K, Takuwa H et al (2013) Measuring the vascular diameter of brain surface and parenchymal arteries in awake mouse. Adv Exp Med Biol 789:419–425
3. Masamoto K, Tomita Y, Toriumi H et al (2012) Repeated longitudinal in vivo imaging of neuro-glio-vascular unit at the peripheral boundary of ischemia in mouse cerebral cortex. Neuroscience 212:190–200
4. Sekiguchi Y, Takuwa H, Kawaguchi H et al (2014) Pial arteries respond earlier than penetrating arterioles to neural activation in the somatosensory cortex in awake mice exposed to chronic hypoxia: an additional mechanism to proximal integration signaling? J Cereb Blood Flow Metab 34:1761–1770
5. Takuwa H, Autio J, Nakayama H et al (2011) Reproducibility and variance of a stimulation-induced hemodynamic response in barrel cortex of awake behaving mice. Brain Res 1369:103–111
6. Grubb S, Cai C, Hald BO et al Precapillary sphincters control cerebral blood flow. 657486(2019):bioRxiv. https://doi.org/10.1101/657486

Potential Biomarker for Triple-Negative Breast Cancer Invasiveness by Optical Redox Imaging

39

Min Feng, He N. Xu, Jinxia Jiang, and Lin Z. Li

Abstract

Predicting tumor metastatic potential remains a challenge in cancer research and in clinical diagnosis. Cancer invasion to neighboring tissues is a significant event in cancer progression to metastasis. Optical redox imaging (ORI) is based on detecting the endogenous fluorescence signals of reduced nicotinamide adenine dinucleotide (NADH) and oxidized flavin adenine dinucleotide (FAD). Previously, we found that ORI can discriminate between cancer and normal tissue specimens from clinical breast cancer patients and can differentiate the relative invasiveness of melanoma and breast tumors. In this study, we aimed to identify ORI biomarkers to differentiate the invasiveness of four triple-negative breast cancer cell lines (TNBC). Using a fluorescence microscope, we acquired NADH and FAD fluorescent signals from cultured MDA-MB-231, MDA-MB-436, HCC1806, and MDA-MB-468 cells. We found that (1) the redox ratio, FAD/(NADH+FAD), differentiated the four TNBC lines; (2) there was a significant difference of invasive potential between MDA-MB-231 and the other three TNBC lines measured by the transwell invasion assay; and (3) there was a positive logarithmic correlation between the redox ratio and the invasive potential, where the most invasive MDA-MB-231 cells had the highest redox ratio and the least invasive MDA-MB-468 cells had the lowest redox ratio. These results suggest that the redox ratio can potentially be used as a biomarker for TNBC invasiveness and prognosis.

Keywords

Optical redox imaging · NADH and FAD · Redox ratio · Triple-negative breast cancer · TNBC · Invasive potential

39.1 Introduction

In 2018, there were about 2.1 million newly diagnosed female breast cancer cases worldwide, and breast cancer is the leading cause of cancer death for female in over 100 countries [1]. It was estimated that 20–30% of patients with node-negative breast cancer will ultimately develop metastatic disease with poor prognosis [2]. Furthermore, the current diagnostic methods can-

M. Feng · H. N. Xu (✉) · J. Jiang · L. Z. Li (✉)
Britton Chance Laboratory of Redox Imaging, Department of Radiology, Perelman School of Medicine, University of Pennsylvania, Philadelphia, PA, USA
e-mail: hexu2@pennmedicine.upenn.edu; linli@pennmedicine.upenn.edu

E. M. Nemoto et al. (eds.), *Oxygen Transport to Tissue XLII*, Advances in Experimental Medicine and Biology 1269, https://doi.org/10.1007/978-3-030-48238-1_39

not accurately predict the metastatic potential of individual tumors. Triple-negative breast cancer (TNBC) is a highly aggressive form of breast cancer and has a poorer prognosis compared to other forms of breast cancer [3]. TNBC is also heterogeneous in many aspects, including its invasiveness. Invasion is one of the key steps of cancer metastasis. Thus, to improve TNBC patient survival, it is important to identify novel biomarkers that can more accurately characterize TNBC invasiveness.

Optical redox imaging (ORI), pioneered by Britton Chance et al., is based on detecting the endogenous fluorescence signals of reduced nicotinamide adenine dinucleotide (NADH) and oxidized flavin adenine dinucleotide (FAD) [4–7]. Recently, ORI has been employed in many cancer studies such as discrimination of cancer aggressiveness [8–10], differentiation among receptor status of breast cancers [11], distinction between clinical biopsies of breast cancer and normal tissues [12], and monitoring therapeutic effects [13, 14]. Previously, Sun et al. showed that the redox ratio differentiated among four breast cancer lines of different molecular subtypes in culture, with the most invasive lines showing the largest redox ratio [15]. In this study, we focused on investigating four TNBC cell lines: MDA-MB-231, MDA-MB-436, HCC1806, and MDA-MB-468. These four TNBC lines represent different molecular subgroups within TNBCs [16] and have different invasive potential. Thus, we selected them as our initial models for the discovery of potential redox biomarkers of invasiveness. We performed ORI of these lines and measured their invasive potentials using the Boyden chamber method. We tested the hypothesis that the redox ratio correlates with the invasive potential of these lines.

39.2 Materials and Methods

TNBC cell lines MDA-MB-231, MDA-MB-436, HCC1806, and MDA-MB-468 were cultured in RPMI 1640 medium (phenol red-free, 11.1 mM glucose, 2.1 mM glutamine, Gibco® catalog no. 11835030) supplemented with 10% FBS and 1% penicillin/strep and maintained at 37 °C and 5% CO_2. Cells (4×10^4, 200 μl) were seeded on 35 mm glass bottom dishes (MatTek, part no. P35GC-1.5-14-C) and incubated for 24 hours as previously described [17]. Approximately 1 hour before imaging, the medium was changed to live cell imaging solution (LCIS, Life Technology®) supplemented with 11 mM glucose and 2.1 mM L- glutamine.

NADH and FAD fluorescence images were obtained under 37 °C with a DeltaVision Deconvolution Microscope System that consists of a xenon lamp as the excitation light source, a 12-bit CCD, an objective of 40X/0.95 NA (image matrix size 512 × 512, bin 2 × 2, and pixel size 0.32 μm), proper excitation/emission filters (NADH: 360 ± 20/455 ± 25 nm; FAD: 470 ± 20/520 ± 20 nm), and an exposure time of 3 s. Three to five fields of view (FOV) were taken for each dish. A customized MATLAB® program was used to extract NADH and FAD signals. Technical details can be found in our previous work [13, 17]. The mean values of FAD, NADH, and redox ratio were averaged across FOVs and then across dishes to obtain the group means and their standard errors (SE).

The Boyden chamber method was employed to measure the invasive potential (IVP) of the TNBC cells as previously described [17, 18]. Each upper chamber of a transwell insert (Corning, catalog No. 3422) was coated with 20 μl Matrigel (Corning, catalog no. CB356238) in a 1:1.5 dilution of Matrigel by FBS-free RPMI 1640 medium. Cells were cultured in serum-free RPMI media for 24 hours and seeded at a density of 5×10^4 cells with 300 μL FBS-free RPMI 1640 medium in the upper chamber. The lower chamber was filled with 500 μL complete RPMI 1640 cell culture medium (containing 10% FBS as chemotactic stimulus). The chambers were incubated at 37 °C for 20 hours. The invaded cells were fixed in methanol and stained with DAPI (300 nM) and tile imaged with a fluorescence microscope to cover the whole area of the chamber membrane. The total numbers of invading cells were quantified using ImageJ (NIH, United States). Triplicate wells were used in each experiment, and the experiment was repeated three times.

One-way ANOVA with post-hoc Tukey multiple comparisons was performed with Prism 8 (GraphPad®) for statistical analysis of the group differences, and $p < 0.05$ was considered statistically significant.

39.3 Results

Figure 39.1 shows the typical redox images for each cell line. The quantitative analysis showed that MDA-MB-231 had the highest FAD intensity while HCC1806 had the lowest FAD intensity among the four TNBC cell lines (Fig. 39.2). On the other hand, MDA-MB-468 had the highest NADH intensity and was significantly different from the other three TNBC cell lines ($p < 0.001$). Furthermore, statistical analysis indicated significant differences in redox ratios among four lines except between HCC1806 and MDA-MB-468. The rank order of the redox ratio from the highest to the lowest was found as follows: MDA-MB-231 > MDA-MB-436 > HCC18 06 > MDA-MB-468.

Based on the total number of cells that invaded through Matrigel-coated membrane, we

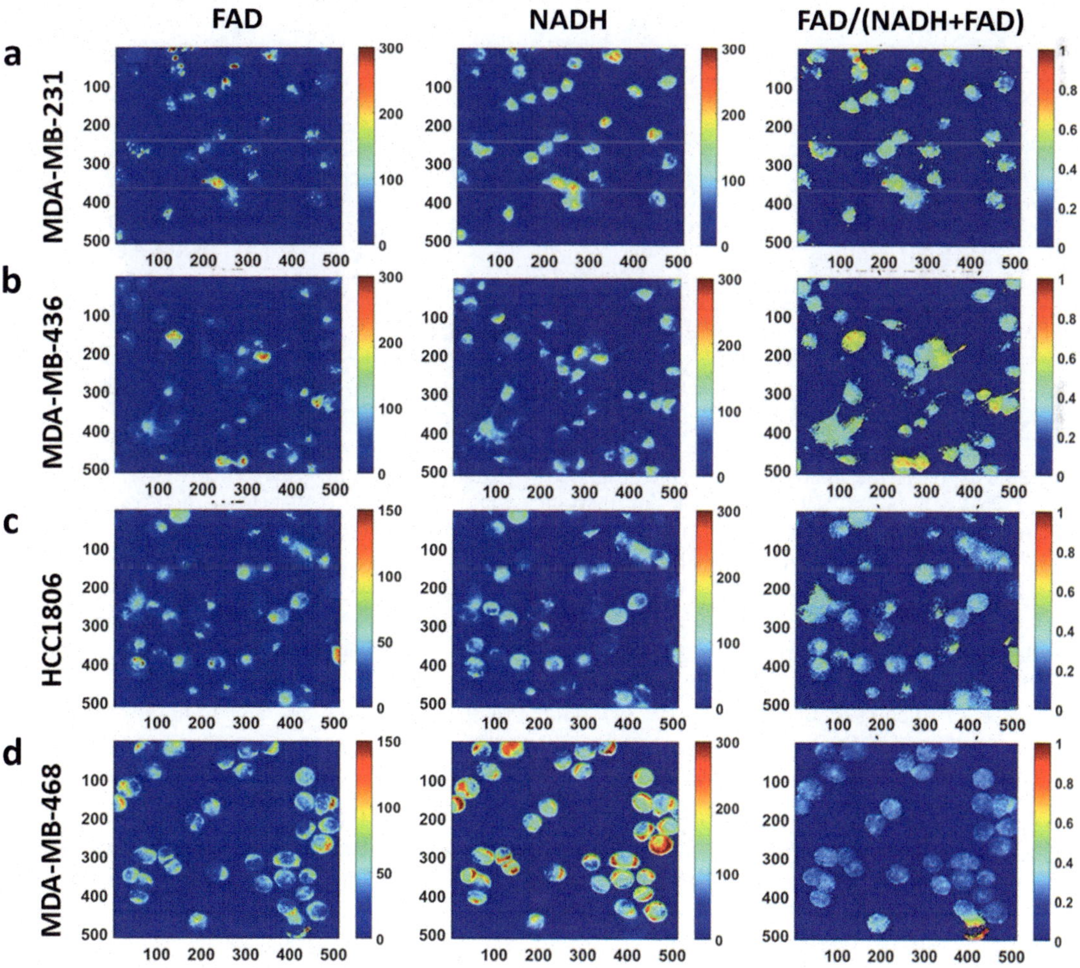

Fig. 39.1 Typical redox images of FAD, NADH, and redox ratio FAD/(NADH+FAD) for (**a**) MDA-MB-231, (**b**) MDA-MB-436, (**c**) HCC1806, and (**d**) MDA-MB-468. The color bars of the FAD and NADH images indicate the signal intensity in arbitrary units. Note that FAD color bars were scaled differently for better displaying of all cells. The color bars of the redox ratio images indicate a range from 0 to 1

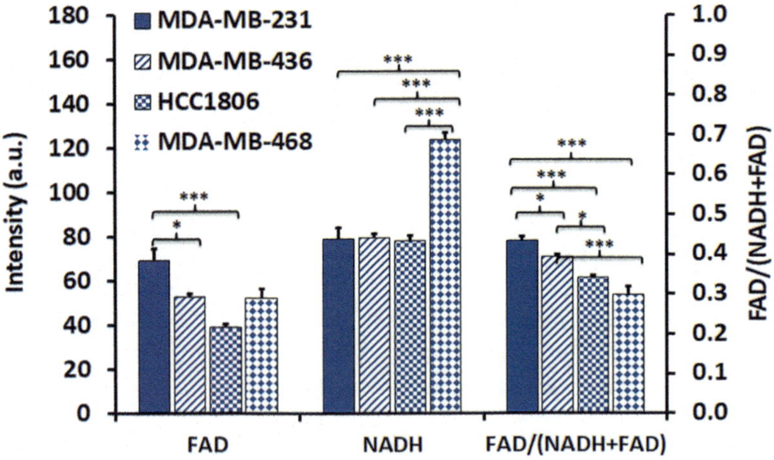

Fig. 39.2 Optical redox imaging quantifications. The left y-axis indicates NADH and FAD intensity in arbitrary units, and the right y-axis indicates FAD/(NADH+FAD) redox ratio. Results are reported as mean ± SE. *$p < 0.05$, **$p < 0.01$, ***$p < 0.001$, $n = 4–9$ dishes

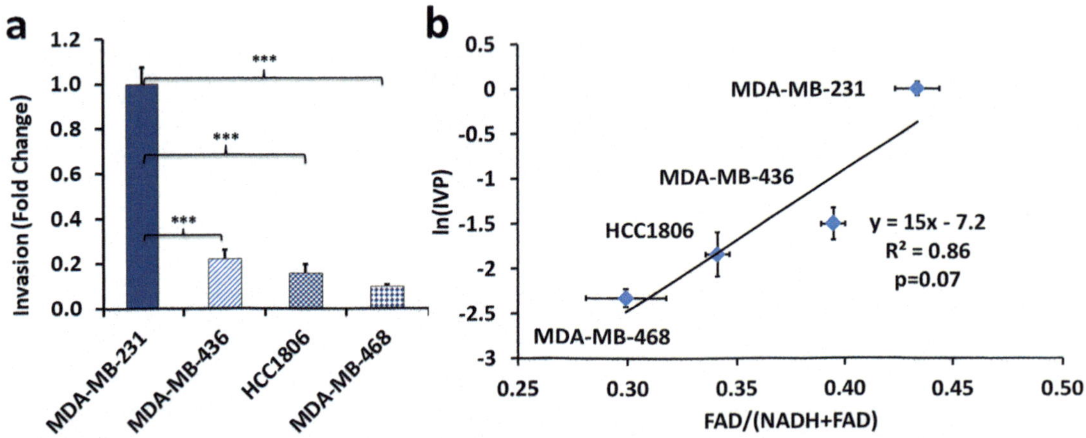

Fig. 39.3 IVP quantification and its correlation with ORI of 4 TNBC lines. (**a**) IVP normalized to that of MDA-MB-231 cells, $n = 6 - 15$ wells. (**b**) Correlation of the logarithm of IVP versus the redox ratio FAD/(NADH+FAD). A trend line, $y = 15x - 7.2$, was generated with a correlation coefficient of $R^2 = 0.86$. Results are reported as mean ± SE. ***$p < 0.001$

found that MDA-MB-231 had a significantly higher invasive potential than the other three TNBC cell lines ($p < 0.001$) (Fig. 39.3a). The IVP of the other three lines were not significantly different. The rank order of the four cell lines from the most invasive to the least invasive was same as the rank order of the redox ratios. A positive linear correlation was found between logarithm of IVP, ln(IVP), and the redox ratio with a borderline significance (Fig. 39.3b; $R^2 = 0.86$; $p = 0.07$).

39.4 Discussion and Conclusions

In this study, we showed that the redox ratios obtained by ORI can differentiate among four TNBC cell lines with different invasiveness. The invasive potential results were consistent with previous studies [15, 19, 20]. Both the redox ratios and the invasive potentials of the four lines exhibited the same rank order, despite the insignificant differences among the invasion of three less invasive TNBC lines. We also found a logarithmic correlation between the invasive potentials and the redox ratios with a borderline significance.

However, this study had several limitations. First, this study has a limited number of TNBC cell lines. Second, redox status may change with metabolic microenvironments such as nutrition levels [15]. Third, the O_2 level in cell culture is quite different from that of tumors in vivo. More studies need to be done in vitro under various microenvironments (including hypoxia) or in tumors in vivo to confirm and generalize the results of this study.

Acknowledgments This work was supported by the NIH Grant R01CA191207 (Li LZ). We thank Allison Podsednik for proofreading the manuscript. We also thank the Cell and Developmental Biology (CDB) Microscopy Core, Perelman School of Medicine, University of Pennsylvania.

References

1. Bray F, Ferlay J, Soerjomataram I et al (2018) Global cancer statistics 2018: GLOBOCAN estimates of incidence and mortality worldwide for 36 cancers in 185 countries. CA Cancer J Clin 68:394–424
2. Cianfrocca M, Goldstein LJ (2004) Prognostic and predictive factors in early-stage breast cancer. Oncologist 9:606–616
3. Dent R, Trudeau M, Pritchard KI et al (2007) Triple-negative breast cancer: clinical features and patterns of recurrence. Clin Cancer Res 13:4429–4434
4. Chance B, Baltscheffsky H (1958) Respiratory enzymes in oxidative phosphorylation: VII. Binding of intramitochondrial reduced pyridine nucleotide. J Biol Chem 233:736–739
5. Chance B, Cohen P, Jobsis F et al (1962) Intracellular oxidation-reduction states in vivo. The microfluorometry of pyridine nucleotide gives a continuous measurement of the oxidation state. Science 137:499–508
6. Chance B, Schoener B, Oshino R et al (1979) Oxidation-reduction ratio studies of mitochondria in freeze-trapped samples. NADH and flavoprotein fluorescence signals. J Biol Chem 254:4764–4771
7. Xu HN, Li LZ (2014) Quantitative redox imaging biomarkers for studying tissue metabolic state and its heterogeneity. J Innov Opt Health Sci 7:1430002
8. Alhallak K, Rebello LG, Muldoon TJ et al (2016) Optical redox ratio identifies metastatic potential-dependent changes in breast cancer cell metabolism. Biomed Opt Express 7:4364–4374
9. Li LZ, Zhou R, Xu HN et al (2009) Quantitative magnetic resonance and optical imaging biomarkers of melanoma metastatic potential. Proc Natl Acad Sci 106:6608–6613
10. Xu HN, Nioka S, Glickson JD et al (2010) Quantitative mitochondrial redox imaging of breast cancer metastatic potential. J Biomed Opt 15:036010
11. Ostrander JH, McMahon CM, Lem S et al (2010) Optical redox ratio differentiates breast cancer cell lines based on estrogen receptor status. Cancer Res 70:4759–4766
12. Xu HN, Tchou J, Feng M et al (2016) Optical redox imaging indices discriminate human breast cancer from normal tissues. J Biomed Opt 21:114003
13. Xu HN, Feng M, Nath K et al (2019) Optical redox imaging of lonidamine treatment response of melanoma cells and xenografts. Mol Imaging Biol 21:426–435
14. Walsh AJ, Cook RS, Manning HC et al (2013) Optical metabolic imaging identifies glycolytic levels, subtypes, and early-treatment response in breast cancer. Cancer Res 73:6164–6174
15. Sun N, Xu HN, Luo Q et al (2016) Potential indexing of the invasiveness of breast cancer cells by mitochondrial redox ratios. Adv Exp Med Biol 923:121–127
16. Lehmann BD, Bauer JA, Chen X et al (2011) Identification of human triple-negative breast cancer subtypes and preclinical models for selection of targeted therapies. J Clin Invest 121:2750–2767
17. Wen Y, Xu HN, Privette Vinnedge L et al (2019) Optical redox imaging detects the effects of DEK oncogene knockdown on the redox state of MDA-MB-231 breast cancer cells. Mol Imaging Biol 21(3):410–416
18. Yan X, Shen H, Jiang H et al (2010) External Qi of Yan Xin Qigong induces apoptosis and inhibits migration and invasion of estrogen-independent breast cancer cells through suppression of Akt/NF-κB signaling. Cell Physiol Biochem 25:263–270
19. Freund A, Chauveau C, Brouillet J-P et al (2003) IL-8 expression and its possible relationship with estrogen-receptor-negative status of breast cancer cells. Oncogene 22:256
20. Thompson EW, Paik S, Brünner N et al (1992) Association of increased basement membrane invasiveness with absence of estrogen receptor and expression of vimentin in human breast cancer cell lines. J Cell Physiol 150:534–544

Optical Redox Imaging Differentiates Triple-Negative Breast Cancer Subtypes

40

Jinxia Jiang, Min Feng, Annemarie Jacob, Lin Z. Li, and He N. Xu

Abstract

Triple-negative breast cancer (TNBC) is a highly diverse group of cancers with limited treatment options, responsible for about 15% of all breast cancers. TNBC cells differ from each other in many ways such as gene expression, metabolic activity, tumorigenicity, and invasiveness. Recently, many research and clinical efforts have focused on metabolically targeted therapy for TNBC. Metabolic characterization of TNBC cell lines can facilitate the assessment of therapeutic effects and assist in metabolic drug development. Herein, we used optical redox imaging (ORI) techniques to characterize TNBC subtypes metabolically. We found that various TNBC cell lines had differing redox statuses (levels of reduced nicotinamide adenine dinucleotide (NADH), oxidized flavin adenine dinucleotide (FAD), and the redox ratio (FAD/(NADH+FAD)). We then metabolically perturbed the cells with mitochondrial inhibitors and an uncoupler and performed ORI accordingly. As expected, we observed that these TNBC cell lines had similar response patterns to the metabolic perturbations. However, they exhibited differing redox plasticity. These results suggest that subtypes of TNBC cells are different metabolically and that ORI can serve as a sensitive technique for the metabolic profiling of TNBC cells.

Keywords

NADH and FAD · Intrinsic fluorescence · Redox plasticity · Triple-negative breast cancer · Metabolic characterization

40.1 Introduction

Triple-negative breast cancer (TNBC) is characterized by the lack of expression of estrogen receptor (ER), progesterone receptor (PR), and human epidermal growth factor receptor 2 (HER2) [1]. This heterogeneous group of tumors constitutes about 15% of all breast cancers and is generally more aggressive, recurrent, and metastatic than other breast cancers [2]. Various studies have investigated the underlying genomic differences in TNBC, and results suggest further characterization by subtyping [3, 4]. One established method of characterization is by analyzing gene expression profiles [4]. This method catego-

J. Jiang · M. Feng · A. Jacob · L. Z. Li · H. N. Xu (✉)
Britton Chance Laboratory of Redox Imaging, Department of Radiology and Johnson Research Foundation, Department of Biochemistry and Biophysics, Perelman School of Medicine, University of Pennsylvania, Philadelphia, PA, USA
e-mail: hexu2@pennmedicine.upenn.edu

E. M. Nemoto et al. (eds.), *Oxygen Transport to Tissue XLII*, Advances in Experimental Medicine and Biology 1269, https://doi.org/10.1007/978-3-030-48238-1_40

rizes TNBC cell lines into the following subtypes: basal-like, immunomodulatory, mesenchymal, mesenchymal stemlike, and luminal androgen receptor. However, altered metabolism is also a hallmark of cancer and can potentially be used in the characterization of TNBC subtypes.

The mitochondrial redox status provides critical information about the energy-linked biological processes in cells and tissues for various types of cancer, including TNBC [5]. Nicotinamide adenine dinucleotide (NADH) and oxidized flavin adenine dinucleotide (FAD) are two coenzymes that play important roles in the mitochondrial electron transport chain (ETC). Pioneered by Chance et al. [6, 7], the redox ratio, calculated by taking the ratio of measured endogenous fluorescence of NADH and FAD, can be used as an indicator of the mitochondrial redox state. Since then, optical redox imaging (ORI) techniques have demonstrated increasing applications in cancer research, such as differentiation among cancer aggressiveness [8–10] and monitoring therapeutic effects [11, 12]. In the present study, we report the use of ORI as a tool in differentiating the mitochondrial redox status among four TNBC cell lines (MDA-MB-231 and MDA-MB-436 mesenchymal-like, MDA-MB468 basal-like 1, HCC1806 basal-like 2) and characterizing their redox plasticity under metabolic modulations. Such characterizations could provide useful information for the metabolic stratification of TNBC cell lines.

40.2 Methods

40.2.1 Cell Culture and Perturbation Drugs

TNBC cell lines MDA-MB-231, MDA-MB-436, MDA-MB-468, and HCC1806 were cultured in RPMI 1640 (Gibco®, Cat No. 11875085) supplemented with 10% fetal bovine serum (Corning®). Cells were maintained at 37 °C and 5% CO_2 and passaged at 80% confluency using 0.25% trypsin-EDTA. Oligomycin (oligo), trifluoromethoxy carbonylcyanide phenylhydrazone (FCCP), rotenone (rot), and antimycin A (aa) (Sigma®) were reconstituted in DMSO (Sigma®) and used at the following final concentrations: oligo (2 μg/mL), FCCP (0.5 μM), rot (1 μM), and aa (1.25 μg/mL).

40.2.2 Live Cell Optical Redox Imaging and Analysis

As detailed previously [11], 80,000 cells were seeded on 35 mm glass bottom dishes (MatTek®) and incubated at 37 °C and 5% CO_2 overnight. Approximately 1 hour before imaging, the medium was replaced with 1 mL live cell imaging solution (Life Technology®) supplemented with 11 mM glucose and 2 mM glutamine (Sigma®), the same as in the RPMI 1640 medium. A DeltaVision widefield microscope was used to collect NADH and FAD fluorescence signals. The excitation band-pass filters for NADH and FAD channels were 360/40 nm and 470/40 nm, respectively; the emission filters of NADH and FAD channels were 455/50 nm and 520/40 nm, respectively. Nine to fifteen dishes were imaged on different days for each cell line with three fields of view (FOV) for each dish with an exposure time of 3 seconds for each channel. For mitochondrial redox plasticity experiments, perturbation drugs were added sequentially in the order of oligo, FCCP, and a mixture of rot and aa (rot/aa), allowing the cells to be pushed to the two redox extremes and the consequent calculation of the cell lines' redox plasticity. The dishes were imaged 3–5 minutes after each drug administration. A customized MATLAB® program was used to extract NADH and FAD signals and the pixel-to-pixel based FAD/(NADH+FAD) ratio, which were first averaged across FOVs and then across individual dishes to obtain the group mean and standard error of the mean (SEM). Heteroscedastic two-tailed t-tests were used for statistical analyses of redox differences among cell lines and the differences before and after a specific treatment. $P < 0.05$ was considered statistically significant.

40.3 Results and Discussion

40.3.1 ORI Differentiates TNBC Cell Lines

We first imaged MDA-MB-231, MDA-MB-436, MDA-MB-468, and HCC1806 cells under normal conditions (Fig. 40.1a). Our quantitative analysis shows MDA-MB-231 exhibiting the highest FAD intensity and MDA-MB-468 exhibiting the highest NADH intensity (Fig. 40.1b). FAD intensity was significantly different ($p < 0.05$) between all cell lines except between MDA-MB-436 and MDA-MB-468. NADH intensity was similar in MDA-MB-231, MDA-MB-436, and HCC1806. Furthermore, we found that MDA-MB-231 exhibits the highest redox ratio of 0.65 ± 0.02, followed by MDA-MB-436, MDA-MB-468, and HCC1806, with the redox ratios of 0.55 ± 0.01, 0.49 ± 0.01, and 0.47 ± 0.01, respectively. The TNBC cell lines significantly differ in their redox ratios, with an exception between MDA-MB-468 and HCC1806, both of which are classified as the basal-like subtype ($p > 0.05$).

40.3.2 ORI Detects Metabolic Changes in TNBC Cell Lines

To show that ORI can reflect the metabolic phenotypes of TNBC cell lines, we sequentially administered oligo, FCCP, and rot/aa and obtained the NADH and FAD fluorescence signals accordingly. Oligo is an inhibitor of the ATP synthase in the ETC, causing a buildup of NADH. FCCP is an uncoupling agent that col-

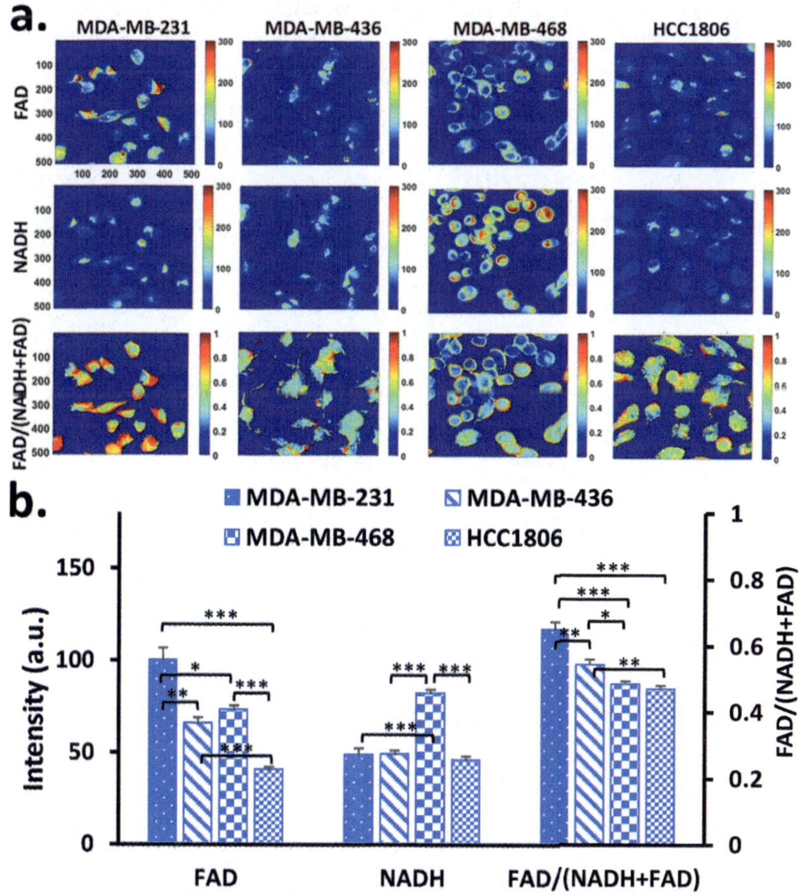

Fig. 40.1 ORI differentiates TNBC cell lines. (**a**) Typical redox images of MDA-MB-231, MDA-MB-436, MDA-MB-468, and HCC1806. FAD and NADH color bar indicates signal intensity in arbitrary unit. FAD/(NADH+FAD) color bar indicates ratio range from 0 to 1. (**b**) Quantification of FAD, NADH fluorescence intensities, and FAD/(NADH+FAD) ratio. Primary y-axis quantifies FAD and NADH signal intensity, and secondary y-axis quantifies the FAD/(NADH+FAD) ratio. Results are reported as mean + SEM. $*p < 0.05$, $**p < 0.001$, $***p < 0.0001$

lapses the proton gradient and disrupts the mitochondrial membrane potential, causing unregulated oxidation of NADH and $FADH_2$ to NAD^+ and FAD, respectively, resulting in decreased NADH and increased FAD. Conversely, rot and aa are inhibitors of complexes I and III, respectively, fully inhibiting respiration, resulting in a maximal NADH signal and decreased FAD. Our results show that FCCP and rot/aa treatments effectively caused a decrease and increase in NADH intensity, respectively, in all four cell lines and an increase and decrease of FAD in three lines except MDA-MB-231 (Fig. 40.2). Furthermore, FCCP and rot/aa also resulted in a significant change in the redox ratios of all four cell lines and induced a more oxidized and a more reduced redox state, respectively. Although oligo administration did induce some significant changes at least in one of the redox indices (FAD, NADH, or the redox ratio) in each cell line, it was not as consistent as those observed from FCCP and rot/aa administration.

40.3.3 TNBC Cell Lines Have Differential FAD and Redox Ratio Plasticity

By taking the difference between the average fluorescence values after FCCP and rot/aa application, we quantified the changes, i.e., the plasticity in NADH, FAD, and the redox ratio, in the TNBC cell lines [11]. Our results showed significant variations in FAD plasticity between the cell lines (Fig. 40.3). MDA-MB-436 and MDA-MB-468 had similar FAD plasticity values of 36 and 38 a.u., respectively, followed by MDA-MB-231 at 17 a.u. and HCC1806 at 6 a.u. No significant differences were found for NADH plasticity across cell lines. Our results also showed that MDA-MB-436 had the largest change in redox ratio, valued at 0.33 a.u., and MDA-MB-231, MDA-MB-468, and HCC1806 had similar changes in redox ratio (0.25, 0.23, and 0.23, respectively).

To our best knowledge, this is the first systematic investigation that reports how ORI differentiates the redox plasticity of TNBC cells. Changes

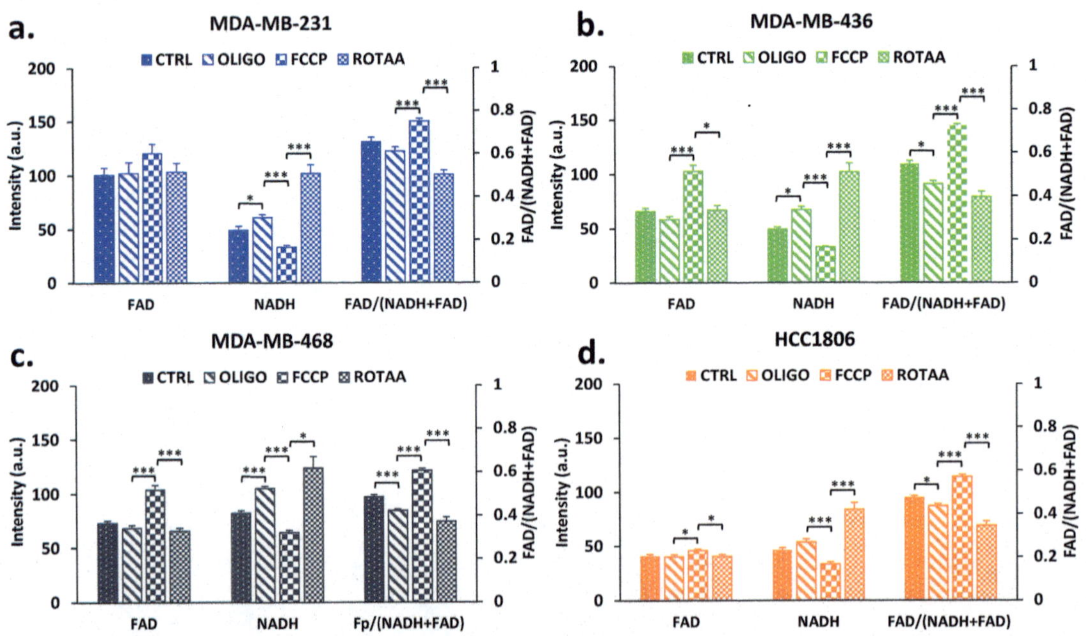

Fig. 40.2 ORI detects metabolic changes in TNBC cell lines. Quantification of FAD, NADH fluorescence intensities, and FAD/(NADH+FAD) ratio for (**a**) MDA-MB-231, (**b**) MDA-MB-436, (**c**) MDA-MB-468, and (**d**) HCC1806 under control conditions, after sequential additions of oligo, FCCP, and rot/aa. Results are reported as mean + SEM. $*p < 0.05$, $***p < 0.0001$

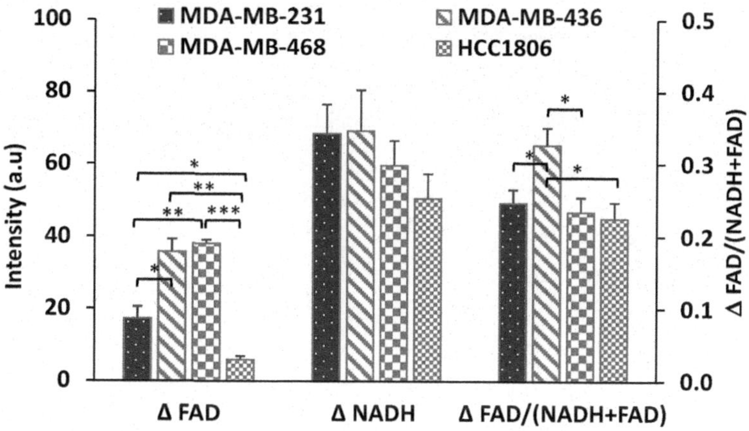

Fig. 40.3 TNBC cell lines have differential redox plasticity. Quantification of FAD, NADH, and redox ratio plasticity. Results are reported as mean + SEM. *$p < 0.05$; **$p < 0.001$, ***$p < 0.0001$

in the redox indices caused by therapeutic interventions could reflect compromised mitochondrial redox plasticity. This information would be helpful in assessing drug effects in vitro, such as screening drugs for developing therapeutic interventions that target the metabolic activities in TNBC cells. Our previous studies have linked the redox ratio of the more oxidized tumor subpopulations to breast tumor and melanoma metastatic risk [9, 10]. Therefore, redox plasticity can also be further investigated to assist in the prediction of different metastatic potential of the TNBC tumors.

In short, the four TNBC lines can be clearly differentiated by ORI, and the underlying mechanisms remain to be elucidated.

Acknowledgments This work was supported by McCabe Pilot Award (H. N. Xu) and NIH Grant R01CA191207 (L. Z. Li). We thank Jeffrey Roman for proofreading the manuscript. We also thank the Cell and Developmental Biology (CDB) Microscopy Core, Perelman School of Medicine, University of Pennsylvania.

References

1. Liedtke C, Mazouni C, Hess KR et al (2008) Response to neoadjuvant therapy and long-term survival in patients with triple-negative breast cancer. J Clin Oncol 26(8):1275–1281
2. Chacon RD, Costanzo MV (2010) Triple-negative breast cancer. Breast Cancer Res 12 Suppl 2:S3
3. Stevens KN, Vachon CM, Couch FJ (2013) Genetic susceptibility to triple-negative breast cancer. Cancer Res 73(7):2025–2030
4. Lehmann BD, Bauer JA, Chen X et al (2011) Identification of human triple-negative breast cancer subtypes and preclinical models for selection of targeted therapies. J Clin Invest 121(7):2750–2767
5. Li LZ, Xu HN, Ranji M et al (2009) Mitochondrial redox imaging for cancer diagnostic and therapeutic studies. J Innov Opt Heal Sci 2(4):325–341
6. Chance B, Schoener B, Oshino R et al (1979) Oxidation-reduction ratio studies of mitochondria in freeze-trapped samples. NADH and flavoprotein fluorescence signals. J Biol Chem 254(11):4764–4771
7. Chance B, Cohen P, Jobsis F et al (1962) Intracellular oxidation-reduction states in vivo. Science 137(3529):499–508
8. Sun N, Xu HN, Luo Q et al (2016) Potential indexing of the invasiveness of breast cancer cells by mitochondrial redox ratios. Adv Exp Med Biol 923:121–127
9. Xu HN, Nioka S, Glickson JD et al (2010) Quantitative mitochondrial redox imaging of breast cancer metastatic potential. J Biomed Opt 15(3):036010
10. Li LZ, Zhou R, Xu HN et al (2009) Quantitative magnetic resonance and optical imaging biomarkers of melanoma metastatic potential. Proc Natl Acad Sci U S A 106(16):6608–6613
11. Xu HN, Feng M, Nath K et al (2018) Optical redox imaging of Lonidamine treatment response of melanoma cells and xenografts. Mol Imaging Biol 21(3):426–435
12. Alam SR, Wallrabe H, Svindrych Z et al (2017) Investigation of mitochondrial metabolic response to doxorubicin in prostate cancer cells: an NADH, FAD and tryptophan FLIM assay. Sci Rep 7(1):10451

Oxygen-Sensing Paramagnetic Probes for Clinical Oximetry

41

M. M. Kmiec, D. Tse, and Periannan Kuppusamy

Abstract

Electron paramagnetic resonance (EPR) oximetry based on lithium naphthalocyanine paramagnetic crystals as oxygen sensors enables direct measurement of the partial pressure of oxygen (pO_2) in tissues. The method uses topical or implantable forms of these oxygen-sensing crystals embedded in a biocompatible siloxane elastomer. This article presents a summary of these sensors for EPR oximetry and their applicability for tissue oxygen measurement in the clinic.

Keywords

Electron paramagnetic resonance (EPR) · Oximetry · OxyChip · SPOTChip · MicroChip · Partial pressure of oxygen (pO_2)

M. M. Kmiec · D. Tse · P. Kuppusamy (✉)
Department of Radiology, Geisel School of Medicine at Dartmouth, Hanover, NH, USA
e-mail: kuppu@dartmouth.edu

41.1 Introduction

Although several methods have been developed to measure oxygen concentration in viable tissues, a suitable technique for direct and repeated quantification of oxygen levels in the clinical setting is not currently available. While electrode-based methods have evolved as the standard for measuring oxygen concentration, they generate analytical artifacts during assay procedures at the freshly probed sites and are not suitable for repeated measurements. Near-infrared and magnetic resonance techniques—such as nuclear magnetic resonance (NMR), blood-oxygen-level-dependent (BOLD) imaging, magnetic resonance imaging (MRI), and Overhauser enhanced magnetic resonance imaging (OMRI)—are noninvasive methods; however, they do not report the absolute values of oxygen concentration (partial pressure of oxygen, pO_2) in the tissues. Electron paramagnetic resonance (EPR) oximetry, closely related to the magnetic resonance techniques, enables direct, accurate, reliable, and repeated measurements of oxygen concentration in tissues [1]. EPR oximetry has been utilized in many preclinical studies to understand the dynamic changes of pO_2 in tumor models and the effect of hyperoxic interventions to enhance tumor response to radiation [2]. In this article, we present a summary of the lithium naphthalocyanine-based oxygen-sensing paramagnetic probes available for EPR-based clinical oximetry.

E. M. Nemoto et al. (eds.), *Oxygen Transport to Tissue XLII*, Advances in Experimental Medicine and Biology 1269, https://doi.org/10.1007/978-3-030-48238-1_41

Table 41.1 Type of oxygen-sensing probes (OxyChips) for in vivo oximetry

Oxygen probe	Shape; size	Usage type	Depth[a] (mm)	Sensors/implant[b]	What is measured
SPOTChip	Film; 3-mm diameter	Sticker	0 (topical)	Single	$TcpO_2$[c]
MicroChip	Cylinder; 0.3 × 1 mm	Implant	1–5	Multiple	Mean pO_2
OxyChip	Cylinder; 0.6 × 5 mm	Implant	5–10	Single	Single pO_2
OxyChip-EL	Wire; 0.4 × > 10 mm	Implant	>10	Multiple	Multiple pO_2

[a]Implantable depth in tissue; [b]readable using single scan; [c]transcutaneous pO_2

41.2 EPR Oxygen Sensors

EPR oximetry requires an exogenous paramagnetic oxygen sensor (probe) to be introduced, i.e., implanted, at the site of measurement [1]. The probe can be customized for specific applications in terms of depth in tissue, oxygen sensitivity (desired resolution of pO_2), oxygen level (desired pO_2 range), and repeated measurements over months or longer at the implant site. Our laboratory has developed and tested a suite of implantable probes for EPR oximetry in preclinical animal models and human subjects. The probes are made with lithium octa-*n*-butoxy-naphthalocyanine (LiNc-BuO) crystals embedded in polydimethylsiloxane (PDMS) elastomer and have been thoroughly characterized and established for oximetry in animal models of diseases [3–5]. The probes are biocompatible and stable with predictable oxygen sensitivity (calibration). The following probes are available for clinical oximetry (Table 41.1): SPOTChip, a skin adhesive film for transcutaneous pO_2 measurements; MicroChip, single or multiple implants for pO_2 measurements in superficial tissues (1–5 mm); OxyChip, a single implant for pO_2 measurements in shallow-depth tissues (1–10 mm); and OxyChip-EL, a single implant for multiple pO_2 measurements in deep tissues (10–100 mm).

41.2.1 SPOTChip for Topical Oximetry

To establish EPR oximetry for monitoring skin oxygenation (transcutaneous pO_2), we have developed an oxygen sensor, termed as "SPOT" (Superficial Perfusion Oxygen Tension) chip [6]. Microcrystals of LiNc-BuO are embedded in PDMS elastomer and assembled into 3-mm-diameter circular films of ~0.06-mm thickness (Fig. 41.1a). One side of the chip is covered with an oxygen-impermeable film, while the other side is permeable to oxygen. The isolation is necessary to ensure that only the oxygen that diffuses through the skin surface is measured, not the oxygen from the ambient environment. The chip is secured to the skin by a medical transfer adhesive. We have demonstrated the functionality of the chip in healthy human subjects with an approved human IRB protocol. The results showed that the chips can be used for pO_2 measurements when applied topically to the region of interest or to multiple anatomical sites. No surgical procedure is required for the placement of the SPOTChip.

41.2.2 MicroChip for Superficial (1–5-mm Depth) Tissue Oximetry

We have fabricated and extensively tested a new form of oxygen sensor called MicroChip (Fig. 41.1b) [7]. The MicroChips were thoroughly characterized for sensitivity, safety, stability, and biocompatibility for measurements in live tissues. The following features were established for MicroChips: (i) linearity of the calibration (EPR signal linewidth vs. pO_2); (ii) stability of EPR characteristic and oxygen sensitivity against autoclaving, exposure to ionizing radiation, and sonication procedures; (iii) mechanical stability and integrity of the chip for retaining the embedded crystals under adverse conditions; (iv) depth sensitivity up to 5 mm for measurements in superficial tissues; (vi) capability for multiple implants (4–10) in a single tissue/tumor and obtaining mean and median pO_2 values using a single scan; (vii) repeated measurements of tissue pO_2 over the long term (8 weeks) studied in animal models; and, (viii) overall, a robust and reliable probe for pO_2 measurements. Using in vitro and in vivo models, we have shown that the MicroChip provides adequate EPR sensitivity, stability, and biocompatibility and enables robust, repeated, and simultaneous measurements from multiple implants (without magnetic field gradients) providing mean and median pO_2 estimates in the implanted region [8]. The MicroChips will be particularly useful for those applications that require repeated measurement of mean/median pO_2 in superficial tissues and malignancies.

41.2.3 OxyChip for Shallow-Depth (<10 mm) Tissue Oximetry

The OxyChips are made by cast molding medical-grade PDMS polymer embedded with LiNc-BuO microcrystals [9]. An example of the OxyChip fabricated using 40% w/w LiNc-BuO is shown in Fig. 41.1b. In vitro evaluation of the OxyChip showed that it is robust and highly oxygen-sensitive (~14 mG/mmHg). The dependence of its EPR linewidth on oxygen is linear in the range 0–100% oxygen and stable over time and after autoclave or irradiation procedure. In vivo efficacy of the OxyChips was evaluated by implanting them in rat femoris muscle and following their response to tissue oxygenation for up to 1 year [9]. The results revealed the preservation of the physical integrity (size and shape) and calibration (oxygen sensitivity) of the OxyChip throughout the implantation period. Further, no inflammatory or unanticipated adverse reactions around the implantation area were observed, thereby establishing its biocompatibility and safety for long-term use. Overall, the results established that the OxyChip is capable of providing long-term oxygen measurements reliably and repeatedly under in vivo conditions.

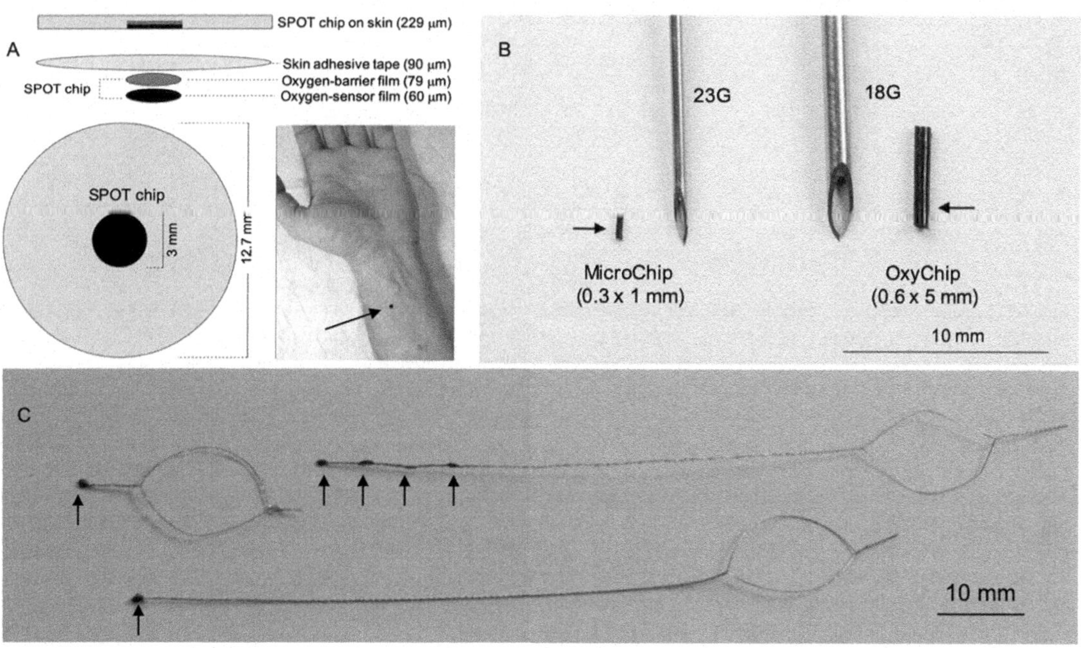

Fig. 41.1 Oxygen-sensing probes. (**a**) SPOTChip for skin oximetry. (**b**) OxyChip and MicroChip for superficial and shallow-depth oximetry, respectively, shown with the needles used for implantation in tissues. (**c**) OxyChip-EL with different lengths and number of sensory elements for deep-tissue oximetry. Arrows point to the oxygen sensor

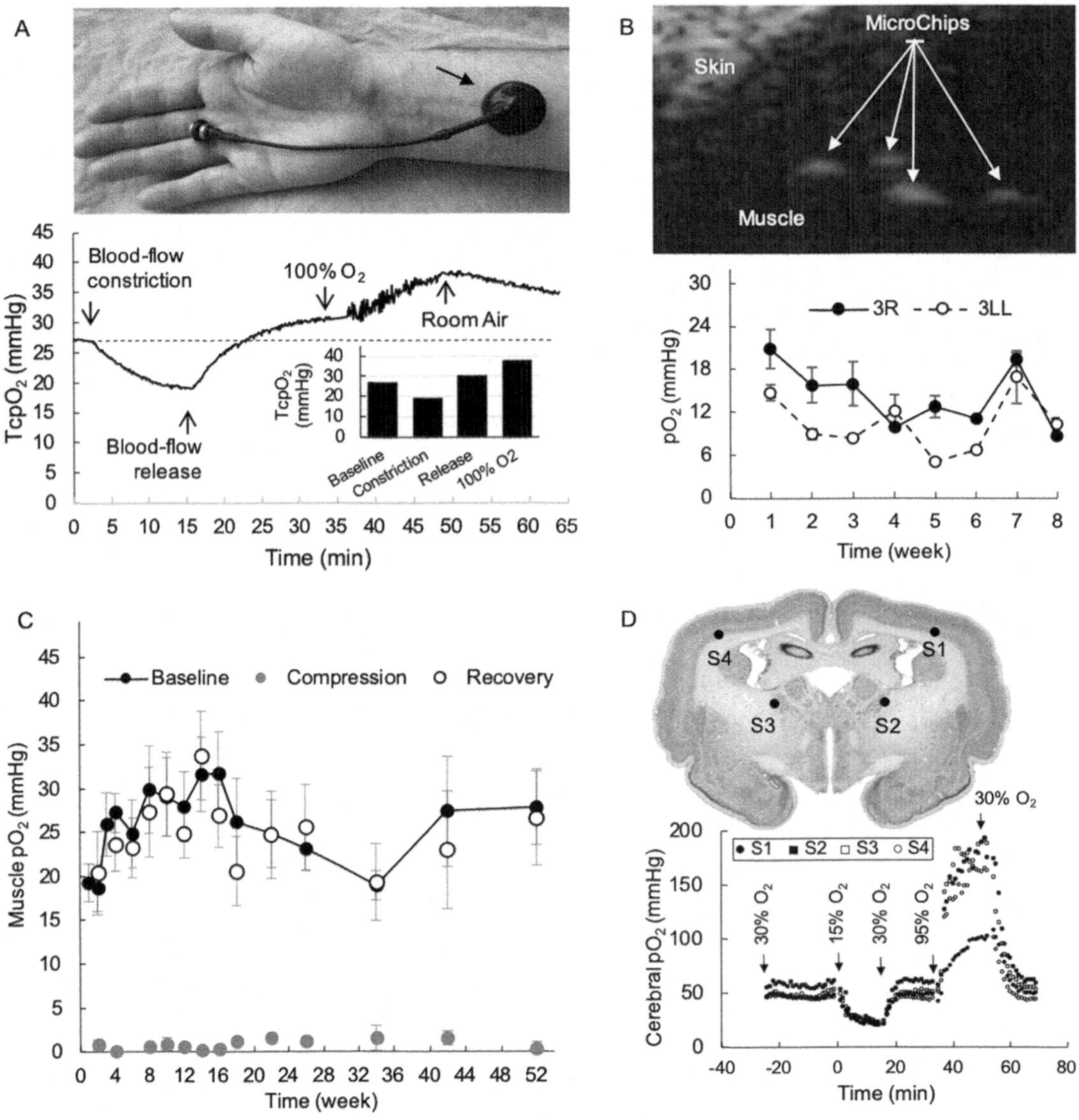

Fig. 41.2 Representative examples of the oxygen sensors in animal models and human subjects. (**a**) Transcutaneous oxygen (pO_2) measurement and dynamic changes of oxygen in the forearm of a healthy volunteer measured using SPOTChip under conditions of normal, blood flow constriction, and hyperoxygen breathing via non-rebreather face mask [6]. The photo shows the placement of a flexible resonator over the SPOTChip. (**b**) Monitoring of leg muscle oxygenation in two mice (3R and 3LL) for period of 8 weeks using four implanted MicroChips [2]. The data represent Mean ± SEM from four MicroChips. The photo shows the ultrasound image of the presence of the four chips in the muscle [2]. (**c**) Average pO_2 (Mean ± SEM) values from 5–8 rats obtained during baseline, compression, and recovery sessions over a 52-week period using OxyChip [9]. The data show that the OxyChip was stable and responsive to changes in muscle pO_2 for up to 1 year. (**d**) Changes in cerebral pO_2 measured in a rabbit subjected to hypoxic and hyperoxic breathing using OxyChip-EL [11]. An OxyChip-EL with four sensory tips (S1–S4) was implanted at two sites in each hemisphere, as shown in the illustration. pO_2 measurements were made on day 21 after sensor placement. Oxygen content in the inhalation gas was varied as indicated. The results show a consistent variation of pO_2 among all four sites on exposure to different oxygen levels

41.2.4 OxyChip-EL for Deep-Tissue (>10 mm) Oximetry

OxyChips, with an extended sensing loop (OxyChip-EL, also known as implantable resonators), are fabricated with one or more oxygen-sensing points (LiNc-BuO in PDMS) incorporated into one end of a twisted-pair transmission line, made of MP35N wire (diameter 0.080–0.125 mm; length >10 mm) attached to a coupling loop (10-mm dia.) on the other end of the transmission line [10]. The coupling loop is designed to be placed subcutaneously to allow inductive coupling to an external surface loop resonator for signal detection (Fig. 41.1c). To avoid any toxicity or mechanical damage, the resonators are further coated with PDMS. Standard in vitro and in vivo biocompatibility tests were carried out to establish the safety and efficacy of the sensor for deep-tissue applications.

41.3 Oxygen Sensor Applications

Some examples of the oxygen-sensing probes for EPR oximetry in mice, rats, rabbits, and human subjects are shown in Fig. 41.2.

41.4 Conclusion

The EPR oximetry with the suite of oxygen-sensing probes based on PDMS-encased LiNc-BuO microcrystals can provide a complete and fully developed platform for clinical oximetry in tissues at any depths, anatomical sites, and duration—an important capability that is not currently available.

Acknowledgments The research was supported by NIH grants R01 EB004031 and P01 CA190193.

References

1. Ahmad R, Kuppusamy P (2010) Theory, instrumentation, and applications of electron paramagnetic resonance oximetry. Chem Rev 110:3212–3236
2. Mast JM, Kuppusamy P (2018) Hyperoxygenation as a therapeutic supplement for treatment of triple negative breast cancer. Front Oncol 8:527
3. Meenakshisundaram G, Eteshola E, Pandian RP et al (2009) Oxygen sensitivity and biocompatibility of an implantable paramagnetic probe for repeated measurements of tissue oxygenation. Biomed Microdev 11:817–826
4. Pandian RP, Parinandi NL, Ilangovan G et al (2003) Novel particulate spin probe for targeted determination of oxygen in cells and tissues. Free Radic Biol Med 35:1138–1148
5. Prabhat AM, Kuppusamy ML, Naidu SK et al (2018) Supplemental oxygen protects heart against acute myocardial infarction. Front Cardiovasc Med 5:114
6. Kmiec MM, Hou H, Lakshmi Kuppusamy M et al (2019) Transcutaneous oxygen measurement in humans using a paramagnetic skin adhesive film. Magn Reson Med 81:781–794
7. Kmiec MM, Tse D, Mast JM et al (2019) Implantable microchip containing oxygen-sensing paramagnetic crystals for long-term, repeated, and multisite in vivo oximetry. Biomed Microdev 21:71
8. Kuppusamy P, Kmiec MM, Tse D et al (2020) Estimation of pO2 histogram from a composite EPR Spectrum of multiple random implants. Biomed Microdev 22:1
9. Hou H, Khan N, Gohain S et al (2018) Pre-clinical evaluation of OxyChip for long-term EPR oximetry. Biomed Microdev 20:29
10. Caston RM, Schreiber W, Hou H et al (2017) Development of the implantable resonator system for clinical EPR oximetry. Cell Biochem Biophys 75:275–283
11. Hou H, Khan N, Gohain S et al (2017) Dynamic EPR oximetry of changes in intracerebral oxygen tension during induced thromboembolism. Cell Biochem Biophys 75:285–294

Evaluation of the Quality of Chest Compression with Oxyhemoglobin Level by Near-Infrared Spectroscopy in a Rat Asphyxia Cardiac Arrest Model

42

Yu Okuma, Lance B. Becker, Tsukasa Yagi, Tai Yin, Takeyuki Kiguchi, Taku Iwami, and Koichiro Shinozaki

Abstract

The real-time evaluation of chest compression during cardiopulmonary resuscitation is important to increase the chances of survival from a cardiac arrest (CA). In addition, cerebral oxygen level measured by near-infrared spectroscopy (NIRS) plays an important role as an indicator of return of spontaneous circulation. Recently, we developed a new method to improve the quality of chest compression using a thoracic pump in conjunction with the classic cardiac pump in a rat asphyxia CA model. This study evaluated the quality of chest compression using NIRS in male Sprague-Dawley rats. NIRS was attached between the nasion and the upper cervical spine, and rats underwent 10 minute asphyxia CA. After CA, we alternately performed three different types of chest compression (cardiac, thoracic, and cardiac plus thoracic pumps) every 30 seconds for up to 4 and a half minutes. We measured the oxyhemoglobin (Oxy-Hb), deoxyhemoglobin (Deoxy-Hb), and tissue oxygenation index (TOI) and compared these values between the groups. Oxy-Hb was significantly different among the groups (cardiac, thoracic, and cardiac plus thoracic, 1.5 ± 0.9, 4.4 ± 0.7, and 5.9 ± 2.1 μmol/L, $p < 0.01$, respectively), while Deoxy-Hb and TOI were not (Deoxy-HB −2.7 ± 1.2, −1.1 ± 3.2, and −1.6 ± 10.1 μmol/L; TOI, 1.8 ± 1.8, 5.5 ± 1.3, and 9.5 ± 8.0%, respectively). Oxy-Hb showed potential to evaluate the quality of chest compression in a rat asphyxia CA model.

Keywords

Cardiac arrest · Oxyhemoglobin (Oxy-Hb) · Cerebral blood oxygenation (CBO) · Near-infrared spectroscopy (NIRS) · Quality of chest compression

42.1 Introduction

Recent guidelines for cardiopulmonary resuscitation (CPR) state that high-quality CPR is the key to improving survival from a cardiac arrest (CA) [1]. Therefore, the real-time evaluation of chest

Y. Okuma (✉) · L. B. Becker · T. Yagi · T. Yin · K. Shinozaki
Feinstein Institute for Medical Research, Northwell Health System, Manhasset, NY, USA

T. Kiguchi · T. Iwami
Kyoto University Health Service, Kyoto, Japan

E. M. Nemoto et al. (eds.), *Oxygen Transport to Tissue XLII*, Advances in Experimental Medicine and Biology 1269, https://doi.org/10.1007/978-3-030-48238-1_42

compression plays an important role in CA [2]. Cerebral blood oxygenation (CBO) has been discussed as a promising indicator of return of spontaneous circulation [3, 4], and CBO measured by near-infrared spectroscopy (NIRS) is used for real-time evaluation of the quality of CPR in clinical settings [5]; however, guidelines have not yet recommended the use of CBO by NIRS for CA due to the lack of clear evidence of its utility [6]. This study was conducted to test the evaluation of quality of chest compression with CBO using NIRS in a rat model. This study is a continuation of a recent study, in which we developed a new method to improve the quality of chest compression using the thoracic pump in conjunction with the classic cardiac pump in a rat asphyxia CA model.

42.2 Methods

42.2.1 Animal Preparation

The Institutional Animal Care and Use Committee (IACUC) of the Feinstein Institute for Medical Research approved these study protocols (2016-047). The details of methods for a rat asphyxia CA model have been described previously [7, 8]. In brief, adult male Sprague-Dawley rats (450–550 g, Charles River Laboratories) were anesthetized with 4% isoflurane (Isosthesia, Butler-Schein AHS) and intubated with a 14-gauge plastic catheter (Surflo, Terumo Medical Corporation). The animals were mechanically ventilated. Anesthesia was maintained with isoflurane 2% at a fraction of inspired O_2 (FIO_2) of 0.3. The left femoral artery was cannulated (sterile polyethylene-50 catheter inserted for 20 mm) for continuous arterial pressure monitoring. A temperature probe was placed in the esophagus for continuous temperature monitoring. The core temperature was maintained at 36.5 ± 1.0 °C during the surgical procedure. The left femoral vein was cannulated with a polyethylene-50 catheter, which was advanced into the inferior vena cava for drug infusion. We attached NIRS (NIRO-200NX, Hamamatsu Photonics, Japan) from the nasion to the upper cervical spine of the rats. The distance between the emission and the detection probes was 3 cm. We examined the mean arterial pressure (MAP), end-tidal carbon dioxide ($ETCO_2$), and oxyhemoglobin (Oxy-Hb)/Deoxyhemoglobin (Deoxy-Hb), and tissue oxygen index (TOI). The NIRS device records the oxygen saturation level (TOI) and the changes in concentration of Oxy-Hb and Deoxy-Hb in real time (100 Hz). We analyzed averaged values over 30 second periods. Oxy-Hb and Deoxy-Hb were collected by modified Beer-Lambert (MBL), and TOI was collected by spatially resolved spectroscopy (SRS) [5]. After instrumentation, neuromuscular blockade was achieved by slow intravenous administration of 2 mg/kg of vecuronium bromide (Hospira, USA). Asphyxia was induced in the rats by switching off the ventilator, and CA occurred 3–4 minutes after asphyxia started. Mechanical ventilation was restarted at an FIO_2 of 1.0, and manual CPR was delivered to CA animals. Chest compressions were performed at a rate of 240–300 per minute.

42.2.2 Cardiopulmonary Resuscitation

The one-side method (cardio pump) involved chest compression vertically performed over the sternum with two fingers at a rate of 240–300 per minutes. The chest compression rate was calculated retrospectively from the record of pressure waveforms of the femoral arterial catheter. The two-side method (thoracic pump) was performed with two fingers horizontally squeezing the chest wall from both sides at the same rate. The three-side chest compression (cardiac plus thoracic pump) was carried out with two fingers of the right hand over the sternum in synchrony with two fingers of the left hand squeezing the chest wall from both sides ([8] Okuma Y – supplement for review only). The three sets of these chest compressions were alternately and randomly tested every 30 seconds, and CPR was performed for up to 4.5 minutes (nine sets of CPR, three for each group). CBO including TOI, Oxy-Hb, and Deoxy-Hb during CPR were compared to the values measured at the end of 10 minutes of asphyxia (baseline). In this experiment, adrenaline was not

Table 42.1 Relationship between mean arterial pressure (MAP), end-tidal carbon dioxide ($EtCO_2$), and cerebral blood oxygenation (CBO) including oxyhemoglobin (Oxy-Hb), Deoxy-Hb, and tissue oxygenation index (TOI)

		Cerebral blood O_2 (CBO)		
	MAP	Oxy-Hb	Deoxy-Hb	TOI
EtCO2	0.48**	0.23**	0.06	0.02
MAP		0.22**	−0.42**	0.31**
Oxy-Hb			−0.93**	0.02
Deoxy-Hb				−0.15*

** $p < 0.01$; * $p < 0.05$

given to the animal to avoid obtaining return of spontaneous circulation (ROSC) from the animals ($n = 5$).

42.2.3 Statistical Analysis

Data are presented as mean and standard deviation (SD). These values were compared between the groups by one-way analysis of variance (ANOVA) with post hoc analysis of the Tukey test. In multiple parameter's comparisons, correlation coefficient (r) values were collected. All statistical analyses were performed with JMP (version 10.1 software; SAS Institute, Cary, NC, USA). p-values less than 0.05 were considered significant.

42.3 Results

ROSC was not achieved in any animals. Oxy-Hb showed a significant correlation with both MAP ($r = 0.218$, $p < 0.0001$) and $EtCO_2$ ($r = 0.2294$, $p < 0.0001$), while Deoxy-Hb and TOI correlated with MAP ($r = -0.4193$, $p < 0.0001$; $r = 0.3125$, $p < 0.0001$, respectively) but not with $EtCO_2$ ($r = 0.0584$, $p = 0.302$; $r = 0.0239$, $p = 0.673$, respectively) (Table 42.1). Likewise, Oxy-Hb identified the differences of three groups (1-side, 2-side, and 3-side, 1.5 ± 0.9, 4.4 ± 0.7, and 5.9 ± 2.1 mmol/L, $p = 0.0008$, respectively), while Deoxy-Hb (1-side, 2-side, and 3-side, −2.7 ± 1.2, −1.1 ± 3.2, and −1.6 ± 10.1 mmol/L, $p = 0.952$, respectively) and TOI (1-side, 2-side, and 3-side, 1.8 ± 1.8, 5.5 ± 1.3, and 9.5 ± 8.0%, respectively, $p = 0.064$) did not (Fig. 42.1).

42.4 Discussion

In our preliminary data, three-side chest compression showed the best performance of CPR compared to the other methods, since the combination of the cardiac and thoracic pumps increased the thoracic pressure [8]. This increased cardiac output and carotid arterial pressure in a rat asphyxia CA model. In the present study, we found that Oxy-Hb identified the differences of the CPR methods and three-side chest compression demonstrated the highest Oxy-Hb level during CPR. This could suggest that Oxy-Hb can serve as an indicator to evaluate the quality of CPR. In addition, Oxy-Hb had a significant correlation with MAP and $EtCO_2$, which are also important indicators of the quality of CPR.

Two different mechanisms of chest compression have been proposed, cardiac pump theory and thoracic pump theory, and both cardiac and thoracic pumps may synergistically contribute to high-quality CPR and subsequently improve survival from cardiac arrest. The three-side method increases intrathoracic pressure and likely stabilizes cardiac hemodynamic status, which may be beneficial to improving the brain function. It is inferred that all CBO parameters including Oxy-Hb, Deoxy-Hb, and TOI increase because of improved cardiac pump effect likewise MAP. On the other hands, only Oxy-Hb reflected thoracic pump effect likewise $EtCO_2$ does. We currently have no data to support this hypothesis, and so future study with larger gyrencephalic species (swine, nonhuman primate, etc.) and measuring the pressure and blood gas in the carotid artery and jugular vein may be crucial to test this hypothesis [8].

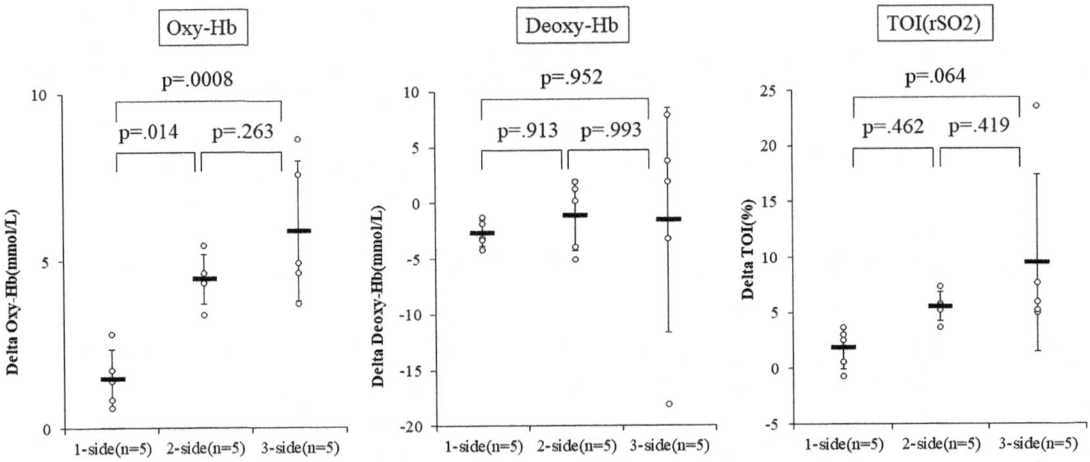

Fig. 42.1 The comparison of differences of cerebral blood oxygenation (CBO) including oxyhemoglobin (Oxy-Hb), Deoxy-Hb, and tissue oxygenation index (TOI) during our original three types of chest compression. The delta is the difference between the current average and the average of the end of the asphyxial period regarded as a baseline. rSO2 regional cerebral tissue oxygen saturation, 1-side one-side chest compression, 2-side two-side chest compression, 3-side three-side chest compression. ##$p < 0.01$; #$p < 0.05$; n.s. not significant

One of the reasons why the current guidelines do not recommend CBO by NIRS during CPR is the lack of evidence showing that CBO can effectively evaluate the quality of CPR. Several parameters of CBO are available by NIRS; however, there is a paucity of data supporting which parameter needs to be used for the evaluation of the quality of CPR.

In this study, we used NIRO instead of the other NIRS devices such as INVOS and regional oximetry. This system does not need to be adjusted for body weight. This is required by other systems, such as SenSmart™, which limits its use to subjects with a body weight over 40 kg. Moreover, in addition to measuring TOI/regional cerebral tissue oxygen saturation (rSO_2), NIRO calculates Oxy-Hb and Deoxy-Hb separately without blood collection at the same time [9]. Oxy-Hb measurement is becoming a hot topic in resuscitation science. The data from a previous Japanese prospective, multicenter observational study suggested that Oxy-Hb might be an indicator of neuroprotection in CA patients, which performance was better than rSO_2 [10]. Our results are consistent with these data, revealing that Oxy-Hb had performed better than TOI or Deoxy-Hb in evaluation of the quality of CPR.

$EtCO_2$ is one of the only indicator suggested to be used during CPR in the guidelines even though multiple studies support the potential use of CBO by NIRS [1]. This opposition is likely due to the fact that TOI/rSO_2 has not shown a good correlation with $EtCO_2$ [11, 12]. Our results are consistent, and TOI/rSO_2 did not have a correlation with $EtCO_2$; however, Oxy-Hb did.

One of the difficulties of NIRS measurements in critically ill patients is a large variability of CBO between individual patients [13, 14]. Taking this into consideration, we adjusted for differences between individuals by comparing the values of CBO in each animal with itself during CA (asphyxiation). This method is applicable in a real clinical setting with patients who have more variability than experimentally controlled animals.

The current study has several limitations. First, our study was preliminary, and larger sample size would be required. Second, the quality of CPR needs to be evaluated by blood flow measurements by other independent systems; however, a real-time measurement of the blood flow is difficult in small rodent models. Therefore, it would be necessary to monitor the blood flow using other animal models such as swine or macaque.

42.5 Conclusion

Oxy-Hb during CPR compared to that of during CA showed the potential to evaluate the quality of CPR in a rat CA model.

References

1. Neumar RW, Shuster M, Callaway CW et al (2015) Part 1: executive summary: 2015 American Heart Association guidelines update for cardiopulmonary resuscitation and emergency cardiovascular care. Circulation 132(18 Suppl 2):S315–S367
2. Lin S, Scales DC (2016) Cardiopulmonary resuscitation quality and beyond: the need to improve real-time feedback and physiologic monitoring. Crit Care 20:182
3. Yagi T, Nagao K, Kawamorita T et al (2016) Detection of ROSC in patients with cardiac arrest during chest compression using NIRS: a pilot study. Adv Exp Med Biol 876:151–157
4. Cournoyer A, Iseppon M, Chauny JM et al (2016) Near-infrared spectroscopy monitoring during cardiac arrest: a systematic review and meta-analysis. Acad Emerg Med 23:851–862
5. Koyama Y, Wada T, Lohman BD et al (2013) A new method to detect cerebral blood flow waveform in synchrony with chest compression by near-infrared spectroscopy during CPR. Am J Emerg Med 31(10):1504–1508
6. Nolan JP, Soar J, Cariou A et al (2015) European Resuscitation Council and European Society of Intensive Care Medicine guidelines for post-resuscitation care 2015: Section 5 of the European Resuscitation Council guidelines for resuscitation 2015. Resuscitation 95:202–222
7. Shinozaki K, Becker LB, Saeki K et al (2018) Dissociated oxygen consumption and carbon dioxide production in the post-cardiac arrest rat: a novel metabolic phenotype. J Am Heart Assoc 7:13
8. Okuma Y, Shinozaki K, Yagi T et al (2019) Combination of cardiac and thoracic pump theories in rodent cardiopulmonary resuscitation: a new method of three-side chest compression. Intensive Care Med Exp 7(1):1–4
9. Yoshitani K, Kawaguchi M, Ishida K et al (2019) Guidelines for the use of cerebral oximetry by near-infrared spectroscopy in cardiovascular anesthesia: a report by the cerebrospinal Division of the Academic Committee of the Japanese Society of Cardiovascular Anesthesiologists (JSCVA). J Anesth 33:167–196
10. Hayashida K, Nishiyama K, Suzuki M et al (2014) Estimated cerebral oxyhemoglobin as a useful indicator of neuroprotection in patients with post-cardiac arrest syndrome: a prospective, multicenter observational study. Criti Care 18:500
11. Singer AJ, Nguyen RT, Ravishankar ST et al (2018) Cerebral oximetry versus end tidal CO2 in predicting ROSC after cardiac arrest. Am J Emerg Med 36:403–407
12. Genbrugge C, De Deyne C, Eertmans W et al (2018) Cerebral saturation in cardiac arrest patients measured with near-infrared technology during pre-hospital advanced life support. Results from Copernicus I cohort study. Resuscitation 129:107–113
13. Prosen G, Strnad M, Doniger SJ et al (2018) Cerebral tissue oximetry levels during prehospital management of cardiac arrest – a prospective observational study. Resuscitation 129:141–145
14. Bouček T, Mlček M, Krupičková P et al (2018) Brain perfusion evaluated by regional tissue oxygenation as a possible quality indicator of ongoing cardiopulmonary resuscitation. An experimental porcine cardiac arrest study. Perfusion 33(1_suppl):65–70

Altered Behavioral Performance in the Neuron-Specific HIF-1- and HIF-2-Deficient Mice Following Chronic Hypoxic Exposure

43

Lei Ma, J. Sebastian Garcia-Medina, Geisa Ortet, Joseph C. LaManna, and Kui Xu

Abstract

Hypoxia-inducible factors (HIFs) are transcriptional regulators that mediate in mice for HIF-1 and HIF-2. The objective of this study was to investigate the effect of neuronal deletion of HIF-1 and HIF-2 in hypoxic adaptation by using the neuron-specific knockout (KO) mice. The floxed control and KO mice were used. Hypoxic mice were kept in a hypobaric chamber at a pressure of 300 torr (0.4 ATM, which was equivalent to 8% oxygen under normobaric condition) for 3 weeks. The littermate, normoxic control mice were housed in the same room next to the chamber to match ambient conditions. Body weights were monitored throughout the 3-week course. Cognitive function was measured using a Y-maze test; motor functions were measured using the rotarod test and the grip strength test. The hematocrit increased significantly at the end of 3-week hypoxic exposure in both control and KO mice. In the Y-maze test, the alternation rate (indicative of sustained cognition) trended lower in the KO mice compared to the controls following hypoxia (%, 51.3 ± 13.1, $n = 6$ vs. 63.2 ± 12.0, $n = 8$). In the rotarod test, the latency (seconds) in the KO mice was significantly lower compared to the controls (50.4 ± 5.7 vs. 77.1 ± 5.0, $n = 3$ each before hypoxia and 66.4 ± 3.4, $n = 6$ vs. 98.1 ± 15.4 after hypoxia, $n = 3$). The grip strength in the KO mice was similar compared to the control mice before hypoxia, but the strength of KO mice trended higher after hypoxic exposure. Our data suggest that deficiency of neuronal HIF-1 and HIF-2 may result in changes in behavioral performance and other adaptative responses to hypoxia.

Keywords

Hypoxia-inducible factors · Chronic hypoxia · Hypoxic adaptation · Cognitive function · Motor function

L. Ma
Department of Physiology and Biophysics, Case Western Reserve University, Cleveland, OH, USA

School of Electronic Information Science and Technology, Nantong University, Nantong, Jiangsu Province, China

J. Sebastian Garcia-Medina · G. Ortet · J. C. LaManna · K. Xu (✉)
Department of Physiology and Biophysics, Case Western Reserve University, Cleveland, OH, USA
e-mail: kxx@case.edu

E. M. Nemoto et al. (eds.), *Oxygen Transport to Tissue XLII*, Advances in Experimental Medicine and Biology 1269, https://doi.org/10.1007/978-3-030-48238-1_43

43.1 Introduction

Hypoxia-inducible factors (HIFs) are transcriptional regulators that respond to decreases in available oxygen in the cellular environment or hypoxic conditions [1, 2]. It regulates the adaptive response to hypoxia, such as angiogenesis, and the resultant increased capillary density that typically occurs over a 3-week time course under normoxic conditions. HIF is hydroxylated by HIF-specific prolyl hydroxylases, which are oxygen sensing. Hydroxylation triggers polyubiquitylation of HIF and targets it for proteasomal degradation by an E3 ubiquitin ligase, the von Hippel-Lindau protein complex. HIF-1 was initially discovered through its ability to activate the erythropoietin (EPO) gene during hypoxia via binding to the enhancer element located in the 3′ flanking region of the gene [3, 4]. Cloning of HIF revealed a heterodimeric protein consisting of two subunits, HIF-1 and HIF-2 [5]. HIF-1 may have an influence on the transcription of vascular endothelial growth factor (VEGF). HIF-2 has emerged as the transcription factor that regulates EPO synthesis which plays a critical role in the regulation of anti-apoptosis and angiogenesis and may have neuroprotection effect. The brain is extremely sensitive to hypoxia. There are large regional changes in local blood flow to account for spatial and temporal heterogeneity of neuronal activity, which is influenced by hypoxic exposure [6].

In this study, we investigated the effect of neuronal deletion of HIF-1 and HIF-2 on hypoxic adaptation by using the neuron-specific knockout (KO) mice. Behavioral tests were performed in order to assess cognitive function and motor function.

43.2 Methods

43.2.1 Animals and Hypoxic Exposure

All procedures were approved by the Institutional Animal Care and Use Committee at Case Western Reserve University. Mice carrying a floxed HIF-1 and HIF-2 allele were crossbred with mice carrying a Cre-recombinase-enzyme-driven neuronally expressed promoter, calcium/calmodulin-dependent kinase (CAMKII)-Cre. All mouse strains were maintained on a C57BL/6 J background. Genotyping was performed using PCR analysis on DNA samples obtained from tail biopsies. Cre (+):HIF-1αF/F:HIF-2αF/F are considered HIF-1 and HIF-2 neuronal knockout mice; littermates with Cre (−):HIF-1αF/F:HIF-2αF/F genotypes were used as controls. All mice were housed and maintained at the animal facility on a 12:12-h light/dark diurnal cycle with unrestricted access to food and water. Hypoxic mice were kept in a hypobaric chamber at a pressure of 300 torr (0.4 ATM, which is equivalent to 8% oxygen at sea level) for 3 weeks. The littermate normoxic control mice were housed in the same room next to the chamber to match ambient conditions. Body weights were monitored throughout the 3-week course.

43.2.2 Behavioral Performance

Cognitive function was measured using a Y-maze test; motor functions were measured using the rotarod and the grip strength test: (1) Y-maze test: This test is based on the innate preference of animals' spontaneous alternations; high alternation rate is indicative of sustained cognition. The animal was allowed to freely explore the three arms for 6 min during which the sequencing and number of arm entries were recorded, and the alternation rate (%) was calculated [7]. (2) Rotarod performance test: The test measures parameters such as riding time or endurance; it also evaluates balance, grip strength, and motor coordination of the subjects [8]. Mice were placed on a rotarod machine (Panlab, Harvard Apparatus), which has a rotating bar that increases in RPM over a set period of time. The rod increased 1 RPM every 3 s, maxing out at 40 RPM. Mice had to increase their speed as well as keep their grip in order to stay on the rotating rod. Time for the mice to fall off the rotarod, as well as the RPM at the time of their fall, was recorded. Three replicates of this test per mouse were performed over the course of a week. (3) Grip strength test: The grip strength meter allows the study of neuromuscular functions in rodents by determining the maximum force displayed by an animal. Mice were placed on a metal grid and allowed to get their footing. After a few seconds, the grid was subsequently flipped upside down. The time for the mice to fall onto the pad below was recorded. The test was ended after 60 s if the mice had not already fallen. Three replicates of this test per mouse were performed. Each test was in the environmental condition and the same operator for all experimental groups under study in order to decrease intersubject variability. The test was used to measure the muscle strength of combined forelimbs and hind limbs with full-grip strength test and forelimbs with a bar-grip strength test [9].

43.2.3 Statistical Analysis

Data are expressed as mean ± SD. Statistical analyses were performed using SPSS V26.0 for Windows. Group comparisons were made by one-way analysis of variance (ANOVA) using Tukey's statistic. The comparison between any two groups was analyzed with a t-test. Significance was considered at the level of $p < 0.05$.

43.3 Results

The body weights for normoxic control and KO mice were 27.3 ± 5.0 (mean ± SD, $n = 8$) and 29.5 ± 1.4 ($n = 4$), respectively. They maintained their body weights during the 3 weeks of exposure. The body weights of control hypoxic mice were decreased significantly starting day 4 of hypoxia compared to the pre-hypoxia values (20.6 ± 2.2 vs. 24.6 ± 4.1, $n = 8$; t-test, $p < 0.05$,) and remained lower till day 14 of hypoxia. The body weights of KO mice decreased about 15 during day 4 to day 14 of hypoxia but did not reach significance at any time point. The baseline hematocrit was 47 ± 4 ($n = 8$) and 49 ± 3 ($n = 4$) in the control and KO groups, respectively. After 3 weeks of hypoxia, the hematocrit was 81 ± 5 ($n = 8$) in the control group and 85 ± 3 ($n = 6$) in the KO groups; the hematocrit was increased significantly at the end of hypoxia in both groups (ANOVA, $p < 0.05$).

As seen in Fig. 43.1a, in the Y-maze test, the control group had a similar alternation rate to the KO group under normoxia (%, 58.3 ± 10.9, $n = 7$ vs. 63.6 ± 21.7, $n = 5$). The alternation rate in the control mice under hypoxia was 63.2 ± 12.0 ($n = 8$), which is similar to its normoxic baseline. In KO mice, the alternation rate trended lower after hypoxia (51.2 ± 13.1, $n = 6$). The number of entries (indicative of activity) was 29.6 ± 9.3 ($n = 7$) in the control normoxic group (Fig. 43.1b), and it was trended lower (ANOVA, $p < 0.05$) in the control hypoxic group 20.5 ± 6.4 ($n = 8$). The KO mormoxic group and KO hypoxic group have similar number of entries (30.2 ± 10.8, $n = 5$ vs. 29.2 ± 13.3, $n = 6$).

As seen in Fig. 43.2, in the rotarod test, the latency (seconds) in the KO mice was significantly lower (ANOVA, $p < 0.05$) under normoxia compared to the controls 50.4 ± 5.7 vs. 77.1 ± 5.0, $n = 3$. After hypoxia, the KO group has significantly lower (ANOVA, $p < 0.05$) latency compared to the control group, 66.4 ± 3 vs. 98.1 ± 15.4, $n = 3$ each. The grip strength (both the full-grip strength and the bar-grip strength) in the KO mice was similar compared to the controls under normoxia. After hypoxia, the strength of KO mice was trended higher compared to its normoxic baseline and was significantly higher compared to the control group for the full-grip strength. There were no significant differences (ANOVA, $p > 0.05$) between any two groups in the full-grip strength and bar-grip strength (Fig. 43.3).

43.4 Discussion

In this study, we investigated the effect of neuronal deletion of HIF-1 and HIF-2 on hypoxic adaptation by using the neuron-specific HIF-1 and HIF-2 knockout mice. In the Y-maze test, the alternation rate was similar in both the WT and KO groups, but we observed significantly increased activity levels represented by increased

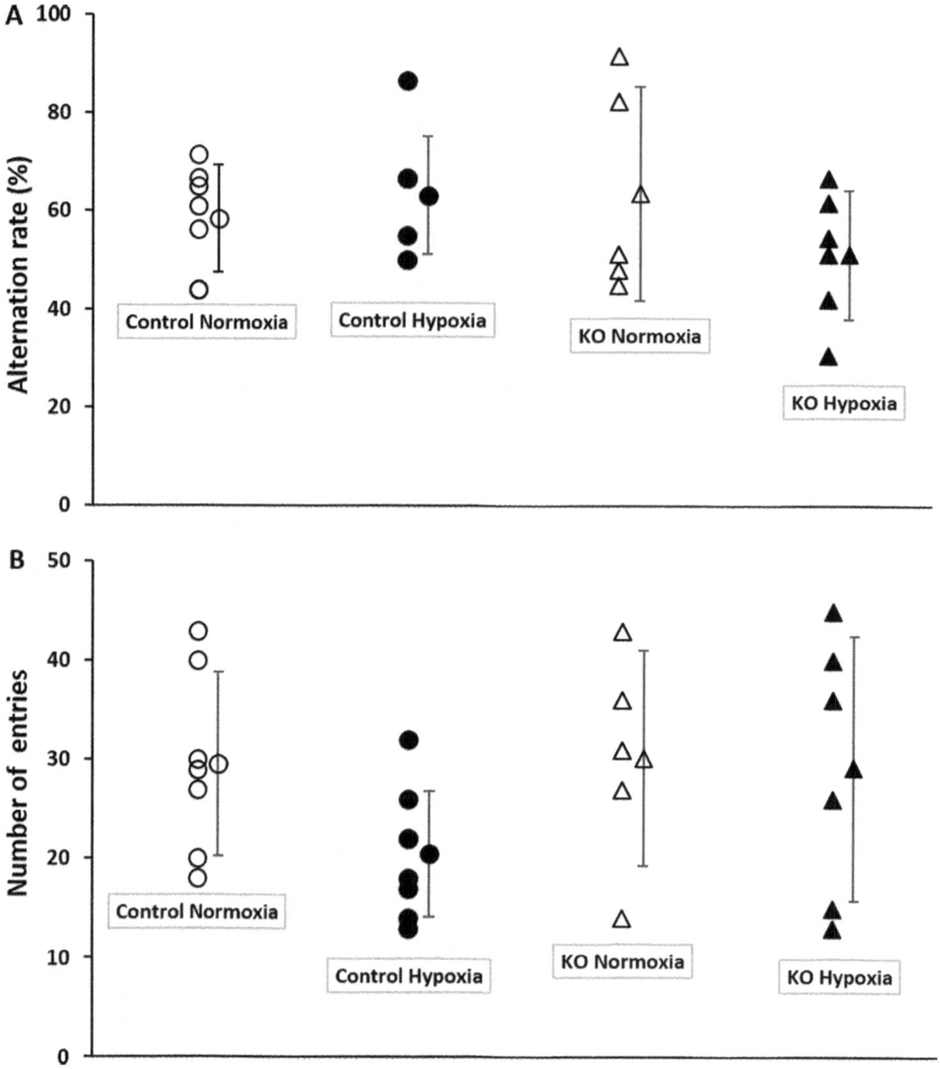

Fig. 43.1 The Y-maze in the control and neuronal HIF-1 and HIF-2 KO mice before and after hypoxia. (**a**) Alternation rate; (**b**) number of entries. Individual data points and mean ± SD (error bar) are presented for each group: control normoxia (empty circle, $n = 7$), control hypoxia (solid circle, $n = 8$), KO normoxia (empty triangle, $n = 5$), and KO hypoxia (solid triangle, $n = 6$). There were no significant differences (ANOVA, $P > 0.05$) between any two groups in alternation rate and number of entries

number of entries after hypoxia stress in the KO mice. The rotarod test shows decreased latency (seconds) in the KO mice compared to the controls before and after hypoxia, suggesting there is an impairment in endurance, balance, grip strength, and motor coordination. The grip strength test could be applied as a supplementary test to differentiate chronic effects on muscular strength. These results suggest that deletion of neuronal HIF-1 and HIF-2 alters the motor function of mice. The limitation of this study is that we only use one test (the Y-maze test) for cognitive function, and the sample size for all tests is very small. In addition, we did not evaluate the cerebral structural changes induced by deficiency of neuronal HIF-1 and HIF-2.

We have shown that the cerebral capillary density was increased after 3 weeks of hypoxia exposure in rat and mouse studies [10, 11]. At the physiological range of ambient oxygen, brain

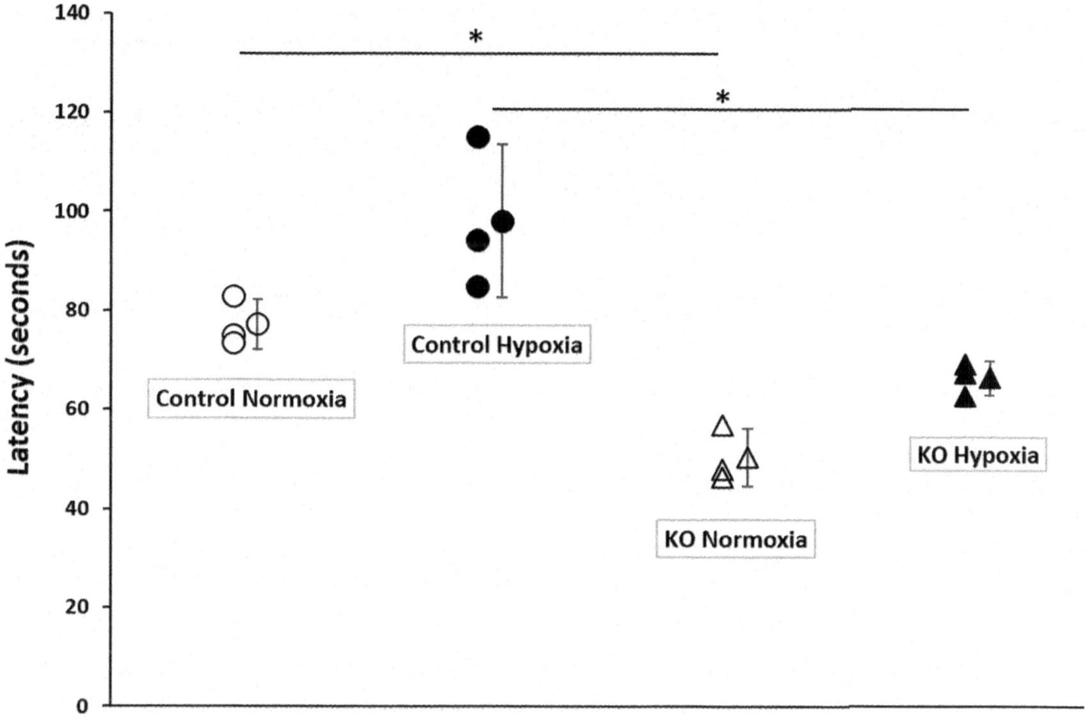

Fig. 43.2 Latency (seconds) in rotarod test in the control and neuronal HIF-1 and HIF-2 KO mice before and after hypoxia. Individual data points and mean ± SD (error bar) are presented for each group: control normoxia (empty circle), control hypoxia (solid circle), KO normoxia (empty triangle), and KO hypoxia (solid triangle); $n = 3$ for each group. * indicates significance (ANOVA, $p < 0.05$) between the control group and hypoxia group under the same exposure condition

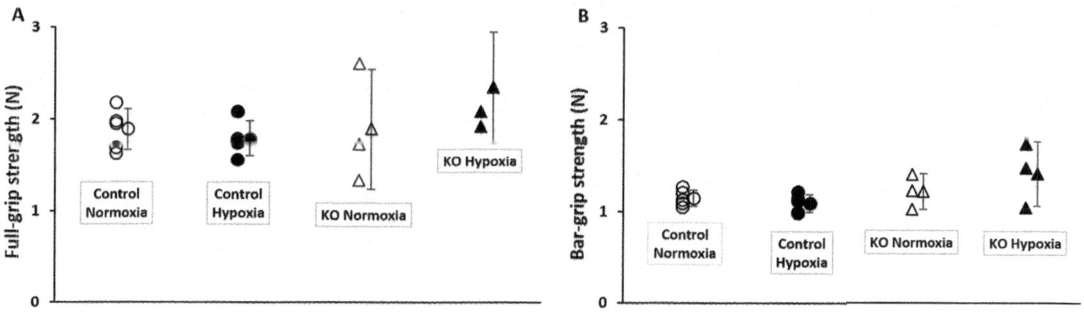

Fig. 43.3 The grip strength performance in the control and neuronal HIF-1 and HIF-2 KO mice before and after hypoxia. (**a**) The full-grip strength (N); (**b**) the bar-grip strength (N). Individual data points and mean ± SD (error bar) are presented for each group: control normoxia (empty circle, $n = 5$), control hypoxia (solid circle, $n = 5$), KO normoxia (empty triangle, $n = 3$), and KO hypoxia (solid triangle, $n = 3$). There were no significant differences (ANOVA, $p > 0.05$) between any two groups in the full-grip strength and bar-grip strength

capillary density is proportional to the fraction of inspired oxygen. The hypoxia-inducible transcription factors, HIF-1 and HIF-2, play an important role in the process of upregulating VEGF [12]. The partial pressure of oxygen in the brain capillary is tightly controlled, and normal brain function is delicately sensitive to continuous and controlled oxygen delivery [13]. HIFs act as a detector of the balance between oxygen delivery and energy demand at the level of the cell redox state, controlling VEGF production that helps determine capillary density in consort with the cyclooxygenase-2/angiopoietin-2 pathway that controls endothelial cell junction mechanical stability. The brain capillary density may be regulated by the incorporation of the HIF-1/VEGF and COX-2/PGE2/Ang-2 pathways, leading to angiogenesis and angiolysis [14].

Our data suggest that deficiency of neuronal HIF-1 and HIF-2 may result in changes in behavioral performance and other adaptative responses to hypoxia. We will further explore the role of HIF-1 and HIF-2 in hypoxic adaptation.

Acknowledgments The study was supported by NIH grant NS 38362. Lei Ma was supported by major program of National Natural Science Foundation of China (61534003).

References

1. Smith TG, Robbins PA, Ratckiffe PJ (2008) The human side of hypoxia-inducible factor. Br J Haematol 141(3):325–334
2. Wilkins SE, Abboun MI, Hancock RL et al (2016) Targeting protein-protein interactions in the HIF system. Chem Med Chem 11(8):773–786
3. Masoud GN, Li W (2015) HIF-1α pathway: role, regulation and intervention for cancer therapy. Acta Pharm Sin B 5(5):378–389
4. Rolf A, Kvietikova I, Gassmann M et al (1997) Oxygen-regulated transferrin expression is mediated by hypoxia-inducible factor-1. J Biol Chem 272(32):20055–20062
5. Freeburg PB, Robert B, St John PL et al (2003) Podocyte expression of hypoxia-inducible factor (HIF)-1 and HIF-2 during glomerular development. J Am Soc Nephrol 14(4):927–938
6. Ratcliffe PJ (2007) HIF-1 and HIF-2: working alone or together in hypoxia? J Clin Invest 117(4):862–865
7. He C, Tsipis T, LaManna JC, Xu K (2016) Environmental enrichment induces increased cerebral capillary density and improved cognitive function in mice. Adv Exp Med Biol 977:175–181
8. Iderberg H, Mccreary AC, Varney MA et al (2015) NLX-112, a novel 5-HT1A receptor agonist for the treatment of l-DOPA-induced dyskinesia: Behavioral and neurochemical profile in rat. Exp Neurol 271:335–350
9. Castro B, Kuang S (2017) Evaluation of muscle performance in mice by treadmill exhaustion test and whole-limb grip strength assay. Bio Protoc 7(8):e2237
10. Ndubuizu OI, Tsipis CP, Li A, LaManna JC (2010) Hypoxia-inducible factor-1 (HIF-1)-independent microvascular angiogenesis in the aged rat brain. Brain Res 1366:101–109
11. Benderro GF, LaManna JC (2014) HIF-1α/COX-2 expression and mouse brain capillary remodeling during prolonged moderate hypoxia and subsequent reoxygenation. Brain Res 1569:41–47
12. Sun X, Tsipis CP, Benderro GF, Xu K, LaManna JC (2014) Defining the role of HIF and its downstream mediators in hypoxic-induced cerebral angiogenesis. Methods Mol Biol 1135:251–260
13. Dore-Duffy P, LaManna JC (2007) Physiologic angiodynamics in the brain. Antioxid Redox Signal 9(9):1363–1371
14. LaManna JC (2018) Cerebral angioplasticity: the anatomical contribution to ensuring appropriate oxygen transport to brain. Adv Exp Med Biol 1072:3–6

44 Effect of Adrenaline on Cerebral Blood Oxygenation Measured by NIRS in a Rat Asphyxia Cardiac Arrest Model

Yu Okuma, Tsukasa Yagi, Tai Yin, Takeyuki Kiguchi, Taku Iwami, Lance B. Becker, and Koichiro Shinozaki

Abstract

Adrenaline is an important pharmacologic treatment during cardiac arrest (CA) for resuscitation. Recent studies suggest that adrenaline increases the likelihood of return of spontaneous circulation (ROSC) but does not contribute to improving neurological outcomes of CA. The mechanisms have not been elucidated yet. A bimodal increase in mean arterial pressure (MAP) is observed after adrenaline injection in rodent CA models (Okuma et al. Intensive Care Med Exp 7(1), 2019). In this study, we focused on alteration of systemic arterial pressure in conjunction with the measurement of cerebral blood oxygenation (CBO) such as oxyhemoglobin (Oxy-Hb), deoxyhemoglobin (Deoxy-Hb), and tissue oxygenation index (TOI) by near-infrared spectroscopy (NIRS). Male Sprague-Dawley rats were used. We attached NIRS between the nasion and the upper cervical spine. Rats underwent 10 minute asphyxia to induce CA. Then, cardiopulmonary resuscitation (CPR) was started, followed by a 20 μg/kg of bolus adrenaline injection at 30 seconds of CPR. This injection accelerated the first increase in MAP, and ROSC was observed with an abrupt increase in CBO. Interestingly, the second increase in MAP, once it exceeded a certain value, was accompanied by paradoxical decreases of Oxy-Hb and TOI while Deoxy-Hb increased. Based on this finding, we compared Oxy-Hb, Deoxy-Hb, and TOI at the first MAP $\approx$ 100 mmHg and the second MAP $\approx$ 100 mmHg. The average of Oxy-Hb and TOI from the 13 animals significantly decreased at the second increase in MAP over 100 mmHg while Deoxy-Hb significantly increased. NIRS identified a decrease in Oxy-Hb after ROSC. These findings may be a clue in understanding the mechanism of how and why adrenaline alters the neurological outcomes of CA post resuscitation.

Keywords

Cardiac arrest · Adrenaline · Cerebral blood oxygenation (CBO) · Near-infrared spectroscopy (NIRS) · Autoregulation

Y. Okuma (✉) · T. Yagi · T. Yin · L. B. Becker · K. Shinozaki
Feinstein Institute for Medical Research, Northwell Health System, Manhasset, NY, USA

T. Kiguchi · T. Iwami
Kyoto University Health Service, Kyoto, Japan

44.1 Introduction

The 2015 International Liaison Committee on Resuscitation (ILCOR) Advanced Life Support (ALS) Guidelines [1] recommended use of intra-

E. M. Nemoto et al. (eds.), *Oxygen Transport to Tissue XLII*, Advances in Experimental Medicine and Biology 1269, https://doi.org/10.1007/978-3-030-48238-1_44

venous adrenaline during resuscitation after cardiac arrest (CA), while recent studies have revealed that adrenaline increased the likelihood of return of spontaneous circulation (ROSC) but did not contribute to improving the neurological outcomes in CA [2, 3]. The mechanisms have not been elucidated yet. A bimodal increase in mean arterial pressure (MAP) is observed after adrenaline injection in rodent CA models [4]. There are a few studies that evaluated the cerebral blood oxygenation (CBO) by near-infrared spectroscopy (NIRS) in swine, but there is no study focused on the relationship between CBO by NIRS and the bimodal increasing in MAP observed in rodent CA models [5]. In this study, we focused on this alteration of the systemic arterial pressure in conjunction with the measurement of cerebral blood oxygenation (CBO) such as oxyhemoglobin (Oxy-Hb), deoxyhemoglobin (Deoxy-Hb), and tissue oxygenation index (TOI) by near-infrared spectroscopy (NIRS). We also tested the effects of adrenaline on both MAP and CBO in sham animals.

44.2 Methods

44.2.1 Animal Preparation

The details of the methods for a rat asphyxia CA model have been described previously [6, 7]. In brief, 12 adult male Sprague-Dawley rats (450–550 g, Charles River Laboratories) were anesthetized with 4% isoflurane (Isosthesia, Butler-Schein AHS) and intubated with a 14-gauge plastic catheter (Surflo, Terumo Medical Corporation). Animals were mechanically ventilated. Anesthesia was maintained with isoflurane 2% at a fraction of inspired O_2 (FIO_2) of 0.3. The left femoral artery was cannulated (sterile polyethylene-50 catheter inserted for 20 mm) for continuous arterial pressure monitoring. A temperature probe was placed in the esophagus for continuous temperature monitoring. The core temperature was maintained at 36.5 ± 1.0 °C during the surgical procedure. The left femoral vein was cannulated with a polyethylene-50 catheter, which was advanced into the inferior vena cava for drug infusion. We attached NIRS (NIRO-200NX, Hamamatsu Photonics, Japan) from the nasion to the upper cervical spine of the rats. The distance between the emission and the detection probes was 3 cm. We examined the mean arterial pressure (MAP), end-tidal carbon dioxide ($ETCO_2$), and Oxy/Deoxy-Hb and TOI. The NIRS device records the oxygen saturation level (TOI) and the changes in concentration of Oxy-Hb and Deoxy-Hb in real time (100 Hz). Data averaged every 20 seconds were used. After instrumentation setup, neuromuscular blockade was achieved by slow intravenous administration of 2 mg/kg of vecuronium bromide (Hospira, USA). Asphyxia was induced in the rats by switching off the ventilator, and CA occurred 3–4 minutes after asphyxia started. We defined CA as a MAP below 20 mmHg; CA was completely untreated during 10 minutes of CA. Mechanical ventilation was restarted at an FIO_2 of 1.0, and manual cardiopulmonary resuscitation (CPR) was delivered to CA animals. Chest compressions were performed at a rate of 240–300 per minute. At 30 seconds after the beginning of CPR, a 20 μg/kg bolus of adrenaline was given to animals through the venous catheter. Following ROSC, defined as a systolic blood pressure above 60 mmHg, CPR was discontinued. If ROSC did not occur by 5 minutes of CPR, resuscitation was terminated. In order to evaluate the dynamics of CBO in post-CPR, we assessed Oxy-Hb, Deoxy-Hb, and TOI 20 seconds before and after the time when MAP reached 100 mmHg. MAP always increased twice after the injection of adrenaline in post-CPR. Six rats underwent sham surgeries including vecuronium and adrenaline administrations but without asphyxia or CPR. The sham animals had one peak of increased MAP after the injection of adrenaline.

44.2.2 Statistical Analysis

Data are shown as mean and SD. The Mann-Whitney U test was used for continuous variables. One-way analysis of variance (ANOVA) was used for the group comparison with post hoc analysis of the Tukey test. We also presented the results of our multiple parameters. All statistical analyses were performed with JMP (version 10.1 software; SAS Institute, Cary, NC, USA). P-values less than 0.05 were considered significant.

44.3 Results

Figure 44.1 shows the trend of MAP, heart rate, TOI, Oxy-Hb, Deoxy-Hb, and EtCO2 in a CA animal and a sham animal. In CA animals, the first peak of increased MAP was observed at ROSC and, it was always followed by the second slow peak of MAP that occurred approximately 10 minutes after ROSC. In CA animals, there was a significant difference in the trend of CBO between the first and the second peak of increased MAP. When animals achieved ROSC and MAP reached 100 mmHg for the first time, Oxy-Hb and TOI increased, but Deoxy-Hb decreased. However, when MAP reached 100 mmHg for the second time, Oxy-Hb and TOI decreased, but Deoxy-Hb increased. This CBO alteration pattern at the second peak was considered paradoxical compared to that of the first peak ($n = 6$). In sham animals, the CBO alteration when MAP increased to 100 mmHg was the paradoxical pattern, in which Oxy-Hb and TOI decreased and Deoxy-Hb increased as MAP increased (Fig. 44.2).

44.4 Discussion

In the present study, we found significantly different patterns of CBO between the first and the second increase in MAP after CPR. The phenomenon of CBO alteration at the second peak of MAP after CPR was similar to that of the effect of adrenaline on sham animals.

It has been accepted that higher Oxy-Hb and rSO2(TOI) suggest improvement in brain function [8, 9]. Because of this, adrenaline is considered damaging to the brain since it paradoxically decreases blood perfusion into the brain. Likewise, after cardiac arrest, adrenaline may decrease brain oxygenation post-CA [5], and it could be harmful even though it is considered necessary for CPR [2, 3].

Adrenaline is referred to as a double-edged sword because it has a beneficial effect on the heart by promoting resuscitation but also has a harmful effect on blood flow to the brain, which in turn is considered to deteriorate neurological outcomes. The mechanisms of altering CBO, cerebral blood flow (CBF), and microcirculation have been poorly understood [3, 10, 11]. A previous study indicated that adrenaline might increase and stabilize CBF under isoflurane [12]. Given our findings that Oxy-Hb and TOI decreased after adrenaline administration, adrenaline might affect the microcirculation in a different way from that for CBF. Previous studies indicated that the vasoactive tone might be incompetent after prolonged CA, resulting in reduced cerebrovascular resistance and increased cerebral microcir-

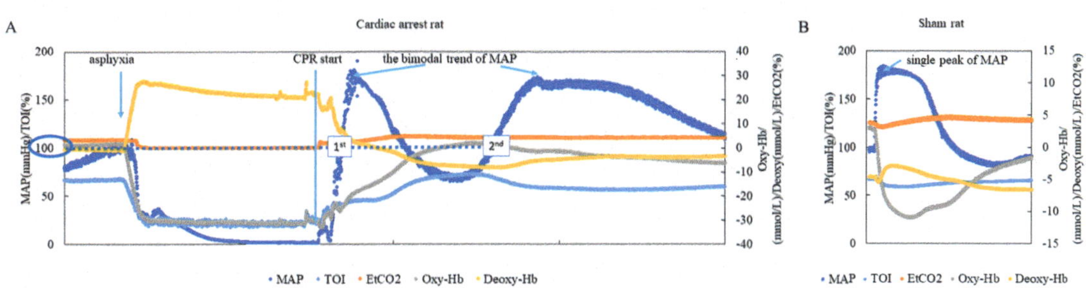

Fig. 44.1 The representative changes in mean arterial pressure (MAP), heart rate, end-tidal carbon dioxide ($EtCO_2$), and cerebral blood oxygenation (CBO) including oxyhemoglobin (Oxy-Hb), Deoxy-Hb, and tissue oxygenation index (TOI): (**a**) a cardiac arrest rat and (**b**) a sham rat. Bimodal peaks in MAP were seen in cardiac arrest, while single peak was observed in sham

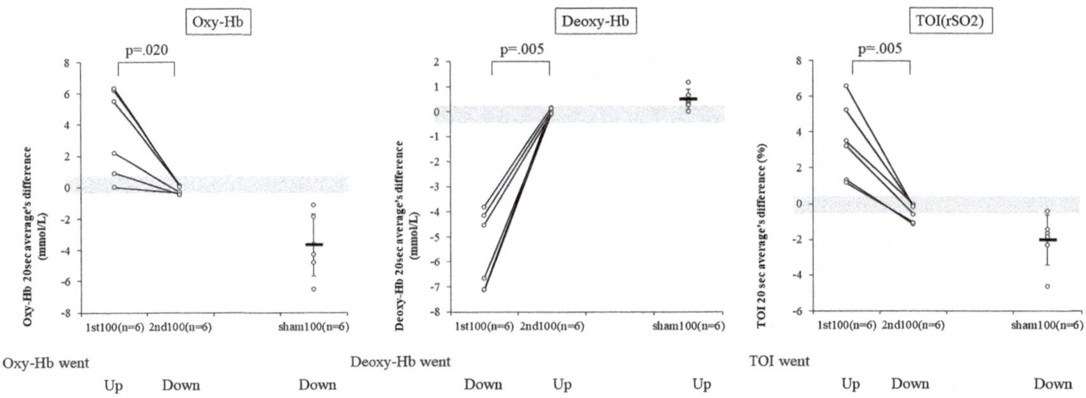

Fig. 44.2 The dynamic trend's comparison of cerebral blood oxygenation (CBO) including oxyhemoglobin (Oxy-Hb), Deoxy-Hb, and tissue oxygenation index (TOI) when mean arterial pressure (MAP) reached 100 mmHg after adrenaline injection in sham model (sham 100) and at the first time (1st 100) and at the second time (2nd 100) in cardiac arrest model. rSO_2 regional cerebral tissue oxygen saturation

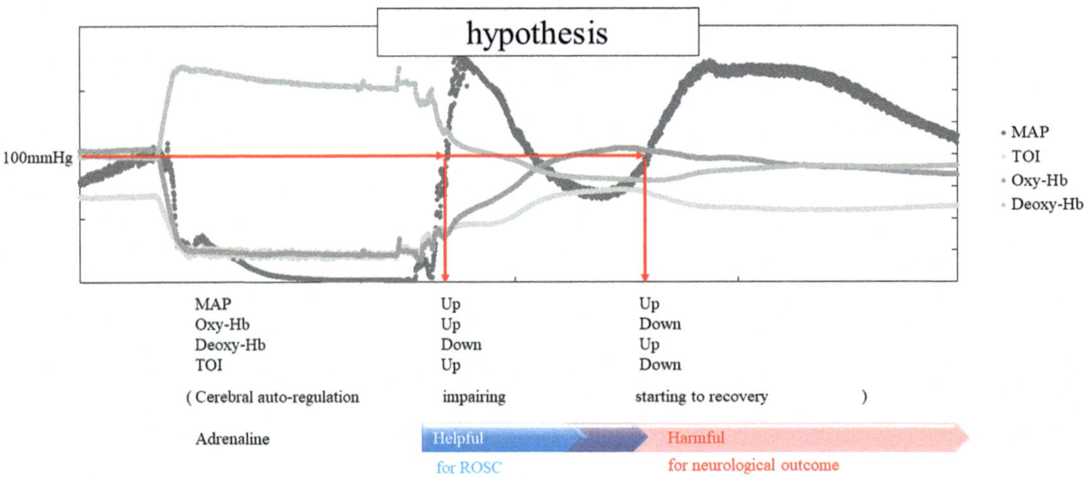

Fig. 44.3 Our hypothesis of adrenaline's effect. MAP mean arterial pressure, Oxy-Hb oxyhemoglobin, Deoxy-Hb deoxyhemoglobin, TOI tissue oxygenation index, ROSC return of spontaneous circulation

culation [13, 14]. Therefore, a linear relationship between MAP and CBO is plausible under conditions of severely devastated cerebral autoregulation as was seen at ROSC [15, 16]. The mechanism that explains the second peak of increased MAP is not clear, but as heart rate also indicated, it may originate from a delayed release of endogenous catecholamine and/or an activation of the sympathetic nervous system that changes the microcirculatory autoregulation [4].

Based on these hypothetical mechanisms and the findings in the present study, we hypothesized that the administration of adrenaline would affect the cerebral microcirculation and CBO (Fig. 44.3), which may depend on the status of cerebral autoregulation. CA is a time-sensitive disorder, so autoregulation in the cerebral microcirculation is heavily impacted by the time after resuscitation [17]. As the cerebral autoregulation recovers, the effect of adrenaline on the cerebral microcirculation alters, and it in turn changes the effect on CBO, which may have a harmful effect on the neurological outcomes.

The current study includes several limitations. First, we did not show a correlation between the CBO by NIRS and the CBF. It is necessary to monitor CBF, but due to technical difficulties in small animal models, further work will be required to better define the relationship of CBO with CBF using larger animal models. Second, the next study needs to examine the effect of exogenous and endogenous adrenaline, which may include additive effects after CA.

44.5 Conclusion

NIRS identified a decrease in Oxy-Hb after ROSC. This phenomenon might be a clue to help understand the mechanism of how and why adrenaline interferes with the improvement of neurological outcomes in post-CA.

References

1. Link MS, Berkow LC, Kudenchuk PJ et al (2015) Part 7: adult advanced cardiovascular life support: 2015 American Heart Association guidelines update for cardiopulmonary resuscitation and emergency cardiovascular care. Circulation 132:S444–S464
2. Hagihara A, Hasegawa M, Abe T et al (2012) Prehospital epinephrine use and survival among patients with out-of-hospital cardiac arrest. JAMA 307:1161–1168
3. Perkins GD, Ji C, Deakin CD, Quinn T et al (2018) A randomized trial of epinephrine in out-of-hospital cardiac arrest. N Engl J Med 379:711–721
4. Neumar RW, Bircher NG, Sim KM et al (1995) Epinephrine and sodium bicarbonate during CPR following asphyxial cardiac arrest in rats. Resuscitation 29:249–263
5. Ristagno G, Tang W, Huang L et al (2009) Epinephrine reduces cerebral perfusion during cardiopulmonary resuscitation. Crit Care Med 37:1408–1415
6. Shinozaki K, Becker LB, Saeki K et al (2018) Dissociated oxygen consumption and carbon dioxide production in the post-cardiac arrest rat: a novel metabolic phenotype. J Am Heart Assoc 7. https://doi.org/10.1161/jaha.117.007721
7. Yu Okuma, Koichiro Shinozaki, Tsukasa Yagi, Kota Saeki, Tai Yin, Junhwan Kim, Lance B. Becker, (2019) Combination of cardiac and thoracic pump theories in rodent cardiopulmonary resuscitation: a new method of three-side chest compression. Intensive Care Medicine Experimental 7 (1)
8. Hallacoglu B, Sassaroli A, Fantini S et al (2011) Cerebral perfusion and oxygenation are impaired by folate deficiency in rat: absolute measurements with noninvasive near-infrared spectroscopy. J Cereb Blood Flow Metab 31:1482–1492
9. Nosrati R, Lin S, Ramadeen A et al (2017) Cerebral hemodynamics and metabolism during cardiac arrest and cardiopulmonary resuscitation using hyperspectral near infrared spectroscopy. Circ J 81:879–887
10. Sigal AP, Sandel KM, Buckler DG et al (2019) Impact of adrenaline dose and timing on out-of-hospital cardiac arrest survival and neurological outcomes. Resuscitation 139:182–188
11. Gough CJR, Nolan JP (2018) The role of adrenaline in cardiopulmonary resuscitation. Crit Care 22:139
12. Myburgh JA, Upton RN, Grant C et al (2002) The cerebrovascular effects of adrenaline, noradrenaline and dopamine infusions under propofol and isoflurane anaesthesia in sheep. Anaesth Intensive Care 30:725–733
13. Lee SK, Vaagenes P, Safar P et al (1989) Effect of cardiac arrest time on cortical cerebral blood flow during subsequent standard external cardiopulmonary resuscitation in rabbits. Resuscitation 17:105–117
14. van den Brule JMD, van der Hoeven JG, Hoedemaekers CWE (2018) Cerebral perfusion and cerebral autoregulation after cardiac arrest. Biomed Res Int 2018:4143636
15. Nishizawa H, Kudoh I (1996) Cerebral autoregulation is impaired in patients resuscitated after cardiac arrest. Acta Anaesthesiol Scand 40:1149–1153
16. Tsuji M, Saul JP, du Plessis A et al (2000) Cerebral intravascular oxygenation correlates with mean arterial pressure in critically ill premature infants. Pediatrics 106:625–632
17. Weisfeldt ML, Becker LB (2002) Resuscitation after cardiac arrest: a 3-phase time-sensitive model. JAMA 288:3035–3038

45 Addition of Drag-Reducing Polymers to Colloid Resuscitation Fluid Enhances Cerebral Microcirculation and Tissue Oxygenation After Traumatic Brain Injury Complicated by Hemorrhagic Shock

Denis E. Bragin, Olga A. Bragina, Lucy Berliba, Marina V. Kameneva, and Edwin M. Nemoto

Abstract

Hemorrhagic shock (HS) is a severe complication of traumatic brain injury (TBI) that doubles mortality due to severely compromised microvascular cerebral blood flow (mvCBF) and oxygen delivery reduction, as a result of hypotension. Volume expansion with resuscitation fluids (RF) for HS does not improve microvascular CBF (mvCBF); moreover, it aggravates brain edema. We showed that the addition of drag-reducing polymers (DRP) to crystalloid RF (lactated Ringer's) significantly improves mvCBF, oxygen supply, and neuronal survival in rats suffering TBI+HS. Here, we compared the effects of colloid RF (Hetastarch) with DRP (HES-DRP) and without (HES). Fluid percussion TBI (1.5 ATA, 50 ms) was induced in rats and followed by controlled HS to a mean arterial pressure (MAP) of 40 mmHg. HES or HES-DRP was infused to restore MAP to 60 mmHg for 1 h (prehospital period), followed by blood reinfusion to a MAP of 70 mmHg (hospital period). In vivo two-photon microscopy was used to monitor cerebral microvascular blood flow, tissue hypoxia (NADH), and neuronal necrosis (i.v. propidium iodide) for 5 h after TBI+HS, followed by postmortem DiI vascular painting. Temperature, MAP, blood gases, and electrolytes were monitored. Statistical analyses were done using GraphPad Prism by Student's t-test or Kolmogorov-Smirnov test, where appropriate. TBI+HS compromised mvCBF and tissue oxygen supply due to capillary microthrombosis. HES-DRP improved mvCBF and tissue oxygenation ($p < 0.05$) better than HES. The number of dead neurons in the HES-DRP was significantly less than in

D. E. Bragin (✉)
Lovelace Biomedical Research Institute,
Albuquerque, NM, USA

University of New Mexico School of Medicine,
Departments of Neurology and Neurosurgery,
Albuquerque, NM, USA
e-mail: dbragin@salud.unm.edu

O. A. Bragina · L. Berliba
Lovelace Biomedical Research Institute,
Albuquerque, NM, USA

M. V. Kameneva
McGowan Institute for Regenerative Medicine,
University of Pittsburgh, Pittsburgh, PA, USA

E. M. Nemoto
Department of Neurosurgery, University of New
Mexico, Albuquerque, NM, USA

E. M. Nemoto et al. (eds.), *Oxygen Transport to Tissue XLII*, Advances in Experimental Medicine and Biology 1269, https://doi.org/10.1007/978-3-030-48238-1_45

the HES group: 76.1 ± 8.9 vs. 178.5 ± 10.3 per 0.075 mm^3 ($P < 0.05$). Postmortem visualization of painted vessels revealed vast microthrombosis in both hemispheres that were 33 ± 2% less in HES-DRP vs. HES ($p < 0.05$). Thus, resuscitation after TBI+HS using HES-DRP effectively restores mvCBF and reduces hypoxia, microthrombosis, and neuronal necrosis compared to HES. HES-DRP is more neuroprotective than lactated Ringer's with DRP and requires an infusion of a smaller volume, which reduces the development of hypervolemia-induced brain edema.

Keywords

Traumatic brain injury (TBI) · Hemorrhagic shock (HS) · Resuscitation fluid (RF) · Hetastarch · Drag-reducing polymer (DRP)

45.1 Introduction

Hemorrhagic shock (HS) is a severe complication of traumatic brain injury (TBI) that frequently occurs in polytrauma and doubles mortality due to severely compromised microvascular cerebral blood flow (mvCBF) and oxygen delivery reduction as a result of hypotension [1–3]. The duration of hypotension is inversely associated with outcome in TBI patients [4]. Current treatments for HS are based on volume expansion with crystalloid or colloid resuscitation fluid (RF) solutions followed by transfusion of donor blood at the hospital. In the case of TBI, this approach is controversial as it does not adequately alleviate impaired mvCBF and thus is not neuroprotective. Moreover, the large volumes infused often exacerbate brain edema [5]. Thus, novel approaches are needed. One of the new possible approaches is the addition of drag-reducing polymers (DRP) to the RF. DRP are linear, blood-soluble, nontoxic macromolecules that in nanomolar concentrations substantially improve rheological properties of blood flow. We previously showed that the addition of DRP to the crystalloid RF (lactated Ringer's) commonly used in the civilian setting significantly improves mvCBF, oxygen supply, and neuronal survival in rats suffering TBI+HS [6]. Here, we evaluate the efficacy of DRP addition to the colloid RF (Hetastarch) preferred for resuscitation in combat casualty settings to compare with lactated Ringer's with DRP.

45.2 Methods

The procedures used in the study have already been described [6] and were conducted according to the approval granted by the Institutional Animal Care and Use Committee of the University of New Mexico and the study Protocol #200640.

The overall design of the study After baseline imaging, TBI was induced and followed by a 1-h hemorrhagic phase, where blood was slowly withdrawn to decrease mean arterial pressure (MAP) to 40 mmHg. In the subsequent 1-h prehospital care phase, resuscitation fluids (HES or HES-DRP) were gradually infused i.v. to increase MAP to ~55 mmHg and CBF (Doppler flux) to ~65% of baseline. In the following 3-h definitive hospital care phase, the withdrawn blood was reinfused to a MAP of 70 mmHg and CBF of ~75% of baseline. In vivo 2PLSM over the pericontusion area of the parietal cortex of the rat brain was performed during the whole study. Monitored variables included cerebral microvascular blood flow velocity, number of perfused capillaries, tissue oxygen supply (NADH fluorescence), and neuronal necrosis (i.v. propidium iodide). The laser Doppler flux was measured via a lateral temporal window using a 0.9-mm-diameter probe (DRT4, Moor Inst., Axminster, UK) in the same region of the brain studied by 2PLSM. Brain and rectal temperatures were monitored and maintained at 38 ± 0.5 °C. Arterial blood gases, electrolytes, hematocrit, and pH were measured hourly (epoc Blood Analysis System, Alere Inc., Waltham, MA, USA). At the end of the experiments, animals were subjected to perfusion with vessel painting.

Surgical preparation Acclimatized male Sprague-Dawley rats (250–300 g) were involuntarily ventilated on isoflurane (2%) in a mix of nitrous oxide (69%) and oxygen (29%) anesthesia. Catheters were inserted into the femoral vein and artery. For TBI and imaging, a craniotomy (5 mm) over the left parietal cortex was filled with agarose in saline (2%) and sealed by a cover glass. The fluid percussion TBI was induced by a pulse from the Pneumatic Impactor connected to the brain through a transducer filled with artificial cerebrospinal fluid (1.5 atm, 50 ms). For HS, blood was slowly withdrawn through the femoral vein.

DRP preparation Polyethylene oxide (PEO, MW ~4000 kDa) was dissolved in saline to 0.1% (1000 ppm), dialyzed against saline using a 50 kD cutoff membrane, diluted in saline to 50 ppm, slow rocked for ~2 h, and then sterilized using a 0.22 μm filter [6]. HES-DRP was prepared before infusion by adding DRP to Hetastarch to reach the final DRP concentration of 0.0005% (5 ppm).

Two-photon laser scanning microscopy Fluorescent serum (i.v. fluorescein isothiocyanate (FITS) dextran, 150 kDa in physiological saline, 5% wt/vol) was visualized using an Olympus BX 51WI upright microscope and water-immersion LUMPlan FL/IR 20X/0.50 W objective. Excitation was provided by a PrairieView Ultima multiphoton microscopy laser scan unit powered by a Millennia Prime 10 W diode laser source pumping a Tsunami Ti: Sapphire laser (Spectra-Physics, Mountain View, CA, USA) tuned to 750 nm center wavelength. Band-pass-filtered epifluorescence (510–530 nm for FITS, 445–475 nm for NADH, and 565–600 for ET) was collected by photomultiplier tubes of the PrairieView Ultima system. Images (512 × 512 pixels, 0.15 um/pixel in the x- and y-axes) or line scans were acquired using PrairieView software. Red blood cell flow velocity was measured in microvessels ranging from 3 to 50 μm diameter up to 500 μm below the surface of the parietal cortex, as described previously [5]. Tissue hypoxia was assessed by measurement of NADH autofluorescence. In offline analyses using NIH ImageJ software, a three-dimensional anatomy of the vasculature in areas of interest was reconstructed from two-dimensional (planar) scans of the fluorescence intensity obtained at successive focal depths in the cortex (XYZ stack).

Animal perfusion and vessel painting At the end of the study, vessel painting was done via cardiac perfusion according to Hughes with 1,1′-dioctadecyl-3,3,3′,3′-tetramethylindocarbocyanine perchlorate (DiI, Invitrogen, USA), which binds preferentially to endothelial cells. The vessel painting included the sequential order for infusion of solutions: (a) PBS (150 ml), (b) 50 ml of DiI (13 μg/ml), and (c) paraformaldehyde (4%, 200 ml). After painting, the brain was extracted from the skull, and all meninges were removed. Imaging was performed using 2PLSM in a custom-made fixed-tissue-imaging chamber.

Statistical analyses were done using GraphPad Prism software 6.0 (La Jolla, CA, USA) by Student's t-test or Kolmogorov-Smirnov test, where appropriate. Differences between groups were determined using a two-way analysis of variance (ANOVA) for multiple comparisons and post hoc testing using the Mann-Whitney U-test.

45.3 Results

Despite unchanged MAP after TBI, cortical CBF, measured by surface laser Doppler probe in the peri-contusional area, fell to 86.9 ± 5.1% from baseline ($P < 0.05$). Capillary flow velocity reduced from 0.75 ± 0.04 mm/s to 0.68 ± 0.04 mm/s, and the number of functioning capillaries reduced from 203 ± 6.5 to 159 ± 5.9 per 0.075 mm^3, leading to tissue hypoxia, reflected by a ~25% increase in NADH autofluorescence ($P < 0.05$ for all, Fig. 45.1).

Subsequent hemorrhagic shock reduced MAP to 41.1 ± 3.6 mmHg and cortical CBF to 46 ± 6.0%, which caused a further reduction of mvCBF and tissue oxygenation, leading to neu-

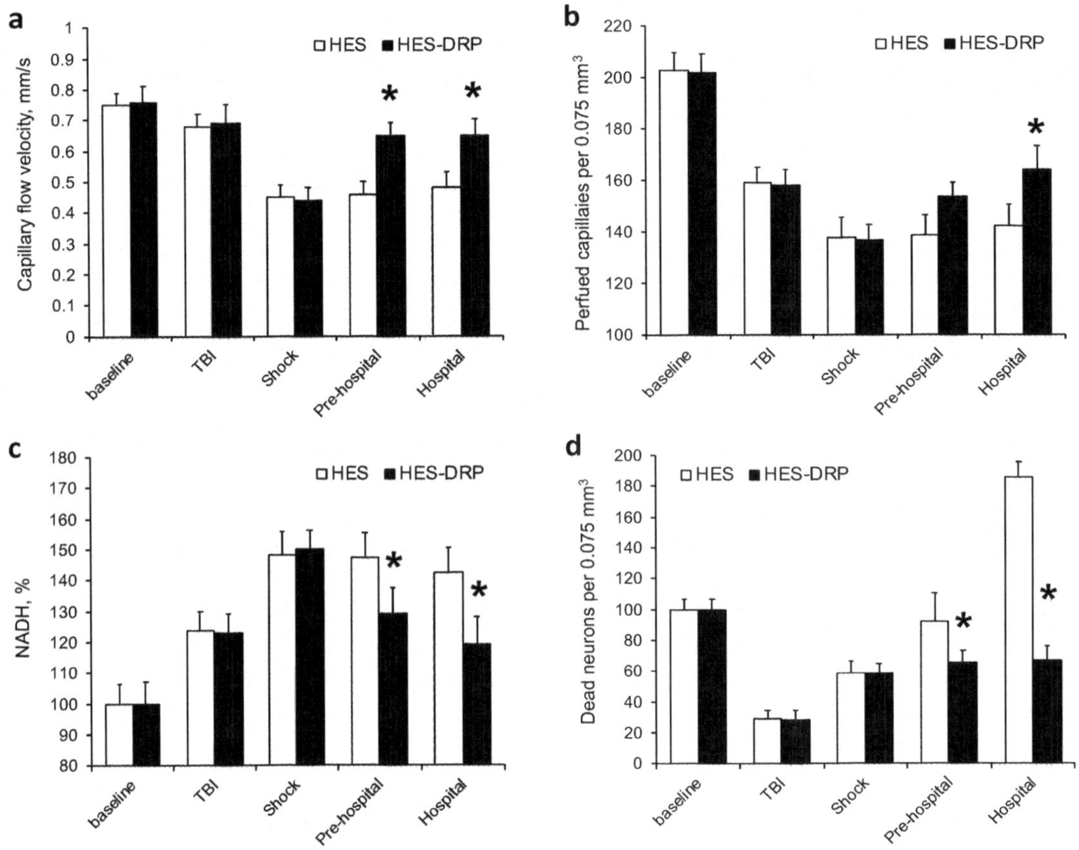

Fig. 45.1 HES-DRP better than HES preserves (**a**) capillary flow velocity, (**b**) the number of perfused capillaries, (**c**) tissue oxygen supply (NADH), and (**d**) neurons. Mean ± SEM; $N = 10$ rats per group, $*P < 0.05$

ronal necrosis with 58.9 ± 5.8 dead neurons per 0.075 mm^3 at the end of the HS phase ($P < 0.05$ for all, Fig. 45.1).

In the prehospital phase, HES, slowly infused in the amount of 4.9 ± 1.7 ml, restored MAP to 54.6 ± 5.2 mmHg and cortical CBF to 59.9 ± 6.8% ($P < 0.05$ from the HS phase). However, no notable changes were observed in mvCBF and tissue oxygenation, which remained at the same level as in the HS phase (Fig. 45.1), while the number of dead neurons increased to 92.3 ± 10.8 per 0.075 mm^3 of brain parenchyma (Fig. 45.1). HES-DRP, infused during *the prehospital phase* in the smaller amount of 2.2 ± 0.4 cml, increased MAP to 46.9 ± 4.3 mmHg, while cortical CBF increased to 66.3 ± 6.5% (Fig. 45.1, $P < 0.05$ from the HES group). In contrast to HES, the infusion of HES-DRP improved mvCBF and tissue oxygenation, i.e., the number of perfused capillaries increased to 153.5 ± 5.7 per 0.075 mm^3, and capillary flow velocity increased to 0.55 ± 0.04, leading to NADH autofluorescence reduction to 129.1 ± 8.4%. Improved oxygen transport to tissue protected neurons from necrosis, as the number of dead neurons showed no significant increase: 65.3 ± 8.1 per 0.075 mm^3 (Fig. 45.1, $P < 0.05$ from the HES group).

During the hospital phase in the HES group, reinfusion of blood increased MAP to 70.2 ± 6.7 mmHg and cortical CBF to 73.8 ± 8.4%. However, as in the prehospital phase, mvCBF and tissue oxygenation in the peri-contusion regions did not change significantly, but there was a trend toward improvement (Fig. 45.1). The number of dead neurons increased to 185.5 ± 10.3 per 0.075 mm^3 of tissue by the end of this phase (Fig. 45.1, $P < 0.05$ from the HES group). In the HES-DRP group, reinfusion of blood during the hospital phase increased MAP to 68.8 ± 5.7 mmHg and cortical CBF to 80.8 ± 6.9%. mvCBF and tissue oxygenation further improved: the number of perfused capillaries increased to 164.3 ± 8.9 per 0.075 mm^3, capillary flow velocity increased to 0.65 ± 0.05, and NADH autofluorescence reduced to 119.3 ± 8.8% (Fig. 45.1, $P < 0.05$ from the HES group). Improved oxygen transport to tissue protected neurons from necrosis, as the number of dead neurons was significantly less than in the HES group: 67.1 ± 8.9 per 0.075 mm^3 (Fig. 45.1, $P < 0.05$ from the HES group).

DiI vessel painting showed a reduction in microvascular density and massive microthrombosis in both hemispheres in rats after TBI with HS. In the injured hemisphere in HES-DRP group, microvascular density was higher than in HES (% vessel/total area*100 was 5.1 ± 0.4 vs. 3.2 ± 0.3, respectively, $p < 0.05$) as opposed to 6.9 ± 0.5 in Sham rats. Contralateral to the injury hemisphere, microvascular density was also reduced (% vessel/total area*100 was 6.2 ± 0.5 vs. 5.1 ± 0.4, in HES-DRP vs. HES, respectively).

45.4 Discussion

In this work, we have evaluated the effects of DRP addition to the colloid resuscitation fluid (Hetastarch). As in our previous work, where we added DRP to the crystalloid resuscitation fluid, it improved microcirculation, tissue oxygen delivery, and neuronal survival (lactated Ringer's) [6]. This is of importance as both crystalloids and colloids do not have any specific protective properties besides temporarily restoring intravascular volume and maintaining appropriate osmotic environment. These fluids rapidly move into the extravascular compartment that exacerbates brain edema and are unable to increase oxygen delivery [5]. Our results showed that DRP added to Hetastarch was more neuroprotective than the DRP added to lactated Ringer's. These results are supported by Kochanek's group who reported better neuroprotective properties of Hetastarch vs. lactated Ringer's [7].

The mechanisms of hemorheological modulation by DRP include increasing the arteriolar blood volume flow via the increase of flow velocity by reduction of flow separations and vortices at vessel bifurcations and decreasing pressure loss across the arterial network due to the viscoelastic properties of DRP [8]. This leads to a rise in precapillary blood pressure, thus enhancing capillary perfusion, countering capillary stasis, and increasing the density of functioning capillaries and the number of red blood cells passing through capillaries to improve tissue oxygenation [8]. Another beneficial property of DRP-RF is that it significantly reduced the amount of fluid required to increase tissue perfusion, which is particularly essential for the traumatized brain. One of the main problems of current resuscitation fluids is the need for the infusion of large volumes that can exacerbate brain edema and cause hemodilution, thereby reducing blood oxygen-carrying capacity that can further compromise oxygenation of the injured brain [5]. Adequate capillary perfusion, which can be restored by HES-DRP, is essential to maintain homeostasis, to remove metabolic waste products which, if allowed to accumulate, exert toxic effects, and to overcome deficits in oxygen delivery.

45.5 Conclusion

Resuscitation after TBI+HS using HES-DRP effectively restores mCBF and better reduces hypoxia, microthrombosis, and neuronal necrosis compared to volume expansion with HES. HES-DRP requires an infusion of a smaller volume to improve tissue perfusion and oxygen delivery, which reduces brain edema formation due to hypervolemia. Colloid-based RF with DRP is more neuroprotective than crystalloid RF.

Acknowledgments Supported by DOD. DB was supported by NIH R01 NS112808.

References

1. Manley G, Knudson MM, Morabito D et al (2001) Hypotension, hypoxia, and head injury: frequency, duration, and consequences. Arch Surg 136(10):1118–1123
2. Navarro JC, Pillai S, Cherian L et al (2012) Histopathological and behavioral effects of immediate and delayed hemorrhagic shock after mild traumatic brain injury in rats. J Neurotrauma 29(2):322–334
3. Chesnut RM, Marshall SB, Piek J et al (1993) Early and late systemic hypotension as a frequent and fundamental source of cerebral ischemia following severe brain injury in the Traumatic Coma Data Bank. Acta Neurochir Suppl 59:121–125
4. Pietropaoli JA, Rogers FB, Shackford SR et al (1992) The deleterious effects of intraoperative hypotension on outcome in patients with severe head injuries. J Trauma 33(3):403–407
5. Ramming S, Shackford SR, Zhuang J et al (1994) The relationship of fluid balance and sodium administration to cerebral edema formation and intracranial pressure in a porcine model of brain injury. J Trauma 37(5):705–713
6. Bragin DE, Lara DA, Bragina OA et al (2018) Resuscitation fluid with drag reducing polymer enhances cerebral microcirculation and tissue oxygenation after traumatic brain injury complicated by hemorrhagic shock. Adv Exp Med Biol 1072:39–43
7. Exo JL, Shellington DK, Bayir H et al (2009) Resuscitation of traumatic brain injury and hemorrhagic shock with polynitroxylated albumin, hextend, hypertonic saline, and lactated Ringer's: effects on acute hemodynamics, survival, and neuronal death in mice. J Neurotrauma 26(12):2403–2408
8. Kameneva MV (2012) Microrheological effects of drag-reducing polymers in vitro and in vivo. Int J Eng Sci 59:168–183

46 Effects of 20-Minute Intensive Exercise on Subjects with Different Working Memory Bases

Weixiang Qin, S. Kojima, S. Morishita, K. Hotta, K. Oyama, and A. Tsubaki

Abstract

Continuous moderate-intensity aerobic exercise improves cognitive function including working memory (WM). We aimed to determine the differences in the effects of exercise on WM based on pre-exercise WM function and oxyhemoglobin (O_2Hb) changes. We enrolled 12 healthy adult males who, after a 4-min rest and warm-up, performed a 20-min exercise regime at a workload corresponding to 50% of maximal oxygen consumption. They performed a pre- and postexercise two-back test, and the reaction times were recorded. Near-infrared spectroscopy was used to monitor the O_2Hb concentration in the left prefrontal cortex during the exercise. Based on the pre-exercise reaction time, the subjects were allocated into either a fast group (FG) or a slow group (SG). The pre- and postexercise changes in the reaction time and time-to-peak O_2Hb were compared. Further, we determined the relationship between the change in the reaction time and time-to-peak O_2Hb. There was no significant change in the reaction time of the FG; however, that in the SG decreased significantly. The time-to-peak O_2Hb in the FG was significantly less than that in the SG. These results showed differences in the changes of reaction time and O_2Hb changes between the FG and SG.

Keywords

Working memory · Oxyhemoglobin · Near-infrared spectroscopy · Two-back test · Moderate-intensity exercise · Prefrontal cortex

46.1 Introduction

Working memory (WM), which is one of the executive function subcomponents, refers to the temporary storage and manipulation of information required for complex tasks such as language comprehension, learning, and reasoning [1]. Moderate-intensity acute aerobic exercise has been shown to have a beneficial effect on WM function [2]. However, some studies have reported individual differences in the degree of exercise-induced WM improvement [3]. Studies have shown that the left prefrontal cortex (L-PFC) plays an important role in WM function [4]. The

W. Qin (✉) · S. Kojima · S. Morishita · K. Hotta · A. Tsubaki
Institute for Human Movement and Medical Sciences, Niigata University of Health and Welfare, Niigata, Japan
e-mail: hwd19005@nuhw.ac.jp

K. Oyama
College of Engineering, Nihon University, Tokyo, Japan

E. M. Nemoto et al. (eds.), *Oxygen Transport to Tissue XLII*, Advances in Experimental Medicine and Biology 1269, https://doi.org/10.1007/978-3-030-48238-1_46

active region of the L-PFC shows an increase in oxygen consumption and blood supply to ensure availability of oxyhemoglobin (O_2Hb) during WM tasks [5, 6]. Functional near-infrared spectroscopy (fNIRS) can be used to measure neuronal activity-dependent changes in hemoglobin dynamics by measuring variations in the light transmitted through the cerebral cortex [7]. Therefore, we used fNIRS to monitor differences in blood flow in the L-PFC in different groups of subjects during exercise and WM testing. We aimed to determine differences in the effect of exercise on WM based on the pre-exercise WM function and O_2Hb changes.

46.2 Methods

We enrolled 12 healthy right-handed adult males (average age ± standard deviation, 22.2 ± 1.5 years). Prior to participating, the participants provided informed consent after receiving an explanation on the purpose and safety of the experiment. The study was approved by the ethics committee of the Niigata University of Health and Welfare.

The main experiment (Fig. 46.1) comprised a 4-min rest and warm-up followed by a 20-min exercise regime at a workload corresponding to 50% of maximal oxygen consumption. The participants performed a pre- and postexercise two-back test, and the reaction times were recorded. We used fNIRS to monitor the concentration of O_2Hb, deoxyhemoglobin (HHb), and total hemoglobin (THb) in the L-PFC.

In the two-back test, which was introduced by Deschuyteneer [8], reaction times were used as measures of the WM updating function (Fig. 46.2). In this test, the participants were required to conduct additions of 0–9, which required 12 calculations. After each calculation, the participants were required to remember the last number of the result. Further, when performing calculations, they were required to use the last numbers of the previous two results before performing the current calculation. We recorded the reaction times in the test as a WM measure.

We performed fNIRS using an eight-channel spectrometer (OMM-3000; Shimadzu Corporation, Japan), with the distance between pairs of emission and detector probes set at 3.0 cm. Based on the International 10/20 system, the Fpz probe was located on the PFC. The collected NIRS data included three measures of cerebral hemoglobin concentration, namely, O_2Hb, HHb, and THb. We used the O_2Hb concentration change for the main statistical analyses because it is considered as the most reliable indicator of changes in regional cerebral blood flow [9]. The time resolution was set at 40 ms. We averaged the O_2Hb data at each channel and applied a 0.1-Hz low-pass filter to reduce heartbeat noise.

In the data analysis, we first calculated the amount of change in the O_2Hb level per minute compared to the resting average. Further, we calculated the time-to-peak O_2Hb for each subject; studies have shown that the time-to-peak O_2Hb represents neuron activation [10, 11]. Next, we calculated the average pre-exercise reaction time. Subjects with a below-average reaction time were allocated to the fast

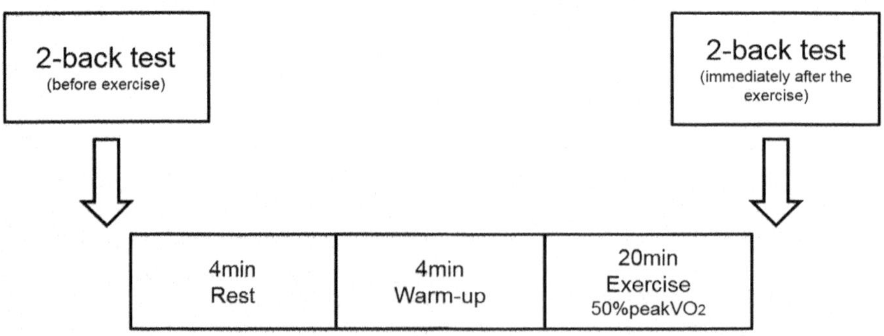

Fig. 46.1 Experimental protocol. A pre- and postexercise two-back test was performed

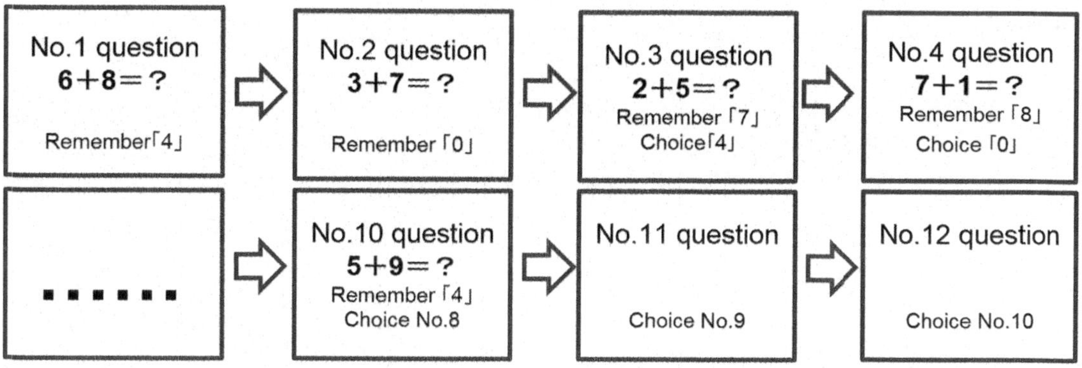

Fig. 46.2 The two-back test protocol showing all the 12 questions in sequence. At each step, the last number of the previous result must be remembered. Subsequently, the last numbers of the two previous results in the sequence should be reported

group (FG) while those with an above-average reaction time were allocated to the slow group (SG). We used the t-test to compare the time-to-peak O_2Hb between the FG and SG. We used one-way ANOVA to compare the pre- and postexercise reaction times between the FG and SG. Finally, we determined the correlation between the time-to-peak O_2Hb and changes in the reaction time (post-pre) using Pearson's correlation coefficient.

46.3 Results

Temporal changes in the O_2Hb, HHb, and THb in the FG and SG are shown in Figs. 46.3 and 46.4, respectively. There was no significant change in the reaction time of the FG (1.87–1.68 s); however, that of the SG significantly decreased (3.08–1.84 s; $p < 0.01$) (Table. 46.1). There was no significant difference in the postexercise reaction between the FG and SG. The time-to-peak O_2Hb in the FG (16.17 ± 3.34 min) was significantly less than that in the SG (18.83 ± 1.07 min) ($p < 0.05$). The time-to-peak O_2Hb was significantly correlated with the reaction time in the FG ($r = -0.84$; $p < 0.05$) (Fig. 46.5) but not in the SG ($r = -0.16$; $p = 0.75$) (Fig. 46.6).

46.4 Discussion

Our findings indicated that the reaction time only significantly improved in the SG. Further, the time-to-peak O_2Hb in the FG (16.17 ± 3.34 min) was significantly less than that in the SG. In addition, the time-to-peak O_2Hb was correlated with the changes of reaction time only in the FG.

A previous MRI study reported that 20 min of aerobic exercise significantly increased neural activity but did not improve performance in the WM task [12]. This previous study suggested that although aerobic exercise can improve neural activity, the improvement of WM function needs further assessment. Our results showed no significant difference in the postexercise reaction time between the FG and SG. This indicates that the improvement effect of the 20-min moderate-intensity exercise had reached its limit. These results are consistent with those of a previous study [13] which, despite using a different WM task with a different duration, reported no significant change in the reaction time after 20-min exercise.

There was a significant difference in the time-to-peak O_2Hb between the FG and SG. This indicates that the speed of O_2Hb changes differed between the FG and SG. However, O_2Hb changes have been reported to affect PFC function [9]. Further, we grouped the participants according to the pre-exercise response time, which seems to indicate that faster O_2Hb changes lead to a faster response time.

The time-to-peak O_2Hb was significantly correlated with the reaction time in the FG but not in the SG. Previous studies have shown that time-to-peak O_2Hb is indicative of cortical activity [10, 11]. Therefore, in the FG, the sooner the O_2Hb peak can be achieved, the greater the improvement of the WM function. Unfortunately, in this study,

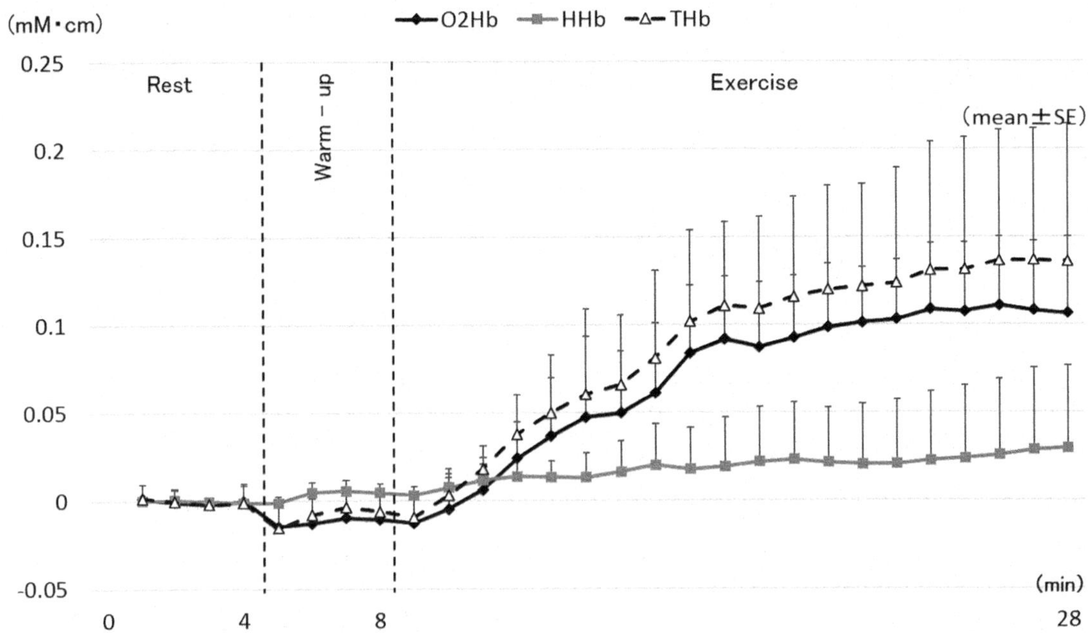

Fig. 46.3 Oxyhemoglobin (O_2Hb), deoxyhemoglobin (HHb), and total hemoglobin (THb) changes in the left prefrontal cortex (L-PFC) per minute in the fast group. Values are presented as mean ± standard error of the mean (SEM)

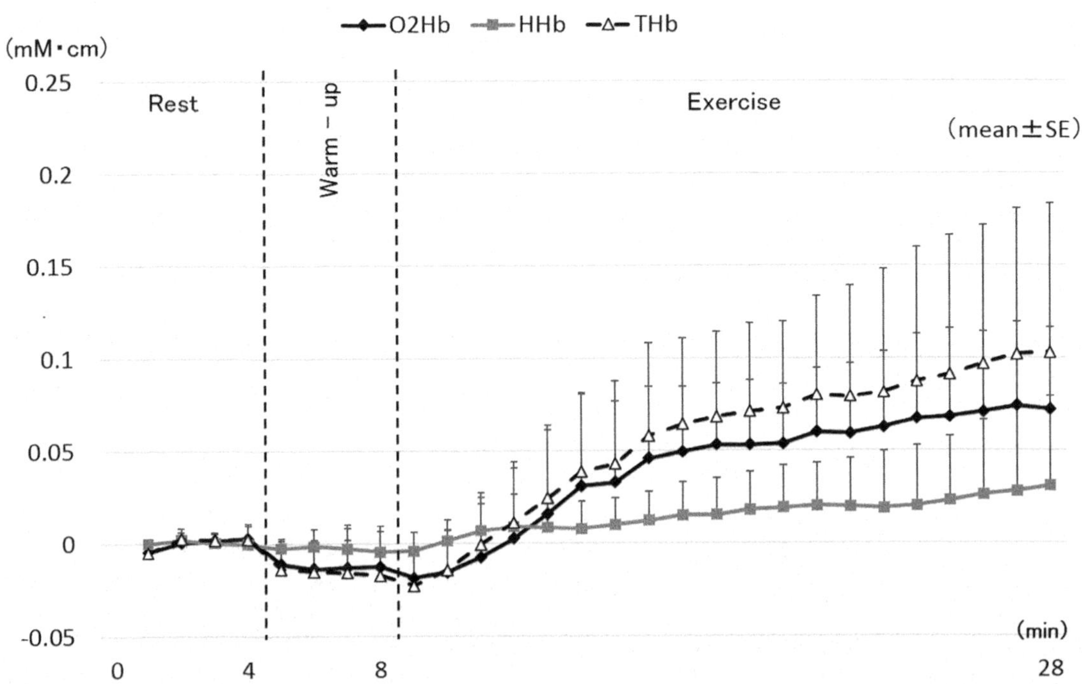

Fig. 46.4 Oxyhemoglobin (O_2Hb), deoxyhemoglobin (HHb), and total hemoglobin (THb) changes in the left prefrontal cortex (L-PFC) per minute in the slow group. Values are presented as mean ± standard error of the mean (SEM)

Table 46.1 Reaction times on the two-back test (mean ± standard error of the mean)

Time point	Reaction time (FG)	Reaction time (SG)
Pre-exercise	1.87 ± 0.54	3.08 ± 0.33
Post-exercise	1.68 ± 0.84	1.84 ± 0.22[a]

[a]Significant difference compared with pre-exercise ($p < 0.05$)

the improvement of the reaction time induced by the 20-min exercise may have reached its limit. Therefore, our correlation findings indicate the possibility that the duration of activation of the PFC neurons may affect WM function, which needs to be further explored.

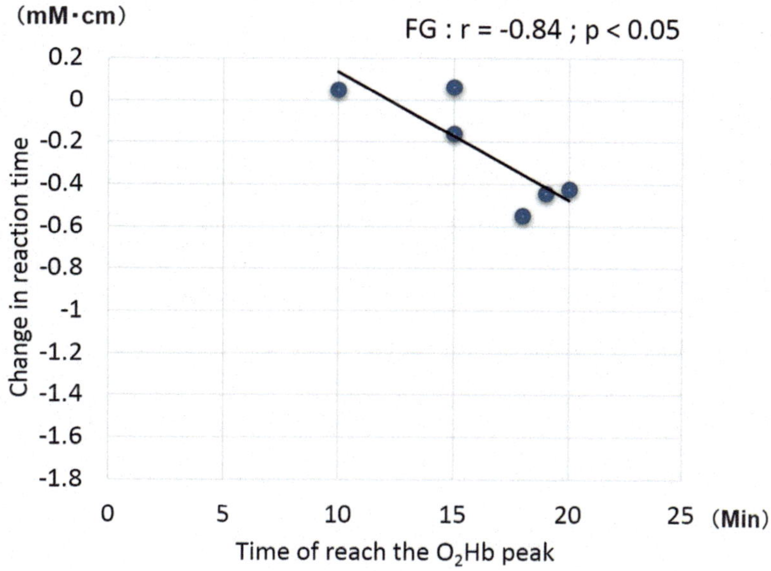

Fig. 46.5 Correlation coefficient between time-to-peak O_2Hb and the change of reaction time (pre- to postexercise) in the fast group

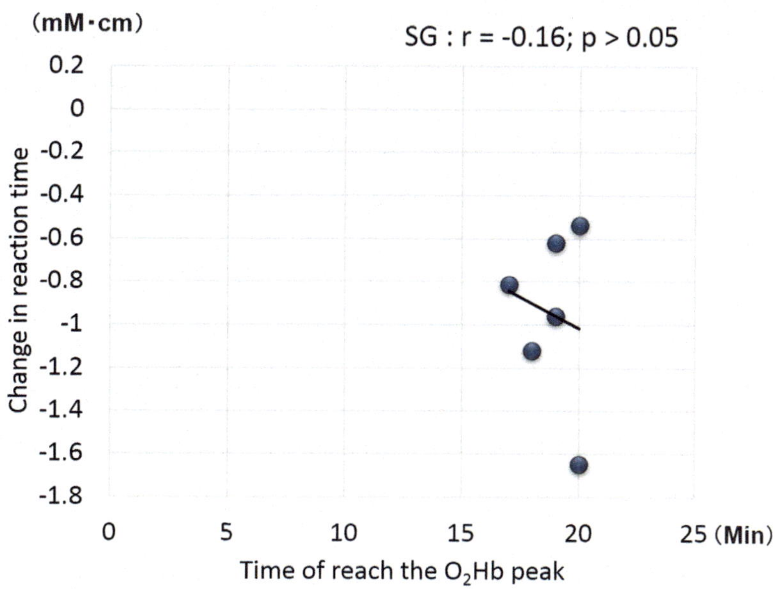

Fig. 46.6 Correlation coefficient between time-to-peak O_2Hb and the change of reaction time (pre- to postexercise) in the slow group

46.5 Conclusions

Our findings showed that the O_2Hb and reaction time changes induced by moderate-intensity 20-min aerobic exercise were different between the FG and SG.

Acknowledgments This study was supported by a Grant-in-Aid for Scientific Research (C) from the Japan Society for the Promotion of Science (A. Tsubaki) and a Grant-in-Aid for Exploratory Research from Niigata University of Health and Welfare (A. Tsubaki).

Disclosure Statement The authors have no disclosures.

References

1. Baddeley A (2010) Working memory. Curr Biol 20:R136–R140
2. McMorris T, Sproule J, Turner A et al (2011) Acute, intermediate intensity exercise, and speed and accuracy in working memory tasks: a meta-analytical comparison of effects. Physiol Behav 102:421–428
3. Sibley BA, Beilock SL (2007) Exercise and working memory: an individual differences investigation. J Sport Exerc Psychol 29:783–791
4. Curtis CE, D'Esposito M (2003) Persistent activity in the prefrontal cortex during working memory. Trends Cogn Sci 7:415–423
5. Tomasi D, Ernst T, Caparelli EC et al (2006) Common deactivation patterns during working memory and visual attention tasks: an intra-subject fMRI study at 4 Tesla. Hum Brain Mapp 27:694–705
6. Banaji M, Mallet A, Elwell CE et al (2008) A model of brain circulation and metabolism: NIRS signal changes during physiological challenges. PLoS Comput Biol 4:e1000212
7. Byun K, Hyodo K, Suwabe K et al (2014) Positive effect of acute mild exercise on executive function via arousal-related prefrontal activations: an fNIRS study. NeuroImage 98:336–345
8. Deschuyteneer M, Vandierendonck A, Muyllaert I (2006) Does solution of mental arithmetic problems such as 2+ 6 and 3× 8 rely on the process of "memory updating"? Exp Psychol 53:198–208
9. Kono T, Matsuo K, Tsunashima K et al (2007) Multiple-time replicability of near-infrared spectroscopy recording during prefrontal activation task in healthy men. Neurosci Res 57:504–512
10. Mirelman A, Maidan I, Bernad-Elazari H et al (2014) Increased frontal brain activation during walking while dual tasking: an fNIRS study in healthy young adults. J Neuroeng Rehabil 11:85
11. Matsuo K, Watanabe A, Onodera Y et al (2004) Prefrontal hemodynamic response to verbal-fluency task and hyperventilation in bipolar disorder measured by multi-channel near-infrared spectroscopy. J Affect Disord 82:85–92
12. Li L, Men WW, Chang YK et al (2014) Acute aerobic exercise increases cortical activity during working memory: a functional MRI study in female college students. PLoS One 9:e99222
13. Yamazaki Y, Sato D, Yamashiro K et al (2018) Inter-individual differences in working memory improvement after acute mild and moderate aerobic exercise. PLoS One 13:e0210053

47 Supine Cycling Exercise Enhances Cerebral Oxygenation of Motor-Related Areas in Healthy Male Volunteers

D. Sato, S. Morishita, K. Hotta, Y. Ito, A. Shirayama, S. Kojima, W. Qin, and A. Tsubaki

Abstract

It has been reported that the cardiovascular response in the supine position is different from that in the sitting position. However, there are few reports on the effects of posture on cerebral oxygenation during exercise. Cycling exercises change oxygenated hemoglobin (O_2Hb) and deoxygenated hemoglobin (HHb) levels in motor-related areas. Therefore, this study compared O_2Hb levels at motor-related areas during recumbent versus supine cycling. Eleven healthy young male performed a 30-min cycling exercise protocol at 50% of the maximal oxygen uptake (VO_2 max) in the recumbent and supine positions. Near-infrared spectroscopy (NIRS) was used to measure exercise-induced O_2Hb and HHb changes in the right (R-PMA) and left premotor areas (L-PMA), supplementary motor area (SMA), and primary motor cortex (M1). In R-PMA, L-PMA and SMA, the O_2Hb obtained during supine cycling was significantly higher than that during recumbent cycling (R-PMA, 0.031 ± 0.01 vs. 0.693 ± 0.01; L-PMA, 0.027 ± 0.01 vs. 0.085 ± 0.013; SMA, 0.041 ± 0.011 vs. 0.076 ± 0.008 mM·cm, recumbent vs. supine position; $p < 0.05$). These results suggest that supine cycling exercise increases R-PMA, L-PMA, and SMA O_2Hb levels in healthy young men.

Keywords

Near-infrared spectroscopy · Oxygenated hemoglobin · Premotor area · Supplementary motor area · Primary motor cortex

47.1 Introduction

It has been reported that the cardiovascular response in the supine position at rest is different from that in the sitting position. Specifically, when comparing both positions at rest, heart rate and blood pressure are higher in the sitting position [1, 2], and cardiac output (CO) increases as the body approaches the supine position [3]. However, there are few reports on the effects of different postures during exercise on cerebral oxygenation.

Cerebral blood flow is redistributed in sites where neural activity occurs, increasing local oxygenation [4]. Mehta et al. used functional

D. Sato · Y. Ito · A. Shirayama
Department of Physical Therapy, Niigata University of Health and Welfare, Niigata, Japan

S. Morishita · K. Hotta (✉) · S. Kojima · W. Qin · A. Tsubaki
Institute for Human Movement and Medical Sciences, Niigata University of Health and Welfare, Niigata, Japan
e-mail: kazuki-hotta@nuhw.ac.jp

E. M. Nemoto et al. (eds.), *Oxygen Transport to Tissue XLII*, Advances in Experimental Medicine and Biology 1269, https://doi.org/10.1007/978-3-030-48238-1_47

magnetic resonance imaging (fMRI) and found that cycling increased blood flow in the premotor cortex (PMA), supplementary motor cortex (SMA), and primary motor cortex (M1) [5]. However, fMRI presents some limitations: (1) different postures cannot be compared in the same subject and (2) poor temporal resolution; therefore, temporal changes during exercise cannot be verified. A near-infrared spectroscopy (NIRS) is used as a means of continuously measuring neural activity in the cerebral cortex during exercise [6].

The purpose of this study was to compare the exercise-induced oxygenation in motor-related cortical areas between the supine and recumbent cycling exercise in right-handed healthy adult men.

47.2 Methods

Eleven subjects (all male, 20.8 ± 0.6 years old, 171.7 ± 6.0 cm, 63.3 ± 6.0 kg) participated in this study. All study participants provided informed consent, and the study design was approved by the Niigata University of Health and Welfare Ethics Committee (approval number 18127-190123).

The exercise task consisted of cycling on a bicycle ergometer (AEROBIKE 75XLII, Combi, Tokyo, Japan). Previously, the subjects had undergone cardiopulmonary exercise testing with supine and recumbent cycling exercise. Maximum oxygen uptake (VO_2 max) was measured using an automated metabolic analyzer (AE-310; Minato Medical Science, Osaka, Japan) followed by recumbent and supine cycling exercise at the intensity of 50% VO_2 max with random order.

A multichannel NIRS imaging system (LABNIRS; Shimadzu Co., Kyoto, Japan) with multiple continuous wavelengths (780, 805, and 830 nm) was used to detect changes in O_2Hb and deoxygenated hemoglobin (HHb) at a sampling rate of 7.4 Hz, based on the modified Beer-Lambert law [7]. The NIRS optodes consisted of eight light-source fibers and eight detectors, which provided 24-channel simultaneous recording. Optodes were arranged in a 4 × 4 fashion in a multichannel probe holder and a 30-mm inter-optode distance was employed to measure cortical tissue oxygenation. Regions of interest included the right (R-PMA) and left premotor areas (L-PMA), supplementary motor area (SMA), and primary motor cortex (M1) [8].

As cardiorespiratory parameters, skin blood flow (SBF) was measured at the forehead using a laser tissue blood flow oxygen monitor (OMEGAFLOW FLO-CI; Omega Wave, Inc). The beat-to-beat mean blood pressure (MAP) was measured on the second finger of the left hand using a continuous blood pressure hemodynamic measurement device (Finometer; Finapress Medical Systems, Amsterdam, The Netherlands). CO was measured using a noninvasive impedance meter (PhysioFlow Q-Link; Manatec Biomedical). End-expiratory carbon dioxide partial pressure ($P_{ET}CO_2$) was measured using an automated metabolic analyzer.

To obtain temporal changes, the O_2Hb, HHb, and SBF values were expressed as changes from the averaged values obtained during the 5 min of rest phase before the exercise. The MAP, CO, and $P_{ET}CO_2$ were averaged every minute. A two-way repeated-measures analysis of variance (ANOVA) was used to test the effects of two factors including time and posture, and interaction between the factors. As a post hoc analysis, paired t-test or Wilcoxon signed-rank sum test were performed to compare between recumbent and supine or at rest and during exercise. In order to compare the exercise-induced cortical oxygenation between recumbent and supine cycling exercise, the average value for the last 20 min of exercise was calculated for each regions as a representative values indicating cortical oxygenation. The level of statistical significance was set at $p < 0.05$. All results are shown as mean ± standard deviation (SD).

47.3 Results

Workload at the 50%VO_2 max, that was employed as an exercise intensity, was significantly lower in supine cycling exercise as compared to recumbent (98.8 ± 12.2 vs. 90.5 ± 12.3

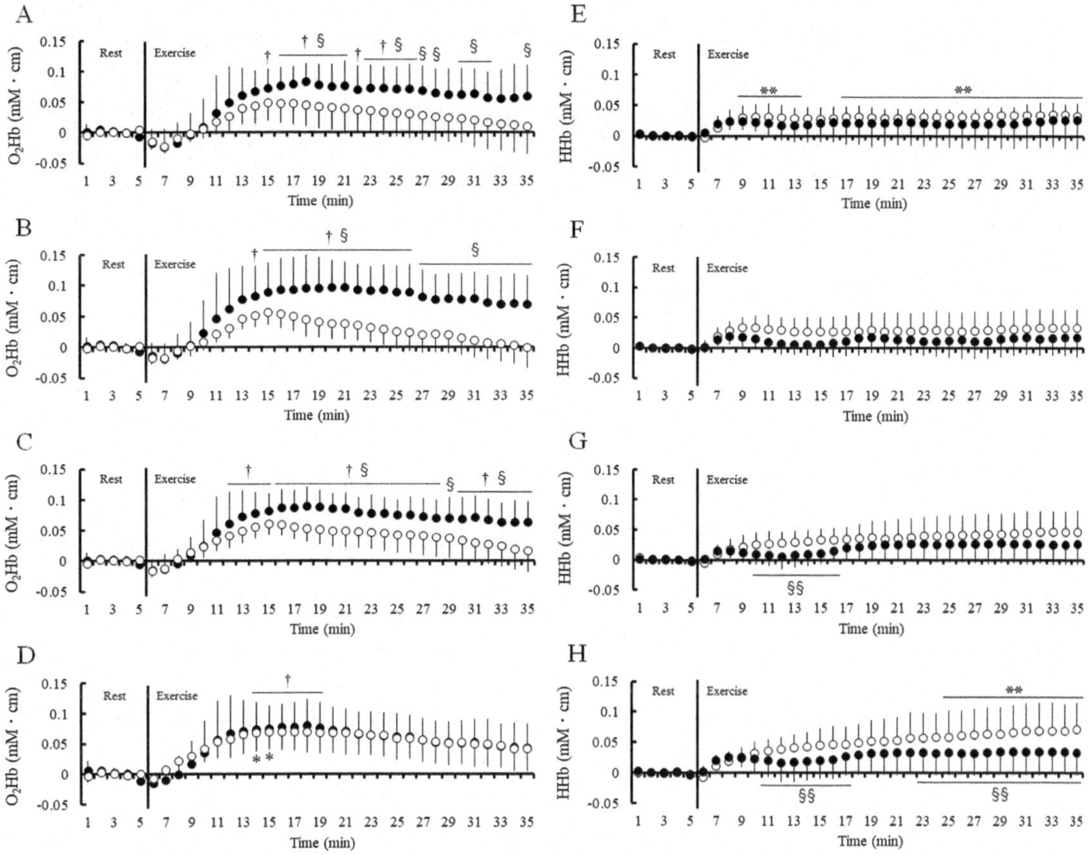

Fig. 47.1 Temporal O_2Hb changes in motor-related cortical area during supine and recumbent cycling exercise. Open and closed circles indicate recumbent and supine cycling exercise, respectively. The O_2Hb and HHb were measured in the right and left PMA, SMA, and M1 areas. Two-way ANOVA (time x posture) revealed a significant main effect of time and posture and significant interaction for the R-PMA of O_2Hb (time, $F = 28.27$; posture, $F = 3.13$; interaction, $F = 5.27$; $p < 0.05$, respectively; **a**), L-PMA of O_2Hb (time, $F = 26.76$; posture, $F = 9.78$; interaction, $F = 5.27$; $p < 0.05$, respectively; **b**), and SMA of O_2Hb (time, $F = 37.56$; posture, $F = 4.64$; interaction, $F = 3.47$; $p < 0.05$, respectively; **c**). For M1 of O_2Hb, while the main effect of time was found to be significant ($F = 27.37$, $p < 0.05$; **d**), neither the main effect of posture nor interaction was found to be statistically significant. Two-way ANOVA (time x posture) revealed a significant main effect of time and posture and significant interaction for the R-PMA of HHb (time, $F = 5.91$; $p < 0.05$; **e**), L-PMA of HHb (time, $F = 4.43$; $p = 0.05$; **f**), SMA of HHb (time, $F = 12.56$; interaction, $F = 1.56$; $p = 0.05$, respectively; **g**), and M1 of HHb (time, $F = 17.62$; interaction, $F = 3.67$; $p = 0.05$, respectively; **h**). R-PMA right premotor area, L-PMA left premotor area, SMA supplementary motor area, M1 primary motor cortex. $^*p < 0.05$ vs. averaged O_2Hb for 5 min of rest before recumbent cycling exercise; $^\dagger p < 0.05$ vs. averaged O_2Hb for 5 min of rest before supine cycling exercise; $^\S p < 0.05$ vs. the same time of recumbent cycling exercise in O_2Hb; $^{**}p < 0.05$ vs. averaged HHb for 5 min of rest before recumbent cycling exercise; $^{\S\S}p < 0.05$ vs. the same time of recumbent cycling exercise in HHb. Mean ± SD

watts, recumbent vs. supine; $p < 0.05$). Figure 47.1 shows O_2Hb and HHb changes in R-PMA, L-PMA, SMA, and M1 (Fig. 47.1) during recumbent and supine cycling exercise. In the right and left PMA and SMA, the O_2Hb significantly increased during supine cycling exercise from the rest ($p < 0.05$, respectively), but not during recumbent cycling exercise (Fig. 47.1a–c). Compared to recumbent, the O_2Hb obtained in those regions was significantly higher during the last 19 min of supine exercise ($p < 0.05$, respectively; Fig. 47.1a–c). Both recumbent and supine cycling exercise increased the O_2Hb in M1 ($p < 0.05$, respectively); however, there was no difference between two types of exercise (Fig. 47.1d). In the R-PMA, the HHb significantly increased during recumbent cycling exercise from the rest ($p < 0.05$), but not during supine cycling exercise (Fig. 47.1e). In the L-PMA, the HHb did not significantly increase during recumbent cycling exercise from the rest and but during supine cycling exercise (Fig. 47.1f). In the SMA, the HHb did not significantly increase during recumbent cycling exercise from the rest but during supine cycling exercise ($p < 0.05$; Fig. 47.1g). In the M1, the HHb significantly increased during recumbent cycling exercise from the rest ($p < 0.05$) and during supine cycling exercise ($p < 0.05$; Fig. 47.1h). The averaged value during exercise was calculated and shown in Fig. 47.2. In the right and left PMA and SMA, the averaged value of O_2Hb for the last 20 min of supine exercise was significantly higher than that of recumbent exercise ($p < 0.05$, respectively), but not in the M1 (Fig. 47.2).

Figure 47.3 shows cardiorespiratory responses during exercise. The SBF, CO, and $P_{ET}CO_2$ significantly increased during both recumbent and supine cycling exercise ($p < 0.05$, respectively; Fig. 47.3). The MAP increased during supine exercise ($p < 0.05$) but did not change during recumbent exercise (Fig. 47.3). As compared to recumbent, the CO was significantly lower during supine exercise ($p < 0.05$, respectively); however, there were no differences in SBF, MAP, and $P_{ET}CO_2$ between recumbent and supine exercise (Fig. 47.3).

47.4 Discussion

One of the major findings in this study was that the O_2Hb in the R-PMA, L-PMA, and SMA increases during supine cycling exercise from the resting values. Furthermore, the O_2Hb in those regions was significantly higher during supine cycling exercise as compared to that obtained during recumbent exercise in healthy men. When considering our results with the previous evidence that cerebral oxygenation could be one of the key for the improvement of cognitive function [9], supine exercise may likely be better therapeutic strategy for cognitive function than the recumbent exercise.

The O_2Hb signal obtained by NIRS is affected by SBF [10]; moreover, systemic cardiovascular changes [11] and changes in blood carbon dioxide partial pressure affect cerebral blood flow [12]. The O_2Hb levels of R-PMA, L-PMA, SMA, and M1 significantly increased during both recumbent and supine positions, while the same time trend was not observed for MAP, SBF, CO, and $P_{ET}CO_2$. This suggests the increase is due to the neural activity of the motor-related areas in each condition and not to changes in cerebral blood flow associated with MAP, SBF, CO, and $P_{ET}CO_2$.

The cortical oxygenation that was found during the 10–30 min period after the start of exercise in this study was also significantly higher in the supine position for the R-PMA, L-PMA, and SMA as compared to those in the recumbent position. The ANOVA did not detect any effects of posture on SBF, MAP, CO, and $P_{ET}CO_2$.

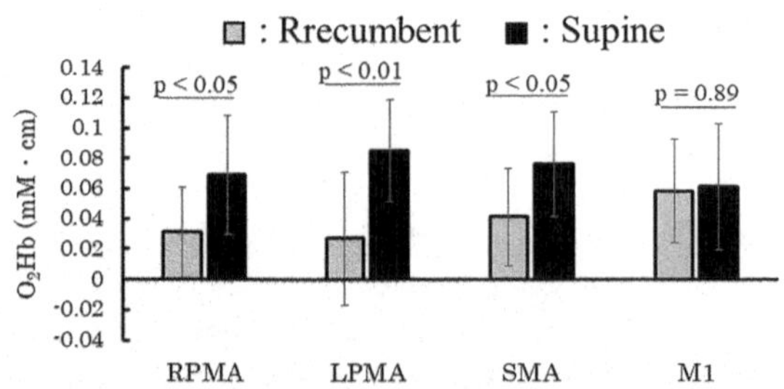

Fig. 47.2 Averaged O_2Hb obtained during the last 20 min of recumbent and supine cycling exercise. Opened and filled bars indicate recumbent and supine cycling exercise. R-PMA right premotor area, L-PMA left premotor area, SMA supplementary motor area, M1 primary motor cortex. §$p < 0.05$ vs. recumbent exercise. Mean ± SD

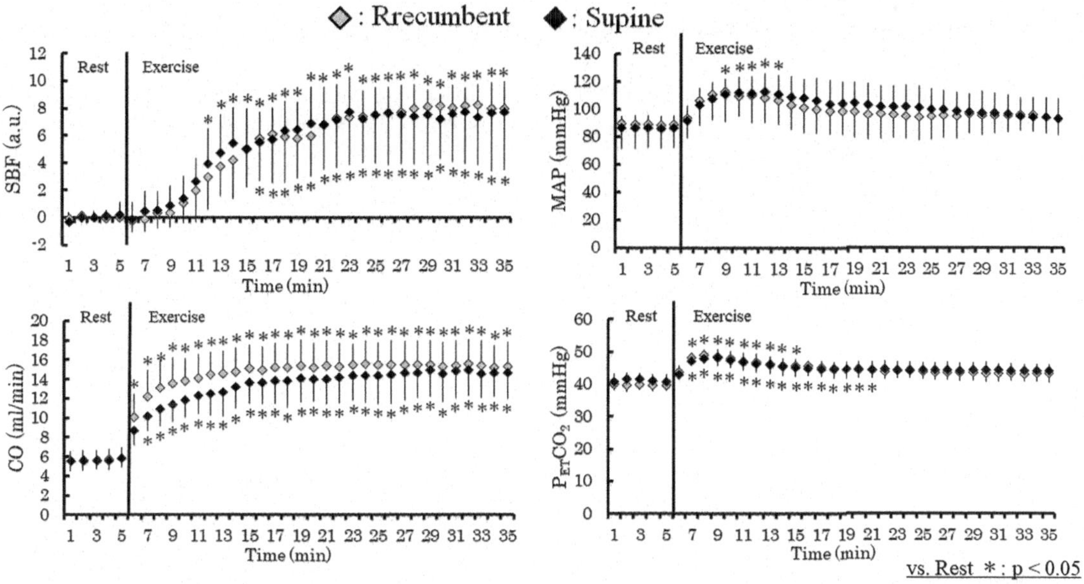

Fig. 47.3 Cardiopulmonary responses during supine and recumbent cycling exercise. Opened and filled circles indicate recumbent and supine cycling exercise, respectively. A significant main effect of time was found in SBF (**a**), MAP (**b**), CO (**c**), and $P_{ET}CO_2$ (**d**) (*F* value was 57.05, 28.27, 87.98, and 50.38 for SBF, MAP, CO, and $P_{ET}CO_2$, $p < 0.05$, respectively). Two-way ANOVA also revealed a significant main effect of posture in MAP ($F = 5.27$, $p < 0.05$) and interaction (time x posture) in CO and $P_{ET}CO_2$ (*F* value was 1.62 and 2.08 for CO and $P_{ET}CO_2$, $p < 0.05$, respectively). MAP tended to have an interaction between time and posture ($F = 1.14$, $p = 0.08$). SBF skin blood flow, MAP mean blood pressure, CO cardiac output, $P_{ET}CO_2$ end-expiratory carbon dioxide partial pressure. $*p < 0.05$ vs. averaged value for 5 min of rest before recumbent cycling exercise; $\dagger p < 0.05$ vs. averaged value for 5 min of rest before supine cycling exercise; $\S p < 0.05$ vs. the same time of recumbent cycling exercise. Mean ± SD

Therefore, cortical oxygenation seems to be independent of exercise-induced cardiorespiratory responses. PMA and SMA are reported to be related to motor program generation and motor learning. The increase in O_2Hb obtained by NIRS has been reported to reflect changes in regional cerebral blood flow associated with neuronal activity in the brain [4]. Studies using positron emission tomography have reported that PMA is active during the early phase of motor learning and SMA is active during well-trained exercise [13]. In the previous studies using NIRS, SMA oxygenation has been reported to occur during the process of motor learning [14]. In this study, subjects performed both recumbent and supine cycling exercises. Interestingly, PMA and SMA were activated by supine exercise, but not by recumbent exercise, suggesting that motor-learning may contribute to SMA oxygenation during supine exercise in healthy men. A previous study reported that middle cerebral artery blood flow is affected by gravity and is higher in the supine than in the upright position [15]. In addition, increased cerebral blood flow has been reported to increase O_2Hb and decrease deoxygenated hemoglobin levels measured by NIRS [16]. Therefore, it is suggested that cerebral blood flow could be higher during supine exercise due to the influence of gravity.

The M1 is an area related to exercise output and control. Previous study reported an oxygenation in M1 during hand grip exercise at the intensity of 20% and 40% of the maximum grip strength [17], and there was no difference in exercise-induced oxygenation in M1 between different exercise intensity. Therefore, M1 activates during voluntary muscle contraction; however, the exercise intensity may not affect the M1 activity. In this study, the exercise intensity of recumbent exercise was significantly higher than that of supine exercise, likely suggesting that different workload of cycle ergometer has no effect on primary motor cortex, which controls motor output.

A 30 min of moderate-intensity (50%VO_2 max) cycling exercise was performed by healthy adult males in this study. In conclusion, supine cycling exercise induced cortical oxygenation in motor-related areas, especially in premotor and supplementary motor areas of healthy male, but recumbent cycling exercise did not.

Acknowledgments This study was supported by a Grant-in-Aid for Exploratory Research from the Niigata University of Health and Welfare.

References

1. Cornelis N, Buys R (2016) The effects of exercise modality on maximal and submaximal exercise parameters obtained by graded maximal exercise testing. Int J Cardiol 222(1):538–547. https://doi.org/10.1016/j.ijcard.2016.07.190
2. Kato S, Yoshitani K, Kubota Y et al (2017) Effect of posture and extracranial contamination on results of cerebral oximetry by near-infrared spectroscopy. J Anesth 31(1):103–110. https://doi.org/10.1007/s00540-016-2275-1
3. Takahashi T, Yamada S, Tanabe K et al (1999) Cardiopulmonary responses at various angles of cycle backrest inclination. J Jpn Phys Ther Assoc 2(1):31–36. https://doi.org/10.1298/jjpta.2.31
4. Lindauer U, Dirnagl U, Fuchtemeier M et al (2010) Pathophysiological interference with neurovascular coupling – when imaging based on hemoglobin might go blind. Front Neuroenerg 2(25). https://doi.org/10.3389/fnene.2010.00025
5. Mehta JP, Verber MD, Wieser JA et al (2009) A novel technique for examining human brain activity associated with pedaling using fmri. J Neurosci Methods 179(2):230–239. https://doi.org/10.1016/j.jneumeth.2009.01.029
6. Hoshi Y (2011) Towards the next generation of near-infrared spectroscopy. Philos Transact A Math Phys Eng Sci 369:4425–4439. https://doi.org/10.1098/rsta.2011.0262
7. Boas DA, Gaudette T, Strangman G et al (2001) The accuracy of near infrared spectroscopy and imaging during focal changes in cerebral hemodynamics. NeuroImage 13(1):76–90. https://doi.org/10.1006/nimg.2000.0674
8. Tsubaki A, Morishita S, Tokunaga Y et al (2018) Changes in cerebral oxyhaemoglobin levels during and after a single 20-minute bout of moderate-intensity cycling. Adv Exp Med Biol 40:127–131. https://doi.org/10.1007/978-3-319-91287-5_20
9. Yanagisawa H et al (2010) Acute moderate exercise elicits increased dorsolateral prefrontal activation and improves cognitive performance with Stroop test. Neuroimage 50(4):1702–1710. https://doi.org/10.1016/j.neuroimage.2009.12.023
10. Miyazawa T, Horiuchi M, Komine H et al (2013) Skin blood flow influences cerebral oxygenation measured by near-infrared spectroscopy during dynamic exercise. Eur J Appl Physiol 113(11):2841–2848. https://doi.org/10.1007/s00421-013-2723-7
11. Katura T, Tanaka N, Obata A et al (2006) Quantitative evaluation of interrelations between spontaneous low-frequency oscillations in cerebral hemodynamics and systemic cardiovascular dynamics. NeuroImage 31(4):1592–1600. https://doi.org/10.1016/j.neuroimage.2006.02.010
12. Querido JS, Sheel AW (2007) Regulation of cerebral blood flow during exercise. Sports Med 37(9):765–782. https://doi.org/10.2165/00007256-200737090-00002
13. van Mier H, Tempel LW, Perlmutter JS et al (1998) Changes in brain activity during motor learning measured with pet. J Neurophysiol 80(4):2177–2199. https://doi.org/10.1152/jn.1998.80.4.2177
14. Hatakenaka M, Miyai I, Mihara M et al (2006) Frontal regions involved in learning of motor skill—a functional NIRS study. NeuroImage 34(1):109–116. https://doi.org/10.1016/j.neuroimage.2006.08.014
15. Ogawa Y, Yanagida R, Ueda K et al (2016) The relationship between widespread changes in gravity and cerebral blood flow. Environ Health Prev Med 21(4):186–192. https://doi.org/10.1007/s12199-016-0513-7
16. Hoshi Y, Kobayashi N, Tamura M (2001) Interpretation of near-infrared spectroscopy signals: a study with a newly developed perfused rat brain model. J Appl Physiol 90(5):1657–1662. https://doi.org/10.1152/jappl.2001.90.5.1657
17. Wriessnegger SC, Kirchmeyr D, Bauernfeind G et al (2017) Force related hemodynamic responses during execution and imagery of a hand grip task: a functional near infrared spectroscopy study. Brain Cogn 117:108–116. https://doi.org/10.1016/j.bandc.2017.06.010

48 What Is the Meaning of an Oxygen Measurement?

Analysis of Methods Purporting to Measure Oxygen in Targeted Tissues

Harold M. Swartz, Ann Barry Flood, Benjamin B. Williams, Brian W. Pogue, Philip E. Schaner, and Peter Vaupel

Abstract

Clinical measurements of O_2 in tissues will inevitably provide data that are at best aggregated and will not reflect the inherent heterogeneity of O_2 in tissues over space and time. Additionally, the nature of all existing techniques to measure O_2 results in complex sampling of the volume that is sensed by the technique. By recognizing these potential limitations of the measures, one can focus on the very important and useful information that can be obtained from these techniques, especially data about factors that can change levels of O_2 and then exploit these changes diagnostically and therapeutically. The clinical utility of such data ultimately needs to be verified by careful studies of outcomes related to the measured changes in levels of O_2.

Keywords

Oxygen measurements · Heterogeneity · Cancer · Clinical outcomes · Oxygen in tissues

48.1 Introduction

The overall goal of this paper is to facilitate clinically effective use of measurements of molecular oxygen (O_2) in tissues, by carefully considering the basis and validity of clinical measurements of O_2 in tissues and how those measurements can be used to advance diagnosis and therapy. While measurements of O_2 in tissues have been an important focus of numerous researchers and a central theme of the International Society for Oxygen Transport to Tissues (ISOTT) since its establishment in 1973, there have been very limited considerations of what

H. M. Swartz (✉)
Department of Radiology, Dartmouth Medical School, Hanover, NH, USA

Department of Radiation Oncology, Dartmouth-Hitchcock Medical Center, Lebanon, NH, USA

Thayer School of Engineering, Dartmouth College, Hanover, NH, USA
e-mail: Harold.Swartz@Dartmouth.edu

A. B. Flood
Department of Radiology, Dartmouth Medical School, Hanover, NH, USA

B. B. Williams · P. E. Schaner
Department of Radiation Oncology, Dartmouth-Hitchcock Medical Center, Lebanon, NH, USA

B. W. Pogue
Thayer School of Engineering, Dartmouth College, Hanover, NH, USA

P. Vaupel
Department of Radiation Oncology, University Medical Center, University of Freiburg, Freiburg, Germany

E. M. Nemoto et al. (eds.), *Oxygen Transport to Tissue XLII*, Advances in Experimental Medicine and Biology 1269, https://doi.org/10.1007/978-3-030-48238-1_48

those measurements mean in terms of quantitatively characterizing the pertinent O_2 levels in tissues. Instead, all too often, when a measurement technique determines that "X" is the amount of O_2 in a given tissue, the assumption is (after taking into account variation due to measurement error) that "X" is a reliable, quantitative representation of the "true" oxygenation status of the tissue and therefore (as clinically appropriate) can be incorporated into plans for therapeutic interventions.

While many have focused on the need to take measurement error into account in interpreting test results, few have examined the biological/clinical meaningfulness of measurements of O_2 in tissues. In this three-part series, we focus on the biological/clinical meaningfulness of O_2 measurements made in living organisms where tissue O_2 is in constant flux. In our previous papers [1, 2], we illustrated the key conclusion by focusing on the inability of electron paramagnetic resonance (EPR) oximetry, using embedded particulates as sensors, to obtain unambiguous measurements of tissue O_2 due principally to complexities associated with the heterogeneity of tissue O_2. We also asserted that all other types of clinically available measurements of O_2 are also unable to resolve the complications introduced by heterogeneity.

In this paper, we delve further into other techniques for measuring O_2 to support our assertion. We emphasize that, to obtain maximum clinical utility of the measurements, it is necessary to consider the goal of the measurements and the limitations of the data that are obtained. We particularly focus on the clinical value of making repeated measurements of O_2, especially in association with strategies/events that potentially change O_2 levels. In this paper, we extend this discussion, providing additional information on such applications to optimize care.

48.2 Analysis of the Ability of Clinically Available Techniques to Measure Absolute Levels of O_2 and/or Resolve Heterogeneity of O_2 Distributions in Tissues

Although there are many techniques that claim to measure O_2 in tissues, only a few actually have the potential to make direct O_2 measurements in the tissues of interest [3, 4]. Techniques that assess O_2 directly include EPR oximetry [5], the Eppendorf electrode [6], and some optical methods based on direct measurements of target molecules in tissues, e.g., phosphorescent quenching of optical sensors placed directly in tissues or as part of a physical probe such as the "OxyLite" [7]. A few other types of measurements measure O_2 directly but only in the vascular system, e.g., optical methods that measure both hemoglobin saturation and total hemoglobin (especially near infrared spectroscopy [NIRS]) [8].

However, the techniques most often used clinically to characterize tissue oxygenation do not in fact measure O_2 directly; instead, they measure "indirect" parameters that can be plausibly linked to actual O_2 levels but only under appropriate circumstances. This latter group of techniques includes positron emission tomography (PET) imaging of glucose derivatives, PET imaging of drugs that localize in hypoxic tissues, and magnetic resonance imaging/nuclear magnetic resonance (MRI/NMR), blood oxygenation level-dependent (BOLD) imaging, MRI perfusion, and laser Doppler flow and measures of metabolites that may be affected by O_2 levels, e.g., lactate and redox intermediates [3, 9].

48.2.1 Direct Measures of O_2 in Targeted Tissues

These are techniques that, while they have the capability of providing direct quantitative measurements of O_2 in homogeneous media, cannot provide such data in tissues in vivo because the volumes that they sense are larger than the volumes of homogeneity of O_2 in actively metabolizing tissues. Consequently, all in vivo measurements of O_2 are inherently "averages." Even neglecting the need to include measures of heterogeneity inside cells, based on the usual volume of cells and assuming that differences are sought for aggregates of three cells, for a measurement of heterogeneity in a 10-mm diameter volume, the spatial resolution needed becomes 8 million voxels. They may not even provide a well-defined averaged pO_2 value within the volume that they sense, because they often have differential sensitivity to some subvolumes due to their proximity to the sensor and sometimes to other factors as well, e.g., EPR is more sensitive to low levels of O_2.

In vivo EPR oximetry in human tissues based on particulates was discussed in some detail in our previous papers [1, 2]. These papers noted that the volume of each unit of measurement was very likely to include subvolumes with significantly different O_2 levels; consequently, each resulting data point will be an average level of O_2. In contrast, EPR imaging oximetry (which is still only in preclinical use) can provide spatially resolved measurements [10, 11]. Nonetheless, the volumes of even the smallest resolvable voxel in the images will still be too large to avoid averaging of the O_2 levels sensed within each voxel.

The Eppendorf electrode has been used clinically to provide direct tissue pO_2 measurements in a track. To create a track, a series of points is obtained by progressing the 200 μm microelectrode through the tissue in a sequence of "Pilgrim steps," i.e., the probe is advanced a prescribed distance and then withdrawn a fraction of that distance to minimize pressure effects. The volume sampled by each point is estimated to be 100–500 cells around the tip of the probe [6]. Therefore, the measurement usually reflects the average of a range of pO_2s, especially in the presence of pathophysiology. The histogram of values of a tumor was thought to be a representative sample of 3–7 tracks through the volume, although this still was only a sampling of the true heterogeneity of the tissue O_2. Nevertheless, in tumors, very useful clinical correlations have been found with the number of points below a threshold value [12]. Note that this does not require that the values be true absolute measurements of O_2. Regardless of its potential advantages, unfortunately, this technique is no longer available clinically. This technique also had some practical limitations, including difficulties to repeat the measurement in a given tissue subvolume because of the local trauma produced from the measurements.

The "OxyLite" technology uses quenching by O_2 of fluorescence with a sensor whose diameter is 230–750 μm [13]. This cross section corresponds to the diameter of a tissue subvolume of 10–75 mammalian cells. Therefore, the sensor will provide an average of the distribution of pO_2 values throughout this volume. It could be used in a manner similar to the Eppendorf electrode to obtain a series of similarly averaged measurements at different locations. Currently, the only version of the oxygen electrode suitable for use in humans is a technique requiring temporary implantation of an oxygen electrode that extends through the skin and is used to monitor severe brain trauma. Such a device, while very useful for its intended purpose, is not suitable for measurements in tumors [14].

Direct injection of phosphorescent agents can provide one way to directly sample tissue O_2, where the signal comes from the phosphorescence lifetime changes that result from excited triplet state quenching of O_2 [15]. High-resolution mapping can be provided, although care must be taken in choosing the probe that localizes in the compartments of interest, as some provide intracellular information, some provide purely extracellular information, and some are simply perivascular in nature [16]. Obviously, a primary limitation of optical methods is the depth of penetration, which is typically limited to just a few millimeters depth, although some X-ray-based methods are now providing imaging through a few centimeters of tissue [17].

Based on the principle that molecular O_2 impacts the relaxation time of nuclei [18, 19], several different approaches have been developed to try to use the power of NMR to measure O_2 in tissues [20]. The direct measurement of O_2 by NMR using isotopes with spin (O^{17} for NMR [21] and O^{15} for PET [22]) is possible, but these are extraordinarily expensive and not suitable for routine clinical use. The most developed has been the use of the relaxation time of fluorine nuclei in fluorinated hydrocarbons injected directly into tissues [23, 24]. The measurements are based on the relaxation time of the F atoms in the emulsion, but the volume of the fluorine containing hydrocarbon is much larger than several capillary networks. Consequently, the data obtained are an average of a range of partial pressures. To date, this approach has not advanced to clinical use. There are a number of other NMR-related approaches that have been suggested using the impact of O_2 on the relaxation of protons [25]. Potentially, these might provide spatially resolved data that could be quite useful. However, it is very unlikely that any could have the resolution to resolve the spatial heterogeneity of O_2 in tissues. Thus, these measurements of O_2 will be similar to the other techniques discussed, i.e., their data will be based on assessing changes in averaged O_2 levels.

48.2.2 Direct Measures of O_2 in the Vascular System

Direct measures of O_2 in the vascular system are based on the known relationship between the O_2 saturation of hemoglobin (Hb) and the ambient pO_2 as shown in the sigmoidal oxygen dissociation curve. However, the vascular system is, by its nature, not uniform with respect to O_2 saturation. Specifically, arterial and venous systems have very different O_2 saturations, while saturation in the capillaries (which is where most O_2 is delivered to the tissue) is in between these extremes, and arterial and venous systems have very different saturations. So, when measurements such as pulse oximetry or NIRS report O_2 saturation, it is important to understand what part of the vascular system is being measured. While these measures may be helpful in assessing response to techniques to increase O_2 availability, they are not measuring the actual increase of oxygen in tissues.

The problem with applying measurements made in blood to tumors (and tissues in general) is that, while the amount of O_2 in the vascular system is an important parameter impacting oxygen levels in the tissue, it is not possible to go directly from measuring O_2 in blood to knowing the O_2 in tissues. That is because O_2 in the tissue is determined by many factors in addition to the potential supply of O_2 from the red blood cells, including many that can affect the delivery of O_2 and/or that can affect the utilization of O_2.

The other type of direct measurement of O_2 in the vascular system is the measurement of blood gases [26]. These are usually done in larger vessels. These measurements have the same limitations as NIRS with regard to being able to provide a measurement of the O_2 in the extravascular tissue compartment.

A related methodology which is widely available, BOLD MRI [27], is sometimes mistakenly thought to provide a direct measurement of O_2 in the vascular system. But because it provides only one parameter, the amount of DeoxyHb, it cannot be used to estimate saturation or pO_2 in the circulatory system. In principle, changes in the amount of the BOLD signal could be used to provide an indication of changing O_2 levels. However, this type of use is limited by the fact that, if the blood volume within the sampled voxels changes, the amount of DeoxyHb will change even if the saturation remains the same. There have been some more recent attempts to use the impact of O_2 on relaxation times of protons [28] directly in tissues, but to date, these have not been able to provide detailed maps resolving the heterogeneity of O_2 in tissues [25].

48.2.3 Indirect Measures of Tissue Oxygen

There are a number of methods used clinically that attempt to provide indications of O_2 levels in tissues, which are based on plausible but indirect relationships to the actual O_2 levels. While these therefore intrinsically do not directly measure O_2 in tissues, because of their widespread availability and, perhaps, some naivete of the clinical users, they are sometimes considered to provide direct measurements of O_2. This simple confusion can be important to their usefulness in clinical applications because, while these techniques may provide valid and quantitative measures of parameters associated with their biological or chemical modes of interaction, their quantitative relationships to O_2 levels may be poorly defined.

The use of molecules such as the nitroimidazoles that selectively localize in hypoxic tissues (O_2 content <1%) has been widely employed, most often using PET labels to indicate their location [29, 30]. The principle is that, with critically low levels of O_2, these can be reduced to reactive intermediates which, if not reoxidized by O_2, can then bind to cellular components [31]. While these probes are widely used and often have been clinically useful, they clearly cannot provide a direct measure of the O_2 content of the tissue. They can, nonetheless, provide a qualitative indication of regions with moderate to good perfusion that were hypoxic at the time that the tracer was delivered.

Another widely used PET clinical imaging technique is based on the observation that many tumors have a high rate of glycolysis and therefore a high uptake of glucose, which can be followed by the use of the imaging agent ^{18}F-fluorodeoxyglucose (^{18}F-FDG) [32]. The amount of uptake is based on a number of different factors including perfusion rate; extent of hypoxia; expression of the Warburg effect, i.e., aerobic glycolysis; number of cells; uptake of glucose analogs; and rate of glycolysis [33]. Clinical use of this technique is widespread and considered clinically useful for a number of contexts, especially in identifying regions where tumor cells are located. Some clinicians even consider areas of high uptake as potentially indicating tumor hypoxia, although the Warburg effect is mainly responsible for the high glucose uptake rates [33]. A major complication is the high rate of false positives, due to many other causes of uptake of the agent [34, 35].

There are also a group of physiological measurements that are sometimes indirectly linked to O_2. Measurements of blood flow, e.g., MRI perfusion [36] and laser Doppler flow [37] are often used clinically to obtain a parameter that is linked to the supply of O_2, but because of the many factors that affect how much O_2 is actually delivered and the impact of utilization on the amount of O_2 is available, these techniques cannot by themselves provide reliable insights into the oxygenation of the tissues. Measurements of metabolites that may be affected by O_2 levels, e.g., lactate and redox intermediates, are frequently used, but their levels are the result of complex interactions that depend on many factors in addition to the amount of available O_2 and therefore cannot reliably indicate O_2levels in tissues. However, these physiological measurements, especially if repeated and related to other parameters can, in some instances, provide some clinical information.

48.3 Discussion

We conclude that, whatever measuring method is employed, the volume that is sensed by the method will always be too large to be homogenous and therefore cannot be truly characterized by a single number. Instead, because of the dynamic heterogeneity of O_2 in living tissues across time and the very small volumes that have uniform O_2, all measurements are fundamentally complex combinations of averages and other types of aggregated and dynamic estimates of O_2 in tissues. Therefore, when such terms as "absolute levels" of O_2 or pO_2 are used to describe in vivo O_2 measurements in blood or other tissues, these terms are not merely inaccurate, but more importantly, they can foster misinterpretations of what is actually occurring in the body. This, in turn, can lead to inappropriate applications of these data to both clinical decision-making and basic science theory. This is because, while the term "absolute" is correctly used to describe gas pressure measured under very controlled conditions, it can connote[1] measurements that are perfect, unbounded, definite, certain, etc., and these meanings, as we have shown, are inaccurate and misleading when applied to the in vivo circumstance. Nevertheless, the practice of using terms like "absolute pO_2" have persisted in the in vivo setting because the techniques that are used, especially when applied in restricted conditions, appear to provide valid measurements of pO_2 or other rigorous parameters *within specific volumes or limited time domains*, so, describing the data as "absolute" gas pressure would seem to be valid. This misinterpretation is further compounded by the knowledge that there are robust data from model systems that appear to indicate that clinical outcomes should be related to tissue O_2. For example, in homogenous cell suspensions where the O_2 can be rigorously controlled, the relationship between radiation sensitivity and pO_2 can be clearly demonstrated.

While we argue that the terminology "absolute" should not be used to describe in vivo O_2 data, we do not argue that these O_2 data are use-

[1]These synonyms are from the thesaurus with Word.

less. Once it is recognized that one cannot obtain unambiguous clinically meaningful direct measurements of O_2 in tissues, the various techniques can be used to provide clinically useful *qualitative* information, e.g., to follow clinically significant changes in O_2 in tissues as a result of disease progression and/or treatment. These can then be exploited to enhance diagnosis and therapy, while keeping in mind the caveats involved in the interpretations of the values obtained from the measurements.

There are a number of significant implications of this conclusion. Clearly, approaches such as predicting the impact of a measured level of O_2on radiation response may be misleading, because the measurements are, in fact, complex aggregates across time and volume, which can reflect the presence of very different distributions and levels of hypoxic and normoxic cells. The implications for "dose painting" are less clear, but these too should be based on understanding what is being painted. While discussions of the potential advantages of increasing dose to more hypoxic regions of tumors have often focused on having "absolute" measures of pO_2, this goal is not only unobtainable but also unnecessary. The really critical issue is to find where there are likely to be more hypoxic cells, and this can be estimated from current techniques. Repeated measurements of changes in O_2 during the course of therapy would be likely to be especially valuable to determine if the treatments were leading to different relative changes in O_2 levels.

Perhaps, the most important implication for cancer is that the most useful clinical value of measurements of direct, or even indirect, measurements of O_2 in tissue is to follow temporal changes that occur by interventions (especially hyperoxic interventions to increase O_2), consequences of therapy (especially the impact from not only radiation but also immunotherapy, chemotherapy, hormone therapy, and surgery), and disease progression. Of course, establishing the clinical value of these measurements of O_2 will ultimately require appropriate studies of the outcomes of therapy using the O_2 measurements to guide choices.

There are similar implications for the use of measurements of O_2 in other diseases. The other most important clinical application is likely to be for peripheral vascular disease, where relative measurements of O_2 may help to identify and follow changes in levels of relatively low oxygenation (for arterial disease) or the location of tissues at risk for diabetic peripheral vascular disease [38]. Such measurements have the potential to very significantly improve clinical outcomes, but as noted for their use in cancer, the ultimate proof of their value needs to come from appropriate studies of outcomes.

48.4 Conclusions

Clinical measurements of O_2 in tissues will inevitably provide data that are, at best, aggregated and will not reflect the inherent heterogeneity of O_2 in tissues over space and time. Additionally, the nature of all existing techniques to measure O_2 results in complex sampling of the volume that is sensed by the technique. By recognizing these potential limitations of the measures, one can focus on the very important and useful information that can be obtained from these techniques, especially data about factors that can change levels of O_2 and then exploit these changes diagnostically and therapeutically. The clinical utility of such data ultimately needs to be verified by careful studies of outcomes related to the measured changes in levels of O_2.

Acknowledgments Major funding is from the National Cancer Institute, PPG Grant P01CA190193. We gratefully acknowledge all the other scientists, clinicians, engineers, and coordinators on the PPG. Disclaimer: HMS and ABF are owners of Clin-EPR, LLC, which manufacturers clinical EPR instruments for investigational use only.

References

1. Swartz HM, Vaupel P, Williams BB et al (2020) 'Oxygen level in a tissue' – what do available measurements really report? Adv Exp Med Biol 1232:145–153
2. Flood AB, Schaner PE, Vaupel P et al (2020) Clinical and statistical considerations when assessing oxygen

levels in tumors: illustrative results from clinical EPR oximetry studies. Adv Exp Med Biol 1232:155–168
3. Springett R, Swartz HM (2007) Measurements of oxygen in vivo: overview and perspectives on methods to measure oxygen within cells and tissues. Antioxid Redox Signal 9:1295–1301
4. Tatum JL, Kelloff GJ, Gillies R (2006) Hypoxia: importance in tumor biology, noninvasive measurement by imaging, and value of its measurement in the management of cancer therapy. Int J Rad Biol 82(10):699–757
5. Swartz HM, Williams BB, Hou H et al (2016) Direct and repeated clinical measurements of pO_2 for enhancing cancer therapy and other applications. Adv Exp Med Biol 923:95–104
6. Vaupel P, Höckel M, Mayer A (2007) Detection and characterization of tumor hypoxia using pO2 histography. Antioxid Redox Signal 9:1221–1235
7. Wen B, Urano M, Humm JL et al (2008) Comparison of Helzel and OxyLite systems in the measurements of tumor partial oxygen pressure (pO2). Radiat Res 169:67–75
8. Scheeren TWL, Schober P, Schwarte LA (2012) Monitoring tissue oxygenation by near infrared spectroscopy (NIRS): background and current applications. J Clin Monit Comput 26(4):279–287
9. Flood AB, Satinsky VA, Swartz HM (2016) Comparing the effectiveness of methods to measure oxygen in tissues for prognosis and treatment of cancer. Adv Exp Med Biol 923:113–120
10. Epel B, Bowman MK, Mailer C et al (2014) Absolute oxygen R1e imaging in vivo with pulse electron paramagnetic resonance. Magn Reson Med 72(2):362–368
11. Hyodo F, Matsumoto S, Devasahayam N et al (2009) Pulsed EPR imaging of nitroxides in mice. J Magn Reson 197:181–185
12. Vaupel P, Mayer A (2007) Hypoxia in cancer: significance and impact on clinical outcome. Cancer Metastasis Rev 26(2):225–239
13. User Manuals for Oxylite products. https://www.oxford optronix.com/support/supp_oxylite.htm. Accessed 1 Oct 2019
14. Stewart C, Haitsma I, Zador Z et al (2008) The new Licox combined brain tissue oxygen and brain temperature monitor: assessment of in vitro accuracy and clinical experience in severe traumatic brain injury. Neurosurgery 63(6):1159–1164; discussion 1164–5
15. Wilson DF, Harrison DK, Vinogradov SA (2012) Oxygen, pH, and mitochondrial oxidative phosphorylation. J Appl Physiol 113(12):1838–1845
16. Esipova TV, Karagodov A, Miller J et al (2011) Two new "protected" oxyphors for biological oximetry: properties and application in tumor imaging. Anal Chem 83(22):8756–8765
17. Pogue BW, Feng J, LaRochelle EP et al (2018) Maps of in vivo oxygen pressure with submillimetre resolution and nanomolar sensitivity enabled by Cherenkov-excited luminescence scanned imaging. Nat Biomed Eng 2(4):254–264
18. Swartz HM, Bennett H, Brown RD III et al (1985) Feasibility of measuring oxygen and redox metabolism in vivo by NMR: effect of paramagnetic materials and their cellular metabolism on relaxation times of protons of water and lipids. Period Biol 87:175–183
19. Bennett HF, Swartz HM, Brown RD III et al (1987) Modification of relaxation of lipid protons by molecular oxygen and nitroxides. Investig Radiol 22:502–507
20. Matsumoto K, Bernardo M, Subramanian S et al (2006) MR assessment of changes of tumor in response to hyperbaric oxygen treatment. Magn Reson Med 56:240–246
21. Zhu X-H, Chen W (2011) In vivo oxygen-17 NMR for imaging brain oxygen metabolism at high field. Prog Nucl Magn Reson Spectrosc 59(4):319–335
22. Hattori N, Bergsneider M, Wu HM et al (2004) Accuracy of a method using short inhalation of ^{15}O-O_2 for measuring cerebral oxygen extraction fraction with PET in healthy humans. J Nucl Med 45:765–770
23. Zhao D, Jiang L, Mason RP (2004) Measuring changes in tumor oxygenation. Methods Enzymol 386:378–418
24. Liu S, Shah SJ, Wilmes LJ et al (2011) Quantitative tissue oxygen measurement in multiple organs using 19F MRI in a rat model. Magn Reson Med 66:1722–1730
25. O'Connor JPB, Naish JH, Jackson A et al (2009) Comparison of normal tissue R-1 and R-2* modulation by oxygen and carbogen. Magn Reson Med 61:75–83
26. Davis MD, Walsh BK, Sittig SE et al (2013) AARC clinical practice guideline: blood gas analysis and hemoximetry. Respir Care 58(10):1694–1703
27. Thulborn KR, Waterton JC, Matthews PM et al (1982) Oxygenation dependence of the transverse relaxation time of water pro-tons in whole blood at high field. Biochim Biophys Acta 714:265–270
28. O'Connor JP, Boult JK, Jamin Y et al (2016) Oxygen-enhanced MRI accurately identifies, quantifies, and maps tumor hypoxia in preclinical cancer models. Cancer Res 76(4):787–795
29. Chapman JD, Franko AJ, Sharplin J (1981) A marker for hypoxic cells in tumors with potential clinical applicability. Br J Cancer 43:546–550
30. Bourgeois M, Rajerison H, Guerard F et al (2011) Contribution of [64Cu] -ATSM PET in molecular imaging of tumour hypoxia compared to classical [18F] -MISO--a selected review. Nucl Med Rev Cent East Eur 14:90–95
31. Sealy RC, Swartz HM, Olive PL (1978) Electron spin resonance--spin trapping: detection of superoxide formation during aerobic microsomal reduction of nitro-compounds. Biochem Biophys Res Commun 82:680–684
32. Lopci E, Grassi I, Chiti A et al (2014) PET radiopharmaceuticals for imaging of tumor hypoxia: a review of the evidence. Am J Nucl Med Mol Imaging 4(4):365–384
33. Vaupel P, Multhoff G (2020) The Warburg effect: historical dogma vs. current rationale. In: Nemoto EM,

Harrison EM, Pias SC, Bragin DE, Harrison DK, LaManna JC (eds) Oxygen transport to tissue XLII, Advances in experimental medicine and biology. Springer International Publishing, Cham
34. Metser U, Even-Sapir E (2007) Increased 18F-Fluorodeoxyglucose uptake in benign, nonphysiologic lesions found on whole-body positron emission tomography/computed tomography (PET/CT): accumulated data from four years of experience with PET/CT. Semin Nucl Med 37:206–222
35. Britton T, Robinson N (2016) Pitfalls and pearls of wisdom in 18F-FDG pet imaging of tumors. J Nucl Med Technol 44:59–64
36. Essig M, Shiroishi MS, Nguyen TB et al (2013) Perfusion MRI: the five most frequently asked technical questions. Am J Roentgenol 200:24–34
37. Briers DJ (2001) Laser Doppler, speckle and related techniques for blood perfusion mapping and imaging. Physiol Meas 22(4):R35–R66
38. The Editors (2012) Peripheral vascular disease in Circulation and the Circulation Subspecialty Journals. Circulation 125:600–611

Part IV

Brain Oxygenation and Function

49

Assessment of Cerebral Blood Oxygenation by Near-Infrared Spectroscopy before and after Resuscitation in a Rat Asphyxia Cardiac Arrest Model

Tsukasa Yagi, Koichiro Shinozaki, Yu Okuma, Tai Yin, Mitsuaki Nishikimi, Takeyuki Kiguchi, Taku Iwami, and Lance B. Becker

Abstract

Clinical investigators have focused on the real-time evaluation of cerebral blood oxygenation (CBO) by near-infrared spectroscopy (NIRS) during cardiopulmonary resuscitation (CPR). A previous study showed that an abrupt increase of oxy-hemoglobin (Hb) level and tissue oxygenation index (TOI) was associated with the timing of return of spontaneous circulation (ROSC). However, it is not clear how TOI alters before and after CPR including a period of cardiac arrest (CA). Therefore, this study aimed to assess CBO with asphyxia CA and its association with CPR to ROSC in rats. Male Sprague-Dawley rats were used. We attached NIRS (NIRO-200NX, Hamamatsu Photonics, Japan) from the nasion to the upper cervical spine in rats. A ten-minute asphyxia was given to induce CA. After CA, mechanical ventilation was restarted, and manual CPR was performed. We examined the mean arterial pressure (MAP), end-tidal carbon dioxide ($ETCO_2$), and Oxy/Deoxy-Hb and TOI. Out of 14 rats, 11 obtained sustained ROSC. After the induction of asphyxia, a rapid drop of TOI was observed, followed by a subsequent increase of Oxy-Hb, Deoxy-Hb, and TOI with CPR. Recent CPR guidelines suggest the use of $ETCO_2$ during CPR since its abrupt increase is a reasonable indicator of ROSC. In this study, abrupt increases in MAP, $ETCO_2$, and TOI were observed at the time of ROSC. TOI can be an alternative to $ETCO_2$ for identifying ROSC after CA, and it also has the capability of monitoring CBO during and after CPR.

Keywords

Cardiopulmonary resuscitation (CPR) · Near-infrared spectroscopy (NIRS) · Return of spontaneous circulation (ROSC) · Tissue oxygen saturation (StO_2) · Cardiac arrest

T. Yagi (✉) · K. Shinozaki · Y. Okuma · T. Yin
M. Nishikimi · L. B. Becker
Feinstein Institute for Medical Research, Northwell Health System, Manhasset, NY, USA

T. Kiguchi · T. Iwami
Kyoto University Health Service, Kyoto, Japan

49.1 Introduction

Cardiac arrest (CA) is a major public health issue worldwide. Despite significant improvements to care for CA, mortality remains high [1]. To

E. M. Nemoto et al. (eds.), *Oxygen Transport to Tissue XLII*, Advances in Experimental Medicine and Biology 1269, https://doi.org/10.1007/978-3-030-48238-1_49

improve CA survival, recent guidelines on cardiopulmonary resuscitation (CPR) indicated that it may be reasonable to use physiologic parameters when feasible to monitor and optimize CPR quality, guide vasopressor therapy, and detect return of spontaneous circulation (ROSC) (Class IIb) [2]. Clinical investigators have focused on the real-time evaluation of cerebral blood oxygenation (CBO) by near-infrared spectroscopy (NIRS) during CPR [3, 4]. A previous study showed that abrupt increases of oxy-hemoglobin (Hb) level and tissue oxygenation index (TOI) were associated with the timing of ROSC [4]. Although there have been studies supporting the use of NIRS during CPR [3–7], the guidelines do not make any statements regarding tissue oxygen saturation (StO_2) or CBO [2] because it is not clear yet how StO_2, including TOI, alters before and after CPR that includes a period of CA. Therefore, this study aimed to assess CBO by using a rat asphyxia CA model to investigate its association with CPR to ROSC. To the best of our knowledge, there have been no reports measuring CBO using NIRS in a rat CA model.

49.2 Methods

The Institutional Animal Care and Use Committee of the Feinstein Institute for Medical Research approved the study protocol. The data that support the findings of this study are available from the corresponding author upon reasonable request.

49.2.1 Animal Surgical Procedure

The details of methods for a rat asphyxia CA model have been described previously [8]. In brief, 34 adult male Sprague-Dawley rats (450–550 g, Charles River Laboratories) were anesthetized with 4% isoflurane (Isosthesia, Butler-Schein AHS) and intubated with a 14-gauge plastic catheter (Surflo, Terumo Medical Corporation). Animals were mechanically ventilated. Anesthesia was maintained with 2% isoflurane at a fraction of inspired O_2 (FIO_2) of 0.3. The left femoral artery was cannulated (sterile polyethylene-50 catheter inserted for 20 mm) for continuous arterial pressure monitoring. A temperature probe was placed in the esophagus for continuous temperature monitoring. The core temperature was maintained at 36.5 ± 1.0 °C during the surgical procedure. The left femoral vein was cannulated with a polyethylene-50 catheter, which was advanced into the inferior vena cava for drug infusion. We attached NIRS (NIRO-200NX, Hamamatsu Photonics, Japan) from the nasion to the upper cervical spine of the rats. The distance between the emission and the detection probes was 3 cm. We examined the mean arterial pressure (MAP), end-tidal carbon dioxide ($ETCO_2$), Oxy/Deoxy-Hb, and TOI. The NIRS device records the oxygen saturation level (TOI) and the changes in concentration of oxygenated hemoglobin (ΔO_2Hb) and deoxygenated hemoglobin (ΔHHb) in real time (100 Hz). Averaged data every 500 msec were used. After instrumentation, neuromuscular blockade was achieved by slow intravenous administration of 2 mg/kg of vecuronium bromide (Hospira, USA). Asphyxia was induced by switching off the ventilator, and CA occurred 3–4 minutes after asphyxia started. We defined CA as a MAP below 20 mmHg; CA was completely untreated for 10 minutes. Mechanical ventilation was restarted at an FIO_2 of 1.0, and manual CPR was delivered to CA animals. Chest compressions were performed at a rate of 240–300 per minute. At 30 seconds after the beginning of CPR, a 20 μg/kg bolus of epinephrine was given to animals through the venous catheter. Following ROSC, defined as a systolic blood pressure above 60 mmHg, CPR was discontinued. If ROSC did not occur by 5 minutes of CPR, resuscitation was terminated.

49.2.2 Statistical Analysis

Data are expressed as means ± standard deviation for continuous variables. Levels of TOI, ΔO_2Hb, and ΔHHb were compared using repeated measures analysis of variance. *P* values ≤0.05 were considered to be statistically significant. All analyses were performed using the SPSS software (version 24.0, J SPSS).

49.3 Results

We monitored CBO by NIRS in 14 rats in CA. Of these, ROSC was observed in 11 rats. After the induction of asphyxia, TOI and ΔO_2Hb rapidly dropped, whereas ΔHHb increased (Fig. 49.1). The values of TOI and ΔO_2Hb were significantly lower during CA than at the start of asphyxia, whereas ΔHHb was significantly higher (TOI: 66.0 ± 5.4, at the start of asphyxia vs. 34.2 ± 10.4 during CA, $p < 0.001$). Towards the end of the 10 minutes of CA period, the level of TOI remained constantly low; ΔO_2Hb kept decreasing; ΔHHb increased at 1–2 minutes after a start of asphyxia and gradually decreased thereafter (Fig. 49.1). This phenomenon was observed until about 8 minutes after starting asphyxia. Figure 49.2 shows the changes in TOI, $ETCO_2$, MAP, ΔO_2Hb, and ΔHHb after starting CPR in a typical case. During CPR, TOI, ΔO_2Hb, and ΔHHb increased in synchrony with chest compressions. An abrupt increase in MAP, $ETCO_2$, and TOI was observed at the time of ROSC (TOI: 36.9 ± 6.8 during CPR vs. 45.9 ± 4.6 at 30 seconds after ROSC, $p < 0.001$). In addition, ΔO_2Hb increased, whereas ΔHHb decreased after ROSC. On the other hand, TOI did not increase in rats without ROSC ($n = 3$).

49.4 Discussion

This study showed that TOI rapidly dropped after induction of asphyxia in a rat CA model. We observed a synchrony of CBO waveforms with chest compression followed by an abrupt increase of TOI at the time of ROSC. Our major finding was the observation of CBO by NIRS during CA, before and after resuscitation in rats. NIRO-200NX has two measurement methods running

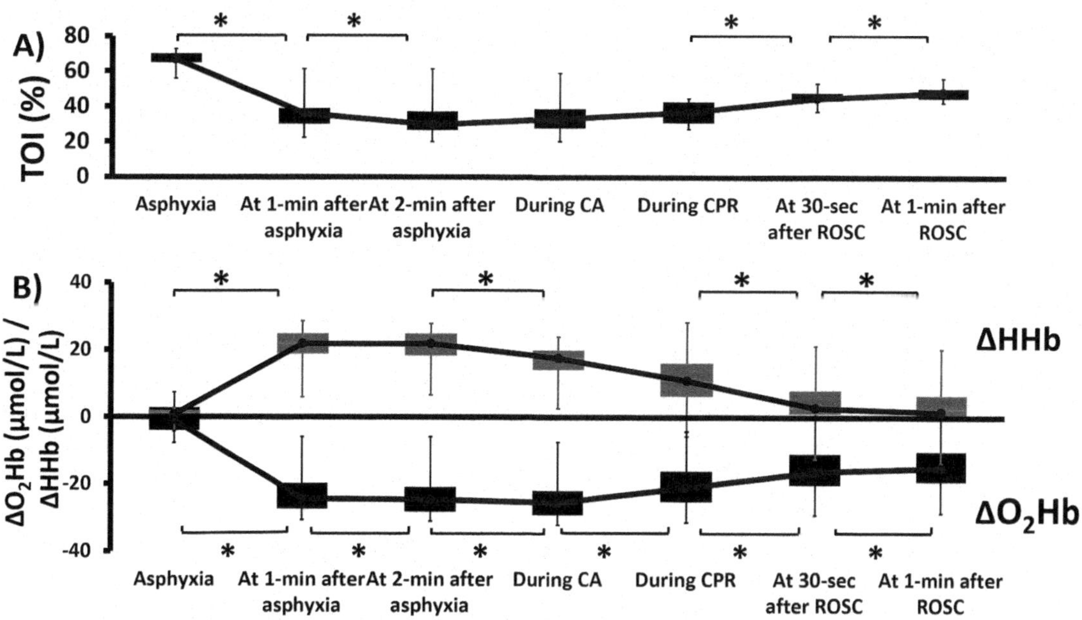

Fig. 49.1 (**a**) Tissue oxygenation index (TOI) and (**b**) the changes in Oxy-hemoglobin (ΔO_2Hb) concentration and Deoxy-Hb (ΔHHb) concentration during cardiac arrest (CA), before and after cardiopulmonary resuscitation (CPR). The number of rats in asphyxia, at 1-minutes after asphyxia, at 2 minutes after asphyxia, during CA was 14. The number of rats during CPR, at 30-seconds after ROSC, and at 1-minutes after ROSC was 11. Asphyxia indicates the time when starting asphyxia (baseline). During CA indicates at 5 minutes after the induction of asphyxia. During CPR indicates before return of spontaneous circulation (ROSC). The asterisk (*) indicates statistical significance ($p < 0.05$)

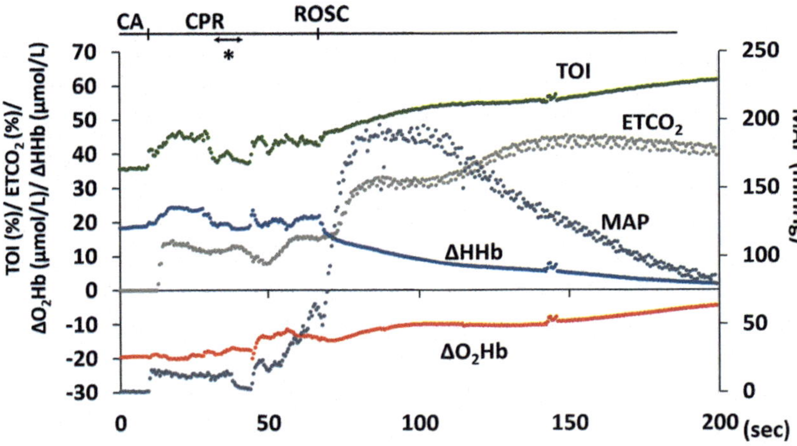

Fig. 49.2 The changes in tissue oxygenation index (TOI), mean arterial pressure (MAP), end-tidal carbon dioxide ($ETCO_2$), Oxy-hemoglobin (ΔO_2Hb), and Deoxy-Hb (ΔHHb) during cardiac arrest (CA) and resuscitation in a typical case. The asterisk symbol indicates the period of the interruption of chest compression due to the administration of epinephrine. ROSC, return of spontaneous circulation; CPR, cardiopulmonary resuscitation

independently of each other: a modified Beer-Lambert (MBL) method and a spatially resolved spectroscopy (SRS) method. Some studies reported that the MBL method may detect mainly shallow layers, and the SRS method may be able to detect deeper layers of the brain [9, 10]. Kakihana et al. showed that excessive exogenous and endogenous epinephrine caused contraction of the scalp blood vessels, and the blood flow and oxygenation of the scalp decreased, because the systolic blood pressure had risen up to 200 mmHg at ROSC in their experiments [10]. Our results were consistent with their findings, and the systolic blood pressure increased to approximately 200 mmHg (Fig. 49.2). Thus, it is plausible that CBO of rats can be measured by NIRO-200NX, which has features of both MBL and SRS.

Recent CPR guidelines suggest a use of $ETCO_2$ during CPR since its abrupt increase is a reasonable indicator of ROSC [2]. However, the guidelines recommended that $ETCO_2$ should not be used in isolation and should not be used in non-intubated patients [2]. In the current study, abrupt increases in MAP, $ETCO_2$, and TOI were observed at the time of ROSC. In clinical settings, it is often difficult to monitor $ETCO_2$ for non-intubated patients and to continuously monitor MAP in CA patients. NIRS, an optical and noninvasive technique, can be used as an alternative to detect ROSC [4] since NIRS does not require intubation for measuring CBO.

Previous experimental porcine CA studies showed that StO_2 decreased during CA [10, 11]. Two studies reported that the StO_2 decrease was rapid, like that observed in the present study [10, 12], but another study reported that it was gradual [11]. One reason for the differences in reports may be the cause of CA, and the capacity of oxygen contents may differ between species. The latter study reported that they induced CA by ventricular fibrillation, while we used an asphyxia CA model.

Some clinical studies reported that initial StO_2 can be applied to patients as a predictor of ROSC [5–7]. However, we could not describe the correlation between the initial StO_2 and ROSC. In a clinical setting, we cannot employ NIRS at the time of sudden cardiac arrest; therefore, no baseline measure of NIRS is available, but we can usually begin the measurement of CBO by NIRS after CPR is initiated. In future studies, it will be necessary to evaluate the association between the value of TOI and the value at the beginning of CPR and to detect ROSC in human beings.

Since our instrument is intended for use in humans and the scull of rats is much smaller than humans, the values of the TOI and O_2Hb and HHb may not be quantitatively correlated with the data from humans. However, comparing the trend in rats is considered legitimate because of its internal standardization.

49.5 Conclusions

In this study, abrupt increases in MAP, $ETCO_2$, and TOI were observed at the time of ROSC. On the basis of these findings, TOI can be an alternative to $ETCO_2$ to detect ROSC after CA and has the potential to monitor CBO during and after CPR.

References

1. Geocadin RG, Callaway CW, Fink EL et al (2019) Standards for studies of neurological prognostication in comatose survivors of cardiac arrest: a scientific statement from the American Heart Association. Circulation 140(9):e517–e542
2. Link MS, Berkow LC, Kudenchuk PJ et al (2015) Part 7: adult advanced cardiovascular life support: 2015 American Heart Association guidelines update for cardiopulmonary resuscitation and emergency cardiovascular care. Circulation 132(18 Suppl 2):S444–S464
3. Koyama Y, Wada T, Lohman BD et al (2013) A new method to detect cerebral blood flow waveform in synchrony with chest compression by near-infrared spectroscopy during CPR. Am J Emerg Med 31(10):1504–1508
4. Yagi T, Nagao K, Kawamorita T et al (2016) Detection of ROSC in patients with cardiac arrest during chest compression using NIRS: a pilot study. Adv Exp Med Biol 876:151–157
5. Tsukuda J, Fujitani S, Morisawa K et al (2019) Near-infrared spectroscopy monitoring during out-of-hospital cardiac arrest: can the initial cerebral tissue oxygenation index predict ROSC? Emerg Med J 36(1):33–38
6. Nishiyama K, Ito N, Orita T et al (2015) Characteristics of regional cerebral oxygen saturation levels in patients with out-of-hospital cardiac arrest with or without return of spontaneous circulation: a prospective observational multicentre study. Resuscitation 96:16–22
7. Takegawa R, Shiozaki T, Ogawa Y et al (2019) Usefulness of cerebral rSO2 monitoring during CPR to predict the probability of return of spontaneous circulation. Resuscitation 139:201–207
8. Shinozaki K, Becker LB, Saeki K et al (2018) Dissociated oxygen consumption and carbon dioxide production in the post-cardiac arrest rat: a novel metabolic phenotype. J Am Heart Assoc 7(13):e007721
9. Al-Rawi PG, Smielewski P, Kirkpatrick PJ (2001) Evaluation of a near-infrared spectrometer (NIRO 300) for the detection of intracranial oxygenation changes in the adult head. Stroke 32(11):2492–2500
10. Kakihana Y, Kamikokuryo C, Furubeppu H et al (2018) Monitoring of brain oxygenation during and after cardiopulmonary resuscitation: a prospective porcine study. Adv Exp Med Biol 1072:83–87
11. Boucek T, Mlcek M, Krupickova P et al (2018) Brain perfusion evaluated by regional tissue oxygenation as a possible quality indicator of ongoing cardiopulmonary resuscitation. An experimental porcine cardiac arrest study. Perfusion 33(1_suppl):65–70
12. Putzer G, Braun P, Strapazzon G et al (2016) Monitoring of brain oxygenation during hypothermic CPR – a prospective porcine study. Resuscitation 104:1–5

Effect of 3-Day and 21-Day Hypoxic Preconditioning on Recovery Following Cerebral Ischemia in Rats

50

Timothy R. Darlington, Joseph C. LaManna, and Kui Xu

Abstract

We have previously reported that in a rat model of chronic hypoxia, HIF-1α and its target genes have significantly accumulated by 3 days of exposure, whereas no significant increase in capillary density has occurred; there is a significant increase in capillary density at 21 days of chronic hypoxic exposure. In this study we hypothesize that by utilizing 3 days and 21 days of hypoxic preconditioning, we would distinguish between the relative neuroprotective contributions of the accumulation of HIF-1α and its target genes and angiogenic adaptation in a rat middle cerebral artery occlusion (MCAO) model. Rats were randomly assigned to either hypoxic precondition groups (3-day and 21-day hypoxia) or normoxic control group. Hypoxic animals were kept in a hypobaric chamber at a constant pressure of 0.5 atmosphere (380 mmHg, equivalent to 10% normobaric oxygen at sea level) for either 3 or 21 days. Normoxic controls were housed in the same room next to the hypobaric chamber. Erythropoietin (EPO) was measured at 3 and 21 days of hypoxia using Western blotting analysis. Infarct volumes were measured following 24 hours of permanent MCAO. We found that EPO is upregulated at 3 days of hypoxia and returns to baseline by 21 days of hypoxia. The infarct volumes following 24-hour MCAO were significantly reduced with 3-day hypoxic preconditioning when compared to normoxic controls (%, 31.8 ± 5, n = 9 vs. 50.1 ± 10.9, n = 7). No significant differences in infarct volume were seen between the normoxic controls and 21-day hypoxic preconditioned rats. We have shown that a 3-day hypoxic preconditioning, but not 21-day hypoxic preconditioning, provides significant neuroprotection against focal ischemia in rats, supporting a larger role for the accumulations of HIF-1α and upregulation of its target genes in the neuroprotection against focal ischemia.

Keywords

Focal ischemia · Neuroprotection · MCAO · Stroke · Infarct volume

T. R. Darlington
Departments of Physiology & Biophysics, Case Western Reserve University, Cleveland, OH, USA

Department of Neurobiology, Duke University School of Medicine, Durham, NC, USA

J. C. LaManna · K. Xu (✉)
Department of Physiology & Biophysics, Case Western Reserve University, Cleveland, OH, USA
e-mail: kxx@case.edu

E. M. Nemoto et al. (eds.), *Oxygen Transport to Tissue XLII*, Advances in Experimental Medicine and Biology 1269, https://doi.org/10.1007/978-3-030-48238-1_50

50.1 Introduction

Hypoxic preconditioning has been shown to be neuroprotective against ischemic insults in experimental studies, for instance, hypoxic preconditioning to be neuroprotective against hypoxia-ischemia in the immature rat brain [1–3]. We have previously showed that short-term hypoxic preconditioning improved survival and recovery following cardiac arrest and resuscitation in rats [4]. Dunn et al. demonstrated that chronic hypoxia exposure provides significant protection against hypoxic/ischemic damage in a rat stroke model [5]. The mechanism behind this neuroprotection is not fully understood.

At the onset of hypoxia, there is an immediate accumulation of hypoxia-inducible factor 1 alpha (HIF-1 α), which acts as a transcription factor once it translocates to the nucleus and dimerizes with hypoxia-inducible factor β (HIF β) [6]. This HIF dimer then binds numerous hypoxia response elements (HREs), causing upregulation of many molecules necessary to restore oxygen and metabolic homeostasis. The target genes include glucose transporter-1 (Glut-1), vascular endothelial growth factor (VEGF), and erythropoietin (EPO), which have been suggested to have neuroprotective qualities [7–10]. The upregulation of these molecules during hypoxia has the potential to prime the tissue for more extreme bouts of hypoxia or ischemia. Many of the molecules that are upregulated during hypoxic exposure play significant roles in angiogenesis [11, 12]. That is, they work to increase the capillary density of tissues, presumably to compensate for the decreased diffusional driving force on oxygen with a decreased intercapillary distance. This could allow for greater collateral circulation and thus greater delivery of oxygen and nutrients to brain tissue during cerebral ischemia, reducing the amount of damage.

We have previously reported that in a rat model of chronic hypoxia, HIF-1α and its target genes have significantly accumulated by 3 days of exposure, whereas no significant increase in capillary density has occurred [11, 13]. Conversely, there is a significant increase in capillary density at 21 days of chronic hypoxic exposure, while HIF-1α and its target genes have returned to baseline levels [11, 13]. In this study, we hypothesized that by utilizing 3 days and 21 days of hypoxic preconditioning, we would distinguish between the relative neuroprotective contributions of the accumulation of HIF-1α and its target genes and angiogenic adaptation in a rat middle cerebral artery occlusion (MCAO).

50.2 Methods

50.2.1 Animals and Hypoxic Preconditioning

The experimental protocol was approved by the Animal Care and Use Committee at Case Western Reserve University. Male Wistar rats (2 months old) purchased from Charles River were allowed to acclimate in the animal resource facility for 1 week before they were used in experiments. Rats were randomly assigned to a normoxic control group, a 3-day hypoxic preconditioning, and a 21-day hypoxic precondition group. Hypoxic animals were kept in hypobaric chambers for either 3 days or 21 days at a constant pressure of 0.5 atmosphere (380 mmHg, equivalent to 10% normobaric oxygen at sea level). The normoxic control rats were housed in the same room to ensure identical ambient conditions [14].

50.2.2 Permanent MCAO and Infarct Volume Analysis

MCAO was induced using the intraluminal monofilament method as previously described [15] with modifications. Anesthesia was induced with 3% isoflurane in 30% O_2 balanced with N_2. Rats were maintained with 1.5% isoflurane in the same gas mixture delivered via a nose cone. Briefly, a 4-0 monofilament with a heat expanded tip was advanced approximately 18 mm from the bifurcation of the common carotid artery into the internal carotid artery. Cerebral blood flow was monitored using a laser Doppler probe, and MCAO was considered successful only if blood flow was reduced by at least 60%. Animals in which cerebral blood flow was not adequately reduced were not included in the analysis. The body temperature was maintained at 37 °C by an infrared heat lamp (250 W, 45 cm above the body) regulated by feedback from a rectal probe during the surgery and until 1 hour postsurgery. Following 24 hours of permanent MCAO, rats were deeply anesthetized using 5% isoflurane and transcardially perfused with saline and 4% paraformaldehyde. Brains were removed and incubated in 4% paraformaldehyde for 24 hours and then cryoprotected in 30% sucrose. The tissue was then embedded in OCT, and 20 μm sections were collected from nine equally spaced brain regions (bregma 4.2 mm to bregma −4.7 mm, [16]) for infarct volume measurement. The thionin stain, which targets nissl substance, was utilized to visualize the infarct in the nine areas for each animal. Bioquant computer software (R&M Biometrics, Nashville, TN) was used to image the sections and measure infarct areas. Infarcts were quantified by determining the percentage of tissue area ipsilateral to the stroke that survived compared to the total area of the contralateral hemisphere in order to take into account any edema that occurred on the ipsilateral side. Infarct volume is represented by the following: infarct volume (%) = (contralateral area − ipsilateral non-infarcted area)/contralateral area × 100.

50.2.3 Western Blot Analysis

Normoxic and hypoxic animals were deeply anesthetized using 5% isoflurane and sacrificed. Brain cortical tissue was collected, frozen in liquid nitrogen, and stored at −80°. Protein (20 μg) from homogenized whole brain tissues was separated on a 12% gel, then transferred to a polyvinylidene difluoride (PVDF) membrane, blocked with 5% bovine serum albumin (BSA), and incubated with EPO primary antibody (1:1000, Santa Cruz Biotechnology, Santa Cruz, CA). Following incubation with the appropriate horseradish peroxidase-conjugated secondary antibody (1:15000, Invitrogen, Camarillo, CA), proteins were detected by chemiluminescence, and densitometry was performed using Image J software [8]. The membrane was stripped and reprobed for β-actin (1:1000, Santa Cruz Biotechnology, Santa Cruz, CA). Optical densities of protein bands were normalized to that of β-actin [15].

50.2.4 Statistical Analysis

Data are expressed as mean ± SD. Statistical analyses were performed using SPSS V26.0 for Windows. Group comparisons were made by one-way analysis of variance (ANOVA) using Tukey's statistic. The comparison between any two groups was analyzed with a *t*-test. Significance was considered at the level of $p < 0.05$.

50.3 Results

Physiological variables were measured before MCAO in the normoxic controls and the hypoxia-preconditioned groups (Table 50.1). The values of body weight and pH were similar in all three groups. The arterial partial pressure of oxygen (P_aO_2) was 121 ± 12 mmHg (mean ± SD, $n = 7$) in the normorxic control group, while the values were significantly higher (ANOVA, $p < 0.05$) in the 3-day preconditioning (142 ± 6, $n = 9$) group and 21-day precondition group (141 ± 9, $n = 7$). The arterial partial pressure of carbon dioxide (P_aCO_2) was significantly lower (ANOVA, $p < 0.05$) in rats which had had hypoxic preconditioning (3 day: 33 ± 4, $n = 9$; 21 day: 36 ± 5, $n = 7$) compared to the normoxic controls (51 ± 6, $n = 7$). The hematocrit was significantly increased (ANOVA, $p < 0.05$) in both 3-day (58 ± 5, $n = 9$) and 21-day (78 ± 4, $n = 7$) hypoxic preconditioned groups compared to the normoxic controls (42 ± 2, $n = 7$).

Protein levels of EPO, a HIF-1 target molecule, were determined using western blot analysis (Fig. 50.1). The EPO level was significantly increased (ANOVA, $p < 0.05$) at 3 days of hypoxia compared to the normoxic controls (optical density normalized to actin, mean ± SD, 0.46 ± 0.12 vs. 0.22 ± 0.02, $n = 3$ each). EPO returned to baseline levels by 21 days of hypoxia (0.23 ± 0.06, $n = 3$).

The infarct volumes were measured in the normoxic controls and the hypoxia-preconditioned groups following a 24-hour permanent MCAO (Fig. 50.2). The infarct volumes were significantly reduced (ANOVA, $p < 0.05$) with 3 days of hypoxic preconditioning when compared to the normoxic controls (%, mean ± SD, 31.8 ± 5.2, $n = 9$ vs. 50.1 ± 10.9, $n = 7$). Interestingly, no significant differences in infarct volume were observed between the 21-day hypoxic preconditioned rats (49.6 ± 10.6, $n = 7$) and normoxic controls.

50.4 Discussion

We have shown that 3, but not 21, days of continuous hypoxic preconditioning provide neuroprotection against focal ischemia in the rat. We further confirmed that EPO, a HIF target gene, is significantly upregulated following 3 days of hypoxic exposure and has returned to baseline levels by 21 days of hypoxia.

This is in agreement with the time course of HIF-1 accumulation during chronic hypoxia. We have previously reported that with chronic hypo-

Table 50.1 Physiological variables before MCAO (mean ± SD)

	Normoxic controls ($n = 7$)	3-Day preconditioning ($n = 9$)	21-Day preconditioning ($n = 7$)
Body weight (g)	289 ± 7	261 ± 8[a]	277 ± 14
pH (unit)	7.36 ± 0.02	7.36 ± 0.03	7.39 ± 0.03
PaO_2 (mmHg)	121 ± 12	142 ± 6[a]	141 ± 9[a]
$PaCO_2$ (mmHg)	51 ± 6	33 ± 4[a]	36 ± 5[a]
Hematocrit (%)	42 ± 2	53 ± 5[a]	78 ± 4[a]

[a]Indicates significant difference vs. Normoxic control group (ANOVA, $p < 0.05$)

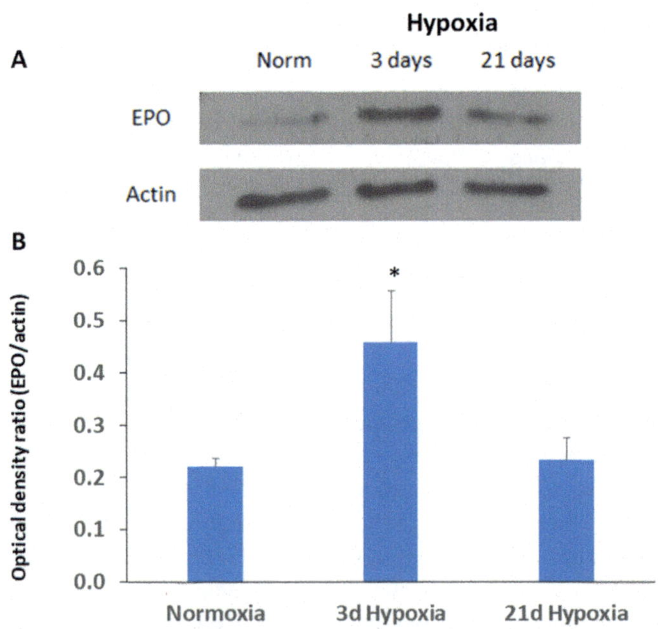

Fig. 50.1 EPO protein level analysis in cortical homogenates following hypoxic exposure. (**a**) Western blot showing EPO and actin bands for normoxic controls (N, $n = 3$) and for animals exposed to hypobaric hypoxia for 3 (3d, $n = 3$) and 21 (21d, $n = 3$) days. (**b**) Optical density ratio normalized to actin. EPO is significantly (ANOVA, $p < 0.05$) increased following 3 days of hypoxia, but returns to about baseline level by 21 day of hypoxic exposure. Values are mean ± SD. *Indicates significant difference (ANOVA, $p < 0.05$) compared to the normoxic control groups

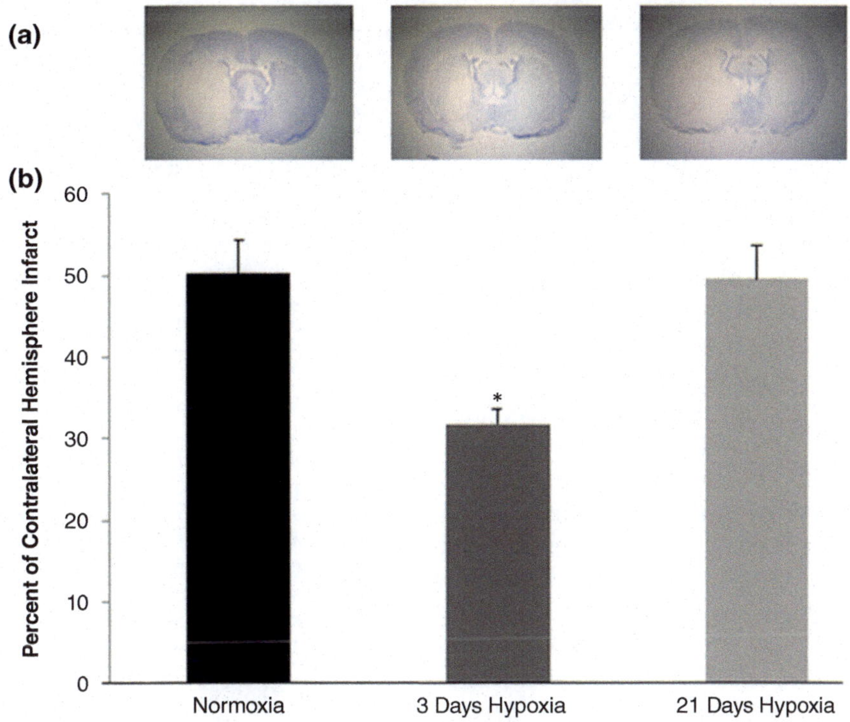

Fig. 50.2 The infarct volumes were measured in the normoxic controls, and the hypoxia-preconditioned groups followed a 24-hour permanent middle cerebral artery occlusion (MCAO). (**a**) Examples of thionin-stained image of normoxic, 3-day, and 21-day hypoxic preconditioned brain section. (**b**) Infarct volume analysis in the normoxic and 3-day and 21-day hypoxic preconditioned groups. Values are mean ± SD. *Indicates significant difference (ANOVA, $p < 0.05$) compared to the normoxic control groups

baric hypoxia, the accumulations of HIF-1α and its target genes (e.g., Epo, VEGF) were significantly increased for the first several days of hypoxic exposure (no significant vascular adaptation has occurred at this point of hypoxic exposure) and returned to baseline levels by 3 weeks when hypoxia-induced angiogenesis (resulting in increased capillary density) is completed [11]. The early accumulation of HIFs during hypoxic exposure leads to upregulation of many HRE genes. Some of these genes are involved in regulating the redox state of the cell, while other genes are involved in regulating the metabolic state of the cell, including the enzymes involved in glycolysis [7–10]. During ischemia, with the reduction of oxygen and glucose availability, it is critical for the cell to shift toward a glycolytic metabolic state and away from an aerobic metabolic state. The upregulation of genes involved in redox and metabolic regulation may protect against ischemia. For example, they may protect cells in the penumbra against the damaging effects of molecules like ROS and glutamate being secreted, which in essence place a higher metabolic demand on already malnourished tissue, from the core of the stroke.

With an increase in capillary density, one might expect some degree of tissue sparing due to increased collateral circulation during stroke. Surprisingly, contrary to the neuroprotection by angiogenesis against reversible focal ischemia shown in previous work [5], in our study hypoxia-induced angiogenesis seems to lend no neuroprotection against permanent focal ischemia. One reason for this discrepancy was the differences in animal models. Dunn group used reversible distal MCAO model, the ischemia time was 60 minutes, and only cortex region was affected. We used permanent proximal MCAO model, the rats underwent 24 hours of ischemia, and both cortex and striatum were affected. During MCAO surgery, they provided higher O_2 in the gas mixture (42% O_2, 56% N_2) compared to the gas mixture we used (30% O_2, 68% N_2). We also observed the other reason that the hematocrit of a 3-week hypoxia animal in the study of Dunn et al. was much lower compared to our 3-week hypoxic animals (%, mean ± SD, 52 ± 7, $n = 15$ vs. 78 ± 4, $n = 7$), which was very close to the values of our 3-day hypoxic group (53 ± 5, $n = 9$). We propose that a portion of the tissue that is lost during permanent stroke is not due to the lack of oxygen and glucose but rather due to a secondary effect of toxic molecules secreted by the core of the stroke. Therefore, tissue that is still receiving blood flow remains susceptible to induced cell death via the release of molecules such as glutamate or radical oxygen species from tissue areas that have lost their blood supply [17–20]. Similar results were found in the rat global ischemia model of cardiac arrest and resuscitation [4]. In conclusion, we have shown that a 3-day hypoxic preconditioning, but not a 21-day hypoxic preconditioning, provides significant neuroprotection against permanent focal ischemia in rats, supporting a larger role for the accumulation of HIF-1α and upregulation of its target genes rather than hypoxia-induced angiogenesis in the neuroprotection against focal ischemia.

Acknowledgments This study was supported by NIH grant NS 38632.

References

1. Feng Y, Rhodes PG, Bhatt AJ (2010) Hypoxic preconditioning provides neuroprotection and increase vascular endothelial growth factor A, preserves the phosphorylation of Akt-Ser-473 and diminishes the increase in caspase-3 activity in neonatal rat hypoxic-ischemic model. Brain Res 1325:1–9
2. Gidday JM, Fitzgibbons JC, Shah AR, Park TS (1994) Neuroprotection from ischemic brain injury by hypoxic preconditioning in the neonatal rat. Neurosci Lett 168(1–2):221–224
3. Vannucci RC, Towfighi J, Vannucci SJ (1998) Hypoxic preconditioning and hypoxic-ischemic brain damage in the immature rat: pathologic and metabolic correlates. J Neurosci 71:1215–1220
4. Xu K, LaManna JC (2014) Short-term hypoxic preconditioning improved survival following cardiac arrest and resuscitation in rats. Adv Exp Med Biol 812:309–315
5. Dunn JF, Wu Y, Zhao Z, Srinivasan S, Natah SS (2012) Training the brain to survive stroke. PLoS One 7(9):e45108
6. LaManna JC (2007) Hypoxia in the central nervous system. Essays Biochem 43:139–151
7. Chateauvieux S, Grigorakaki C, Morceau F, Dicato M, Diederich M (2011) Erythropoietin, erythropoiesis and beyond. Biochem Pharmacol 82:1291–1303
8. Ma Y, Qu Y, Fei Z (2011) Vascular endothelial growth factor in cerebral ischemia. J Neurosci Res 89:969–978
9. Dore-Duffy P, LaManna JC (2007) Physiologic angiodynamics in the brain. Antioxid Redox Signal 9:1363–1371
10. Semenza GL (2003) Targeting HIF-1 for cancer therapy. Nat Rev Cancer 3:721–732
11. Chavez JC, Agani F, Pichiule P, LaManna JC (2000) Expression of hypoxia-inducible factor-1alpha in the brain of rats during chronic hypoxia. J Appl Physiol 89(5):1937–1942
12. Harik N, Harik SI, Kuo NT, Sakai K, Przybylski RJ, LaManna JC (1996) Time-course and reversibility of the hypoxia-induced alterations in cerebral vascularity and cerebral capillary glucose transporter density. Brain Res 737:335–338
13. Xu K, LaManna JC (2006) Chronic hypoxia and the cerebral circulation. J Appl Physiol 100(2):725–730
14. Xu K, Puchowicz MA, LaManna JC (2004) Renormalization of regional brain blood flow during prolonged mild hypoxic exposure in rats. Brain Res 1027(1–2):188–191
15. Puchowicz MA, Zechel JL, Valerio J, Emancipator DS, Xu K, Pundik S, LaManna JC, Lust WD (2008) Neuroprotection in diet-induced ketotic rat brain after focal ischemia. J Cereb Blood Flow Metab 28(12):1907–1916
16. Palkovits M, Brownstein MJ (1988) Maps and guide to microdissection of rat brain. Elsevier, New York
17. Harris RJ, Symon L (1984) Extracellular pH, potassium, and calcium activities in progressive ischaemia of rat cortex. J Cereb Blood Flow Metab 4:178–186
18. Choi DW (1988) Calcium-mediated neurotoxicity: relationship to specific channel types and role in ischemic damage. Trands Neurosci 11:465–469
19. Dawson V, Dawson TM, London ED, Bredt DS, Snyder SH (1991) Nitric oxide mediates glutamate neurotoxicity in primary cortical cultures. Proc Natl Acad Sci U S A 88:6368–6371
20. Pacher R, Beckman JS, Liaudet L (2007) Nitric oxide and peroxynitrite in health and disease. Physiol Rev 87:315–424

51

Time Series Tracking of Cerebral Microvascular Adaptation to Hypoxia and Hyperoxia Imaged with Repeated In Vivo Two-Photon Microscopy

Takuma Sugashi, Tomoya Niizawa, Hiroki Suzuki, Hiroyuki Takuwa, Miyuki Unekawa, Yutaka Tomita, Iwao Kanno, and Kazuto Masamoto

Abstract

The present study describes methodological aspects of image analysis for angiographic image data with long-term two-photon microscopy acquired for the investigation of dynamic changes in the three-dimensional (3D) network structure of the capillaries (less than 8 μm in diameter) in the mouse cerebral cortex. Volume images of the identical capillaries over different periods of days up to 32 days were compared for adaptation under either chronic hypoxia (8–9% O_2) or hyperoxia (40–50% O_2). We observed that the median diameters of measured capillaries were 5.8, 8.4, 9.0, and 8.4 μm at 0, 1, 2, and 3 weeks during exposure to hypoxia, respectively ($N = 1$, $n = 2193$ pairs at day 0), and 5.4, 5.7, 5.4, 6.0, and 6.1 μm measured weekly up to 32 days under hyperoxia ($N = 1$, $n = 1025$ pairs at day 0). In accordance with these changes in capillary diameters, tissue space was also observed to change in a depth-dependent manner under hypoxia, but not hyperoxia. The present methods provide us with a method to quantitatively determine three-dimensional vascular and tissue morphology with the aid of a computer-assisted graphical user interface, which facilitates morphometric analysis of the cerebral microvasculature and its correlation with the adaptation of brain cells imaged simultaneously with the microvasculature.

Keywords

Brain microcirculation · Optical imaging · 3D Image analysis · Animal experiments · Machine learning

T. Sugashi (✉) · T. Niizawa · H. Suzuki
Department of Mechanical Engineering and Intelligent System, University of Electro-Communications, Tokyo, Japan

H. Takuwa · I. Kanno
Department of Functional Brain Imaging, National Institute of Radiological Sciences, Chiba, Japan

M. Unekawa · Y. Tomita
Department of Neurology, Keio University School of Medicine, Tokyo, Japan

K. Masamoto
Department of Mechanical Engineering and Intelligent System, University of Electro-Communications, Tokyo, Japan

Department of Functional Brain Imaging, National Institute of Radiological Sciences, Chiba, Japan

Center for Neuroscience and Biomedical Imaging, University of Electro-Communications, Tokyo, Japan
e-mail: masamoto@mce.uec.ac.jp

E. M. Nemoto et al. (eds.), *Oxygen Transport to Tissue XLII*, Advances in Experimental Medicine and Biology 1269, https://doi.org/10.1007/978-3-030-48238-1_51

51.1 Introduction

The cerebral cortex consists of several layers formed with multiple cell types. Due to variable activities and cellular densities across the layers, energy demand in the cortex varies depending on the layer [1]. To meet local heterogeneity of tissue demand, cerebral microvessels must play a key role in balancing blood supply to the cortex. Because oxygen delivery to tissue relies on red blood cells (RBCs) flowing in blood, it is important to know the entire pathway of RBCs through three-dimensional networks of the cortical microcirculation from artery to vein. We have previously quantified morphological features and number densities of the penetrating arteries and veins that are solely responsible for supplying and draining blood in the cortex, respectively, using two-photon microscopic angiography [2]. However, considering the fact that the major compartments for oxygen exchange between brain cells and blood take place in capillaries, it is further needed to quantitatively determine the capillary morphology in the brain tissue where tens of thousands of capillaries are present within 1 mm cubic tissue volume.

In the present study, we aimed to quantify volume images of the cortical capillaries acquired from repeated imaging of longitudinal two-photon laser scanning fluorescence microscopy (2PLSM) in single animals. To overcome sampling bias and resolve the layer dependency of the longitudinal adaptation of cortical microvasculature, the present study has developed a novel method for computer-assisted quantification of vascular network morphology and structural changes by tracking the volume images of microvasculature and tissue structure repeatedly measured in the identical locations of the cortex.

51.2 Methods

Experimental protocols were approved by the Institutional Animal Care and Use Committee of the National Institute of Radiological Sciences and University of Electro-Communications. A portion of the imaging data was reanalyzed from the previously published report [3]. Briefly, six C57BL/6 male mice (8–12 weeks) were anesthetized with isoflurane (3–4% for induction, 2–3% for surgery, and 1% for experiments). A closed cranial window (3–4 mm in diameter) was attached on the left parietal cortex after removing the skull [4]. On the day of the imaging experiments, sulforhodamine 101 (5–10 mM in saline) was intraperitoneally injected to the animal to label blood plasma [5]. The cortical microvasculature was imaged through a band pass filter of 610/75 nm with 2PLSM (TCS SP5MP, Leica Microsystems, Germany) and excited at 900 nm Ti:Sapphire laser (MaiTai HP, Spectra-Physics, CA). The pixel intensity was represented with a 12-bit gray scale, and each image consisted of 1024 by 1024 pixels with an in-plane pixel resolution of 0.45 μm. In each location, z-stack images were acquired to a depth of 800 μm from the cortical surface with a step size of 5 μm.

To correct the 2PLSM point spread functions in biological tissues, a phantom model with a mixture of fluorescent and latex beads of known size was used to adjust a binarization threshold according to a signal-to-noise ratio (SNR) within the region of interest (ROI) in the image. All slice images were reconstructed into a 3D volume matrix with the aid of MatLab-R2018b software. In preprocessing, a median filter (a kernel radius of 4.4 pixel) was applied to all 2D slice images. Then, a 3D Gaussian filter (σ = 3.8 pixel for XY-plane and 0.85 pixel for Z-axis) was also applied to enhance blood vessels, and a contrast noise level was adjusted over depths.

After extracting the vessel regions, each vessel was automatically segmented by dividing the vessels at the branch points, and a segment length was measured (Fig. 51.1a). A signal level was defined as the average of pixel intensities around the center point of the vessel (3 × 3 × 3 voxels), and a noise level was the mode value of the measured pixel intensity over the pixels within the ROI (i.e., an intensity equivalent to the background intensity in the slice image). The diameter of the vessel was then measured at each center position by taking account of the SNR for correction of the binarization threshold.

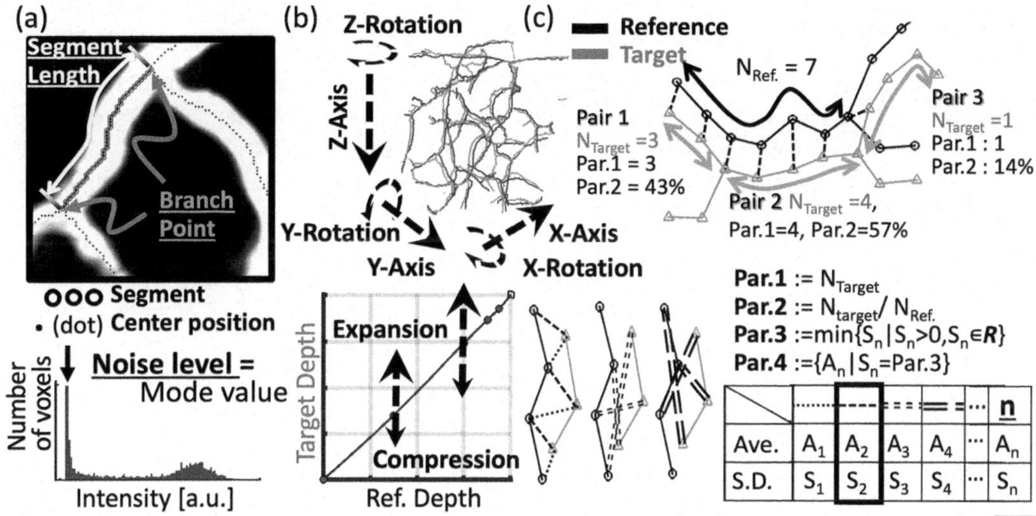

Fig. 51.1 Explanation on the measured parameters. (**a**) A gray dot indicates the center position of the vessel segment (white). The segment was defined as a portion of the vessel from the branch to the branch or from/to the end point. The segment length was measured by summing the Euclidean distances from the end to the other end in each segments. (**b**) The custom-written GUI allows free movement of the 3D-reconstructed images, taken at the different days, with seven degrees of freedom (i.e., X, Y, Z-axes, their rotations, and expansion and compression (right) in the Z-direction. (**c**) The SVM classifier was used to determine the identical segments measured over different days. To this end, the following four parameters (Par.) were measured: (i) the number of the center positions in the target segment (N_{Target}), (ii) a ratio of the number of the center positions in the reference (N_{Ref}) and target segments, (iii) the minimum value of the standard deviation (S_n) of the difference in the number of the center positions, and (iv) the mean value of their distances (A_n)

For analysis of the long-term structural changes in capillaries from repeated imaging with 2PLSM, manual alignment of the image registration was first performed with a graphical user interface (GUI). The custom-written GUI allows free movement of the reconstructed images with seven degrees of freedom (i.e., X, Y, Z-axes, their rotations, and expansion or compression in the Z-direction; see Fig. 51.1b) with regard to the original vessel positions, rotation, and sizes measured at day 0. We maintained spatial misalignment between the target segment taken on different days and the control one measured at day 0 as less than 5 μm. Positional deviations over time were evident along the X, Y, Z-axis, and also rotational deviations occurred around the three axes, depending on the depth, largely due to the fixation difference among the animals under the microscope over different days. There were also deformations of the vessel network structures in the Z-direction during hypoxia adaptation, probably due to expansion and/or compression of the brain tissue.

Computer-aided technology using a machine learning classifier with a support vector machine (SVM) with a Gaussian kernel (radial basis function: RBF) [6–8] was used to identify one thousand vessel segments over long-term images taken at different days. Moreover, whether true or false segments were selected at different days was evaluated by referring to the day 0 image. As the training data, the volume data for one measurement were used to track identical segments at day 0 and other days, and a total of 5807 pairs of the segments were used for manual judgment of the correctness. Candidates of the possible pairs at different days were picked from the points in selecting the segments which were the closest to the original segment to be tracked. Then, the following four parameters were calculated as the input parameters to SVM classifier (Fig. 51.1c): the number of duplications in the true-pair segments, a ratio of the duplications to the number of center positions of the day 0 segments, the minimum standard deviation of the difference in the number the center positions, and the mean value of their differences.

Finally, by using the GUI, the data for each segment were manually inspected and tracked across different days of the measurements with the aid of the SVM classifier. Three-dimensional reconstructions of the vascular and tissue volumes were also conducted with a 1 μm/voxel-resolution based on the measurements of all the vascular diameters.

51.3 Results

The accuracy of the SVM classifier for the true pairs of the segments was 84% with the error of 16% which were determined by comparing with the manual classification. For the false pair segments, the accuracy of 88% with the error of 12% was achieved, resulting in the overall accuracy of 86% for the SVM classifier. It took about 6 hours to identify 5807 pairs for creating training data. With the assistance of the SVM classifier described in the present study, the time necessary to distinguish the identical segments in two images (e.g., longitudinal images taken at day 0 and day 7) consisting of about 4000–5000 segments can be shortened to about 30 minutes.

After identifying the identical vascular segments which were taken from repeated imaging of longitudinal 2PLSM at the identical locations, the diameter changes over cortical depths of 0–500 μm were quantitatively compared for the different groups of the mice adapted either to hypoxia or hyperoxia (Fig. 51.2a). Two weeks after the exposure to hypoxia or hyperoxia, the capillary diameter increased for hypoxia (1.5 times), but not for hyperoxia. A representative result shows that a median value of the capillary diameter was 5.8, 8.4, 9.0, and 8.4 μm at days 0, 7, 14, and 21 under hypoxia, respectively (n = 2193, 1231, 859, and 1094 segments identical over days from day 0), and that was 5.4, 5.7, 5.4, 6.0, and 6.1 μm at day 0, 7, 14, 21, and 32 under hyperoxia, respectively (n = 1025, 593, 361, 294, and 407 segments identified).

Additionally, a long-term change in tissue space was also compared. As represented in Fig. 51.2b, a mode value of tissue space (i.e., the Euclidian distance from the nearest vessel edge to all pixels in tissue, except for the inside of the vessel) was about 13 μm under normal conditions. After hyperoxia adaptation, no detectable changes in tissue space were evident, but hypoxia caused a slight shrinkage of tissue space which accounts for a 4 μm shift in the mode value.

51.4 Discussion

A 3D capillary network in the mouse cortex was automatically analyzed in a segment-basis manner with the aid of SVM by tracking the identical segments over longitudinal volume images obtained with repeated 2PLSM. To help visual inspection and facilitate the automated analysis for large-scale 2PLSM image data, the present study developed a Matlab-based software (Matlab R2018b) which will be available to the public. We also distribute the software upon request.

With regard to technical considerations, there are some unsolved problems in the present tracking algorithm, which should be improved in future work. First, an automatic classification of the present method relies on the accuracy of the classifier made by the training data. For this reason, large volume data sets are needed to further improve the accuracy of the classifier. Secondly, since Euclidian distances between tissue and vessel regions were used to track the identical capillary segments for longitudinal 2PLSM images, a shift of the vessel location due to morphological changes in tissue and motion artifacts during the image sessions critically affects the accuracy of tracking. To minimize the errors, visual inspection and manual alignment are currently needed in preprocessing.

To overcome these limitations, it might be better to utilize a parameter unaffected by the spatial relationship of target pairs which are identical over the different image sessions. For example, all capillary locations should be estimated and allocatable once the locations of the penetrating arteries and/or veins are assigned, because the penetrating arteries and veins are maintained relatively stable for long-term imaging and could be

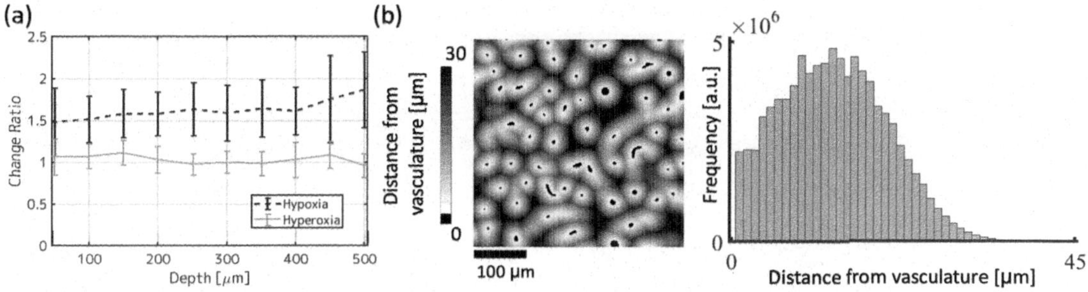

Fig. 51.2 Capillary adaptation and tissue space measurements. (**a**) A comparison of capillary diameter responses to hypoxia (black) and hyperoxia. Relative change in capillary diameter for the tracked segments, measured at day 14, was plotted over depths (at day 14 relative to day 0). (**b**) A representative parenchymal vascular image with Euclidian distance from the vessel edges to all pixels in tissue (gray scale), except for the inside of the vessel segments. Vasculature (black objects in the left) was three-dimensionally reconstructed using the measured diameter data, and a histogram of the distance from the vasculature (right) was calculated for all voxels in tissue segments over cortical depths of 0–500 μm

therefore used as a landmark for the image alignment.

In the future, an extension of the present method is expected for automated analysis of large-scale 2PLSM angiographic image data scanned from a typical 1 mm cubic volume, which will be beneficial for further understanding the balancing mechanisms of the blood supply in local and global regions of the cerebral cortex.

Acknowledgments This study was partially supported by KAKENHI (JP201710551 to TS and 19 K07795 to KM).

References

1. Zilles K, Wree A (1995) In: Paxinos G (ed) Cortex: areal and laminar structure, in: the rat nervous system, 2nd edn. Academic Press, San Diego, pp 649–685
2. Sugashi T, Yoshihara K, Kawaguchi H, Takuwa H, Ito H, Kanno I, Yamada Y, Masamoto K (2014) Automated image analysis for diameters and branching points of cerebral penetrating arteries and veins captured with two-photon microscopy. Adv Exp Med Biol 812:209–215
3. Yoshihara K, Takuwa H, Kanno I, Okawa S, Yamada Y, Masamoto K (2013) 3D analysis of intracortical microvasculature during chronic hypoxia in mouse brains. Adv Exp Med Biol 765:357–363
4. Tomita Y, Kubis N, Calando Y, Tran Dinh A, Méric P, Seylaz J, Pinard E (2005) Long-term in vivo investigation of mouse cerebral microcirculation by fluorescence confocal microscopy in the area of focal ischemia. J Cereb Blood Flow Metab 25(7):858–867
5. Masamoto K, Tomita Y, Toriumi H, Aoki I, Unekawa M, Takuwa H, Itoh Y, Suzuki N, Kanno I (2012) Repeated longitudinal in vivo imaging of neuro-gliovascular unit at the peripheral boundary of ischemia in mouse cerebral cortex. Neuroscience 212:190–200
6. Kecman V, Huang T-M, Vogt M (2005) Iterative single data algorithm for training kernel machines from huge data sets: theory and performance. In: Wang L (ed) Support vector machines: theory and applications. Springer-Verlag, Berlin, pp 255–274
7. Christianini N, Shawe-Taylor JC (2000) An introduction to support vector machines and other kernel-based learning methods. Cambridge University Press, Cambridge
8. Hastie T, Tibshirani R, Friedman J (2008) The elements of statistical learning, 2nd edn. Springer, New York

52 Environmental Enrichment Improved Cognitive Performance in Mice under Normoxia and Hypoxia

Sahej Bindra, Joseph C. LaManna, and Kui Xu

Abstract

The mammalian brain modulates its microvascular network to accommodate tissue energy demand in a process referred to as angioplasticity. There is an aging effect on cognitive function and adaptive responses to hypoxia. Hypoxia-induced angiogenesis is delayed in the aging mouse brain. Additionally, it has been shown that environmental enrichment provides an environment that fosters increased physical activity and sensory stimulation for mice as compared to standard housing; this stimulation increases neuronal activity and consequently brain oxygen demand. In this study, we investigated the effect of environmental enrichment and chronic hypoxia on cognitive performance in the young (2–4 months old) and the aged mice (17–21 months old). Mice were placed in a non-enriched or an enriched environment for 4 weeks under normoxia followed by 3 weeks of hypobaric hypoxia (~0.4 atm, equivalent to 8% normobaric oxygen at sea level). Cognitive function was evaluated using the Y-maze and the novel object recognition tests in the enriched or non-enriched mice under normoxic or hypoxic conditions. In Y-maze, a high alternation rate is indicative of sustained cognition as the animals must remember which arm was entered last, so as not to re-enter it. Novel object recognition is based on the natural tendency of rodents to investigate a novel object instead of a familiar one; a higher novel object exploration rate is indicative of better cognitive function. The young mice showed a significantly higher alternation rate (%, 63 ± 7 vs. 48 ± 10, $n = 8$ and 10, respectively) in the Y-Maze test as compared to the aged mice. Under normoxia, the enriched mice showed an improved alternation rate (%, 63 ± 10, $n = 10$) in Y-Maze test and a higher novel object exploration rate (%, 68 ± 10 vs. 52 ± 10) compared to the non-enriched controls. Similar results were observed for both young and aged mice following hypoxic exposure. Our data suggests that environmental enrichment improved the cognitive performance in the young and aged mice under normoxic and hypoxic conditions.

Keywords

Hypoxic adaptation · Behavioral performance · Aging · Chronic hypoxia · Cognitive function

S. Bindra
Hathaway Brown High School,
Shaker Heights, OH, USA

J. C. LaManna · K. Xu (✉)
Department of Physiology & Biophysics, Case Western Reserve University, Cleveland, OH, USA
e-mail: kxx@case.edu

E. M. Nemoto et al. (eds.), *Oxygen Transport to Tissue XLII*, Advances in Experimental Medicine and Biology 1269, https://doi.org/10.1007/978-3-030-48238-1_52

52.1 Introduction

The mammalian brain modulates its microvascular network to accommodate tissue energy demand in a process referred to as angioplasticity. There is an aging effect on cognitive function [1] and adaptive responses to hypoxia [2]. Exposure to hypoxia is shown to lead to the initial doubling of cerebral blood flow (CBF). The CBF returns to the baseline due to increasing hemoglobin, which is represented by a saturation curve and increasing hematocrit due to erythropoietin upregulation [3, 4]. The brain capillary density increases (angiogenesis) as a response to chronic hypoxia. Hypoxia-inducible factors (HIFs) are factors that mediate the response of cells and tissues based on changes in tissue oxygenation [5]. Previous studies have showed that hypoxia-induced angiogenesis in the brain is delayed in aged mice, which is due to the decrease of HIF accumulation in response to hypoxia [2].

Environmental enrichment provides an environment that facilitates increased physical activity and sensory stimulation compared to standard housing for the mice. This increases neuronal activity and brain oxygen demand. We have reported that young mice living under environmental enrichment were shown to have a much higher capillary density in the brain as opposed to the non-enriched mice [6]. We hypothesize that environmental enrichment leads to improved cognitive performance and better adaptation to hypoxia. In this study, we investigated the effect of environmental enrichment and hypoxia on cognitive performance in the young (2–4 months old) and the aged mice (17–21 months old).

52.2 Methods

52.2.1 Animals, Environmental Enrichment, and Hypoxic Exposure

The experimental protocol was approved by the Animal Care and Use Committee at Case Western Reserve University. The young mice (2–4 months old) and the aged mice (17–21 months old) were randomly placed into the environmental enrichment (EE) and non-enriched (NE) control groups, respectively. Enrichment cages were supplied with various toys of different size, shape, and texture to promote visual/sensory stimulation and physical activity through climbing, burrowing, and exploration [6]. Toys were cycled between enrichment cages approximately every 3 days throughout the time course of the experiment. Groups of three mice were housed in each enrichment cage to prevent overcrowding/competition and monitored on a daily basis. The non-enriched control mice were maintained in standard housing devoid of enrichment and monitored on a regular schedule. Cognitive function was evaluated before and after 4 weeks of enrichment. Hypoxic animals were kept in hypobaric chambers for 21 days at a constant pressure of 0.4 atmosphere (~300 mmHg, equivalent to 8% normobaric oxygen at sea level). The normoxic control mice were housed in the same room to ensure identical ambient conditions.

52.2.2 Measurement of Cognitive Function

Cognitive function was evaluated using the Y-maze test and the novel object recognition test. (1) Y-maze test: The test is based on the innate preference of animals' spontaneous alternations. A high alternation rate is indicative of sustained cognition as the animals must remember which arm was entered last, so as not to re-enter it. Testing occurred in a Y-shaped maze with three silver-collared metal arms at a 120° angle from each other. After introduction to the center of the maze, the animal was allowed to freely explore the three arms for 6 min. The sequencing and number of arm entries were recorded, and the alternation rate (%) was calculated [6]. (2) Novel object recognition test: this test is based on the natural tendency of rodents to investigate a novel object instead of a familiar one. Each animal was allowed a 10-min training session with exposure to two identical toy bricks placed in the back left and right corners of the arena. After the training session, the animal was returned to its home cage for a 30-min retention interval. For testing, each animal was lowered into the testing arena in which one familiar object was replaced with differently shaped toy bricks. Each session was video-recorded, and the animal was given 10 min to explore. The frequency and duration of inspecting the objects were recorded. The novel object exploration rate (%) was calculated as the time spent with the novel object divided by the total time spent exploring either object [6].

52.2.3 Statistical Analysis

Data are expressed as mean ± SD. Statistical analyses were performed using SPSS V26.0 for Windows. The comparison between any two groups was analyzed with a *t*-test, and significance was considered at the level of $p < 0.05$.

52.3 Results

The Y-maze test and novel object recognition test were used to evaluate cognitive function in the young and aged mice with or without environmental enrichment, under normoxia or hypoxia. As seen in Fig. 52.1, without environmental enrichment, the alternation rate decreased significantly in the aged mice compared to the young mice (%, 53.2 ± 13.4, $n = 9$ vs. 65.7 ± 4.9, $n = 6$). The environmental enrichment increased the alternation rate in the young and the aged normoxic mice and the young hypoxic mice. The alternation rate was treaded lower in all hypoxic groups compared to their respective normoxic controls. In the object recognition test (Fig. 52.2), the novel object exploration rate in the EE groups trended higher compared to the NE groups; the novel object exploration rate in the hypoxic groups trended lower compared to the normoxic groups. There was no significance between any two groups.

52.4 Discussion

Our results show that cognitive function declines with age and that environmental enrichment improves the cognitive performance in mice under normoxia or hypoxia. The results found in this study are consistent with our previous studies [6], in which higher capillary density was found in the environmentally enriched mice. Seo et al. reported that the enriched environment enhances angiogenesis and motor performance through the fibroblast growth factor-2 pathway in mice following chronic hypoxic-ischemic brain injury [7]. An enriched environment has been shown to prevent hypobaric hypoxia-induced memory impairment and neurodegeneration in rats [8]. In addition, studies have shown that environmental enrichment provided protection in animals subjected to neonatal hypoxia ischemia [9]. Regardless of oxygen conditions, we observed that being in an enriched environment allows for increase cognitive function. These data support that there are ways to combat the physiological effects of hypoxia by means of enrichment, for example, and also the effects it has upon the body and cerebral capillaries. Having that enriched environment strengthens the body against oxygen depletion and provides a better defense against serious implications of hypoxia.

In conclusion, our data suggests that cognitive function declines with age and environmental enrichment improves cognitive performance in both young and aged mice under normoxic and hypoxic conditions. Our data also suggest that lifestyle factors such as environmental enrichment are important to delay or prevent age-related cognitive deficits in elderly.

Acknowledgments This study was supported by NIH grant NS 38632.

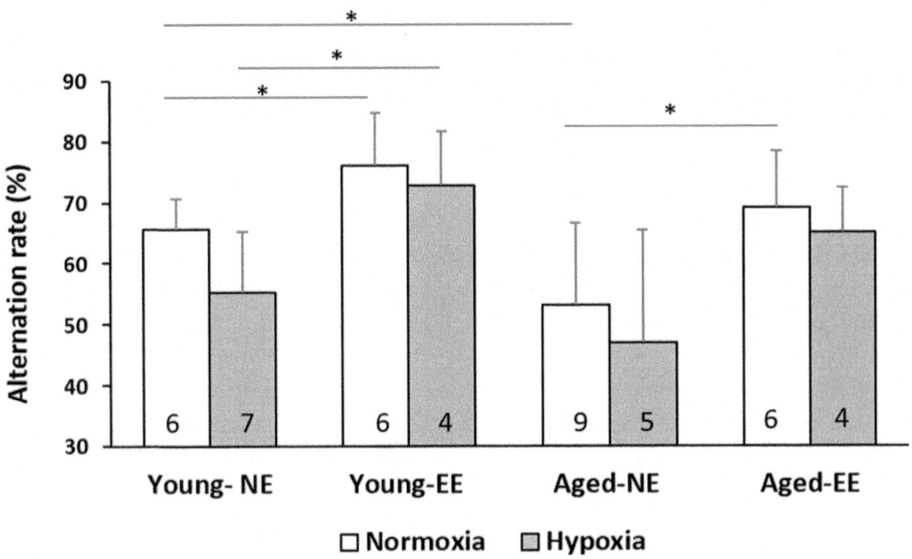

Fig. 52.1 Alternation rate (%) in the Y-maze test. Values are mean ± SD. *Indicates significant difference (t-test, $p < 0.05$). NE non-enriched, EE environmentally enriched. The number of animals of each group is indicated on the each bar

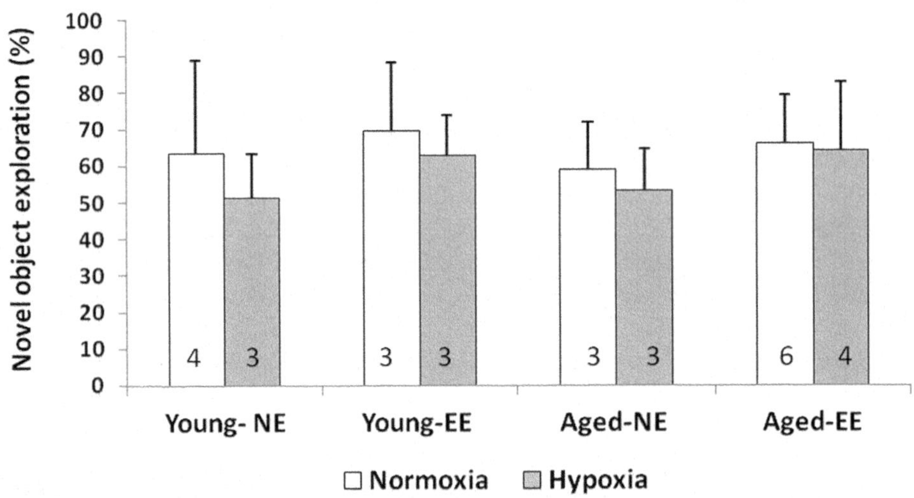

Fig. 52.2 The novel object exploration rate (%) in the novel object recognition test. Values are mean ± SD. NE non-enriched, EE environmentally enriched. The number of animals of each group is indicated on the each bar. There was no significance between any two groups

References

1. Mora F (2013) Successful brain aging: plasticity, environmental enrichment, and lifestyle. Dialogues Clin Neurosci 15(1):45–52
2. Benderro G, LaManna JC (2011) Hypoxia-induced angiogenesis is delayed in aging mouse brain. Brain Res 1389:50–60
3. Xu K, Puchowicz MA, LaManna JC (2004) Renormalization of regional brain blood flow during prolonged mild hypoxic exposure in rats. Brain Res 1027(1–2):188–191
4. Xu K, LaManna JC (2006) Chronic hypoxia and the cerebral circulation. J Appl Physiol 100(2):725–730
5. LaManna JC (2007) Hypoxia in the central nervous system. Essays Biochem 43:139–151
6. He C, Tsipis T, LaManna JC, Xu K (2016) Environmental enrichment induces increased cerebral capillary density and improved cognitive function in mice. Adv Exp Med Biol 977:175–181

7. Seo JH, Yu JH, Suh H et al (2013) Fibroblast growth factor-2 induced by enriched environment enhances angiogenesis and motor function in chronic hypoxic-ischemic brain injury. PLoS One 8(9):e74405
8. Jain V, Baitharu I, Prasad D et al (2013) Enriched environment prevents hypobaric hypoxia induced memory impairment and neurodegeneration: role of BDNF/PI3K/GSK3 pathway coupled with CREB activation. PLoS One 8(5):e62235
9. Durán-Carabali LE, Arcego DM, Odorcyk FK, Reichert L, Cordeiro JL, Sanches EF, Freitas LD, Dalmaz C, Pagnussat A, Netto CA (2018) Prenatal and early postnatal environmental enrichment reduce acute cell death and prevent neurodevelopment and memory impairments in rats submitted to neonatal hypoxia ischemia. Mol Neurobiol 55(5):3627–3641

Effect of Prolonged Pressure on Hemodynamics of Sacral Tissues Assessed by Diffuse Optical Imaging: A Pilot Study

53

B. Day and L. Pollonini

Abstract

Pressure injuries (PIs) are wounds resulting from prolonged pressure exerting on the skin and underlying tissues over bony prominences (e.g., lower back, heels, shoulders) in bed-bound patients and wheelchair users. Minimizing pressure has long been considered the most effective preventative method, and current guidelines require visual skin inspection and repositioning every two hours. However, these strategies are often applied deficiently and do not adequately prevent PIs from becoming penetrating wounds. Recent studies attribute the development of PIs to cell deformation, inflammatory, and ischemic damages that cumulatively propagate from the microscale (death of few cells) to the macroscale (tissue necrosis) within one to several hours. Although the nature of the PI pathogenesis is complex and multifactorial, measuring tissue alterations in real-time may elucidate the origination mechanism and ultimately allow detecting PIs at the earliest stage. In this pilot study, we evaluated the ability of diffuse optical imaging (DOI) to assess hemodynamic changes resulting from prolonged pressure on the sacral tissues in five healthy volunteers laying immobile in a supine position for 2 hours. A thin, body-conforming optical imaging probe encompassing 256 optodes arranged in a regularly spaced grid over a 160 × 160 mm area was used to construct DOI volumetric images representing changes of oxyhemoglobin (HbO_2) and deoxyhemoglobin (HHb) concentration from a zeroed baseline. After 2 hours of continuous body weight pressure, hemodynamic images in all subjects were substantially dissimilar from their individual baseline. We also found that hemodynamic similarity computed pairwise across subjects exhibited a high value and limited variability around the mean, thus denoting a consistent level of image similarity across subjects. These preliminary results indicate that prolonged pressure causes distinctive hemodynamic patterns that can be effectively investigated with DOI and that monitoring functional changes over time holds potential for clarifying the development mechanisms of PIs.

Keywords

Diffuse optical tomography · Near-infrared spectroscopy · Tissue hemodynamics · Pressure injuries · Wearable sensors

B. Day
Department of Engineering Technology, University of Houston, Houston, TX, USA

L. Pollonini (✉)
Department of Engineering Technology, University of Houston, Houston, TX, USA

Electrical and Computer Engineering, University of Houston, Houston, TX, USA
e-mail: lpollonini@uh.edu

E. M. Nemoto et al. (eds.), *Oxygen Transport to Tissue XLII*, Advances in Experimental Medicine and Biology 1269, https://doi.org/10.1007/978-3-030-48238-1_53

53.1 Introduction

Pressure injuries (PIs), also known as pressure ulcers, are wounds localized to the skin and/or underlying tissues that develop as a result of prolonged pressure exerted by a bony prominence (most frequently sacrum and heels) or a medical device. Although all populations with limited mobility are at risk of developing PIs, the highest rates are found in non-ambulatory patients who have no self-ability to reposition their body, especially those who are bed-bound recovering from trauma, surgery, or acute illness in intensive care units (ICUs), terminally ill patients, and wheelchair users. The prevention, assessment, and treatment of PIs are universally considered part of nursing care, and since minimizing the pressure over bony prominences has long been considered the most effective method of PI prevention, patients at high risk of PIs need to be repositioned every 2 hours or less and receive a visual skin inspection by nursing staff to detect any newly developing PIs. Despite the recommended guidelines, the PI prevalence remains high (i.e., 2.5 million cases annually in the US alone, resulting in 60,000 deaths [1]). To avoid these issues, effective methods for detecting PIs as early as possible are needed.

Recent studies attribute the development of PIs to a series of cascading, additive, and damaging events consisting of weight-related cell deformation damage, followed by an inflammatory response-related damage and culminated in an ischemic damage [2]. These adverse events may originate within minutes of one another but then progress at different rates, cumulatively producing damage that propagates from the microscale (death of few cells) to the macroscale (necrosis of tissue) within one to several hours. Despite the complexity of the PI pathogenesis, measuring tissue alterations in real time may elucidate the origination mechanism and ultimately allow detecting PIs at the earliest stage.

In this pilot study, we evaluated the ability of diffuse optical imaging (DOI), i.e., an imaging technique based on near-infrared spectroscopy (NIRS), to assess hemodynamic changes resulting from prolonged pressure on the sacral tissues of healthy individuals. Briefly, NIRS measures the optical absorption of two dominant chromophores in human tissues, i.e., oxygenated hemoglobin (HbO_2) and deoxygenated hemoglobin (HHb) by illuminating the tissue with near-infrared (NIR) light and detecting the light that is partially backscattered by optically turbid tissues like skin, fat, muscle, and bone. Since applying pressure on a slab of tissue significantly affects its hemodynamics by occluding small vessels (capillaries, arterioles and venules), NIRS can measure the effect of such pressure as soon as it manifests [3]. In the last decade, a few studies correlated NIRS-derived tissue oxygenation parameters to PI risk [4], although these were not designed to investigate the disease mechanism. In order to capture hemodynamic events of interest that may relate to the clinical development of PIs, we relied on DOI to (1) measure hemodynamics on a large area of tissue and at different of depths around a bony prominence and (2) monitor structural features of such hemodynamic changes from the moment pressure is applied and continuously over time.

53.2 Methods

Building on our previous design of a small-sized imaging system for detecting vascular occlusion during surgery [5], we developed a DOI probe embedding 128 emitters (dual-wavelength LEDs at 680 and 780 nm) and 128 detectors (silicon photodiodes) arranged alternatively on a 10-mm regularly spaced grid (total field of view: 150 × 150 mm). To follow the curvature of the body (critical for wearability), the probe was built on a flexible printed circuit board (PCB) covered with a layer of optically clear, biocompatible silicone for safe and comfortable application to the human skin. Optical absorption measurements were taken at both wavelengths and in dark condition (LEDs off) to subtract any background contribution. A total of 1736 optical channels with source-detector separations of 10 mm (480 channels), 22 mm (840 channels), and 30 mm (416 channels) were used to reconstruct tomographic images of changes of HbO_2

and HHb with NIRFAST, i.e., a finite-element method often utilized for functional brain imaging [6, 7]. Hemodynamic images were reconstructed for a volume of 168 × 168 × 12 mm with a voxel size of 1 mm^3.

To assess the quality of optical readings and to conduct a preliminary assessment of hemodynamics in soft tissues exposed to prolonged pressure, we asked five healthy volunteers (four males, age 24.6 ± 4.4 yr., weight 71.2 ± 13.9 kg.) to lay supine on a cushioned bed for 2 hours, thus matching the time period for body repositioning recommended to avoid PI formation. The optical probe was manually placed on the sacral region with the sacrum prominence located in an approximate central position. Hemodynamic images were collected every minute after the body weight pressure was applied onto the sacral tissues for a total of 120 minutes.

The effect of 2 hour body weight pressure on the sacral tissues was assessed in terms of patterns of hemodynamic activity (increase or decrease of HbO_2 and/or HHb from baseline) measured over time. We used the structural similarity (SSIM) index [8] as a measure of similarity between two volumetric hemodynamic images, where SSIM = 1 indicates perfectly overlapping activity patterns (e.g., co-located hemodynamically active volumes) while SSIM = 0 indicates maximally dissimilar activity patterns (e.g., a hemodynamically active volume in one image co-located to an inactive volume in the second image). For each individual subject, we quantified the similarity of activation volumes, separately for HbO_2 and HHb, captured 1 minute after baseline (i.e., reference image) and every minute after ($HbO_{2\,t=N}$ vs. $HbO_{2\,t=1}$, $HHb_{t=N}$ vs. $HHb_{t=1}$). We also evaluated the similarity over time between activity patterns of different hemoglobin species ($HbO_{2\,t=N}$ vs. $HHb_{t=N}$) within each subject. Across different subjects selected pairwise, we quantified the similarity between hemodynamic patterns within species measured at the same time during the experiment ($HbO_{2\,sbj=X,\,t=N}$ vs. $HbO_{2\,sbj=Y,\,t=N}$, $HHb_{sbj=X,\,t=N}$ vs. $HHb_{sbj=Y,\,t=N}$). To avoid saturation effects in computing SSIM, all hemodynamic images were normalized to the maximum activation value (either positive or negative) measured over the entire experiment. In addition, we chose to mask the hemodynamic image background (i.e., voxels with less than 10% of peak activation value) to avoid considering spatially overlapping, inactive areas that would have resulted in an overestimation of SSIM. To present these results concisely, we computed the average and standard deviation of SSIM values computed for all comparisons of interests.

53.3 Results

The similarity of hemodynamic changes evaluated over time within each subject is shown in Fig. 53.1. Expectedly, the SSIM values at the start of the experiment approached unity, as hemodynamic images acquired only few minutes apart were structurally very similar. Subsequently, the average SSIM decreased with the passage of time due to pressure-induced hemodynamic activity that increasingly differed from the initial pattern. Also, the variability of SSIM around the mean value increased over time, reflecting subject-specific downtrend rates.

A decreasing SSIM trend was also observed when HbO_2 image patterns were compared to HHb patterns within the same individual (Fig. 53.2). However, similarity across species decreases less compared to similarity within species (Fig. 53.1), confirming the physiological relation between co-located HbO_2 and HHb activities.

The hemodynamic similarity computed pairwise across subjects and then averaged is shown in Fig. 53.3. The initial SSIM value was found to be lower than the corresponding within-subject value due to intersubject differences between hemodynamic patterns. The mean SSIM for HbO_2 slightly increased during the first 30 minutes and reached a plateau thereafter, whereas the SSIM for HHb was essentially constant over time. The SSIM trends also exhibited a limited variability around the mean value, thus denoting a consistent level of image similarity across subjects.

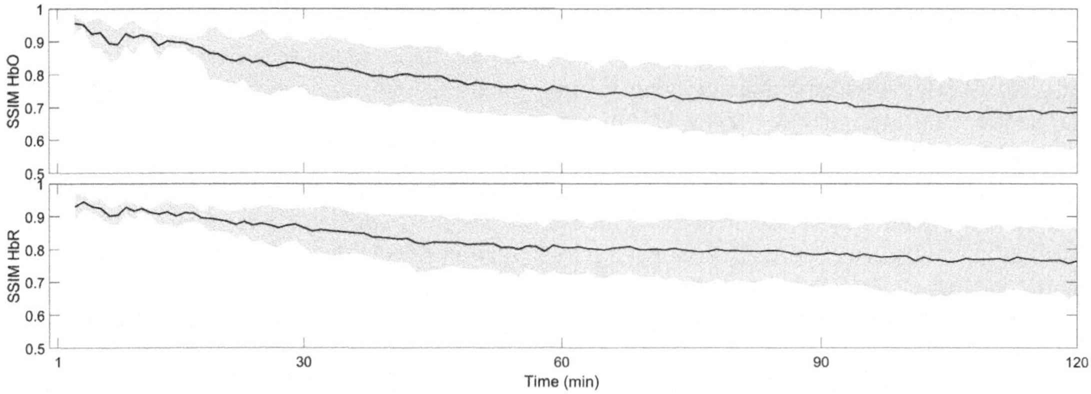

Fig. 53.1 Structural similarity index of time-evolving HbO_2 (top) and HHb (bottom) images using the subject-specific initial hemodynamic image as reference. Mean (black line) and standard deviation (gray bands) computed across all subjects

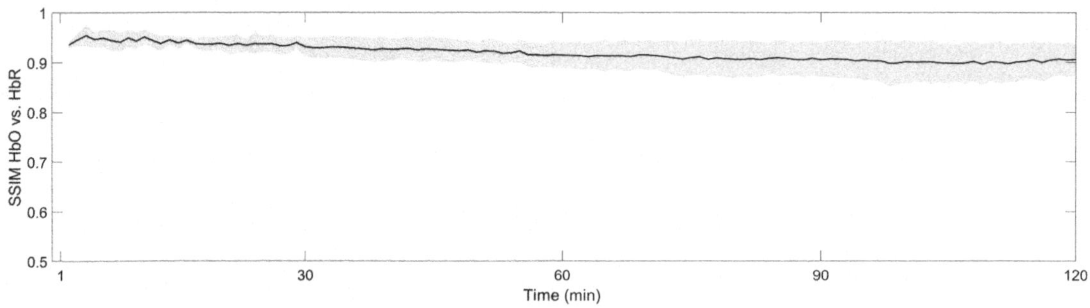

Fig. 53.2 Structural similarity index between HbO_2 and HHb images acquired simultaneously within a subject. Mean (black line) and standard deviation (gray bands) computed across subjects

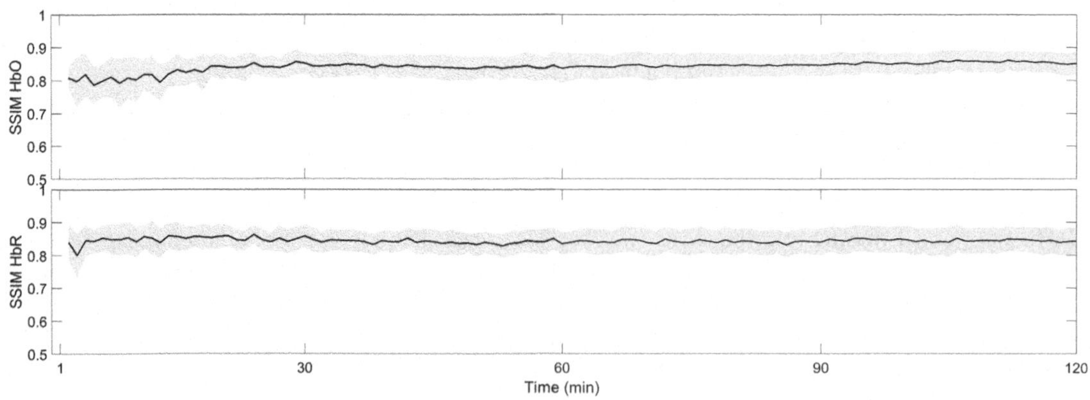

Fig. 53.3 Structural similarity index of time-evolving HbO_2 (top) and HHb (bottom) images computed across two different subjects. Mean (black line) and standard deviation (gray bands) computed across all pairwise combination of subjects

53.4 Discussion

To the best of our knowledge, this is the first study assessing the effect of a prolonged (i.e., 2 hour) body weight pressure on the hemodynamics of sacral tissues minute by minute. Although we designed the study around the overarching hypothesis, supported by a strong physiology rationale, that capillary occlusions induced locally by the sacrum pressing onto the interfacing muscle and skin would cause the tissue hemodynamics to change over time, the novelty of our imaging approach made this study partly exploratory in nature, as the measurements of specific patterns of hemodynamic activity were unprecedented. Diffuse optical imaging provides rich information about tissue hemodynamics, i.e., it delivers tomographic images for HbO_2 and HHb concentrations, separately and independently, that may locally increase or decrease as a function of time, making the summarization and interpretation of those images inherently challenging.

To address this matter, we evaluated such complex image features with structural similarity index (SSIM) that is a quantitative measure that reflects, with both fidelity and simplicity, hemodynamic changes over time within the individual subject and also across subjects with different anatomy and physiology.

Our results show that, in all subjects, body weight pressure induced hemodynamic changes that began immediately after pressure exertion and continued throughout the 2-hour experiment, thus confirming the overarching hypothesis. This was particularly evident at the individual subject level, where the hemodynamic activity patterns of individual Hb species departed quite substantially from their initial pattern. Still at the subject level, the similarity across species changed only moderately over time, thus suggesting that, from a hemodynamic imaging perspective, HbO_2 and HHb may provide some redundant information about the effect of prolonged pressure. More interestingly, the similarity of hemodynamic pattern across subjects was fairly high and stable over time, which indicates that subjects exhibited consistent image features.

53.5 Conclusion

This pilot study shows that diffuse optical imaging is a valid tool for investigating hemodynamic effects of prolonged pressure. In the longer term, DOI could elucidate the origination mechanism of PIs and potentially lead to their early detection.

Acknowledgments This material is based upon work supported by the National Science Foundation under Grants No. 1803826 and No. 1919269, by the Houston Methodist Hospital and the University of Houston Technology Gap Fund.

References

1. Gould LJ, Bohn G, Bryant R et al (2019) Pressure ulcer summit 2018: an interdisciplinary approach to improve our understanding of the risk of pressure-induced tissue damage. Wound Repair Regen 27(5):497–508
2. Gefen A (2018) The future of pressure ulcer prevention is here: detecting and targeting inflammation early. EWMA J 19:7–13
3. Jayachandran M, Rodriguez S, Solis E et al (2016) Critical review of noninvasive optical technologies for wound imaging. Adv Wound Care 5:349–359
4. Li Z, Zhang M, Wang Y et al (2011) Wavelet analysis of sacral tissue oxygenation oscillations by near-infrared spectroscopy in persons with spinal cord injury. Microvasc Res 81:81–87
5. Pollonini L, Forseth KJ, Dacso CC et al (2015) Self-contained diffuse optical imaging system for real-time detection and localization of vascular occlusions. In: 2015 37th Annual International Conference of the IEEE Engineering in Medicine and Biology Society (EMBC). IEEE, pp 5884–5887
6. Dehghani H, Eames ME, Yalavarthy PK et al (2009) Near infrared optical tomography using NIRFAST: algorithm for numerical model and image reconstruction. Commun Numer Methods Eng 25(6):711–732
7. Zeff BW, White BR, Dehghani H et al (2007) Retinotopic mapping of adult human visual cortex with high-density diffuse optical tomography. Proc Natl Acad Sci U S A 104:12169–12174
8. Simoncelli EP, Sheikh HR, Bovik AC, Wang Z (2004) Image quality assessment: from error visibility to structural similarity. IEEE Trans Image Process 13:600–612

54 In Phantom Validation of Time-Domain Near-Infrared Optical Tomography Pioneer for Imaging Brain Hypoxia and Hemorrhage

J. Jiang, S. Lindner, A. Di Costanzo-Mata, C. Zhang, E. Charbon, M. Wolf, and A. Kalyanov

Abstract

The neonatal brain is a vulnerable organ, and lesions due to hemorrhage and/or ischemia occur frequently in preterm neonates. Even though neuroprotective therapies exist, there is no tool available to detect the ischemic lesions. To address this problem, we have recently designed and built the new time-domain near-infrared optical tomography (TD NIROT) system – Pioneer. Here we present the results of a phantom study of the system performance. We used silicone phantoms to mimic risky situations for brain lesions: hemorrhage and hypoxia. Employing Pioneer, we were able to reconstruct accurately both position and optical properties of these inhomogeneities.

Keywords

Time-domain near-infrared optical tomography (TD NITOR) · Diffuse optical tomography · Tissue optical properties reconstruction · Tissue oxygenation · Preterm brain imaging

54.1 Introduction

The brain of extreme preterms is subject to injuries due to the too low or too high oxygenation in the brain tissue. Both hemorrhage and ischemia occur frequently in preterm neonates. Happening early in life, they often lead to long-term disabilities. Despite an improved survival rate (~80%), up to 25% of extremely preterm infants develop cerebral palsy or a low IQ, and a significant cognitive delay is present in ~12% by school age [1, 2]. Neuroprotective therapies exist and are available to clinicians. However, there is no tool that can detect ischemia or hypoxia at the bedside. Cranial ultrasound (cUS) is frequently applied in

J. Jiang · A. Di Costanzo-Mata · M. Wolf
A. Kalyanov (✉)
Biomedical Optics Research Laboratory (BORL), Department of Neonatology, University of Zurich and University Hospital Zurich, Zurich, Switzerland
e-mail: alexander.kalyanov@usz.ch

S. Lindner
Biomedical Optics Research Laboratory (BORL), Department of Neonatology, University of Zurich and University Hospital Zurich, Zurich, Switzerland

Advanced Quantum Architecture (AQUA) laboratory, School of Engineering, EPFL Lausanne, Lausanne, Switzerland

C. Zhang
Applied Quantum Architectures, Delft University of Technology, Delft, the Netherlands

E. Charbon
Advanced Quantum Architecture (AQUA) laboratory, School of Engineering, EPFL Lausanne, Lausanne, Switzerland

Applied Quantum Architectures, Delft University of Technology, Delft, the Netherlands

E. M. Nemoto et al. (eds.), *Oxygen Transport to Tissue XLII*, Advances in Experimental Medicine and Biology 1269, https://doi.org/10.1007/978-3-030-48238-1_54

neonatology, because the fontanel provides a window to the brain. Although cUS provides anatomical images of the brain and cerebral blood flow velocity (CBFV), it is insensitive to hypoxia (low tissue oxygen saturation (StO_2)). A lesion can be identified only once the tissue degraded. MRI measures cerebral blood flow (CBF), e.g., by arterial spin labeling, but StO_2 cannot be determined, and the method is rarely applied in intensive care [3, 4], because it is not bedside, and requires a risky transport of the vulnerable patient.

The most promising noninvasive method so far is near-infrared spectroscopy (NIRS) [5–8], which measures the StO_2, which reflects the proportion of hemoglobin carrying oxygen in the field of view of NIRS. Even though NIRS provides StO_2 values of brain tissue, the technology lacks spatial resolution. Thus, it cannot provide a full picture of cerebral StO_2, since the hypoxia of brain is a localized event [9].

Another approach is time-domain near-infrared optical tomography (TD NIROT) which provides 3D images of StO_2. In TD NIROT, a set of light sources and detectors is arranged over the tissue. Light intensity and photon time-of-flight (ToF) between emission and detection are measured for each source-detector pair [10, 11]. The measured data is then fed into an image reconstruction method based on a physical model for light propagation in tissue. It has been shown that, using short source detector distances and photons with "long" TOFs, TD NIROT is able to reach a depth of 60 mm [12].

State-of-the-art NIROT technology is currently based on photomultiplier tubes [13]. Due to the bulkiness of such systems, the number of detectors that can be used in a system is limited to a few dozen [13, 14], and it would be impossible to increase this number by a factor of 10. The next generation of detectors – single-photon avalanche photodiodes (SPADs) – enables a significant increase in the number of detectors, which leads to better spatial resolution [15–17].

To benefit from this new technology, we have recently designed and built the new TD NIROT system – Pioneer [18]. It aims at imaging the brain of preterm neonates with a high spatial resolution and at detecting hypoxia and bleeding. Here the aim was to study the system performance in a silicone phantom that mimics risky situations for brain lesions: hemorrhage and hypoxia. These are characterized by different optical properties and location.

54.2 Methods

Pioneer is a TD NIROT system based on a time-of-flight camera with 1024 pixels (Fig. 54.1). Each pixel comprises a SPAD with 116 ps time resolution and an unprecedented sensitivity of 12% at 800 nm. This camera chip was specifically designed for NIROT by Biomedical Optics Research Laboratory, University of Zurich and University Hospital Zurich, Switzerland (BORL) and Advanced Quantum Architecture laboratory, School of Engineering, EPFL Lausanne, Switzerland (AQUA) [19]. Pioneer is equipped with a super continuum laser (SuperK Extreme-15, NKT, Denmark) connected through optical fibers to 11 light sources arranged in a circle around the field of view (FoV) (Fig. 54.1). Altogether, we employed almost 4000 source-detector pairs. Emission wavelength can be set in a wide NIR range (650–950 nm); consequently, the system enables multispectral tomography of tissue. Thus, detection of multiple chromophores, such as oxy- and deoxyhemoglobin, fat, water, etc., is possible. Three wavelengths were employed in this work: 689 nm, 802 nm, and 838 nm. For more details on Pioneer, consult our previous publications [18, 20, 21].

We created a silicone phantom with an inclusion to test the system. The phantom has a cylindrical shape: Ø110 × 62 mm^3. It is large enough to ensure the absence of influence from boundaries on the light propagation. The inclusion, a Ø10 × 30 mm^3 cylinder, was located at 15 mm depth at the center of the phantom (Fig. 54.2a). This phantom was manufactured in two steps: (i) the inclusion of desired shape was made out of silicone with certain inks added to achieve the optical properties [22]; (ii) after curing, the inclusion was placed in the mold for the phantom and fixed at the chosen location by fishing rope; then the mold was filled with silicone with bulk optical properties.

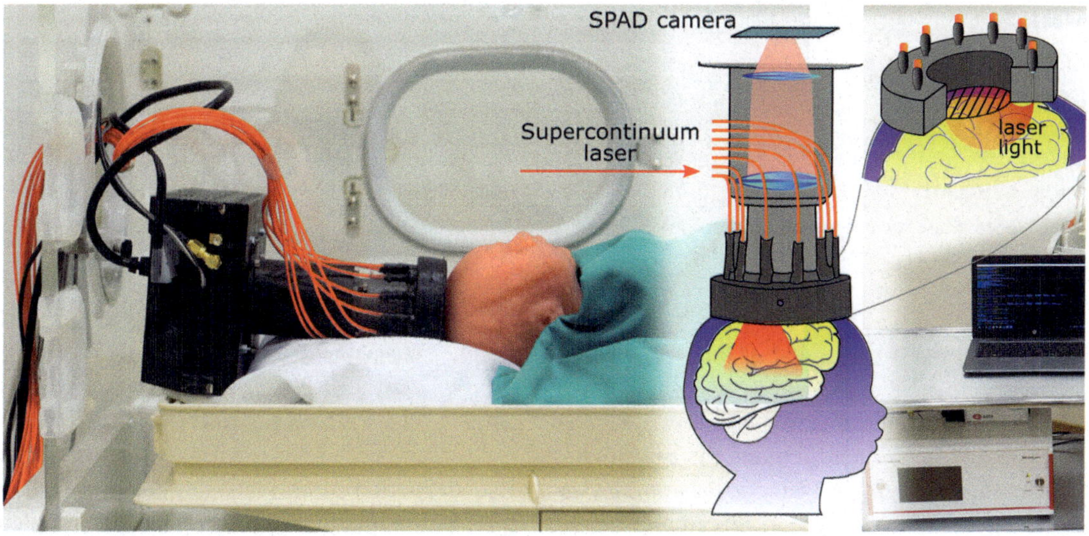

Fig. 54.1 Pioneer tomography setup. The image shows schematic of Pioneer probe design (center), the actual sensor placed inside neonatology intensive care unit (NICU) and applied to dummy baby head (left), and the overview of the whole system including bulky components placed next to the NICU (right)

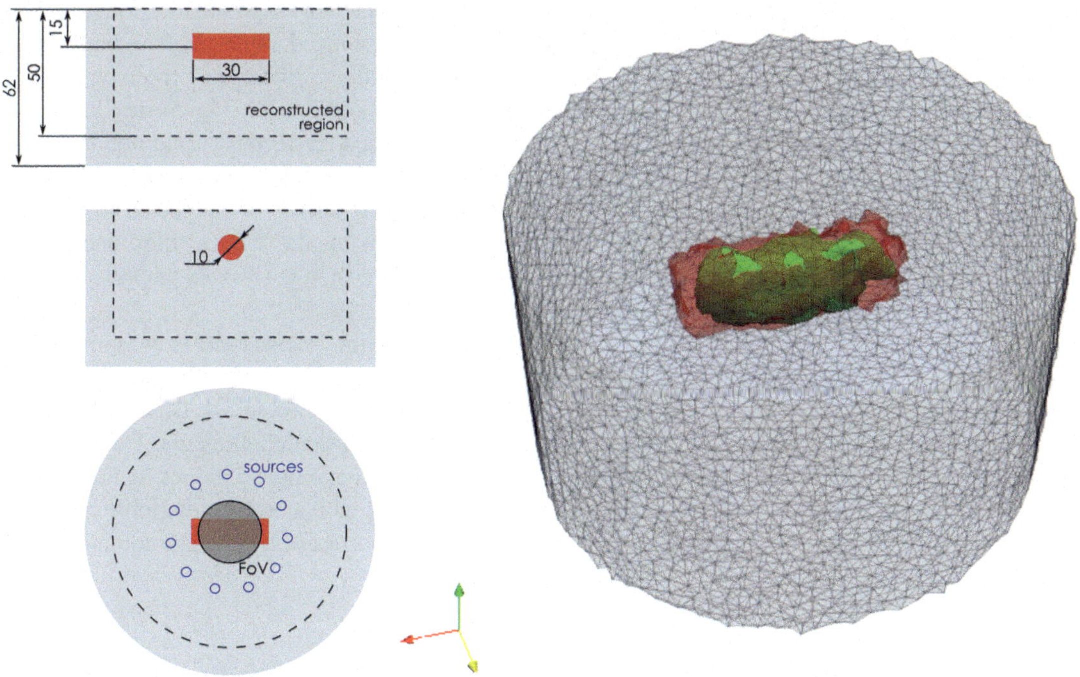

Fig. 54.2 Schematic of silicone phantom with inclusion (left) and reconstructed 3D image (center and right): ground truth in red, reconstructed inhomogeneity in green

Once cured, we removed fishing rope from the phantom. Due to its flexibility and elasticity, the silicone expanded into the cavities and completely closed them.

Optical properties of the bulk and the inclusion were measured with frequency domain NIRS Imagent (ISS; USA) [23]. We give these values in Table 54.1. Absorption of the bulk was

Table 54.1 Optical properties of the phantom and the MC reconstructed values

λ	Inclusion	Contrast	μ_s' [cm^{-1}]	μ_a bulk [cm^{-1}]			μ_a of inclusion [cm^{-1}]		
[nm]	Type		Bulk/inclusion	Target[b]	Meas	Diff	Target[b]	Meas	Diff
689	Hemorrhage	7×	8.1/9.5	0.055	0.050	**−10%**	[a]0.366	0.320	**−14%**
802	–	3×	6.9/8.3	0.055	0.054	**−2%**	0.187	0.187	**0%**
838	Hypoxia	2×	6.7/8.0	0.055	0.069	**21%**	0.124	0.162	**24%**

μ_s' reduced scattering coefficient, μ_a absorption coefficient
[a]Measured with ±15% accuracy due to high μ_a
[b]±10% error

constant at the wavelengths of interest, whereas absorption of the inclusion was wavelength dependent. It enabled us to achieve various contrasts between the inclusion and the surrounding media (see Table 54.1). Namely, the contrast varied from 2× (hypoxia) to 7× (hemorrhage) depending on the wavelength. This high contrast is typical for hemorrhage lesion due to the high concentration of hemoglobin. Despite the wavelength-dependent absorption spectra of the inclusion, we did not aim at modeling an actual spectrum of tissue but rather created a model for several distinct cases of lesion. We also produced a homogeneous phantom with the same bulk optical properties and used it as a reference in the reconstruction, i.e., scaled simulated signal by the one measured on the homogeneous phantom to correct for artifacts related to hardware (e.g., intensity and time offset related to different sources). Alternatively, wavelength normalization method can be used instead, as it was recently reported [26, 27]. However, we did not employ the method in this work.

We performed two types of reconstructions. First, we reconstructed spatial distribution of absorption coefficient within the phantom based on 689 nm data. We chose this wavelength due to the highest contrast. This reconstruction was performed in the NIRFAST package for Matlab (finite element method FEM) [24]. Next, we segmented the model based on this reconstruction. All nodes with absorption below a certain threshold were assigned to segment 1 (bulk), whereas nodes above the threshold were assigned to segment 2 (inclusion). The threshold was set as 50% difference between maximum and minimum reconstructed absorption. Finally, we performed a hard prior reconstruction on the segmented mesh at all three wavelengths based on MCX (Monte Carlo MC) [25][28].

54.3 Results and Discussion

54.3.1 No-Prior Reconstruction

Reconstruction of an inclusion position without prior information is not trivial, since the problem is ill posed. Nevertheless, Pioneer provides a rich set of data, which enable us to reconstruct the inclusion inside the phantom.

The reconstructed inhomogeneity agrees with the inclusion in both shape and location (Fig. 54.2). However, we noticed a mismatch on both sides of the cylinder due to its length exceeding the field-of-view (FoV) of Pioneer (Fig. 54.2a). Please note that we reduced the reconstructed region as compared to the real phantom IN order to achieve faster reconstruction. This is not expected to affect the reconstruction quality since the reconstructed region is large enough to avoid the influence from boundaries.

The no-prior reconstruction was run on the data acquired at 689 nm. At this wavelength, the phantom has 6.7× contrast between bulk and inclusion absorption coefficients. This contrast is well within physiological values. A hemorrhage, i.e., a volume with a high hemoglobin concentration, has a contrast of a factor 50 compared to the bulk tissue.

54.3.2 Region-Based Reconstruction

In a region-based reconstruction, the problem is simplified by implementing a known geometry and structure of the object. Such information can be employed by the no-priors reconstruction. An area with similar optical properties is treated as a single region. Therefore, the number of unknowns is limited by the number of regions. In our case, we had only two regions (bulk and inclusion).

We performed a MC reconstruction of absorption for three wavelengths: 689, 802, and 838 nm. The results are presented in Table 54.1. We achieved good agreement for shorter wavelengths at which the contrast between the inclusion and the bulk was high: 6.7× at 689 nm and 3.4× at 802 nm. At 838 nm, the contrast was only 2.3×. Here we observed an offset. It has to be considered that the true values were measured with an error of ±10%.

As expected, a priori structural information enabled accurate reconstruction of optical properties. The low contrast case, which imitated hypoxia, demonstrated an increased relative error (Table 54.1), whereas, the error was ≤10% for the high contrast cases, which is similar to a hemorrhage.

54.4 Conclusions

The new high-resolution time-domain near-infrared optical tomography system Pioneer was built and tested on a silicone phantom. We were able to achieve good agreement in the geometry and optical properties between the reconstructed image and the ground truth. Thus, an important step in the translation of Pioneer to detect ischemia and hemorrhage in the brain of preterms was mastered.

Acknowledgments This research was supported by Swiss Cancer Research grant KFS-3732-08-2015, the Swiss National Science Foundation project 159490, the National Competence Center in Biomedical Imaging (NCCBI), and CONACyT by the CVU-627802. MW declares that he is founder and president of the board of OxyPrem AG.

References

1. Fischer N, Steurer MA, Adams M et al (2009) Survival rates of extremely preterm infants (gestational age <26 weeks) in Switzerland: impact of the Swiss guidelines for the care of infants born at the limit of viability. Arch Dis Child Fetal Neonatal Ed 94:F407–F413
2. Hutchinson EA, De Luca CR, Doyle LW et al (2013) School-age outcomes of extremely preterm or extremely low birth weight children. Pediatrics 131:e1053–e1061
3. Tortora D, Mattei PA, Navarra R et al (2017) Prematurity and brain perfusion: arterial spin labeling MRI. Neuroimage Clin 15:401–407
4. De Vis JB, Hendrikse J, Petersen ET et al (2015) Arterial spin-labelling perfusion MRI and outcome in neonates with hypoxic-ischemic encephalopathy. Eur Radiol 25:113–121
5. Scholkmann F, Kleiser S, Metz AJ et al (2014) A review on continuous wave functional near-infrared spectroscopy and imaging instrumentation and methodology. Neuroimage 1:6–27
6. Hyttel-Sorensen S, Pellicer A, Alderliesten T et al (2015) Cerebral near infrared spectroscopy oximetry in extremely preterm infants: phase II randomised clinical trial. BMJ 350:g7635
7. Alderliesten T, van Bel F, van der Aa NE et al (2018) Low cerebral oxygenation in preterm infants is associated with adverse neurodevelopmental outcome. J Pediatr 207:109–116
8. van Bel F, Mintzer JP (2018) Monitoring cerebral oxygenation of the immature brain: a neuroprotective strategy? Pediatr Res 84:159–164
9. Guo T, Duerden EG, Adams E et al (2017) Quantitative assessment of white matter injury in preterm neonates. Association with outcomes. Neurology 88:614–622
10. Zhao H, Gao F, Tanikawa Y et al (2007) Time-resolved diffuse optical tomography and its application to in vitro and in vivo imaging. J Biomed Opt 12:062107
11. Gibson AP, Hebden JC, Arridge SR (2005) Recent advances in diffuse optical imaging. Phys Med Biol 50:R1–R43
12. Pifferi A, Contini D, Mora AD et al (2016) New frontiers in time-domain diffuse optics, a review. J Biomed Opt 21:091310
13. Yamada Y, Suzuki H, Yamashita Y (2019) Time-domain near-infrared spectroscopy and imaging: a review. Appl Sci 9(6):1127
14. Hebden JC, Austin T (2007) Optical tomography of the neonatal brain. Eur Radiol 17:2926–2933
15. Dalla Mora A, Contini D, Arridge S et al (2015) Towards next-generation time-domain diffuse optics for extreme depth penetration and sensitivity. Biomed Opt Express 6:1749–1760
16. Villa F, Lussana R, Bronzi D et al (2014) CMOS imager with 1024 SPADs and TDCs for single-photon timing and 3-D time-of-flight. IEEE J Sel Top Quant 20(6):364–373
17. Sawosz PL, Kacprzak M, Zolek NS et al (2010) Optical system based on time-gated, intensified charge-coupled device camera for brain imaging studies. J Biomed Opt 15:1–7, 7
18. Kalyanov A, Jiang J, Lindner S, et al (2018) Time domain near-infrared optical tomography with time-of-flight spad camera: the new generation. Optical Society of America, City, p OF4D.5
19. Lindner S, Zhang C, Antolovic IM, et al (2018) A novel 32 × 32, 224 mevents/s time resolved SPAD image sensor for near-infrared optical tomography. Optical Society of America, City, p JTh5A.6

20. Kalyanov A, Jiang J, Lindner S, et al (2018) TR NIROT system 'Pioneer' for preterm brain imaging: in-phantom tests, City
21. Di Costanzo Mata A, Jiang H, Lindner S, et al (2018) Time-resolved NIROT Pioneer system for imaging of human tissue and preterm-infant brain oxygenation, City
22. Tomm N, Ahnen L, Isler H et al (2018) Characterization of the optical properties of color pastes for the design of optical phantoms mimicking biological tissue. J Biophotonics 12(4):e201800300
23. Hueber DM, Fantini S, Cerussi AE, et al (1999) New optical probe designs for absolute (self-calibrating) NIR tissue hemoglobin measurements. SPIE
24. Dehghani H, Srinivasan S, Pogue BW et al (2009) Numerical modelling and image reconstruction in diffuse optical tomography. Philos Transact A Math Phys Eng Sci 367:3073–3093
25. Fang Q, Boas DA (2009) Monte Carlo simulation of photon migration in 3D turbid media accelerated by graphics processing units. Opt Express 17:20178–20190
26. Stanislaw Wojtkiewicz, Anna Gerega, Marta Zanoletti, Aleh Sudakou, Davide Contini, Adam Liebert, Turgut Durduran, Hamid Dehghani, (2019) Self-calibrating time-resolved near infrared spectroscopy. Biomedical Optics Express 10 (5):2657
27. Jingjing Jiang, Aldo Di Costanzo Mata, Scott Lindner, Chao Zhang, Edoardo Charbon, Martin Wolf, Alexander Kalyanov, (2020) Image reconstruction for novel time domain near infrared optical tomography: towards clinical applications. Biomedical Optics Express 11 (8):4723
28. Jingjing Jiang, Martin Wolf, Salvador Sánchez Majos, (2016) Fast reconstruction of optical properties for complex segmentations in near infrared imaging. Journal of Modern Optics 64 (7):732–742

Online Noninvasive Assessment of Human Brain Death by Near-Infrared Spectroscopy with Protocol of O_2 Inspiration

55

Boan Pan, Jiangbo Pu, Ting Li, Mingliang Zhao, and Xiping Yang

Abstract

Brain death is the irreversible loss of all the functions of the brain and brainstem. Compared to traditional diagnostic methods of brain death, near-infrared spectroscopy (NIRS) is a noninvasive, objective, cost-effective, and safe way of assessment of brain death. Eighteen brain dead patients and 20 healthy subjects were studied by NIRS, with a multiple-phase protocol at varied fractions of inspired O_2 (FIO_2). We found that the changes in the concentration ratios of oxyhemoglobin to deoxyhemoglobin ($\Delta[HbO_2]/\Delta[Hb]$) in the cerebral cortex of brain dead patients were significantly higher than those of healthy subjects, and its low-to-high FIO_2 phase was most sensitive, with a recommended threshold in the range 1.40–1.50. Our study indicated that NIRS is a promising technology for assessing brain death. The success of this application potentially offers a supplementary technique for the assessment of brain death in real time in order to be able to promptly offer quality-assured donor organs.

Keywords

Near-infrared spectroscopy · Brian death · Noninvasive assessment · Protocol of O_2 inspiration · Monte Carlo

55.1 Introduction

Brain death is defined as permanent loss of brain and brain stem function. Current clinical organ transplantation mostly depends on the organs of brain dead patients, which account for more than 22% of total organ donation in many countries [1].

As being well-recognized standards for diagnosing brain death, there is no spontaneous breathing, irreversible deep coma is identified, there is a lack of a brain stem reflex, and no brain electrical activity can be identified for a continuous period of 72 hours [2]. Recently, some novel methods were reported to evaluate brain death. Transcranial Doppler (TCD) is a widely

B. Pan
Institute of Biomedical Engineering, Chinese Academy of Medical Sciences & Peking Union Medical College, Tianjin, P. R. China

Science and Technology on Electronic Information Control Laboratory, Chengdu, P. R. China

J. Pu · T. Li (✉)
Institute of Biomedical Engineering, Chinese Academy of Medical Sciences & Peking Union Medical College, Tianjin, P. R. China
e-mail: liting@bme.cams.cn

M. Zhao · X. Yang
Department of Neurosurgery, Characteristic medical center of the Chinese People's Armed Police Force, Tianjin, P. R. China

E. M. Nemoto et al. (eds.), *Oxygen Transport to Tissue XLII*, Advances in Experimental Medicine and Biology 1269, https://doi.org/10.1007/978-3-030-48238-1_55

researched monitoring method for brain death; however, it is prone to false-negatives of brain death caused by brain injury [3]. Computed tomography angiography (CTA) is another novel method for brain death evaluation, but with relatively low sensitivity [4]. An ideal method to assess brain death should be noninvasive, sensitive, universally available, simple to perform at the bedside, timely, and free from any side effects of drugs and other factors [5]. However, none of the existing methods meet these criteria.

Near-infrared spectroscopy (NIRS) is capable of evaluating cerebral hemodynamics noninvasively and continually [6, 7]. It has been applied to a number of monitoring and evaluation studies, such as shock and brain function activity [8, 9].

In this study, we attempted to assess brain death with our portable NIRS instrument. Prior to the test, we used a Monte Carlo simulation to theoretically investigate the difference between the high and low oxygen concentrations in the brain. Then we investigated $\Delta[HbO_2]$ (the concentration changes in oxyhemoglobin) and $\Delta[Hb]$ (the concentration changes in deoxyhemoglobin) in the region around the forehead of medically evaluated brain dead patients and healthy subjects (with no brain damage). A protocol with varied fractions of inspired O_2 (FIO_2) was designed to be incorporated into the experiments. A potential distinguishing method between the two groups was proposed based on the results of the tests.

55.2 Methods

We developed a NIRS oximeter [10–12] to monitor the hemodynamics in the prefrontal cortex of the brain dead patients and healthy subjects. The instrumentation details can be found in Ref. [11]. Briefly, 2 dual-wavelength near-infrared LED light sources (735 and 850 nm) and 16 detectors were integrated into the flexible probe; the control module and the software on the computer were designed to control the whole device (Fig. 55.1a). Then, we calculated [Hb] and $\Delta[HbO_2]$ from the light intensities with the modified Beer-Lambert law [13, 14].

Approved by the Human Subjects Institutional Review Board at the University of Electronic Science and Technology of China, our experiment protocol (Fig. 55.1b) included four stages and lasted 2.5 hours. Twenty healthy subjects and 18 brain dead patients were recruited from the intensive care unit (ICU) for this study. In the experiment, the protocol consisted of 1-hour preparation, half-hour measurement at 60% FIO_2 (I, high oxygen), half-hour measurement at 40% FIO_2 (II, low oxygen), and half-hour measurement at 60% FIO_2 (III, high oxygen).We regarded the "I" and "II" stage as the "I–II" phase (i.e., the high-low stage in a high-low-high protocol) and the "II" and "III" phase as the "II–III" phase (i.e., the low-high stage in a high-low-high protocol). We did the high-low-high experiments for each patient and collected $\Delta[Hb]$ and $\Delta[HbO_2]$ in different phases.

The Monte Carlo simulation was utilized to compute light propagation in the visible Chinese human (VCH) [15] to explore if there is difference between detected light intensities from human brains at different levels of blood oxygenation with respect to brain death. A previously developed and fully tested Monte Carlo modeling software for light propagation in 3D voxelized media (MCVM) was employed [16]. 10^8 photons MCVM simulation were performed on each of the brain models.

55.3 Results

The signal sensitivity distribution (SSD) (Fig. 55.2b) at the three head models all showed a high penetration depth of the light, in close accordance with the previous theoretical studies [16]. As expected, the normalized light intensity at the head models at different blood oxygenation levels showed a dramatic distinction (Fig. 55.2c). The normalized light intensities were 0.09 ± 0.01 (mean ± standard deviation) in low oxygen content conditions, 0.24 ± 0.05 in normal oxygen content conditions, and 0.85 ± 0.06 in high oxygen content conditions.

Figure 55.3a shows the hemodynamic changes of the mean values of 38 subjects during high-

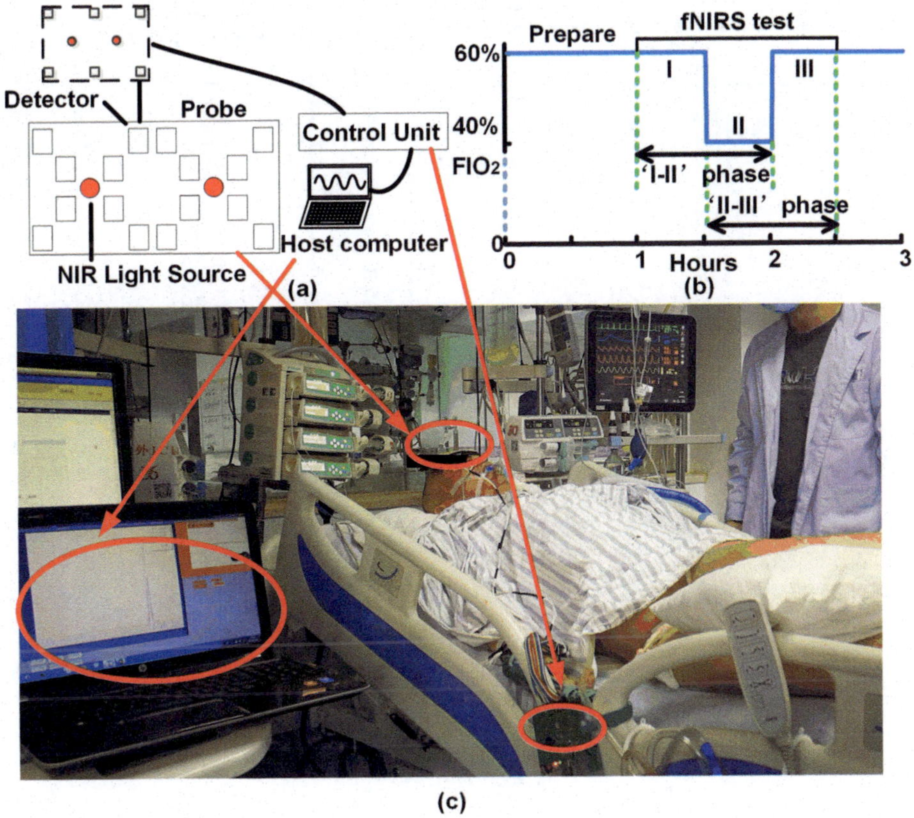

Fig. 55.1 The experiment device and protocol. (**a**) The NIRS system comprised a probe, a control module, and the software in a computer. (**b**) Timeline of the measurement. (**c**) Testing on a subject

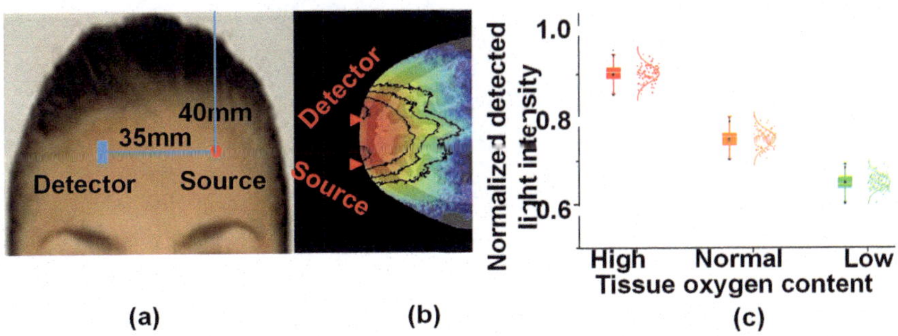

Fig. 55.2 The VCH head model and simulation settings. (**a**) Placement of the light source and detector. (**b**) A slice of the spatial sensitivity profile in simulation. (**c**) The detected light intensity of low, normal and high oxygen content tissue in Monte Carlo simulation experiment

low-high experiments. An obvious decline in $\Delta[HbO_2]$ (−26.30 μM maximum) and relatively small elevation in $\Delta[Hb]$ (12.20 μM maximum) were observed while the FIO_2 was changing from high to low (Fig. 55.3a). After the FIO_2 returned back to high level, $\Delta[HbO_2]$ and $\Delta[Hb]$ gradually recovered to similar baseline levels. More importantly, the changes in $\Delta[HbO_2]$ were much larger than $\Delta[Hb]$ in the brain dead patient in phases "I–II" and "II–III," while the variations of the two parameters were less in the healthy subjects. Figure 55.3b displays the statistics of the

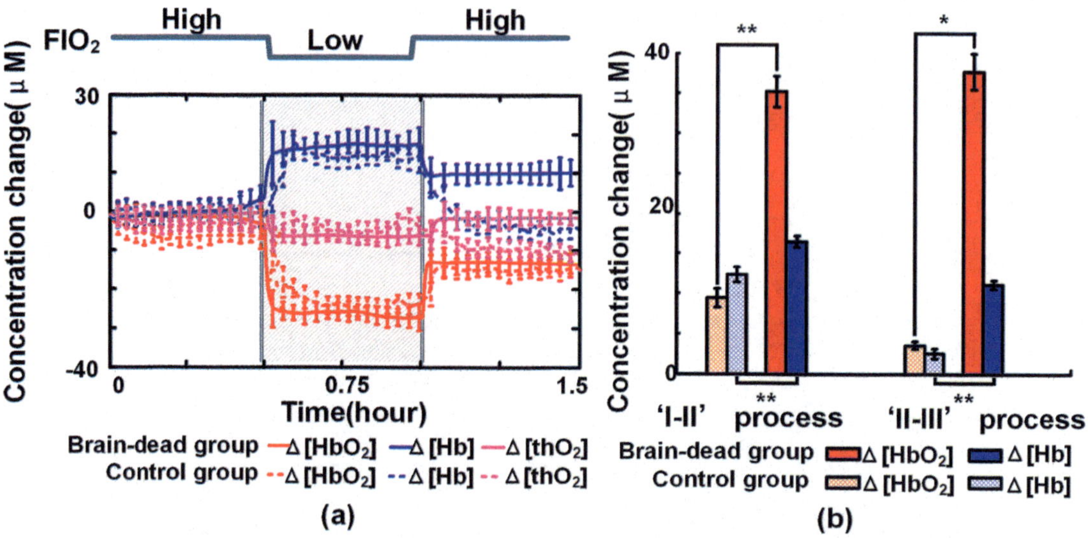

Fig. 55.3 Blood oxygen response in the course of FIO_2 experiment. (**a**) The mean response over 38 subjects during the high-low-high experiment. (**b**) Summary results of $\Delta[HbO_2]$ and $\Delta[Hb]$ variations in phases "I–II" and "II–III" in different groups. *$P < 0.05$, **$P < 0.01$, ***$P < 0.001$ (*t*-test)

Fig. 55.4 The means and standard deviation bar of $\Delta[HbO_2]/\Delta[Hb]$ during the phase "I–II" and "II–III." ***$P < 0.001$ (*t*-test)

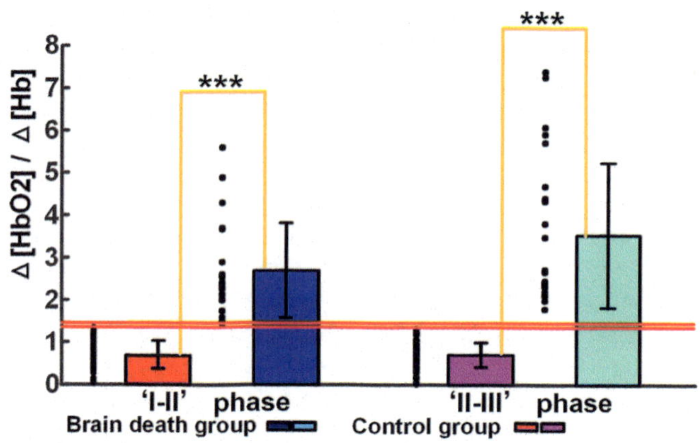

$\Delta[HbO_2]$ and $\Delta[Hb]$ variations in phases "I–II" and "II–III" in the different groups, which also support the same findings. We performed t-tests for $\Delta[HbO_2]$ and $\Delta[Hb]$ from the control and brain dead groups at each stage, with the resulting p values indicating significant differences. The results show that the ratio $\Delta[HbO_2]/\Delta[Hb]$ may be a way to evaluate brain death.

The value of $\Delta[HbO_2]/\Delta[Hb]$ during the "I–II" phase and "II–III" phase is shown in Fig. 55.4. In "I–II" phase, the mean values of $\Delta[HbO_2]/\Delta[Hb]$ are 2.74 ± 1.25 in the brain dead group and 0.79 ± 0.18 in the control group ($p = 0.0011$). The comparable values are 3.45 ± 1.83 and 0.76 ± 0.17 in "II–III" phase ($p = 0.0009$). Apparently, phase "II–III" serves better than phase "I–II" to distinguish the two groups. Phase "II–III" is an optimal monitoring phase in assessing brain death.

55.4 Conclusions

In this study, we attempted to evaluate the performance of our portable NIRS instrument in assessing brain death. A NIRS oximeter with 2 sources and 16 channels was employed to measure $\Delta[HbO_2]$ and $\Delta[Hb]$ in brain dead patients ($n = 18$) and healthy subjects ($n = 20$). Significant differences were found between these groups.

NIRS usually measures metabolism which occurs in the deeper brain. We utilized the Monte Carlo simulation to obtain the photon pathway of this NIRS setup, and the result suggested that the light intensities detected from human brains are different at different levels of blood oxygenation. Also, it is confirmed that the photons received by the detectors include enough transcranial information.

The results of comparing brain oxygenation in brain dead patients and healthy subjects show that the combined indicator $\Delta[HbO_2]/\Delta[Hb]$ was found to be sensitive in distinguishing the two groups with a threshold range (1.40–1.50). We compared the two phases of FIO_2 stimuli. The "II–III" phase is a promising stage to evaluate brain death, because the $\Delta[HbO_2]/\Delta[Hb]$ between control and brain dead groups in "II–III" phase was significantly larger than that of the "I–II" phase, as can be seen in Fig. 55.4.

In the future, we propose using non-contact probes to make measurements in more patients (who have severe injuries on the head) to enlarge the statistical power.

In summary, we investigated the blood oxygenation dynamics in the region around the forehead for brain death assessment. The values of $\Delta[HbO_2]/\Delta[Hb]$ are greater than 1.50 in most brain dead patients and less than 1.40 in most healthy subjects. The result is better expressed in the "II–III" phase. It showed that $\Delta[HbO_2]/\Delta[Hb]$ in the "II–III" phase may provide a biomarker for brain death evaluation. It is also expected we will develop a non-contact design in the near future, which would allow the comfortable and flexible design of the above NIRS devices to study brain metabolism. This study paves the way to evaluating brain death and other brain dysfunction problems with NIRS.

Acknowledgments This study was supported by the National Key R&D Program of China (No. 2018YFC2001100), National natural Science Foundation of China (No. 81971660), financial support from the program of China Scholarships Council (No. 201908110204), Beijing major science and technology projects (No. Z191100010618004), Tianjin Special Branch Plan High Level Innovation Team Grant and Tianjin Key Project Grant (18JCZDJC32700).

References

1. Nakagawa TA, Ashwal S, Mathur M, Mysore M (2012) Guidelines for the determination of brain death in infants and children: an update of the 1987 task force recommendations & mdash; executive summary. Ann Neurol 71:573–585
2. Wijdicks EFM (2002) Brain death worldwide accepted fact but no global consensus in diagnostic criteria. Neurology 59:20
3. Frampas E, Videcoq M, De KE et al (2009) CT angiography for brain death diagnosis. Am J Neuroradiol 30:1566
4. Welschehold S, Boor S, Reuland K et al (2012) Technical aids in the diagnosis of brain death: a comparison of SEP, AEP, EEG, TCD and CT angiography. Deutsches Arzteblatt Int 109:624–630
5. Shemie SD, Dhanani S (2014) Brain death. Pediatr Critical Care Med 1:481–495
6. Li T, Li Y, Lin Y, Li K (2017) Significant and sustaining elevation of blood oxygen induced by Chinese cupping therapy as assessed by near-infrared spectroscopy. Biomed Opt Express 8:223
7. Pierro ML, Hallacoglu B, Sassaroli A, Kainerstorfer JM, Fantini S (2014) Validation of a novel hemodynamic model for coherent hemodynamics spectroscopy (CHS) and functional brain studies with fNIRS and fMRI. NeuroImage 85:222–233
8. Li T, Duan M, Li K, Yu G, Ruan Z (2015) Bedside monitoring of patients with shock using a portable spatially-resolved near-infrared spectroscopy. Biomed Opt Express 6:3431–3436
9. Yamaki T, Nozaki M, Sakurai H, Takeuchi M, Soejima K, Kono T (2006) The utility of quantitative calf muscle near-infrared spectroscopy in the follow-up of acute deep vein thrombosis. J Thrombosis Haemostasis 4:800–806
10. Fang X, Li H, Liu W, Li Y, Li T (2019) A parallel mode optimized GPU accelerated Monte Carlo model for light propagation in 3-D voxelized bio tissues. IEEE Access 7(1):81593–81598
11. Li T, Zhong F, Pan B, Li Z, Huang C, Deng Z (2017) A brief review of OPT101 sensor application in near-infrared spectroscopy instrumentation for intensive care unit clinics. Sensors 17:1701
12. Fang X, Pan B, Liu W, Wang Z, Li T (2018) Effect of scalp hair follicles on NIRS quantification by Monte Carlo simulation and visible Chinese human dataset. IEEE Photonics J 10(5):3901110
13. Gobrecht A, Bendoula R, Roger JM, Bellonmaurel V (2015) Combining linear polarization spectroscopy and the representative layer theory to measure the Beer-Lambert law absorbance of highly scattering materials. Anal Chim Acta 853:486
14. Bhatt M, Ayyalasomayajula KR, Yalavarthy PK (2016) Generalized Beer-Lambert model for near-infrared light propagation in thick biological tissues. J Biomed Opt 21:076012

15. Wu L, Lin Y, Li T (2017) Effect of human brain edema on light propagation: a Monte Carlo modeling based on the visible Chinese human dataset. IEEE Photonics J 9(5):1–1

16. Li T, Gong H, Luo Q (2011) Visualization of light propagation in visible Chinese human head for functi4onal near-infrared spectroscopy. J Biomed Opt 16:045001

56 Not Removing the Glossy White Cover from Adhesive INVOS Neonatal Sensors Affects the Oxygenation Measurement

Mathias Lühr Hansen, Daniel Ostojic, Stefan Kleiser, Gorm Greisen, and Martin Wolf

Abstract

The randomized clinical trial, SafeBoosC III, evaluates the effect of treatment guided by cerebral tissue oximetry monitoring in extremely preterm infants. Treatment should be considered, when cerebral oxygen saturation (StO_2) drops below a predefined hypoxic threshold. This threshold value differs between different brands of instruments. To achieve high external validity, in this pragmatic trial all commercially available cerebral tissue oximeters have been accepted, provided their specific hypoxic threshold value has been determined in phantom studies. Since most companies produce sensors with an adhesive surface on the patient-contacting side, in the phantom studies these sensors were applied according to the specifications, i.e., the glossy cover was removed from the sensor. However, since the skin of preterm infants is particularly fragile, some neonatologists keep this cover on the adhesive sensors, to avoid the risk of skin injury when removing the sensor. Therefore, the aim of this study was to determine whether keeping this cover on leads to different StO_2 values. To evaluate the effect of the cover, we performed multiple deoxygenations in a blood-lipid phantom and compared an INVOS neonatal sensor (Medtronic), with and without the cover, to a reference oximeter (OxiplexTS, ISS). As expected, the relationship of the StO_2 between the INVOS neonatal sensor and OxiplexTS was linear ($r^2 = 0.999$) with and without cover, but the cover influenced the linear equation: $StO_{2\_INVOS\_cover} = 1.133*StO_{2\_ISS} + 7.1$ as opposed to $StO_{2\_INVOS\_nocover} = 1.103*StO_{2\_ISS} + 12.0$. Furthermore, the hypoxic SafeBoosC III threshold differed as well: 60.3% with cover and 63.8% without cover. In conclusion, keeping the adhesive cover on an INVOS neonatal sensor results in lower measured values. At the hypoxic threshold, this is more than 3% (from 60.3% to 63.8%), and therefore, if clinicians keep the cover on the sensor, they need to be aware of this difference.

Keywords

Safeboosc · Near-infrared spectroscopy · Cerebral tissue oxygenation · Brain oxygenation · Blood-lipid phantom · Liquid phantom · Neonates

M. L. Hansen (✉) · G. Greisen
Department of Neonatology, Rigshospitalet, University of Copenhagen, Copenhagen, Denmark

D. Ostojic (✉) · S. Kleiser · M. Wolf
Biomedical Optics Research Laboratory (BORL), Department of Neonatology, University Hospital Zürich, University of Zürich, Zurich, Switzerland
e-mail: Daniel.Ostojic@usz.ch

E. M. Nemoto et al. (eds.), *Oxygen Transport to Tissue XLII*, Advances in Experimental Medicine and Biology 1269, https://doi.org/10.1007/978-3-030-48238-1_56

56.1 Introduction

Near-infrared spectroscopy (NIRS) is a noninvasive technology to monitor tissue oxygenation, by using near-infrared light [1]. It provides a value of tissue oxygen saturation (StO_2), expressed as the ratio of oxygenated to total hemoglobin in the tissue under the sensor [1]. It is possible to monitor StO_2 of various tissues, but so far, it has mostly been used to assess cerebral StO_2 [2–4]. In neonatology, despite lacking clear evidence of positive effects on patient-relevant outcomes [5], clinical usage of cerebral NIRS monitoring is growing [1, 6]. SafeBoosC-III is a randomized clinical trial evaluating the effect of treatment guided by cerebral NIRS monitoring in extremely preterm infants [7]. In SafeBoosC III, treatment should be considered when the cerebral StO_2 drops below a predefined hypoxic threshold. The primary end-point of the trial is survival without severe brain injury. Since SafeBoosC III is a pragmatic trial aiming for a high external validity, all NIRS devices approved for clinical use in newborns are allowed in the trial. However, previous studies have shown that different NIRS devices differ in absolute StO_2 values [8, 9], i.e., the value of the hypoxic threshold differs between different brands of instruments. A previous study has found the StO_2 normal range in preterm babies to be between 55% and 85% with the INVOS adult SomaSensor [10]. For the purpose of SafeBoosC, hypoxic thresholds corresponding to 55% with the INVOS adult SomaSensor have been determined in a blood lipid phantom for most commercially available NIRS devices [11, 12]. The majority of NIRS sensors are produced with an adhesive surface on the patient-contacting side to make skin attachment easier. However, since the skin of extremely preterm infants is fragile [13], some clinicians within and outside the SafeBoosC organization have previously kept the cover on the adhesive sensors during NIRS monitoring outside of SafeBoosC context, to avoid the risk of skin injury when the sensor is repositioned or removed (personal communication). In the phantom studies [11, 12], sensors were tested according to the specifications, without the cover. Although unexpected, it is possible that the cover affects the measurement of StO_2 and hence the hypoxic threshold. The aim of this study was to evaluate the effect of not removing the cover from an adhesive sensor when measuring cerebral StO_2.

56.2 Methods

We compared the INVOS 5100C with Cerebral/Somatic Oximetry Infant-Neonatal sensor (Medtronic, Inc. Minneapolis, MN, USA), with and without cover, to the Oxiplex TS (ISS, Inc., Champaign, IL, USA) as a reference oximeter [11, 12]. The phantom design and setup was previously described [11]. Human blood from recently expired human erythrocyte concentration bags and Intralipid were added, to obtain a hemoglobin concentration of 40 μM and a scattering coefficient (at 834 nm) of 5.3 cm^{-1}. Both parameters remained unchanged throughout the measurement. We performed a total of four deoxygenations, where the sensor's response to oxygenation changes was measured simultaneously. For deoxygenation one, two INVOS sensors—one with a cover (S1) and one without (S2)—and the Oxiplex TS were attached to the phantom windows (Fig. 56.1). The INVOS sensor without cover (S2) served as a control measure of the hypoxic threshold and sensitivity to oxygenation changes, since we already know these values from previous experiments [11]. Before deoxygenation two, the two INVOS sensors (S1 and S2) had the window switched (Fig. 56.1) to assess a potential effect of sensor positioning. Before deoxygenation three, the cover was removed from S1, i.e., both sensors were without a cover (Fig. 56.1). Before deoxygenation four, the INVOS sensors (S1 and S2) were once again switched back to their starting positions (Fig. 56.1) and remained without the cover. The primary analysis was a linear regression between the INVOS neonatal sensor with cover (S1) and the Oxiplex TS (Fig. 56.2). Finally, we compared the sensitivity and hypoxic threshold for S1 during deoxygenation one and two (with cover) and deoxygenation three and four (without cover). The hypoxic

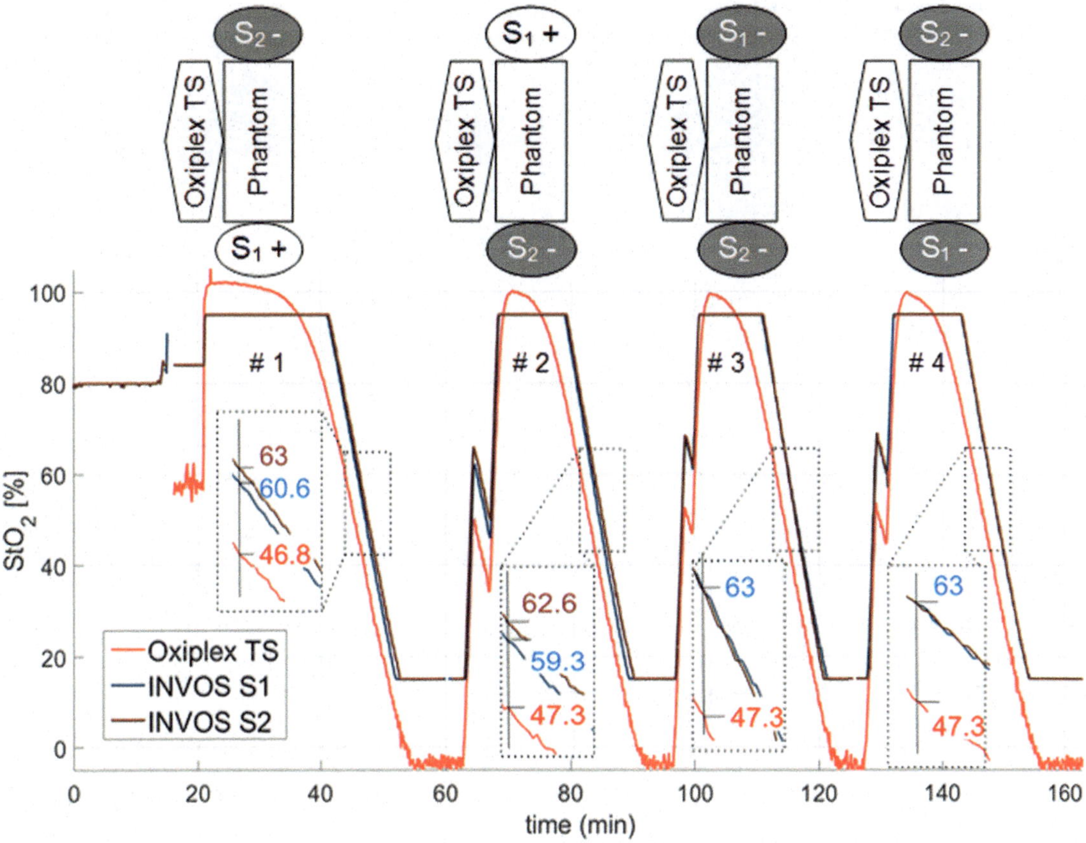

Fig. 56.1 Time series of the four deoxygenations and corresponding phantom setup. For each deoxygenation, there is a time series (bottom) of the StO_2 values in synchronized time, and an illustration of the phantom setup (top). S1 INVOS neonatal sensor with cover initially, S2 INVOS neonatal sensor without cover (control sensor). '+' with cover, '–' without cover

threshold and sensitivity for the control sensor (S2) were calculated as well, to ensure that the values were consistent and similar to those previously reported [11]. To quantify intersensor variation, measurements during deoxygenations three and four, with both sensors lacking a cover, were considered (Table 56.1). Data processing methods were the same as previously used in [11, 12].

56.3 Results

Figure 56.1 shows the time series for the four deoxygenations. The relationship between S1 and Oxiplex TS was linear ($R^2 = 0.999$) both with and without the cover. Table 56.1 shows the coefficients for the linear fits, i.e., the sensitivity to oxygenation changes, as well as the hypoxic thresholds. The sensitivity to oxygenation changes differed depending on the cover. The hypoxic thresholds were determined for StO_2 = 47% for the OxiplexTS, which corresponds to 55% with the INVOS Adult SomaSensor [11]. Based on the linear fits (Table 56.1) and the threshold of the OxiplexTS of 47%, we calculated the hypoxic threshold for S1. This threshold depended on the cover: with the cover, it was 60.3% and without the cover 63.8%. The repositioning of the sensors only had a minor effect on these values (Table 56.1). Also, the intersensor variation was small (Table 56.1). These data show that phantom measurements are a highly reproducible way of testing NIRS instrumentation.

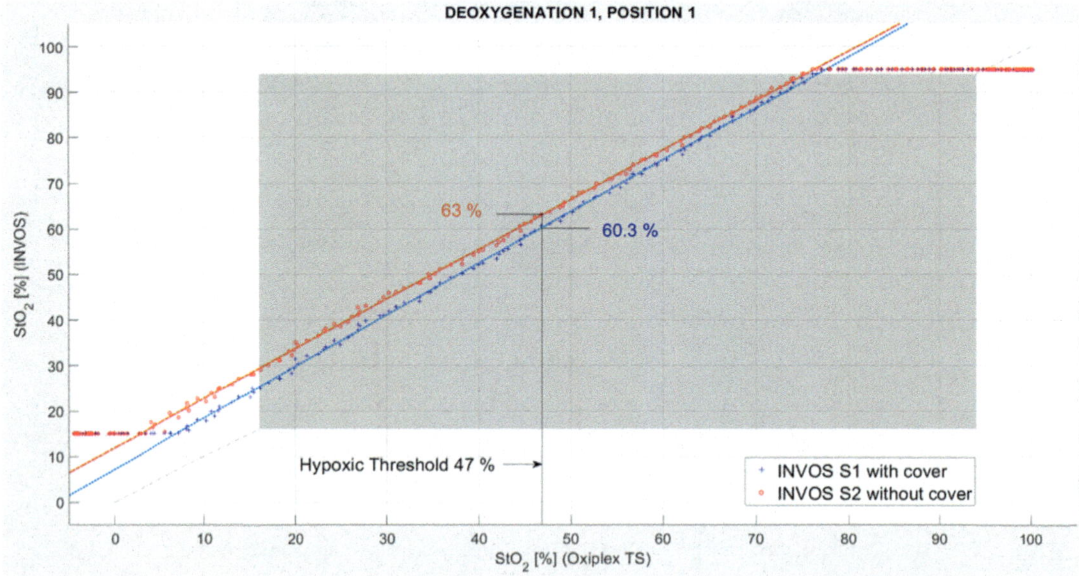

Fig. 56.2 INVOS neonatal sensor and Oxiplex TS linear correspondence with and without cover

Table 56.1 Overview of the four deoxygenations

Sensor	Position	Deoxygenation	Cover	a	b	StO_2% Oxiplex TS 47%
S1	1	1	+	1.133	7.067	60.324
S1	2	2	+	1.144	6.708	60.468
S1	2	3	–	1.086	12.020	63.047
S1	1	4	–	1.103	11.992	63.836
S2	2	1	–	1.089	11.823	63.013
S2	1	2	–	1.092	12.466	63.797
S2	1	3	–	1.152	8.410	62.548
S2	2	4	–	1.105	12.173	64.124

The table includes position in the phantom setup, status on cover (+ with and – without cover), linear coefficients (a = slope, b = intercept, $StO_2(INVOS) = a*StO_2(OxiplexTS) + b$) and hypoxic thresholds corresponding to an StO_2 of 47% with Oxiplex TS (corresponding to the hypoxic threshold of 55% as defined by the INVOS with the small adult sensor)

56.4 Discussion

The main finding of this study is that keeping the glossy white cover on an INVOS neonatal sensor during cerebral oxygenation monitoring decreases the hypoxic threshold by more than 3%. This is an unexpected finding. Furthermore, although the relationship to the reference oximeter, Oxiplex TS [12], is linear, the slope also deviates by ~3%. How can this surprising result be explained? Since the algorithm of the INVOS neonatal sensor is not published, we can only speculate why the absolute StO_2 values are lower when the cover is on. We suggest the following possible reasons: (a) light is channeling through the adhesive (light piping) when the cover is taken off, i.e., the cover reduces light piping by the adhesive, (b) the cover's scattering is higher at low wavelengths, and/or (c) the very high scattering of the cover (~60 cm^{-1}) behaves optically like a mirror and creates a boundary condition more similar to an infinite geometry. An explanation must take into account that, at high StO_2, the difference between the measurement with and without the cover is smaller. This indicates that mainly the lowest wavelengths of the INVOS are affected and means that the slope of intensity versus distance at this wavelength must be steeper with a cover. A more infinite boundary condition (option c) would lead to a decrease in the steepness of the slope and is, therefore, unlikely. A higher scattering at lower wavelength (option b) might increase the slope at a lower wavelength. However, when we measured the scattering of the cover, the scattering was strong (~60/cm, approximately ten times higher than the scattering of tissue), but no wavelength dependency was visible. It must be kept in mind that this high scattering was at the detection limit of our spectrometer. Thus, a more likely explanation seems to be the light channeling effect. A major strength in this study is the experimental setup. By performing multiple deoxygenations and changing sensor position as well as cover status, we were able to quantify the effect of sensor position as well as intersensor variance with high precision. Both had little effect on sensitivity and oxygenation values (Table 56.1). Furthermore, we used a dynamic in vitro phantom, which has the advantage of controllable optical properties, minimal variations, and the possibility to test the device's reactions to oxygenation changes for a wide range of StO_2 [11]. This would not be possible if the experiments had been performed in vivo in neonates. Frequency domain NIRS, such as OxiplexTS, is acceptable as a reference, since it accurately measures the total concentrations of O_2Hb (oxyhaemoglobin) and HHb (deoxyhemoglobin). Additionally, it enables monitoring of variations in scattering [14]. In conclusion, keeping the adhesive cover on an INVOS neonatal sensor results in lower measured values. At the hypoxic threshold, this is more than 3% (from 60.3% to 63.8%), and therefore, if clinicians keep the cover on the sensor, they need to be aware of this difference.

References

1. Green MS, Sehgal S, Tariq R (2016) Near-infrared spectroscopy: the new must have tool in the intensive care unit? Semin Cardiothorac Vasc Anesth 20:213–224
2. Taillefer MC, Denault AY (2005) Cerebral near-infrared spectroscopy in adult heart surgery: systematic review of its clinical efficacy. Can J Anaesth 52:79–87
3. Dullenkopf A, Frey B, Baenziger O et al (2003) Measurement of cerebral oxygenation state in anaesthetized children using the INVOS 5100 cerebral oximeter. Pediatr Anesth 13:384–391
4. Hyttel-Sørensen S, Pellicer A, Alderliesten T et al (2015) Cerebral near infrared spectroscopy oximetry in extremely preterm infants: phase II randomised clinical trial. BMJ 350:1–11
5. Hyttel-Sørensen S, Greisen G, Als-Nielsen B, Gluud C (2017) Cerebral near-infrared spectroscopy monitoring for prevention of brain injury in very preterm infants. Cochrane Database Syst Rev 9(9):CD011506
6. Hunter CL, Oei JL, Suzuki K et al (2018) Patterns of use of near-infrared spectroscopy in neonatal intensive care units: international usage survey. Acta Paediatr 107:1198–1204
7. Hansen ML, Pellicer A, Gluud C, et al (2019) Cerebral near-infrared spectroscopy monitoring versus treatment as usual for extremely preterm infants. A protocol for the SafeBoosC phase III randomized clinical trial. Manuscr Submitt Publ
8. Hessel TW, Hyttel-Sorensen S, Greisen G (2014) Cerebral oxygenation after birth – a comparison of INVOS® and FORE-SIGHT™ near-infrared spectroscopy oximeters. Acta Paediatr Int J Paediatr 103:488–493
9. Dix LML, van Bel F, Baerts W, Lemmers PMA (2013) Comparing near-infrared spectroscopy devices and their sensors for monitoring regional cerebral oxygen saturation in the neonate. Pediatr Res 74:557–563
10. Hyttel-sørensen S, Austin T, Van BF et al (2013) Clinical use of cerebral oximetry in extremely preterm infants is feasible. Dan Med J 60(1):A4533
11. Kleiser S, Nasseri N, Andresen B et al (2016) Comparison of tissue oximeters on a liquid phantom with adjustable optical properties. Biomed Opt Express 7:2973
12. Kleiser S, Ostojic D, Andresen B et al (2018) Comparison of tissue oximeters on a liquid phantom with adjustable optical properties: an extension. Biomed Opt Express 9:86
13. Greisen G, Leung T, Wolf M (2011) Has the time come to use near-infrared spectroscopy as a routine clinical tool in preterm infants undergoing intensive care? Philos Trans R Soc A Math Phys Eng Sci 369:4440–4451
14. Ostojic D, Kleiser S, Nasseri N et al (2018) In vitro comparisons of near-infrared spectroscopy oximeters: impact of slow changes in scattering of liquid phantoms. Adv Exp Med Biol 1072:375–379

Probe Design Optimization for Time-Domain NIROT "Pioneer" System for Imaging the Oxygenation of the Preterm Brain

57

A. Di Costanzo-Mata, J. Jiang, S. Lindner, C. Zhang, E. Charbon, M. Wolf, and A. Kalyanov

Abstract

In preterm infants, there is a risk of life-lasting impairments due to hemorrhagic/ischemic lesions. Our time-domain (TD) near-infrared optical tomography (NIROT) system "Pioneer" aims at detecting both disorders with high spatial resolution. Successfully tested on phantoms, "Pioneer" entered the phase of improvements and enhancements. The current probe (A-probe) was adapted for an optoacoustics instrument. A new probe (B-probe) optimized for TD measurements is required. Our aim is to determine the optimal arrangement of light sources in the B-probe to increase the sensitivity and the resolution of Pioneer and to improve the ability of the system to detect both ischemia and hemorrhage. To do this, we simulated TD-NIROT signals in NIRFAST, a MATLAB-based package used to model near-infrared light propagation through tissue. We used 16 × 16 detector array, with ~2.2 mm distance between the detectors. Light sources were arranged around the field of view (FoV). We performed forward simulations of light propagation through a "homogeneous case" (HC) tissue (μ'_s = 5.6 cm^{-1}, μ_a = 0.07 cm^{-1}). Next, we simulated light propagation through "inhomogeneous case" -tissue' (IC) tissue by adding ischemia ($\mu_a = \mu_a \cdot 2.5$ cm^{-1}) or hemorrhage ($\mu_a = \mu_a \cdot 50$ cm^{-1}) to HT as a spherical inclusion of 5 mm radius at different depths in the FoV center and identified the source location that provides the higher contrast on the FoV: $\max_{i \in I}$ ($FoVContrast_{SOURCE}$). It was found that sources located closer to the FoV center generate greater contrast for late photons. This study suggests the light sources in B-probe should be closer to the FoV center. The higher sensitivity is expected to lead to a higher image quality.

A. Di Costanzo-Mata (✉) · J. Jiang · M. Wolf
A. Kalyanov
Biomedical Optics Research Laboratory (BORL), Department of Neonatology, University of Zurich and University Hospital Zurich, Zurich, Switzerland
e-mail: aldo.dicostanzomata@usz.ch

S. Lindner
Biomedical Optics Research Laboratory (BORL), Department of Neonatology, University of Zurich and University Hospital Zurich, Zurich, Switzerland

Advanced Quantum Architecture (AQUA), Laboratory, School of Engineering, EPFL Lausanne, Lausanne, Switzerland

C. Zhang
Applied Quantum Architectures, Delft University of Technology, Delft, the Netherlands

E. Charbon
Advanced Quantum Architecture (AQUA) Laboratory, School of Engineering, EPFL Lausanne, Lausanne, Switzerland

E. M. Nemoto et al. (eds.), *Oxygen Transport to Tissue XLII*, Advances in Experimental Medicine and Biology 1269, https://doi.org/10.1007/978-3-030-48238-1_57

Keywords

Near-infrared optical tomography (NIROT) · Time-domain imaging · Tissue oxygenation · Time-domain simulations · Time-domain NIROT

57.1 Introduction

Worldwide, ~15 million infants are born preterm every year, and this number is rising. This represents ~10% of the total births [1]. Preterm infants are delicate, and in particular, the brain is vulnerable to lesions, and these do not heal well. Long-term cognitive, sensory, motor, and/or behavioral impairments affect up to ~50% of preterm born patients at school-age [2]. In addition, these lifetime disabilities may lead to significant healthcare costs [3]. Brain lesions are probably often caused by hypoxia or hyperoxia, which may lead to hemorrhage and infarction and ultimately white matter injuries (WMI).

Magnetic resonance imaging (MRI) is a powerful neuroimaging tool for detecting brain structural lesions, i.e., white matter injury [4]. Nonetheless, MRI is unable to detect hypoxia or ischemia causing the WMI. In addition, MRI requires a risky transport of these delicate patients. Therefore, a bedside method is required. Ultrasound (US) is a bedside instrument and detects hemorrhagic lesions immediately. However, US is unable to measure oxygenation and detect hypoxia.

Near-infrared spectroscopy (NIRS) detects hyperoxia, hypoxia, or ischemia, but it is not spatially specific. Near-infrared optical tomography (NIROT) is still at the research stage, but has the potential to fulfill all the requirements, i.e., to become a bedside tool able to measure the oxygenation with high-spatial resolution [5]. Therefore, it is expected to the early detect and possibly prevent hemorrhage, hypoxia, and ischemia.

Recently, we introduced "Pioneer" as a time-domain (TD) NIROT imaging system [6]. Tests detecting ischemic-like inclusions inside phantoms have been successful. Now, "Pioneer" has entered the phase of improvements and enhancements.

The current Pioneer probe (A-probe setup) comprises a ring structure with 11 sources ~23 mm away from the field-of-view (FoV) center. The FoV has 32 × 32 SPAD detectors array (camera), with ~1.1 mm distance between the detectors. The A-probe was adapted from a multimodal optoacoustic-NIROT instrument [7].

A new optimized Pioneer probe (B-probe) is required to increase the sensitivity to the late-arriving photons (LAPs) [8], which will enable higher image quality and sensitivity to deep hemorrhage, hypoxia, or ischemia.

The aim is to investigate the optimal arrangement of light sources in the B-probe to increase the sensitivity for LAPs, hemorrhage, and hypoxia.

57.2 Method

The metric which we used to identify which source locations will enhance the signal sensitivity was the contrast ratio between the time-point spread functions (TPSF) and, in particular, the LAPs, from a simulated "healthy" tissue, i.e., a homogeneous case (HC), against tissue including a localized ischemia or hemorrhage, an inhomogeneous case (IC).

The light propagation in tissue was simulated by NIRFAST [9]. A mesh was generated to mimic tissue and to implement the FoV of Pioneer (detectors set). The mesh has dimensions of 100 × 100 × 50 mm ("xyz-axis") with 0.6 mm nodal distance. Virtual detectors (D) were placed as a 16 × 16 squared grid at "$z = 0$" and centered over the "xy-axis." Detectors were separated by 2.2 mm between them $\{D \in N^{256} | D = (1, \cdots, 256)\}$. Nine virtual sources (S) were placed covering an octant external to the FoV $\{S \in N^{9} | S = (1, \cdots, 9)\}$ (Fig. 57.1a). The mesh optical properties were $\mu'_s = 5.6\ \text{cm}^{-1}$ and $\mu_a = 0.07\ \text{cm}^{-1}$, which are optical properties of an infant's head for the HC [10]. Ischemia ($\mu_{a\ ischemia} = \mu_{a\ HC} \cdot 2.5$) and hemorrhage ($\mu_{a\ hemorrhage} = \mu_{a\ HC} \cdot 50$) were modeled as spherical inclusions of 10 mm diam-

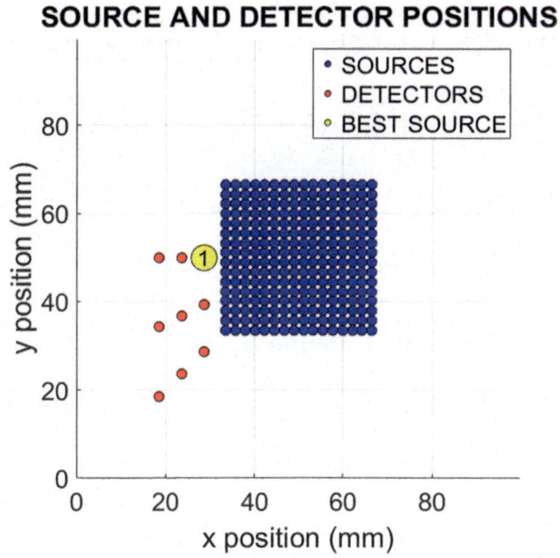

Fig. 57.1 Simulated mesh sources and detector positions. In blue, 16 × 16 squared grid of detector array with 2.2 mm separation distance between them. In red, nine sources with 5 mm x-axis equidistant separation between them. Highlighted in yellow, the selected source locations yielding a greater contrast for different ischemic inclusion depth (Table 57.1) and for hemorrhagic inclusions (Table 57.2)

eter. Mesh simulations with these inclusions represent the IC. Each IC mesh has an inclusion placed at a different depth below the center of the FoV.

NIRFAST TD computational modeling generated TPSF data for the HC and IC. The simulations covered a 6 ns time window with a sampling rate of 0.1 ns, resulting in 61 time-bins (TB), $\{TB \in R^{61} | TB = (0, 0.1, \cdots, 6)\}$. We considered the LAPs to be present in the time-bins from TB_{29} = 2.8 ns to TB_{61} = 6 ns, $\left\{LAPs \in I^{33} \mid LAPs = (29, \cdots, 61)\right\}$. The LAP's interval represents the photons reaching ~15 mm depth and below [11].

To calculate the intensity I over the time interval of the LAPs, we employ

$$I_{TPSF_{S,D,TB}}\left(LAPs\right) = \sum_{LAPs} TPSF_{S,D,TB_{LAPs}}, \quad (57.1)$$

where S is the selected source, D is the selected detector, and TPSF represents the simulated TD data matrix $\{TPSF_{S,D,TB} \in R^{9,256,61}\}$.

The contrast C represents a percentage difference between the IC intensity (I_{IC}) and the HC intensity (I_{HC}) in the time interval of the LAPs:

$$C_{S,D}\left(LAPs\right) = 1 - \frac{I_{IC_{S,D,TB}}\left(LAPs\right)}{I_{HC_{S,D,TB}}\left(LAPs\right)}. \quad (57.2)$$

The FoV contrast (FoVC) is the summated contrasts from all the detectors regarding a single source S in the time interval of the LAPs:

$$FoVC_S\left(LAPS\right) = \sum_{D} C_{S,D}\left(LAPs\right) \quad (57.3)$$

The FoVC yielding the greatest value, among the $FoVC_S(LAPS)$ vector's values, determines the "selected source S" that generates the greater contrast for our Pioneer system (selected $S = \max_{S \in I}\left(FoVC_S\left(LAPS\right)\right)$). Such a "selected S" xyz-location is retrieved from the mesh design parameters (Fig. 57.1). Finally, we calculate the Euclidian distance of the "selected S" against the closest boundary to the FoV perimeter and to the FoV center. Such distances identify the location where the sources generate a higher system sensitivity to a deep inclusion below the FoV center.

57.3 Results

The simulations have sources placed from 21.43 mm to 44.44 mm away from the FoV center and 5.05 mm to 21.11 mm away from the FoV perimeter (edge). According to the index value obtained from $\max_{S \in I}\left(FoVC_S\left(LAPS\right)\right)$, the most sensitive contrast for LAPs is for the sources near the FoV perimeter and to the FoV center. The "selected source" metrics for different ischemic inclusion depth are in Table. 57.1 and for hemorrhagic inclusions in Table 57.2 (Fig. 57.1).

To generate data diversity, three lines of three sources were simulated. The sources had 5 mm separation between them and away from the FoV in the x-axis. Each line of sources had an angular displacement of ∠22.5° starting at ∠180° relative to the FoV center. It was observed that sources located near the FoV perimeter deliver a higher $FoVC_S(LAPS)$ values (Fig. 57.2a), and the highest $FoVC_S(LAPS)$ was for the source nearest to the FoV center (Fig. 57.2b).

Table 57.1 Selected source S data table for ischemic inclusion at different depths (Fig. 57.1)

Inclusion depth	Selected S#	Max ($C_{S\#,D}$(LAPs))	S-FoV center dist.	S-FoV edge dist.	$FoVC_S$(LAPS)
10 mm	1	80.3%	21.43 mm	5.05 mm	~76.95
20 mm	1	72.2%	21.43 mm	5.05 mm	~66.19
25 mm	1	61.1%	21.43 mm	5.05 mm	~48.43
30 mm	1	39.0%	21.43 mm	5.05 mm	~30.64

Table 57.2 Selected source S data table for hemorrhagic inclusion at different depths (Fig. 57.1)

Inclusion depth	Selected S#	Max ($C_{S\#,D}$(LAPs))	S-FoV center dist.	S-FoV edge dist.	$FoVC_S$(LAPS)
10 mm	1	84.59%	21.43 mm	5.05 mm	~96.96
20 mm	1	87.43%	21.43 mm	5.05 mm	~85.79
30 mm	1	55.47%	21.43 mm	5.05 mm	~42.77
40 mm	1	14.41%	21.43 mm	5.05 mm	~11.06

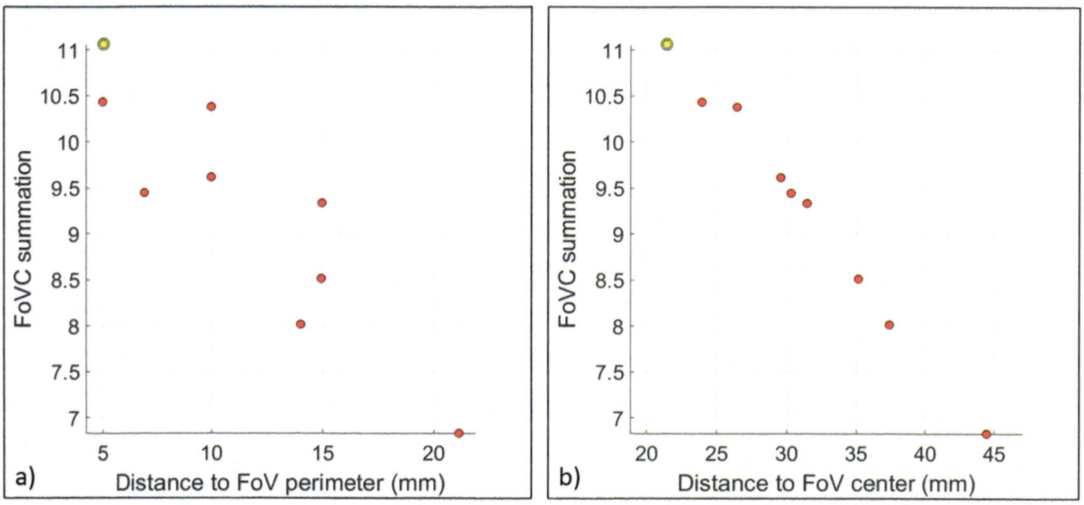

Fig. 57.2 Plot of summated contrast ratio (FoVC) for a hemorrhagic inclusion 40 mm deep (**a**) versus the distance of each source from the perimeter of the FoV (**b**) versus the distance of each source from the center of the FoV. Each source is represented as a red dot. In yellow is the selected source yielding a greater contrast

57.4 Discussion

Pioneer time-domain data enables to resolve deeper anomalies (~3 cm) in tissues, with short S-D distances (~2 cm), which is not possible by continuous-wave (CW) NIROT. This depth resolution is relevant, because tissue consists of layers with different optical properties (skin, skull, muscle, brain) and because it enables to obtain the optical properties of the layer of interest (e.g., the brain). This layered structure was not represented in our phantoms. However, due to the high contrast of the lesions (e.g., hemorrhage is 50 times more absorbant than the surrounding tissue), the difference between the other tissue layers may be neglected as a first approximation. The A-probe had a comparably long distance to the FoV of the detectors. For the B-probe, the sources were close (~5 mm) to the FoV perimeter. This small distance yielded the greatest contrast for all 1024 detectors. In addition, in the A

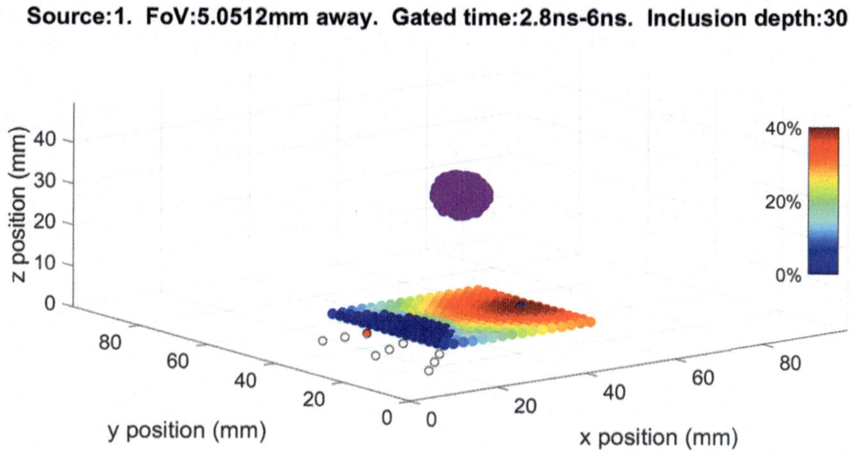

Fig. 57.3 Simulated contrast map in the field of view for an ischemic inclusion 30 mm deep for the source ~5 mm away from the detector edge and ~21.5 mm from the FoV center yielding the highest contrast ratio

probe a high number of 700 detectors was not sensitive to the light, i.e., inactive. The higher contrast and number of active detectors provides a higher signal-to-noise ratio and more information for the image reconstruction. The A-probe showed a contrast of ~20% for ischemia 30 mm deep using ~330 detectors [6]; with the B-probe, we achieved a contrast ~39% using 1024 detectors.

57.5 Conclusion

To achieve a high contrast for the LAPs, the B-probe sources must be close to the FoV perimeter and the center for ischemic or hemorrhage deep inclusions (Fig. 57.3). The higher sensitivity is expected to lead to a higher image quality.

Acknowledgments This research was supported by Swiss Cancer Research grant KFS-3732-08-2015, the Swiss National Science Foundation project 159490 and CONACyT by the CVU-627802. MW declares that he is president of the board and co-founder of OxyPrem AG.

References

1. Anderson P et al (2003) Neurobehavioral outcomes of school-age children born extremely low birth weight or very preterm in the 1990s. JAMA 289(24):3264–3272
2. World Health Organization (2018) Preterm birth. https://www.who.int/news-room/fact-sheets/detail/preterm-birth. Accessed 24 Jun 2019
3. Fanaroff AA et al (2007) Trends in neonatal morbidity and mortality for very low birthweight infants. Am J Obstet Gynecol 196(2):147–1e1
4. Lee YA (2017) White matter injury of prematurity: its mechanisms and clinical features. J Pathol Transl Med 51(5):449
5. Boas DA et al (2001) Imaging the body with diffuse optical tomography. IEEE Signal Process Mag 18(6):57–75
6. Di Costanzo-Mata A et al (2018) Time-resolved NIROT 'Pioneer' system for imaging oxygenation of the preterm brain: preliminary results. In: Ryu P, Lee S, Harrison D, LaManna J (eds) The 46th annual meeting of the International Society on Oxygen Transport to Tissue Proceedings. Springer, Cham, p 2018
7. Ahnen L et al (2017) Development and validation of a sensor prototype for near-infrared imaging of the newborn brain. In: Halpern H, LaManna J, Harrison D, Epel B (eds) Oxygen transport to tissue XXXIX. Advances in experimental medicine and biology, vol 977. Springer, Cham
8. Proskurin SG (2011) Using late arriving photons for diffuse optical tomography of biological objects. Quantum Electron 41(5):402
9. Jermyn M et al (2013) Fast segmentation and high-quality three-dimensional volume mesh creation from medical images for diffuse optical tomography. J Biomed Opt 18(8):086007
10. Arri SJ et al (2011) Precision of cerebral oxygenation and hemoglobin concentration measurements in neonates measured by near-infrared spectroscopy. J Biomed Opt 16(4):047005
11. Torricelli A et al (2005) Time-resolved reflectance at null source-detector separation: improving contrast and resolution in diffuse optical imaging. Phys Rev Lett 95(7):078101

Part V

Interstitium, Lymphatics and Blood

Effect of Blood Flow on Hemoglobin and Myoglobin Oxygenation in Contracting Muscle Using Near-Infrared Spectroscopy

58

B. Koirala, G. M. Saidel, A. Hernández, L. B. Gladden, and N. Lai

Abstract

Insufficient O_2 delivery to, and uptake by skeletal muscle can produce mobility limitations for patients with chronic diseases. Near-infrared spectroscopy (NIRS) can be used to noninvasively quantify the balance between skeletal muscle O_2 delivery and utilization during contraction. However, it is not clear how the oxygenated or deoxygenated NIRS signal should be used to assess muscle O_2 changes. This issue is related to the fact that the contributions of hemoglobin (Hb) and myoglobin (Mb) cannot be distinguished. This conundrum can be resolved by quantitative analysis of experimental data by computer simulations with a mechanistic, mathematical model. Model simulations distinguish dynamic responses of the oxygenated (HbO_2, MbO_2) and deoxygenated (HHb, HMb) contributions to the NIRS signal components ($HbMbO_2$, HHbMb). Simulations of muscle O_2 uptake and NIRS kinetics correspond closely to published experimental data (Hernández et al., J Appl Physiol 108: 1169–1176, 2010). Simulated muscle O_2 uptake and oxygenation kinetics with different blood flows indicate (1) faster O_2 delivery is responsible for slower muscle oxygenation kinetics; (2) Hb and Mb contributions to the $HbMbO_2$ are similar (40–60%); and (3) Hb and Mb contributions to the HHbMb are significantly different, 80% and 20%, respectively. The effect of slow blood flow kinetics on oxygenated Hb and Mb contributions is minimal. However, the effect on the imbalance between O_2 delivery and utilization rates causes significant overshoots and undershoots of deoxygenated Hb and Mb contributions. Model analysis in combination with NIRS measurements and

B. Koirala
Department of Electrical and Computer Engineering and Institute of Biomedical Engineering, Old Dominion University, Norfolk, VA, USA

G. M. Saidel
Department of Biomedical Engineering, Case Western Reserve University, Cleveland, OH, USA

A. Hernández
Office of Research and Economic Development, University of California, Merced, Merced, CA, USA

L. B. Gladden
Department of Kinesiology, Auburn University, Auburn, AL, USA

N. Lai (✉)
Department of Electrical and Computer Engineering and Institute of Biomedical Engineering, Old Dominion University, Norfolk, VA, USA

Department of Biomedical Engineering, Case Western Reserve University, Cleveland, OH, USA
e-mail: nlai@odu.edu

E. M. Nemoto et al. (eds.), *Oxygen Transport to Tissue XLII*, Advances in Experimental Medicine and Biology 1269, https://doi.org/10.1007/978-3-030-48238-1_58

information on hemodynamic and microvascular distribution can help to determine the use of NIRS signal in evaluating the factors limiting exercise tolerance in health and disease states.

Keywords

Computational modeling · NIRS · Metabolic flux · Exercise · Oxygen delivery

58.1 Introduction

Imbalance between oxygen delivery and utilization in skeletal muscle produces significant mobility limitations for patients with chronic diseases. NIRS has been used to evaluate noninvasively the balance between these two physiological variables in contracting muscle [1, 2]. The interpretation of the NIRS signals (oxygenation and deoxygenation) depends on microvascular and extravascular O_2 concentration changes in response to blood flow and O_2 utilization rate kinetics. Mb and Hb in oxygenated (HbO_2, MbO_2) and deoxygenated (HHb, HMb) forms contribute to the oxygenated ($HbMbO_2$) and deoxygenated (HHbMb) NIRS signals.

It is unclear how $HbMbO_2$ or HHbMb from NIRS signals could be used to evaluate muscle O_2 extraction [1]. Some consider only HHbMb kinetics because the blood flow to the skin affects the $HbMbO_2$ signal resulting in a reoxygenation of the signal during contraction [3]. However, HHbMb signal is minimally affected by these changes. To avoid effects of skin blood flow in studying NIRS signals, an animal model of muscle oxidative metabolism [4] can be used, allowing simultaneous venous O_2 content and NIRS signal measurements during contraction.

Since these responses depend on muscle O_2 utilization and delivery rates, the relative contributions to $HbMbO_2$ and HHbMb can be quantitatively distinguished by analyzing experimental NIRS data. Using computer simulations with a mechanistic, mathematical model, we can analyze the underlying transport and metabolic processes that affect O_2 utilization in contracting skeletal muscle [5, 6].

We validate the model by comparison of simulations with experimental venous O_2 and NIRS signal responses from contracting skeletal muscle. The simulated outputs are compared to experimental $HbMbO_2$ and HHbMb kinetics obtained from contracting dog skeletal muscle under fast and slow blood flow kinetics [4].

58.2 Methods

Our mechanistic model of O_2 transport and metabolism [5] simulates vascular and extravascular oxygenation in contracting muscle. By comparison to NIRS data, we can quantify changes of muscle blood volume and contributions of Hb and Mb to the NIRS signals [6]. We used this approach to analyze the effects of blood flow kinetics on the NIRS signals measured in contracting dog gastrocnemius [4].

The O_2 transport and utilization dynamics in capillary and extravascular tissue of contracting muscle are modeled with dynamic mass balance equations of O_2 in the blood domain and O_2, ADP, and PCr in the tissue domain. This model incorporates the metabolic fluxes of ATPase, oxidative phosphorylation, and creatine kinase [5]. At the onset of contraction, the dynamic response of blood flow is represented by an exponential function, and permeability surface area is considered a function of blood flow [7]. The model simulates concentrations of free and bound O_2 to Hb and Mb in capillary and tissue, respectively. Blood domain contributions to the NIRS signal have three compartments: arterial, capillary, and venous [6]. The change in muscle oxygenation during contraction incorporates the oxygenated Hb and Mb concentrations within the whole muscle as

$$HbO_2(t) = f_{bl}(t)[C^B_{O_2,cap} f_{cap}(t) + C^B_{O_2,art} f_{art}(t) + C^B_{O_2,ven} f_{ven}(t)]/4 \quad (58.1)$$

$$MbO_2(t) = f_{tis}(t) C^B_{O_2,c}/4 \quad (58.2)$$

where $C^B_{O_2,art}$, $<C^B_{O_2,cap}>$, $C^B_{O_2,ven}$, and $C^B_{O_2,c}$ are the bound O_2 concentrations in arteries, spatially averaged capillaries, veins, and muscle cells. f_{art}, f_{ven}, and f_{cap} are the arterial, capillary, and venous volume fractions in blood; f_{bl} and ($f_{tis} = 1 - f_{bl}$) are the vascular and extravascular volume fractions in muscle. Equations (58.1) and (58.2) can be rewritten in terms of oxygenated heme groups of Hb and Mb ($C_{oxy,\,x}$) as

$$HbO_2(t) = f_{bl}(t)[C_{oxy,cap}\, f_{cap}(t) + C_{oxy,art}\, f_{art}(t) + C_{oxy,ven}\, f_{ven}(t)] \quad (58.3)$$

$$MbO_2(t) = f_{tis}(t)\,C_{oxy,tis} \quad (58.4)$$

These equations can be used to calculate deoxygenated Hb and Mb heme groups (*HHb*, *HMb*) in muscle as

$$HHb(t) = f_{bl}(t)[C_{deoxy,cap}\, f_{cap}(t) + C_{deoxy,art}\, f_{art}(t) + C_{deoxy,ven}\, f_{ven}(t)] \quad (58.5)$$

$$HMb(t) = f_{tis}\left(C_{c,Mb} - C^B_{O_2,c}\right)/4 = f_c\, C_{deoxy,tis} \quad (58.6)$$

where in blood compartments (x = cap, art, ven) $C_{deoxy,\,x} = C_{b,\,Hb} - C_{oxy,\,x}$. The $f_{bl}(t)$ is related to the change of total heme concentration $\Delta HbMb_{tot}(t)$ normalized by the maximal change measured during contraction ($\Delta HbMbO_{2,\,max}$) by NIRS [6]:

$$f_{bl}(t) = f^R_{bl} + \frac{\left[\dfrac{\Delta HbMb_{tot}(t)}{\Delta HbMbO_{2,\max}}\right]_{exp}\left[\Delta HbMbO_2(t)\right]_{mod}}{C_{b,Hb} + C_{c,Mb}/4} \quad (58.7)$$

Here, f^R_{bl} is the resting blood volume fraction; $C_{b,\,Hb}$ and $C_{c,\,Mb}$ are the Hb and Mb concentrations in blood and tissue, respectively. The vascular volume changes during contraction affect arterioles, capillary, and venules and tissue volume fractions [6]. The simulated oxy-/deoxygenated Hb and Mb concentrations contributing to the NIRS signals are

$$HbMbO_2(t) = HbO_2(t) + MbO_2(t); \quad HHbMb(t) = HHb(t) + HMb(t) \quad (58.8)$$

Hb and Mb contributions to the $HbMbO_2$ and *HHbMb* signals are quantified as

$$y_{HbO_2}(t) = \frac{HbO_2(t)}{HbMbO_2(t)}; \quad y_{MbO_2}(t) = \frac{MbO_2(t)}{HbMbO_2(t)} \quad (58.9)$$

$$y_{HHb}(t) = \frac{HHb(t)}{HHbMb(t)}; \quad y_{HMb}(t) = \frac{HMb(t)}{HHbMb(t)} \quad (58.10)$$

where $y_{HbO2}(t)$ and $y_{MbO2}(t)$ are the fraction of oxygenated Hb and Mb in the oxygenated heme group; $y_{HHb}(t)$ and $y_{HMb}(t)$ are the fractions of deoxygenated Hb and Mb in the deoxygenated heme group. To compare NIRS oxygenation and deoxygenation responses to contraction with those simulated, the changes in oxygenated ($\Delta HbMbO_2$) and deoxygenated ($\Delta HHbMb$) signals are normalized by the maximal oxygenated signal change during contraction ($\Delta HbMbO_{2,\,max}$)

$$\Delta HbMbO_{2,N}(t) = \frac{\Delta HbMbO_2(t)}{\Delta HbMbO_{2,\max}} \quad (58.11)$$

$$\Delta HHbMb_N(t) = \frac{\Delta HHbMb(t)}{\Delta HbMbO_{2,\max}} \quad (58.12)$$

58.3 Results

The mathematical model was tested by comparing simulated muscle O_2 uptake (not shown) and NIRS kinetics and experimental data obtained for two different contracting bouts (B1, B2) [4].

Table 58.1 Concentration of oxygenated and deoxygenated heme groups in whole muscle (HbO_2, MbO_2, HHb, HMb) and skeletal muscle compartments ($C_{oxy,\,x}$, $C_{deoxy,\,x}$) (x = art, cap, ven, tis) and their volume fractions at rest

Compartment	Volume fraction [%]	$C_{oxy,\,x}$ [μM]	$C_{deoxy,\,x}$ [μM]	HbO_2 or MbO_2 [μM]	HHb or HMb [μM]
Arterial	0.5	2360	100	11.8	0.3
Capillary	0.75	2150	500	14.8	1.2
Venous	3.75	2250	300	80.9	9.9
Myocytes	95	80	3	74.1	2.2

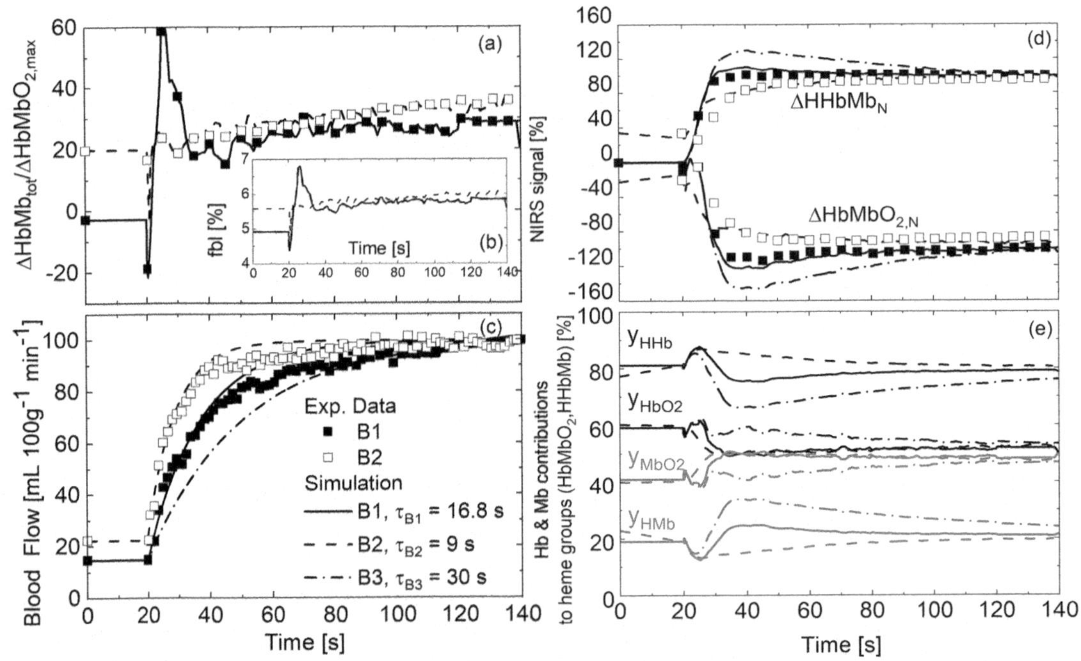

Fig. 58.1 Model inputs and output for bouts 1, 2, and 3 of muscle contraction: (**a**) kinetics of the total NIRS signal normalized (input); (**b**) blood volume fraction (output); (**c**) blood flow kinetics (input). Effects of blood flow kinetics on (**d**) simulated (output) and experimental NIRS signals normalized; and (**e**) simulated Hb (black lines) and Mb (gray lines) contributions to $HbMbO_2$ and $HHbMb$ (output)

B1 is a prior bout of muscle contraction followed by 2 minutes of rest and a second bout of contraction (B2). The sum of the oxygenated and deoxygenated NIRS signal ($\Delta HbMb_{tot}/\Delta HbMbO_{2,\,max}$) kinetics (Fig.58.1a) is used to quantify the blood volume changes indicated by f_{bl} (Fig.58.1b) during contraction. The kinetics of muscle blood volume ($\Delta HbMb_{tot}/\Delta HbMbO_{2,\,max}$), and flow (Fig. 58.1c) as well as the metabolic (related to O_2 uptake at steady state) parameters are model inputs for simulations of $\Delta HbMbO_2$ and $\Delta HHbMb$ kinetics (normalized) (Fig.58.1d) [4]. The blood flow time constant in the first bout is larger ($\tau_{B_1} = 16.8$ s) than the second one ($\tau_{B_2} = 9$ s), whereas the amplitude of blood flow and O_2 uptake are the same in both bouts. Simulated oxygenated and deoxygenated kinetics based on Hb and Mb contributions follow closely those measured by NIRS. The faster the blood flow kinetics, the slower the NIRS kinetics (Fig.58.1d) [4]. A third bout (B3) was simulated with the same conditions of B1 except blood flow time constant that was greater ($\tau_{B_3} = 30s$). Under this condition, a concomitant undershoot of the oxygenated and an overshoot of the deoxygenated signals were observed.

The effect of blood flow kinetics on Hb and Mb contributions to the $HbMbO_2$ and $HHbMb$ (Fig. 58.1e) are simulated for all bouts. At the onset of contraction, an overshoot of the deoxy-/oxygenated Hb contributions and an undershoot of the deoxy-/oxygenated Mb contribution are observed. Hb and Mb contribute similarly to the $HbMbO_2$ ($y_{HbO2}(t)$ and $y_{MbO2}(t)$): approximately 40% for Mb and 60% for Hb at rest. In contrast, the contributions of Hb and Mb to the deoxygenated NIRS signals ($y_{HHb}(t)$ and $y_{HMb}(t)$) are 70–80% and 20–30%, respectively. Table 58.1 shows the concentration of oxygenated and deoxygenated heme groups in the vascular and extravascular domains and whole muscle at rest.

Under normal or fast O_2 delivery (B1 and B2) during muscle contraction, when NIRS signal approaches to a plateau ($\Delta HbMbO_{2,\,max}$), y_{MbO2} reaches 50% in less than 10s. In the presence of O_2 delivery impairment (B3), y_{MbO2} kinetics is slower than that observed for B1 and B2, while y_{HMb} reaches its peak. Specifically, at 40s, in the presence of a $\Delta HbMbO_{2,\,N}$ undershoot of 60% of the plateau ($\Delta HbMbO_{2,\,max}$), y_{MbO2} remains close to the rest value (40%), while y_{HMb} increases from 20% to 37%.

58.4 Discussion

Our mathematical model predicts the effects of blood flow kinetics on the oxygenated and deoxygenated kinetics by NIRS. For the same O_2 demand, fast muscle O_2 delivery slows both oxygenated and deoxygenated kinetics. An imbalance between muscle O_2 delivery and utilization rate kinetics is responsible for the observed trend. Hb and Mb contributions (y_{HbO2}, y_{MbO2}) to the $HbMbO_2$ at rest and during contraction differ from those (y_{HHb}, y_{HMb}) to the $HHbMb$. The effect of blood flow kinetics on y_{HbO2} and y_{MbO2} kinetics was minimal, while that on y_{HHb} and y_{HMb} determined overshoots and undershoots.

Simulations predict that in the presence of fast blood flow kinetics, an abundant muscle O_2 delivery in relation to its utilization (Fig. 58.1d) is the main cause for slow muscle oxygenation and deoxygenation responses to contraction. To further establish the relationship between blood flow and NIRS kinetics, model simulation shows that slow muscle O_2 delivery causes undershoots and overshoots of oxygenated and deoxygenated kinetics, respectively (Fig. 58.1e).

At rest, the contribution of Hb and Mb (y_{HbO2} and y_{MbO2}) to the oxygenated heme groups is similar (Fig. 58.1e). These contributions depend on heme concentration in the vascular and extravascular domains and on their volume fractions (Table 58.1). Thus, high heme concentration in blood domains with low volume fraction (<5%) or low heme concentration in tissue domain with high f_{tis} (95%) resulted in a similar concentration of oxygenated heme group in muscle. The Hb contribution to the deoxygenated signal is higher than that of Mb. This is mainly related to the O_2 saturation of Hb (predominately in venous blood, 89%) compared to Mb (96.2%) that leads to a higher HHb than HMb (Table 58.1).

At the onset of contraction, the abrupt increase of y_{HbO2} and y_{HHb} observed for both bouts 1 and 2 (Fig. 58.1e) is due to the increase in blood volume detected by NIRS measurement (Fig. 58.1a). This is quantified by the model with an increase of the vascular fraction f_{bl} (Fig.58.1b). The size of the microvascular and extravascular volume fractions determines the amplitude of the changes in Hb and Mb contributions to the NIRS signal. During contraction, the Hb and Mb kinetics are affected by the interplay between O_2 delivery (convection and diffusion) and utilization. An impaired O_2 delivery represented by slow blood flow kinetics was associated to a slow y_{MbO2} and fast y_{HMb} kinetics during the first 20s of muscle contraction. Under this condition, the deoxygenation rate in tissue was faster than that in blood domain. Tissue oxygenation increased only when the O_2 delivery was enough to balance the O_2 utilization.

In conclusion, the contribution of Mb to the NIRS signals is significant. This is consistent with other experimental [2] and computational studies [6, 8]. Quantitative analysis indicates that oxygenated and deoxygenated kinetics are similarly affected by blood flow kinetics in the absence of confounding factor as blood flow to the skin. Hb and Mb contributions to the oxygenated and deoxygenated heme groups significantly changes with O_2 delivery. These contributions are relevant in the interpretation of NIRS signal used to evaluate chronic disease in which O_2 delivery is impaired. Approaches that combines NIRS with model simulation and devices quantifying hemodynamic and microvascular distribution can help to overcome NIRS inability to distinguish Hb/Mb contributions.

Acknowledgments Supported in part by the Department of Electrical and Computer Engineering of Old Dominion University and grant from the National Institute of Arthritis and Musculoskeletal and Skin Diseases (NIH-NIAMS) - K25AR057206.

References

1. Grassi B, Quaresima V (2016) Near-infrared spectroscopy and skeletal muscle oxidative function in vivo in health and disease: a review from an exercise physiology perspective. J Biomed Opt 21(9):091313
2. Davis ML, Barstow TJ (2013) Estimated contribution of hemoglobin and myoglobin to near infrared spectroscopy. Respir Physiol Neurobiol 186:180–187
3. Grassi B, Pogliaghi S, Rampichini S, Quaresima V, Ferrari M, Marconi C, Cerretelli P (2003) Muscle oxygenation and pulmonary gas exchange kinetics during cycling exercise on-transitions in humans. J Appl Physiol (1985) 95(1):149–158
4. Hernández A, McDonald JR, Lai N, Gladden LB (2010) A prior bout of contractions speeds VO_2 and blood flow on-kinetics and reduces the VO_2 slow-component amplitude in canine skeletal muscle contracting in situ. J Appl Physiol 108:1169–1176
5. Lai N, Saidel GM, Grassi B, Gladden LB, Cabrera ME (2007) Model of oxygen transport and metabolism predicts effect of hyperoxia on canine muscle oxygen uptake dynamics. J Appl Physiol (1985) 103(4):1366–1378
6. Lai N, Zhou H, Saidel GM, Wolf M, McCully K, Gladden LB, Cabrera ME (2009) Modeling oxygenation in venous blood and skeletal muscle in response to exercise using near-infrared spectroscopy. J Appl Physiol (1985) 106(6):1858–1874
7. Spires J, Gladden LB, Grassi B, Goodwin ML, Saidel GM, Lai N (2013) Distinguishing the effects of convective and diffusive O_2 delivery on VO_2 on-kinetics in skeletal muscle contracting at moderate intensity. Am J Physiol Regul Integr Comp Physiol 305(5):R512–R521
8. Spires J, Lai N, Zhou H, Saidel GM (2011) Hemoglobin and myoglobin contributions to skeletal muscle oxygenation in response to exercise. Adv Exp Med Biol 701:347–352

Magnetoresistance Properties of Red Blood Cells in Plasma Combined with Several Magnetic Beads Passing Two Cu Electrodes

59

Jong-Gu Choi, Byeong-Uk Kang, and Sang-Suk Lee

Abstract

In recent years, research has been intensively carried out on the applicability of magnetic beads (MBs) and magnetic nanoparticles coupled to biological objects such as red blood cells (RBCs). The magnetoresistance (MR) of a solution of RBCs and MBs (RBCs+MBs) was evaluated when MBs migrated in the presence or absence of an external magnetic field. The pattern of distribution of the MBs, which were homogeneously suspended in deionized distilled water, varied depending on the magnitude of the external magnetic field applied between the Cu electrodes connected to the two terminals. As the magnitude of the external magnetic field is increased or decreased, MBs are split on both sides and evenly mixed, respectively. The ratios (ΔMR/MR) versus an external magnetic field for the solutions of only MBs and a mixed RBCs+MBs were −33.4% and −27.4% at ±30 Oe and ±46 Oe of coercive fields, respectively. These results show that a solution of RBCs+MBs can act like a high-resolution biosensor that detects the oxygenation state of RBCs.

Keywords

Magnetic bead (MB) · Red blood cell combined with magnetic beads (RBC+MBs) · Deionized distilled water (ddH_2O) · Magnetoresistance (MR) curve

59.1 Introduction

Oxyhemoglobin and deoxyhemoglobin in the red blood cell (RBCs) are diamagnetic and paramagnetic, respectively, and those show very weakly behavior even in the strong magnetic field. In addition, the RBCs have a normal circular membrane, and the oxygen deficiency causes the RBCs of the abnormally ellipsoidal membrane to be combined with the magnetic beads (MBs). Therefore, studying the characteristics of the RBCs combined with MBs (RBCs+MBs) in response to the magnetic properties will provide information about the oxygen state of the blood. MBs can be used to analyze specific molecular species that selectively react by combining biological cognitive systems and physicochemical signal transducers [1]. MBs are approximately 1 μm in diameter and can be detected at their target location by using a magnetoresistance (MR) sensor. Thus, they can be used to develop a high-resolution nanobiosensor with magnetic separation properties and enough sensitivity to measure

J.-G. Choi · B.-U. Kang · S.-S. Lee (✉)
Department of Oriental Biomedical Engineering, College of Health Sciences, Sangji University, Wonju, Republic of Korea
e-mail: sslee@sangji.ac.kr

E. M. Nemoto et al. (eds.), *Oxygen Transport to Tissue XLII*, Advances in Experimental Medicine and Biology 1269, https://doi.org/10.1007/978-3-030-48238-1_59

the signal from a single MB [2]. In particular, a technique for removing offset signals caused by self-resistance has been reported when measuring a weak MB signal, using a planar Hall sensor [3].

The core of MBs consists of magnetite (Fe_3O_4), which is applied as nanoparticles in cancer research [4]. MBs will offer a different surface charge and charge distribution which will influence their binding property to DNA, RNA, and proteins. This property of MBs can be applied to methods such as purification, biomolecule adsorption, and protein separation [5]. The RBCs were combined with MBs in such a way that 7–9 MBs were positioned in the center part or at the edge part of one RBC by organic chemical binding [6]. In one study, the characteristics of deformed RBC membranes (containing Fe-hemoglobin) were analyzed by the giant magnetoresistance-spin valve (GMR-SV) device, which is a highly sensitive magnetic sensor [7]. In this study, we investigated the MR of a suspension of RBCs+MBs in deionized distilled water (ddH_2O), by applying an external magnetic field.

59.2 Materials and Methods

MBs used in this study are SiMAG-Silanol (Si-OH) from chemicell GmbH (Berlin, Germany) and have a negatively charged silica surface. The average diameters of MBs and RBCs are about 1 μm and 7 μm, respectively [8]. MBs with a Fe_3O_4 core are suspended at a concentration of 50 mg/ml in 2.5 ml of autoclaved ddH_2O [8]. The human RBCs used in this study have been obtained from normal plasma and have not undergone centrifugation. Two copper wires with a diameter of 1 mm and a separated distance of 3 mm were used for the two electrodes, which were installed at the center lower half position of a micro-centrifuge tube of 1.5 ml with a diameter of 8.0 mm that contained 1.2 ml blood and 0.3 ml MB solution, as shown in Fig. 59.1a. Thus, the total volume of the solution was 1.5 ml, and the concentration ratio was 4:1. The RBCs in plasma show sedimented solids over time, as shown in Fig. 59.1c. Figure 59.1b, d shows the even distribution of MBs and RBCs+MBs after manually inverting the tubes to mix the contents evenly. The resistance values change based on the distribution area of the RBCs+MBs when the magnetic field is applied with respect to resistance measurement geometry parallel to two Cu-wire electrodes.

The MR ratio obtained by changing the resistance values as the MBs move is shown in Fig. 59.2. The middle panel of Fig. 59.2 is a digital multimeter (DMM) that measures resistance by connecting the Cu electrode to the two terminals. The RBCs+MBs in the tube moved either left or right, according to the magnetic field. A two-probe MR measurement system is used at up to ±1200 Oe to observe the change in resistance values in the external magnetic field when passing through the channel between the two Cu electrodes.

The instrument is a Keithley 197 Autoranging Microvolt DMM that can be connected to two or four terminals to measure multiple resistance values simultaneously. The resistance measurement is DC-based for two terminals, and the current of the electromagnet generating the external magnetic field is also DC-based. The external magnetic field changes slowly (with frequency in milli Hz range) from +1200 Oe to −1200 Oe and returns to +1200 Oe during one cycle. To obtain the MR curve, as shown in the right panel of Fig. 59.2, where resistance values change with the motion of the MBs, an electromagnetic coil, 150 mm in diameter, was placed so that an external magnetic field could be applied uniformly, as shown in the left panel of Fig. 59.2.

The applied external magnetic field holds the tube containing RBCs with MBs solution horizontally, and the measurement range is ±1200 Oe with a major MR curve. The coercivity (H_c) and MR ratio (%) obtained from the MR curve were investigated by increasing the sweeping frequency to 0.7 mHz (10^{-3} Hz), 3.7 mHz, and 10.7 mHz [9].

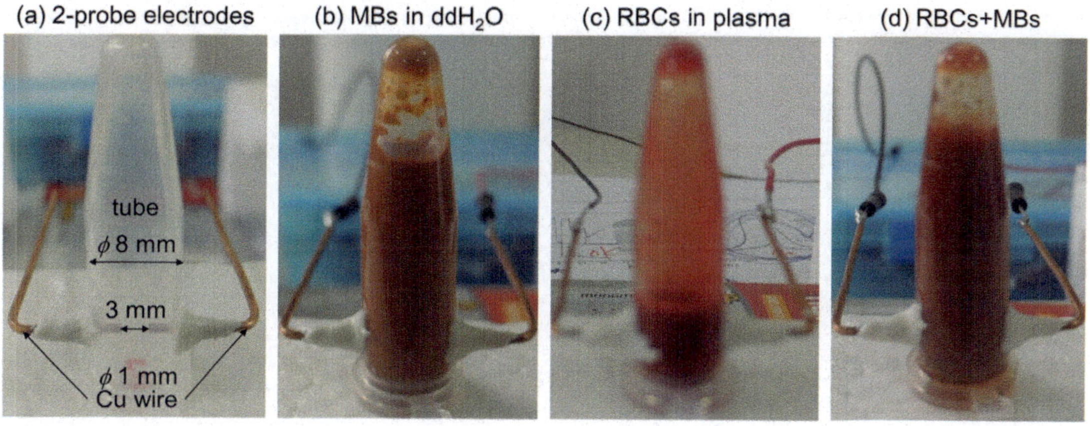

Fig. 59.1 The photographs for three different status contained of RBCs and MBs: (**a**) 2-probe Cu electrodes and vacant tube, (**b**) evenly mixed MBs in ddH_2O, (**c**) only pure RBCs in plasma, and (**d**) RBCs combined with MBs evenly in all volume of tube

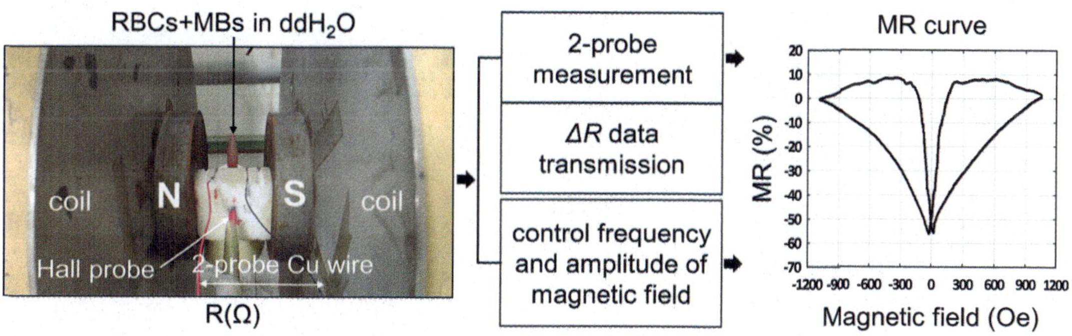

Fig. 59.2 Schematic of 2-probe MR measurement system with a control frequency and amplitude of magnetic field for RBCs in plasma combined with MBs immersed in ddH_2O

59.3 Experimental Results and Discussion

MBs are superparamagnetic and very sensitive to external magnetic fields. The schematic diagram of the reaction of a RBCs+MBs solution in the cylindrical tube according to the three types of external magnetic field intensity is shown in Fig. 59.3. Figure 59.3a shows one state where RBCs+MBs are balanced evenly when no external magnetic field is applied. Depending on the magnitude of the external magnetic field, RBCs+MBs cluster on opposite walls of the tube and are separated from each other. As the magnitude of the external magnetic field increases, MBs move farther toward the sides [10]. The area without MBs is much larger as shown in Fig. 59.3c than Fig. 59.3b. MBs are separated from each other by moving between the two terminals of the Cu electrodes; therefore, the difference in the area occupied by blood plasma and ddH_2O is expected to change the resistance value.

Figure 59.4 shows the MR curves for the solution of MBs in ddH2O, measured by Cu electrodes connected to the two terminals, under an the external magnetic field with a range of ±1200 Oe and frequency of 3.7 mHz. When the external magnetic field range was ±1200 Oe, the MR ratio was negative. The MR curve starts at +1200 Oe and goes beyond 0 Oe to −1200 Oe and again from −1200 Oe to 0 Oe for 270s at 3.7 mHz. Depending on the MR ratio measured

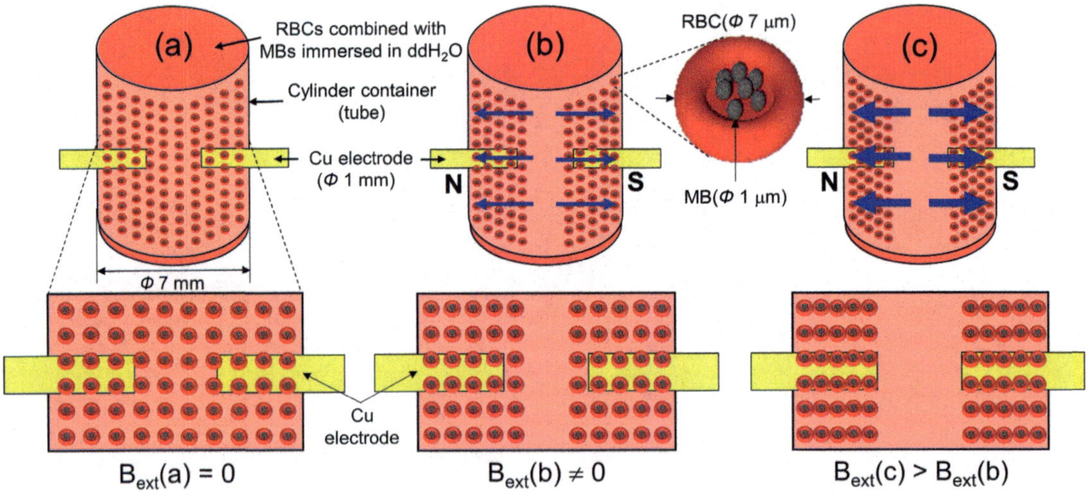

Fig. 59.3 The different three distributed status of RBCs in plasma and MBs in ddH_2O inside of cylinder container with two Cu electrodes: (**a**) $B_{ext} = 0$, (**b**) $B_{ext} \neq 0$, and (**c**) $B_{ext}(c) > B_{ext}(b) \neq 0$ applied the external magnetic field used by the electromagnet

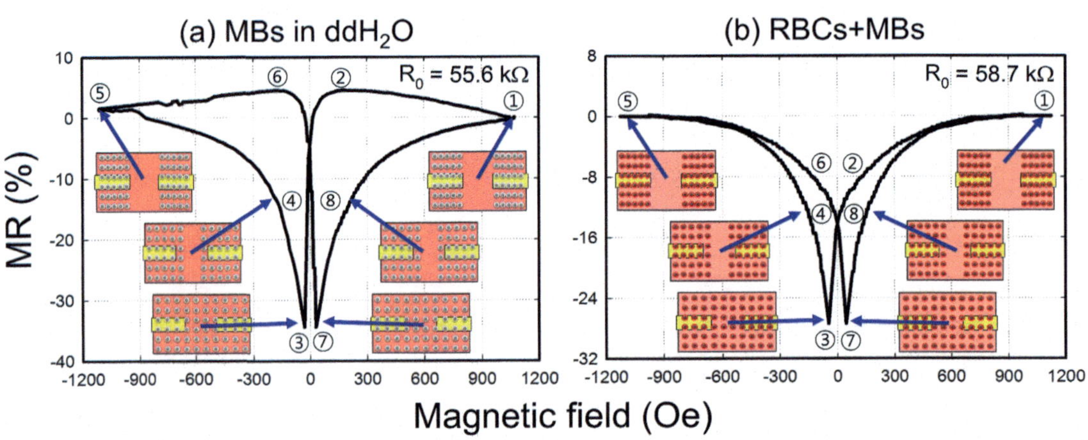

Fig. 59.4 MR curves for (**a**) only MBs and (**b**) mixed RBCs+MBs in ddH_2O inside of cylinder container according to different distributed status with a sweeping step order of +1200 Oe → 0 Oe → −1200 Oe → 0 Oe → +1200 Oe corresponding to one cycle of ①→②→③→④→⑤→⑥→⑦→⑧→①

while an external magnetic field is applied, the changed results are shown in Fig. 59.4a.

MBs were significantly separated by clustering to two sides between the Cu electrodes connected to the two terminals. At the magnetic field of 1200 Oe, the resistance value was 55.6 kΩ. Subsequently, the resistance value gradually decreased to −30 Oe beyond the region of 0 Oe. In the second step, MBs between the two electrodes connected to Cu were distributed evenly, and the resistance value was 37.0 kΩ. As shown in the MR curve of Fig. 59.4a, H_c is approximately ±30 Oe, and the MR ratio is −33.4%. It is a large MR ratio having the hysteresis property which allows MBs to be distributed evenly between two Cu electrodes, as shown in Fig. 59.3a.

The MR curve for RBCs+MBs solution in Fig. 59.4b compared to 59.4a shows the MR ratio decreased by about 6%, but the value of H_c was significantly different. Here, H_c is approximately ±46 Oe, which corresponds to the hysteresis curve, and the MR ratio is −27.4%. The MR curves observed at different frequencies show that the MR ratio decreases as the frequency increases to 10.7 mHz. As a result, hysteresis might have been induced by the balance and distribution of MBs coupled to RBCs.

To obtain the MR curve shown in Fig. 59.4b, MBs coupled to RBCs are moved into the solution in the tube that is placed between the Cu electrodes connected to the two terminals, corresponding to the stages during one cycle. This phenomenon is similar to that shown in the MR curve with a GMR-SV, which corresponds to the magnetized spin array in a multilayer structure [7]. When the magnetized spin arrays of ferromagnetic materials, which form pinned and free layers in a multilayer structure, are in parallel and in antiparallel states, the device shows (due to the spin-dependent scattering effect) minimum and maximum resistance values. This result shows the possibility of detecting the oxygenated states of the hemoglobin using MR measurements.

59.4 Conclusions

MBs with surface silanol groups (Si-OH) on Fe_3O_4 and a human RBC have average diameters of approximately 1 μm and 7 μm, respectively. The states of RBCs+MBs passing through a channel between the two Cu electrodes are differentially distributed when an external magnetic field of ±1200 Oe is applied to the cylindrical tube containing RBCs in plasma combined with MBs in distilled water. The maximum MR ratio obtained from MR curve was about −27.4% with coercive field ±46 Oe for 3.7 mHz external magnetic field. The distribution of MBs coupled with RBCs is affected by a small variation of the external magnetic field. This result suggests the possibility to develop a biosensor of detecting the oxygenated states of the hemoglobin using MR measurements using a solution of RBCs+MBs.

Acknowledgments This paper is the result of a study which was funded by the Sangji University Research Program.

References

1. Johansen PL, Fenaroli F, Evensen L, Griffiths G, Koster G (2016) Optical micromanipulation of nanoparticles and cells inside living zebrafish. Nat Commun 7:10974, 1–10974, 8
2. Parkin SS, Kaiser C, Panchula A et al (2004) Giant tunneling magnetoresistance at room temperature with MgO (100) tunnel barriers. Nat Mat 3:862–867
3. Kim H, Reddy V, Kim KW et al (2014) Single magnetic bead detection in a microfluidic chip using planar hall effect sensor. J Magnetics 19:10–14
4. Wang X, Zhang R, Wu C, Dai Y, Song M, Gutmann S, Gao F, Lv G, Li J, Li X, Guan Z, Fu D, Chen B (2007) The application of Fe_3O_4 nanoparticles in cancer research: a new strategy to inhibit drug resistance. J Biomed Mater Res 80A:852–860
5. Neumann J, Brinkmann R (2005) Boiling nucleation on melanosomes and microbeads transiently heated by nanosecond and microsecond laser pulses. J Biomed Optics 10:024001–024012
6. Choi JG, Kim SH, Lee SS (2018) Use of a turn coil and channel above a GMR-SV device to observe and measure the properties of deoxidized red blood cells coupled to magnetic beads. Adv Exp Med Bio 1072:345–349
7. Bento D, Rodrigues RO, Faustino V et al (2018) Deformation of red blood cells, air bubbles, and droplets in microfluidic devices. Micromachines 9:151–169
8. http://www.chemicell.com/products/microparticles/simag-basic/index.html
9. Choi JG, Jung HM, Lee SS (2017) Fabrication and usage of a multi-turn μ-coil and a PR channel combined with a dual-type GMR-SV device. J Magnetics 22:649–653
10. Choi JG, Kang BU, Lee SS (2019) Magnetic resistance characteristics depending on magnetic field of magnetic bead solution in deionized distilled water. J Korean Magn Soc 29:123–128

Measurement of Tissue Oxygen as a Novel Approach to Optimizing Red Blood Cell Quality Assessment

60

Paul W. Buehler, Ann Barry Flood, and Harold M. Swartz

Abstract

The effectiveness of blood transfusions can be impacted by storage and extensive processing techniques that involve treatment of red blood cells (RBCs) with pathogen reduction technologies (e.g., UV-light and chemical treatment), ex vivo stem cell derivation/maturation methods, and bioengineering of RBCs using nanotechnology. Therefore, there is a need to have methods that assess the evaluation of the effectiveness of transfusions to achieve their intended purpose: to increase oxygenation of critical tissues. Consequently, there has been intense interest in the development of techniques targeted at optimizing the assessment of RBC quality in preclinical and clinical settings. We provide a critical assessment of the ability of currently used methods to provide unambiguous information on oxygen levels in tissues and conclude that they cannot do this. This is because they are based on surrogates for the true goal of transfusion, which is to increase oxygenation of critical organs. This does not mean that they are valueless, but it does indicate that other methods are needed to provide direct measurements of oxygen in tissues. We report here on the initial results of a method that can provide direct assessment of the impact of the transfusion on tissue oxygen: EPR oximetry. It has the potential to provide such information in both preclinical and clinical settings for the assessment of blood quality posttransfusion.

Keywords

Red blood cell transfusion · Tissue oxygen measurements · Electron paramagnetic resonance (EPR) oximetry · Preclinical study

60.1 Introduction

Variability in the quality of donor blood (red blood cells [RBCs] and blood components [platelets, white blood cells, and plasma]) is inevitable, due to the impact of the donor's genetics, gender, diet, drug therapy, environmental exposures, and

P. W. Buehler (✉)
Department of Pathology, Department of Pediatrics, Center for Blood Oxygen Transport and Hemostasis, University of Maryland School of Medicine, Baltimore, MD, USA
e-mail: pbuehler@som.umaryland.edu

A. B. Flood
Radiology, Geisel School of Medicine at Dartmouth College, Hanover, NH, USA

H. M. Swartz
Radiology, Geisel School of Medicine at Dartmouth College, Hanover, NH, USA

Radiation Oncology, Dartmouth-Hitchcock Medical Center, Lebanon, NH, USA

E. M. Nemoto et al. (eds.), *Oxygen Transport to Tissue XLII*, Advances in Experimental Medicine and Biology 1269, https://doi.org/10.1007/978-3-030-48238-1_60

disease states. These are among the factors that affect posttransfusion effective circulation time (for transfused RBCs), clotting function (for transfused platelets and plasma), and attenuation of infection (for transfused white blood cells).

Additionally, most whole blood and derivatives of whole blood undergo processing and storage prior to administration to patients. While current criteria for storage specify factors such as temperature and length of storage, there is a well-recognized need to extend the period of time that blood can be safely and effectively utilized. Numerous preclinical and clinical studies suggest that processing and storage conditions can impact the clinical effectiveness of transfusions [1]. Consequently, whole blood and RBC processing techniques have advanced to include more extensive methodologies beyond that of testing additive preservation solutions for storage (e.g., anticoagulant/preservative solutions: AS-1, AS-3, AS-5, CDPA-1). Innovative techniques can involve processing of donor blood and RBCs using novel storage conditions (e.g., anaerobic storage under Argon gas) and pathogen reduction technologies that apply ultraviolet (UV) light and/or chemical treatment to reduce the risk of transfusion transmitted disease. Further, new RBCs are being developed for universal transfusion, obviating the need for blood typing. Approaches to developing novel RBCs include maturation from progenitor cells (stem cell-derived RBCs) and the bioengineering of synthetic RBCs (nanoparticle-based biomaterials).

The US Food and Drug Administration's (FDA) current acceptance criteria for investigational RBC products apply to the evaluation of collection systems, processing, storage devices, anticoagulants, and additive solutions that effect RBC integrity. Tests used to qualify investigational RBC products are performed on the day of collection, pre- and post-processing, and at the proposed expiration date (e.g., 42 days for RBC units) at two independent laboratories using in vitro tests to assess the concentration of some RBC metabolites (e.g., adenosine triphosphate and 2,3-diphosphoglycerate [2,3-DPG]). In vitro testing also includes the accurate documentation of total and extracellular "free" hemoglobin levels to determine percent hemolysis, which must not exceed 1% with 95% confidence that 95% of the product meets or exceeds this expectation.

Currently, in vivo testing primarily involves the 24-hour posttransfusion recovery (PTR) of autologous transfused chromium-51-labeled RBCs. PTR is conducted in at least 20 volunteers performed by two laboratories. The expectation for 24-hour recovery is that the mean number of chromium-51-labeled transfused cells remaining in circulation is ≥75% of the total RBCs transfused. While PTR is currently the standard for the evaluation of RBC quality within the context of processing and storage, some have challenged the criteria and have demonstrated that PTR can be influenced by factors such as blood donor differences, volume of RBC infused, and disease state [2–4]. Extensively processed RBC products such as RBCs exposed to pathogen reduction technologies (e.g., UV-light and chemical treatment) typically involve more extensive evaluation. This may include conduct of immunogenicity studies and later phase clinical trials in patients requiring RBC transfusions to demonstrate both efficacy and safety of novel RBC products compared to predicate donor cells.

Thesis of this paper: Underlying these criteria and studies is the universally agreed-upon purpose of transfusing RBCs in patients with extensive blood loss: to provide oxygen to the tissues in a timely and effective manner. Therefore, direct in vivo measurement of *tissue oxygenation* to evaluate RBC quality may offer advantages to better assess the effectiveness of storage conditions, improve the understanding of the effect of more advanced processing, and ultimately monitor tissue oxygenation to make decisions on the optimization of blood transfusion.

In October 2016, the US FDA, Department of Defence, and the National Institutes of Health (NIH) held a workshop on new red blood cell product regulatory science [5]. While several topics of interest were covered, a central and important theme was the use and interpretation of measurements of tissue oxygen in preclinical and clinical evaluation of novel blood products.

Subsequently, in April 2018, the NIH held a related public workshop entitled Toward

Minimally Invasive or Noninvasive Approaches to Assess Tissue Oxygenation Pre- and Posttransfusion [6]. This workshop focused entirely on techniques to evaluate tissue oxygen to determine the need for and effectiveness of blood transfusions. Techniques presented and discussed included phosphorescence quenching, blood oxygen-dependent magnetic resonance imaging (BOLD-MRI), and photoacoustic tomography as well as electron paramagnetic resonance (EPR) oximetry.

The timing and substance of these workshops suggests an interest in incorporating measurements of tissue oxygenation into the evaluation and understanding of blood quality and transfusion effectiveness. Here we summarize our evaluation of the ability of various techniques in current use to provide direct measurements of oxygen in tissue. Further, we discuss the initial proof of concept to directly measure oxygen partial pressure (pO_2) by EPR oximetry in muscle tissue following transfusion of differing quality RBC preparations.

60.2 Overview of Methods to Measure Oxygen in Tissues to Assess the Efficacy of RBC Preparations

Several methods have been used to assess transfusion efficacy in clinical settings to provide a measure of general tissue oxygenation of various organs. Those that have been frequently applied in animals and/or humans include nitroimidazole hypoxic markers [7], BOLD MRI [8, 9], MRI perfusion/diffusion [10], hypoxia molecule detection [5], positron emission tomography [11], phosphorescence quenching [12], *n*ear-*i*nfra*r*ed *s*pectroscopy (NIRS) [13, 14], and blood gas analysis [15]. These will be briefly compared and contrasted in the context of their potential usefulness for assessing transfusion efficacy.

The analysis of the suitability of techniques to provide assessment of tissue oxygen can be conveniently viewed by considering the parameters that are being measured and their direct/indirect relationship to assessing oxygen in various tissues. These are (1) direct measurements of oxygen in the blood/circulatory system, (2) indirect measurements of oxygen in muscle and other tissues that are potential surrogates for direct measurements, and (3) direct measures of oxygen in muscle and other tissues [16].

Direct measurements of oxygen in the blood/circulatory system: Techniques that directly measure oxygen in the blood/circulatory system are based on measurements in the capillary and peripheral arterial/venous compartments of hemoglobin (Hb), O_2 saturation (SpO_2), and/or total hemoglobin [17]. The techniques usually use NIRS, but direct measurements of blood gases are also possible.

While these techniques assess oxygen in blood, neither NIRS nor blood gas techniques provide direct pO_2measurements in tissues. Instead, they assess the supply of oxygen before it diffuses into and is consumed by tissues. However, assuming the goal is assessing whether transfusions result in increasing oxygen in vulnerable tissues, there are many possible sources of variation that preclude going reliably from knowing the level of oxygen in the circulation to knowing the level of oxygen in the tissues. While translation of SpO_2measurements to the effective off-loading of O_2 from RBC Hb and myoglobin within localized tissue sites is critical to understanding O_2 delivery and the processes that maintain or restore O_2 homeostasis, without more direct information on tissue oxygen it remains poorly defined.

The widely available technique BOLD MRI sometimes is thought to be another method to measure oxygen in the circulatory system, but actually it only measures total deoxyhemoglobin in large vessels. However, without a simultaneous measure of total hemoglobin, it is not possible to calculate the oxygen tension in the vascular compartment with this method. Even relative changes in BOLD do not necessarily provide information on oxygen changes in the vascular system. Two unaccounted for factors are critical to the utility of BOLD to estimate oxygen levels: (1) the amount of deoxyhemoglobin, which reflects the oxygen levels in the blood, and (2) the volume of blood contained within the physiologic system that is being evaluated.

The other methods noted above do not measure oxygen directly but instead measure parameters that are related indirectly to the actual levels of oxygen except for some uses of phosphorescent quenching. The use of "hypoxic cell markers" such as nitroimidazole hypoxic markers [7] indicates the amount of marker that is retained in the tissues at the time that the marker is administered. But this process depends on many factors including blood flow, rate of reduction by the enzymes that produce the reactive intermediate that can bind to cells, the oxygen tension, and washout. It usually is not possible to know all of these parameters, and even if one could, the results give only a one-time picture of a very dynamic process.

MRI perfusion/diffusion [10] measurement provides important information on the dynamics of the functions of the vascular systems but in themselves has no clear quantitative relationship to the actual oxygen levels in the tissues.

There are several techniques that utilize positron emission tomography [7] to measure intermediates such as glucose analogs or hypoxic cell markers whose uptake is influenced by tissue oxygen levels. However, there is no straightforward relationship, due to the many variables that can affect localization such as perfusion, washout, and tissue binding.

There are also a number of molecular markers such as HIF-1α, whose quantity is affected by oxygen. Again, the relationship is not straightforward because of their dependency on a number of other processes in addition to the amount of oxygen.

There are some methods that can directly measure O_2 within tissue sites. Those that can make repeated measurements are likely to be most useful, because the processes of interest are dynamic, and time-dependent changes are probably the most useful parameters for evaluating the adequacy of the oxygenation provided by RBC transfusions. The most widely used technique clinically was the oxygen electrode [18], but it is no longer available for clinical use. Additionally, because of its invasive nature, it could not be used for repeated measurements.

In preclinical studies, the use of techniques based on fluorescence quenching of oxygen (OxyLite) is demonstrated, and the OxyLite technique has been used fairly widely [19]. However, like the oxygen electrode, it is invasive for long-term repeated measurements and has not advanced into clinical use.

Some oxygen-dependent NMR relaxation techniques using molecules whose relaxation rate is directly proportional to oxygen have been suggested, especially based on fluorine-containing hydrocarbons, but these also have not advanced to clinical use [20].

The most promising technique for preclinical and clinical direct measurements of oxygen may be electron paramagnetic resonance (EPR) oximetry using particulates as the oxygen sensors. This is a minimally invasive technique that directly measures oxygen and allows for continuous and repeated assessment of tissue oxygenation based on a one-time injection of O_2-sensitive biocompatible material (e.g., lithium octa-n-butoxynaphthalocyanine [LiNc-BuO] crystals encased in polydimethylsiloxane [an "OxyChip"] or suspended paramagnetic carbon particles ["India ink"]) in one or more tissues [21, 22]. This material then allows for noninvasive repetition of measurements over acute (hours) and chronic (months and years) temporal intervals. Moreover, EPR oximetry has demonstrated its broad application in proof-of-concept studies in animals, fostering drug development across a wide range of hypoxic and ischemic disorders [22–24]. The technique is uniquely applicable to clinical tissue pO_2 measurements in cancer and peripheral vascular disease [25–27]. Based on these key features, EPR oximetry provides an intriguing method for application to monitoring the efficacy of RBC transfusion in both preclinical and clinical settings [28].

60.3 EPR Measurements of Impact of RBC Preparations on Oxygen in Tissues: A Rat Blood Loss/Transfusion Experiment

The Dartmouth College Animal Care and Use Program approved the use of animals and the experimental protocol. Male Lewis rats (Charles

River Laboratory, Wilmington, MA), each weighing 300–400 g, were assigned to donor or treatment groups. The donor animals were divided into three donor groups: (1) fresh RBCs (1-day refrigerator storage) ($n = 10$ donor rats), (2) 7-day RBC refrigerator storage ($n = 10$ donor rats), and (3) 14-day RBC refrigerator storage ($n = 10$ donor rats). The transfused animals ($n = 28$) had their oxygen levels in skeletal muscle measured continuously during blood loss, transfusion, and post-transfusion using one of four treatments: (1) transfusion with fresh blood (1 day storage time RBCs, $n = 7$), (2) transfusion with blood stored for 7 days ($n = 7$), (3) transfusion with blood stored for 14 days ($n = 7$), and (4) transfusion with 5% albumin (non-oxygen carrying control group (i.e., receiving the same osmotic pressure but without RBCs), $n = 7$). All RBC recipient animals received RBCs in plasma (45% hematocrit).

Animals were anesthetized by nose-cone breathing of 2–2.5% isoflurane in 30% oxygen and standard clinical EPR probes (consisting of OxyChips, 5.0 mm × 0.6 mm) implanted in the biceps femoris (3–4 mm from the surface of the skin) of the left hind limb using an 18-G angiocatheter 5–21 day prior to EPR measurements. The synthesis and physicochemical characterization of LiNc-BuO microcrystals as well as their formulation into implantable cylindrical OxyChips have been described previously [22, 29]. OxyChips were from the same manufacturing batch and calibrated before implantation into the rat hind limb biceps femoris muscle, and the EPR spectra reflect the average pO_2 on the surface of each OxyChip. Prior to implantation, OxyChips were heat sterilized at 121 °C for 30 minutes.

Results of the study have been published in detail [30] and are reviewed briefly here. Figure 60.1 (modified from the publication) shows the muscle pO_2 as a function of time during the phases of blood loss, transfusion, and post-transfusion. Note: the data presented for fresh blood and albumin are identical in both Fig. 60.1a, b; Fig. 60.1a (7 day), b (14 day) is separated to emphasize that the patterns and magnitude for the two storage lengths are essentially identical.

As expected, when fresh blood (day 1) was used, muscle pO_2 was restored to baseline levels during transfusion (and the apparent decrease posttransfusion is not significant). Transfusions done with 7-day and 14-day old blood showed three findings: (1) tissue pO_2 for 7-day- and 14-day-old RBCs did not differ from each other; (2) however, both resulted in lower oxygen content in the muscles during both the transfusion and post-transfusion phase of the study compared to fresh blood; and (3) as expected, the use of both fresh and stored RBCs resulted in higher tissue pO_2 compared to when the control transfusion of albumin was administered.

Red blood cell metabolic changes occur during refrigerator storage [1]. Metabolic parameters such as 2,3-DPG and ATP ultimately impact red blood cell hemoglobin oxygen equilibrium and the morphology of the red cell membrane, respectively. To examine these parameters, separate in vitro experiments were performed on Lewis rat red blood cells at days 1, 7, and 14 of refrigerator storage. 2,3-DPG and ATP were normal at the start of storage (day 1). At days 7 and 14 of storage, both 2,3-DPG and ATP decreased significantly compared to day 1. 2,3-DPG and ATP were similarly decreased at days 7 and 14 compared to the start of refrigerator storage. Oxygen binding and dissociation measurements as well as electron microscopy studies of RBC morphology demonstrated nearly identical results at days 7 and 14 of refrigerator storage. Further, the in vitro observations at day 7 and day 14 were consistent with the results observed in the rat transfusion experiment, i.e., as shown in Fig. 60.1, pO_2measurements made in muscle at day 7 and day 14 were equally inferior compared to the tissue oxygenation of day 1 blood. These combined observations suggest that by day 7 both oxygen dissociation and tissue perfusion may be altered in the rat transfusion model, due to impaired allosteric oxygen off-loading at tissue sites (i.e., 2,3-DPG depletion) and by impaired flow of morphologically impaired RBCs (i.e., ATP reduction). Day 1 RBCs demonstrated normal disc morphology; however, by days 7 and 14, RBCs demonstrated echinocyte morphologies consistent with impaired blood flow [31].

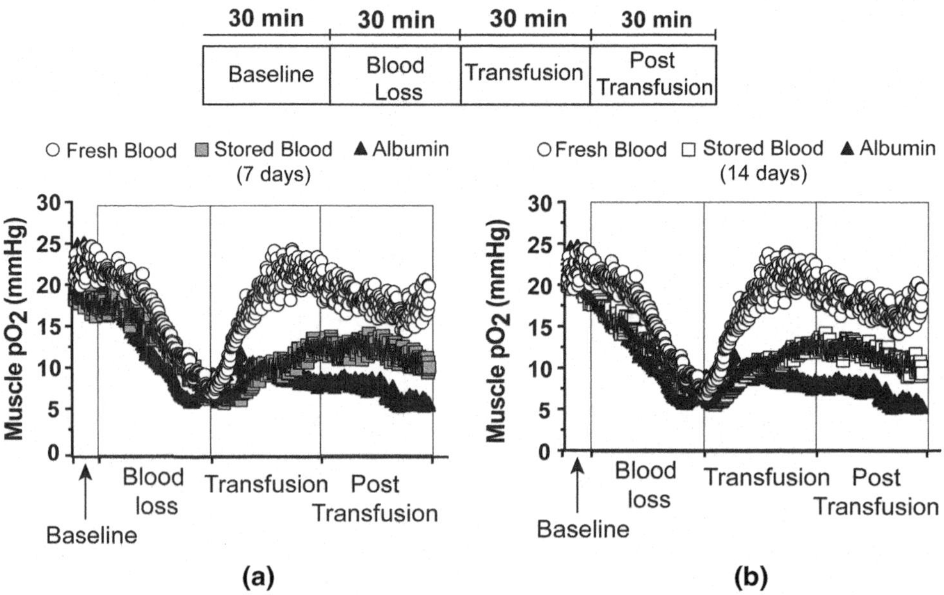

Fig. 60.1 Comparing measurements of pO_2 in rat muscle during baseline, blood loss, RBC transfusion, and post-transfusion: (**a**) (left) compares fresh blood, RBCs stored 7 days, and a control (albumin). (**b**) (right) presents the same data for fresh blood and the control but compared to RBCs stored 14 days

60.4 Discussion and Conclusions

Our initial studies in preclinical proof of concept suggest that EPR oximetry is a useful approach to detect posttransfusion tissue pO_2 differences following acute blood loss and administration of different RBC preparations in Lewis rats [30]. We expect that adapting our current normal animal model, as well as animal models involving genetic anemia, vascular disease, and hemorrhaged animals, all of which predispose animals to a basal reduction in perfusion, will be relevant to clinical situations. Additionally, EPR oximetry is available for minimally invasive clinical applications; therefore, tissue pO_2 measurements made to determine the effectiveness of transfusions are in fact feasible. Based on our preclinical proof-of-concept study, which specifically evaluated in vitro red blood cell changes under refrigerator storage and then tested tissue oxygen measurements using EPR oximetry in a Lewis rat model of blood loss and transfusion, we have defined a preclinical approach to test differences in processed blood and tissue oxygenation following transfusion. We plan to further test this approach in additional animal models (e.g., genetic anemias and polytrauma with hemorrhagic shock) where tissue oxygenation and transfusion can be more extensively scrutinized. These studies will add to the rigor and reproducibility of our existing results and further define the relevance of EPR oximetry within the context of understanding blood quality and transfusion effectiveness. Translating these findings to the application of clinical EPR in the assessment of transfusion remains the ultimate goal of this research.

As described above, there are many techniques other than EPR oximetry that are widely available for use clinically or used in preclinical models that can provide potentially clinically useful insights into the status of tissue oxygenation. However, many of these techniques only provide indirect evidence on the actual impact of transfusions on tissue oxygenation, which is an important limitation for the purposes discussed here. In this context, another potentially important role for EPR oximetry could be to provide a standard for determining the circumstances where these more indirect but more widely available techniques can provide the information needed for clinically useful decision-making. That is, by comparing these measures under specified conditions to direct measurements made by EPR, one can determine how well each indirect measure reflects the actual tissue oxygenation in circumstances relevant for assessing RBC quality for transfusion.

Acknowledgements FDA/CBER/OBRR internal funds were allocated for the EPR studies described and we would like to thank Dr. Jay Epstein for supporting these efforts. The comments and contributions of the authors are an informal communication and do not bind or obligate FDA.

Disclosure of conflicts of interest: ABF and HMS are co-owners of Clin-EPR, LLC which manufactures EPR instruments for investigational use.

References

1. Yoshida T, Prudent M, D'Alessandro A (2019) Red blood cell storage lesion: causes and potential consequences. Blood Transfus 17(1):27–52
2. Dumont LJ, AuBuchon JP (2008) Evaluation of proposed FDA criteria for the evaluation of radiolabeled red cell recovery trials. Transfusion 48(6):1053–1060
3. Francis RO, Mahajan S, Rapido F et al (2019) Re-examination of chromium-51 labeled posttransfusion red blood cell recovery method. Transfusion 59(7):2264–2275
4. Roussel C, Buffet PA, Amireault P (2018) Measuring post-transfusion recovery and survival of red blood cells: strengths and weaknesses of chromium-51 labeling and alternative methods. Front Med 15(5):130
5. Vostal JG, Buehler PW, Gelderman MP et al (2018) Proceedings of the Food and Drug Administration's public workshop on new red blood cell product regulatory science 2016. Transfusion 58(1):255–266
6. National Institutes of Health (2018) Towards minimally-invasive or non-invasive approaches to assess tissue oxygenation pre- and post-transfusion workshop 2018, April 23–24, Neuroscience Center, Bethesda. https://www.nhlbi.nih.gov/events/2018/tissue-oxygenation-workshop. Last Accessed 10 Nov 2019
7. Parliament MB, Wiebe LI, Franko AJ (1992) Nitroimidazole adducts as markers for tissue hypoxia: mechanistic studies in aerobic normal tissues and tumour cells. Br J Cancer 66:1103–1108
8. Jacobi B, Bongartz G, Partovi S et al (2012) Skeletal muscle BOLD MRI: from underlying physiological concepts to its usefulness in clinical conditions. J Magn Reson Imaging 35:1253–1265
9. Stacy MR, Caracciolo CM, Qiu M et al (2016) Comparison of regional skeletal muscle tissue oxygenation in college athletes and sedentary control subjects using quantitative BOLD MR imaging. Physiol Rep 4(16):e12903
10. Duong TQ (2013) Magnetic resonance imaging of perfusion-diffusion mismatch in rodent and non-human primate stroke models. Neurol Res 35:465–469
11. Rojas-Quijano FA, Tircso G, Tircsone Benyo E et al (2012) Synthesis and characterization of a hypoxia-sensitive MRI probe. Chem 18:9669–9676
12. Ferguson SK, Harral JW, Pak DI et al (2018) Impact of cell-free hemoglobin on contracting skeletal muscle microvascular oxygen pressure dynamics. Nitric Oxide 76:29–36
13. Dhabangi A, Ainomugisha B, Cserti-Gazdewich C et al (2016) Cerebral oximetry in ugandan children with severe anemia: clinical categories and response to transfusion. JAMA Pediatr 170:995–1002
14. Podbregar M, Gavric AU, Podbregar E et al (2016) Red blood cell transfusion and skeletal muscle tissue oxygenation in anaemic haematologic outpatients. Radiol Oncol 50:449–455
15. Vallet B, Robin E, Lebuffe G (2010) Venous oxygen saturation as a physiologic transfusion trigger. Crit Care 14:213
16. Springett R, Swartz HM (2007) Measurements of oxygen *in vivo*: overview and perspectives on methods to measure oxygen within cells and tissues. Antioxid Redox Signal 9(8):1295–1301
17. Ostojic D, Kleiser S, Nasseri N et al (2018) Hemoglobin spectra affect measurement of tissue oxygen saturation. In: Raghavachari R, Liang R (eds) SPIE BiOS. SPIE Digital Library, San Francisco, pp 1–6
18. Vaupel P, Mayer A, Höckel M (2004) Tumor hypoxia and malignant progression. Methods Enzymol 381:335–354
19. Braun RD, Lanzen JL, Snyder SA et al (2001) Comparison of tumor and normal tissue oxygen tension measurements using OxyLite or microelectrodes in rodents. Am J Physiol Heart Circ Physiol 280:H2533–H2544
20. Mason RP, Zhao D, Pacheco-Torres J et al (2010) Multimodality imaging of hypoxia in preclinical settings Q. J Nucl Med Mol Imaging 54:259–280
21. Flood AB, Wood VA, Swartz HM (2017) Using India ink as a sensor for oximetry: evidence of its safety as a medical device. Adv Exp Med Biol 977:297–312
22. Hou H, Khan N, Nagane M et al (2016) Skeletal muscle oxygenation measured by EPR oximetry using a highly sensitive polymer-encapsulated paramagnetic sensor. Adv Exp Med Biol 923:351–357
23. Khan N, Hou H, Swartz HM et al (2015) Direct and repeated measurement of heart and brain oxygenation using in vivo EPR oximetry. Methods Enzymol 564:529–552
24. Hou H, Krishnamurthy Nemani V, Du G et al (2015) Monitoring oxygen levels in orthotopic human glioma xenograft following carbogen inhalation and chemotherapy by implantable resonator-based oximetry. Int J Cancer 136:1688–1696

25. Swartz HM, Williams BB, Jarvis LA et al (2013) Repeated monitoring of tumor oxygen while breathing carbogen to determine the therapeutic potential of hyperoxic therapy. Pract Radiat Oncol 3:S23–S24
26. Swartz HM, Hou H, Khan N et al (2014) Advances in probes and methods for clinical EPR oximetry. Adv Exp Med Biol 812:73–79
27. Williams BB, Hou H, Coombs R et al (2016) EPR oximetry for investigation of hyperbaric O_2 pretreatment for tumor radiosensitization. Adv Exp Med Biol 923:367–374
28. Swartz HM, Williams BB, Zaki BI et al (2014) Clinical EPR: unique opportunities and some challenges. Acad Radiol 21:197–206
29. Pandian RP, Parinandi NL, Ilangovan G et al (2003) Novel particulate spin probe for targeted determination of oxygen in cells and tissues. Free Radic Biol Med 35:1138–1148
30. Hou H, Baek JH, Zhang H et al (2019) Electron paramagnetic resonance oximetry as a novel approach to measure the effectiveness and quality of red blood cell transfusions. Blood Transfus 17(4):296–306
31. Lim HWG, Wortis M, Mukhopadhyay R (2002) Stomatocyte-discocyte-echinocyte sequence of the human red blood cell: evidence for the bilayer- couple hypothesis from membrane mechanics. Proc Natl Acad Sci U S A 99(26):16766–16769

Gene Expression of *Prox-1* and *Hif-1a* in Primo Vessels Inside Lymph Vessels of the Rabbit

61

Jun-Young Shin, Jong-Gu Choi, Sungchul Shin, Sujung Yeo, and Sang-Suk Lee

Abstract

The gene expression of *Prox-1* and *Hif-1a* for the isolated primo vessels (PVs) and composite lymphatic vessels (LVs) containing PVs (LVs + PVs) was investigated by RNA-sequencing (Seq) and quantitative polymerase chain reaction (qRT-PCR) analysis. RNA-Seq on the passed 10 samples on RNA-QC for two experimental groups with PVs and PVs + LVs proceeded to the library construction stage automatically and analyzed differentially expressed genes (DEGs). From the real-time qRT-PCR analysis data, we found the marker genes of *Prox-1* and *Hif-1a* were enriched and decreased in an isolated PVs compared to LVs, respectively. Based on mRNA transcriptional data, *Prox-1* and *Hif-1a* were increased and decreased in PVs compared to LVs + PVs under lipopolysaccharide (LPS) treatment and relieved by acupuncture electric stimulation (AES), respectively. This finding indicates that high and low levels of *Prox-1* and *Hif-1a* may be involved in the function of PVs and that pathophysiological and physiological condition could progress into inflamed lymphatic endothelial cells expanding the PV within the LV.

Keywords

Primo vascular system (PVS) · Differentially expressed gene (DEG) · RNA-sequencing (Seq) · Quantitative reverse transcription-polymerase chain reaction (qRT-PCR)

J.-Y. Shin · J.-G. Choi · S.-S. Lee (✉)
Department of Oriental Biomedical Engineering, College of Health Sciences, Sangji University, Wonju, Republic of Korea
e-mail: sslee@sangji.ac.kr

S. Shin
Department of Animal Biotechnology, College of Biology Sciences, Sangji University, Wonju, Republic of Korea

S. Yeo
Department of Meridian and Acupuncture, College of Korean Medicine, Sangji University, Wonju, Republic of Korea

61.1 Introduction

In living organisms, the primo vascular system (PVS) comprising primo vessels (PVs) is one of the most important organs aimed at maintaining homeostasis and assisting in the recovery of the body by stimulating a state of control so the body reacts when exposed to disease [1]. A microscopic observation study characterized PVs as thread-like structures orientated on the longitudinal axis on the surface of the mammalian organ and a very small vessel floating in the lymph vessels (LVs) [2]. In stereo microscopic images of rabbits, the PV appears as a transparent and thick thread in

E. M. Nemoto et al. (eds.), *Oxygen Transport to Tissue XLII*, Advances in Experimental Medicine and Biology 1269, https://doi.org/10.1007/978-3-030-48238-1_61

contrast to the organ itself and the LV [3]. The middle and bundle part of the thread-like structure is the primo node. In green fluorescence microscope images, nuclei are present in the inner and outer walls of the PV [4]. Thus, the PV is composed of a nucleus containing cell spheres, and the primo microcells can function as meridians [2].

To understand the PV function, it is necessary to know protein expression. Thus, we will identify gene expression levels, based on which we aim to establish a strategy for the development of protein antibodies. The protein coding genes such as the prospero homeobox protein 1 (*Prox-1*) and hypoxia inducible factor 1 alpha subunit (*Hif-1a*) are typical lymphocyte markers [5, 6]. *Hif-1a* is regarded as the major transcription factor which can control cellular and developmental reaction to hypoxia. This indicates that inflammatory conditions are hypoxic conditions that suppress oxygen supply. LVs normally grown from the cardiovascular system to the immune system are activated by inflammatory agents, such as lipopolysaccharide (LPS) [7]. However, gene expression in the PV caused by the activation of inflammatory cells and PVs is not known. Further, an important part of this study is to isolate a small PV found in a LV with high purity.

Our research investigates the analysis of the expression of genes in the lymphocytes of healthy rabbits in a stable state. This research includes a comparative gene expression analysis of the PV in the LV of an inflammation-induced rabbit by LPS treatment and of rabbits treated with acupuncture electrical stimulation (AES) [8]. The experimental results of the RNA-sequencing (RNA-Seq) and qRT-PCR analysis suggest that gene expressions of *Prox-1* and *Hifl-a* are specifically contained in the PV. Further scientific studies will be performed to investigate the impact and nature of this finding.

61.2 Materials and Methods

Ten-week-old New Zealand female rabbits (approximately 1.8 kg) were supplied from the DaeHan Biolink Company (Eumseong, Chungbuk, Republic of Korea). All animal protocols were approved by the Institution of Animal Care and Use Committees (IACUC) of Sangji University [4, 7, 8]. All experiments were conducted with the approval of the Animal Ethics Review Committee of Sangji University. The rabbits used in the anatomical experiment were anesthetized by injecting 3.0 mL of a mixture of Zoletil® (2.5 mL) and Rompun® (0.5 mL) into the leg muscle of each rabbit. Especially because the Zoletil reagent is classified as a controlled substance, we obtained approval from the Ministry of Food and Drug Safety, Republic of Korea. All anatomical procedures were performed in a general anesthetic environment.

In this study, 200 μg/kg of LPS was injected into the lymphatic node near the abdominal vein of the rabbit. Total applied stimulation time of square waveform was 540 second with the frequency of 66.7 kHz and the power of 920 μW by using AES of model GP-302N applied to two meridian points of the Joksamni (ST36) and Hapgok (LI04). Immediately following injection of alcian blue (AB) solution and staining, the PV was observed inside the LV of the rabbit. Experimental procedures were performed in the order of LPS injection, disease induction, AES treatment, relief therapy, AB staining, PV extraction, structural image acquisition, RNA-Seq experiments, and real-time quantitative reverse transcription polymerase chain reaction (RT-PCR) analysis.

Figure 61.1a shows an image of LVs before LPS injection and AB staining in the lymphatic node near the abdominal vein of a test rabbit, while Fig. 61.1b indicates staining observed following LPS injection and AB staining, with identification of a PV from observing the morphological structure with an optical stereo microscope. LPS and AB stain were injected into the lymphatic node and subsequently spread to the small-sized LVs according to the lymphatic flow system.

An example of AB-stained PVs in LVs is shown in Fig. 61.1c. The PV clearly shows as a long thread shape. Injection of AB stain into the lymphatic node largely flows along the lymphatic system connected to the lymphatic node, and only the PV is stained. The diameter of the LV

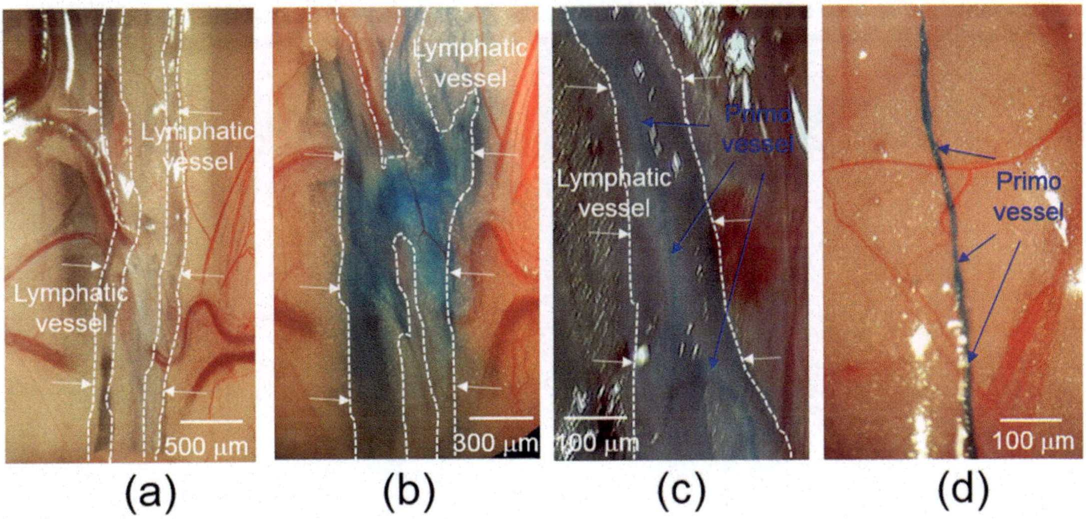

Fig. 61.1 Images of LVs in the vena cava of a rabbit (**a**) before and (**b**) after LPS injection and AB staining. Images of (**c**) floating PVs inside a LV and (**d**) an isolated PV. Dotted white lines and white arrows indicate LVs, and blue arrows indicate PVs

ranges from several hundred micrometers to several millimeters, but the diameter of the observed PV was very small, mostly several tens of micrometers. Figure 61.1d shows an image of an isolated PV stained with AB separated from the LV and stretched in a thread-like shape.

61.3 Differentially Expressed Genes (DEGs) of *Prox-1* and *Hifl-a* in PV

The primo circulatory system was successfully isolated from the lymphatic endothelium by AB staining of lymphatic nodes (Fig. 61.1a, b). An important goal of this study was to successfully isolate PVs from LVs. After stable RNA extraction from small primo tissues, certain genes were investigated. We examined the expression of two lymphatic genes, including *Prox-1* and *Hif-1a* in rabbits. Determination of RNA extraction yield and purity from a small PV were performed by the measurement of candidate gene expression using qRT-PCR. The work described in our study design was carried out over 14 days in three steps of rabbit preparation, dissection, and PCR analysis. A floating PV inside a LV and an isolated PV extracted from LV are shown in Fig. 61.1c, d, respectively, as images of LVs after LPS and AB injection in the vena cava lymphatic node of a rabbit.

Figure 61.2a shows the DEG analyses for the three genes obtained from RNA-Seq data for i) the pure PVs and ii) LVs including PVs of ten rabbits. Fragments per kilobase of exon per million (FPKM) as expression level is the average of duplicated experiments (at least two per experiment). FPKMs of *Prox-1* and *Hif-1a* were increased in LVs including PVs, when compared with pure PVs. On the other hand, FPKMs of *Gapdh* were markedly increased in pure PVs.

From Fig. 61.2b, we found the following *Prox-1* and *Hif-1a* genes by qRT-PCR analysis expressed in PVs were up- and downregulated compared to PV + LV, respectively. Comparative expression of target genes normalized to *Gapdh* between sample types is shown in Fig. 61.2b and includes significantly increased expression in *Prox-1*(2.38-fold). We also found decreased expression of *Hif-1a* (0.90 fold) in PV compared to that found in PV + LV.

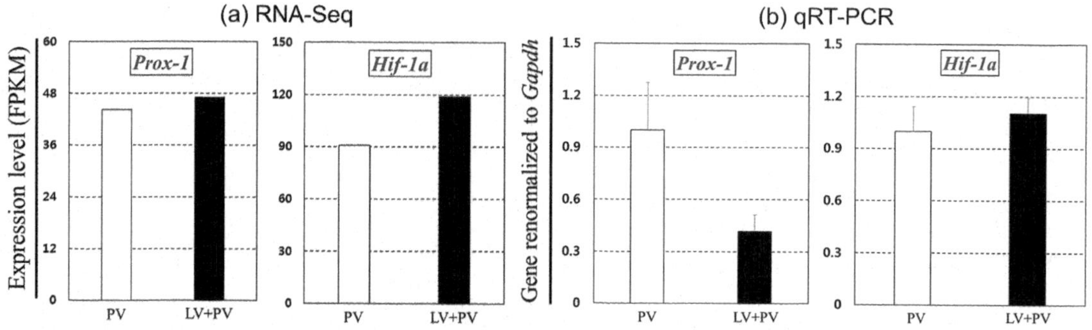

Fig. 61.2 (**a**) DEG analysis of *Prox-1* and *Hif-1a* by RNA-Seq data. Expression level (FPKM) of gene markers in PV (□) and LV + PV (■). FPKM; fragments per kilobase of exon per million. (**b**) Expression of two different genes (*Prox-1* and *Hif-1a*) in PV (□) and LV + PV (■) by qRT-PCR analysis. The p-value for each gene expression is <0.05

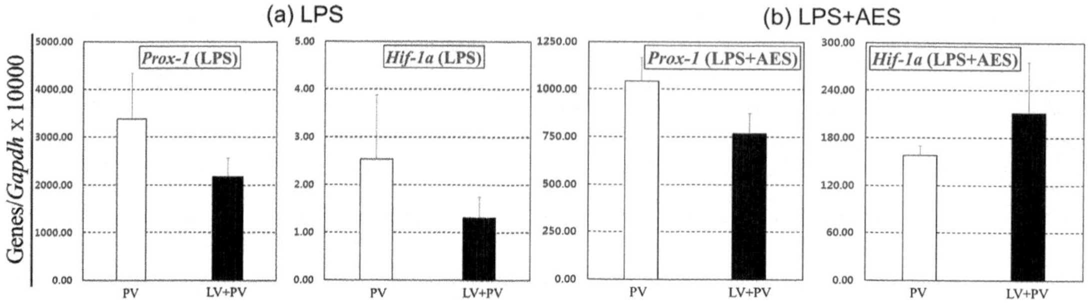

Fig. 61.3 Gene expressions of *Prox-1* and *Hif-1a* markers in PV (□) and LV + PV (■) (**a**) under LPS inflammation (**b**) by AES and LPS treatment were revealed. The p-values for only PV and PV + LV under LPS and LPS + AES are of <0.01 and <0.001, respectively

61.4 *Prox-1* and *Hif-1a* Gene Expression Analysis of PV in LV of LPS- and AES-Treated Rabbits

The changes in gene expression of PV in LV activated by LPS or conconavalin inflammation are unknown [9]. It has been proved that the AES treatment effect is stimulated through meridian system, but it is also unknown what kind of genetic material is expressed and changed. PCR analysis demonstrated augmented expression of *Prox-1* (1.5-fold) and *Hif-1a* (2.5-fold) in the PV compared with the LV including PV under LPS treatment, as shown in Fig. 61.3a. *Prox-1* is a central transcription factor in lymphatic endothelial cells (LEC) [5, 6]. Both *Prox-1* and *Hif-1a* also showed higher expression in the PV than in the LV. Plots of target gene expression normalized to *Gapdh* showing upregulation of the genes, *Prox-1* in PVs versus PVs and LVs. Stable RNA extraction from small PVs was performed under stringent sterile conditions. We also found that expression of *Hif-1a* was increased in LPS-treated PVs compared to that found in LVs (a factor of 2.5 times higher), suggesting a central role for primo circulation in inflammation.

We were demonstrably able to successfully isolate pure PVs from the LVs and confirm stable RNA extraction of the small PVs. Genes in PVs with increased expression following LPS treatment may be useful in investigating the etiology of diseases involving PVs and for further study of primo biology. In normal rabbits, the expression of *Prox-1* gene is greater in PV than LV, but the one of *Hif-1a* gene is less in PV than LV, as shown in Fig. 61.2b. The gene expressions of *Prox-1* and *Hif-1a* are markedly increased in PV in rabbits treated with LPS, as shown in Fig. 61.3a. However, their expressions were significantly reduced when the AES was applied to two acupoints ST36 and LI04 after inflammation. It suggests inactivation of these genes by acupuncture. Two genes as representative markers for LEC displayed a significant difference in PV in terms of AES.

Hif-1a is regarded as the major transcription factor which can control cellular and developmental reaction to hypoxia. It is known that upregulation of *Hif-1a* can regenerate damaged tissues having a repair response [6]. It has also been shown that the function of *Hif-1a* in angiogenesis and cancerous environments has already been elucidated, and LVs are also regulated by *Hif-1a* [6]. Our data in Fig. 61.3b showed gene expression of *Prox-1* was similar to the case of LPS treatment. On the other hand, gene expression of *Hif-1a* was decreased remarkably in PV. It is statistically significant in acupoint stimulation and strongly suggests that AES may induce therapeutic effects in PV due to *Prox-1* gene rather than *Hif-1a*. PCR data continuously showed the importance of PV in LV.

61.5 Conclusions

We have successfully isolated pure primo vasculature from the lymphatic endothelium and have been able to extract stable RNA of small PVs. Two marker gene expressions of *Prox-1* and *Hif-1a* for the isolated PVs and composite PVs LVs + PVs were investigated by RNA-Seq and qRT-PCR analysis. The DEGs analyzed by using RNA-Seq experiments showed that *Prox-1* and *Hif-1a* genes were decreased in pure PVs compared to LVs including PVs. From the real-time qRT-PCR analysis data, we found the marker gene of *Prox-1* was enriched in isolated PVs compared to LVs. On the other hand, *Hif-1a* gene was decreased in isolated PVs compared to LVs. Based on mRNA transcriptional data stressed under LPS treatment and relieved by AES, *Prox-1* and *Hif-1a* were increased and decreased in PVs compared to LVs + PVs after those treatments, respectively. These genes on PVs are remarkably influenced under LPS and AES treatment, and it could be useful for investigating the pathogenesis of diseases involving the primo vasculature and further studying primo biology.

Acknowledgments This work was supported by the National Research Foundation of Korea (NRF) funded by the Korea government (Ministry of Science and ICT) under Grant No. 2016R1E1A2A01953467.

References

1. Lee BS, Lee BC, Park JE et al (2014) Primo vascular system in human umbilical cord and placenta. J Acupunct Meridian Stud 7:291–297
2. Bae KH, Kwon HM, Soh KS (2015) DNA budding of primo microcells. J Acupunct Meridian Stud 8:103–104
3. Soh KS (2009) Bonghan circulatory system as an extension of acupuncture meridians. J Acupunct Meridian Stud 2:93–106
4. Noh YI, Rho M, Yoo YM et al (2012) Isolation and morphological features of primo vessels in rabbit lymph vessels. J Acupunct Meridian Stud 5:201–205
5. Wigle JT, Oliver G (1999) Prox1 function is required for the development of the murine lymphatic system. Cell 98:769–778
6. Tsuchida S, Arai Y, Takahashi KA et al (2014) HIF-1α-induced HSP70 regulates anabolic responses in articular chondrocytes under hypoxic conditions. J Orthop Res 32:975–980
7. Lee HR, Rho M, Hong YJ et al (2015) Primo vessel stressed by lipopolysaccharide in rabbits. J Acupunct Meridian Stud 8:301–306
8. Shin JY, Ji JO, Choi DW et al (2019) Expression of genes in primo vasculature floating in lymphatic endothelium under lipopolysaccharide and acupuncture electric stimulation. J Acupunct Meridian Stud 12:3–10
9. Kataru RP, Kim H, Jang C, Choi DK, Koh BI, Kim M et al (2011) T lymphocytes negatively regulate lymph node lymphatic vessel formation. Immunity 34:96–107

On the Feasibility of Pulse Wave Velocity Imaging for Remote Assessment of Physiological Functions

62

Gennadi Saiko, M. Dervenis, and A. Douplik

Abstract

Introduction: Pulse wave velocity imaging (PWVi) is a novel technology developed by our group for real-time assessment of ischemia. The objectives of this proof-of-concept study included (1) remote detection of blood flow pulse and (2) assessing the feasibility of pulse wave velocity (PWV) imaging. *Methods*: PWVi is based on a 12-bit RGB camera (Basler acA-2000-165uc) capturing videos at up to 1000 fps. Videos of the hands of healthy individuals were taken, segmented, and processed to assess pulse wave velocity (PWV) and photoplethysmographic (PPG) signals. *Results*: PWV and PPG waveforms were readily collected for multiple segments. The PWVi device performed well, even without an external source of illumination. Mean PWV of 341.3 (±151.0) cm/s was obtained. *Conclusions*: PWVi is a portable, accessible, and cost-effective technology for assessing physiological parameters remotely.

Keywords

Wound healing · Tissue imaging · Blood flow pulse · Remote PPG

G. Saiko (✉)
Swift Medical Inc., Toronto, ON, Canada
e-mail: Gennadi.saiko@swiftmedical.com

M. Dervenis
Department of Physics, Ryerson University, Toronto, ON, Canada

A. Douplik
Department of Physics, Ryerson University, Toronto, ON, Canada

iBEST, Keenan Research Centre of the LKS Knowledge Institute, St. Michael Hospital, Toronto, ON, Canada

62.1 Introduction

A "pulse wave" occurs during the contraction of the left ventricle; as blood is released from the left ventricle into the systemic circulatory system, pressure increases inside the aorta and radiates distally throughout the arteries and arterioles. The speed at which the pulse wave travels through the arteries can reveal key information about the health of the arteries, including elasticity, stiffness, and even potential calcification and stenosis as well as the viscosity of the blood [1, 2].

Pulse waves can be monitored in the clinic to address certain vascular issues, such as cardiovascular disease [3, 4] using photoplethysmography (PPG) [5]. PPG works by measuring the absorption of light through tissue. In a typical scenario, PPG measurements are collected at a single wavelength, usually within infrared range (700–900 nm), at which hemoglobin (Hb) absorbs light at a reduced level, in transmission

E. M. Nemoto et al. (eds.), *Oxygen Transport to Tissue XLII*, Advances in Experimental Medicine and Biology 1269, https://doi.org/10.1007/978-3-030-48238-1_62

or reflectance set up. Common heart rate monitors use transmission PPG to measure heart rate through the tip of the finger, earlobe, or septum of the nose. Reflectance PPG can, however, be measured anywhere on the skin.

As the PPG sensor is usually placed onto the skin, it requires the patient to hold a still position, and the method is very sensitive to motion artifacts. However, the main obstacle to obtaining good quality, i.e., highly reproducible, data by PPG is related to the fact that the sensor is mechanically fixed to the skin and hence introduces a certain external pressure factor, which in turn affects the PPG signal.

A remote PPG (rPPG) can be implemented without direct contact between a PPG sensor and skin. By measuring a diffuse reflectance from the skin at a distance, it is possible to determine the PPG signal over a large area, albeit with much lower signal intensity and certain artifacts [6–8].

Various data collection rPPG schemas have been proposed. McDuff et al. [9] recovered pulse wavefront morphology, including systole-diastole time using a digital camera at 30 frames per second (fps) located at 3 m from a subject's face. Kumar et al. [10] developed similar technology for noncontact vital sign monitoring in the facial region, which they called DistancePPG.

Previous work has also shown that rPPG can be used to determine pulse transit time (PTT) [11], the time it will take for a pulse wave to travel between two spots of the body. Knowing the distance between the spots and PTT, it is also possible to detect pulse wave velocity (PWV) – the parameter that can be used for ischemia monitoring [3, 12].

Existing technologies for ischemia monitoring, such as the brachial-ankle pulse wave velocity (baPWV) based on the difference in time a pulse takes to arrive from the heart to both the brachium and ankle, have been used as a diagnostic tool with regard to coronary artery disease (CAD) [13, 14]. As the existing methods are usually a point measurement, the results may vary significantly depending on the particular area selected for data collection and measurement geometry such as in the case of Doppler anemometry [15].

In addition to baPWV, other geometries for PTT/PWV evaluation have been proposed. Simultaneous measurement of ECG and rPPG of the facial region was proposed to estimate PTT and blood pressure [16]. Simultaneous measurement of PPG signal on the palm and forehead was used to determine PTT and systolic blood pressure [17].

To overcome the existing limitations for ischemia diagnostics, our group developed the rPPG technology in imaging mode, termed pulse wave velocity imaging (PWVi), which makes it distinctive and more robust in terms of collected data statistics as the data is collected from an area instead of a single point. This device works in a similar manner to rPPG, but by spatially resolving several plethysmographic signals over a single skin area, facilitating measurement of PTT and pulse wave velocity (PWV) in imaging mode.

PWVi has the capacity to determine pulse wave velocity, pulse transit time (PTT), and perform plethysmographic waveform analysis within a single area. The objectives of this proof-of-concept study included (1) remote detection of blood flow pulse and (2) assessing the feasibility of pulse wave velocity (PWV) imaging.

62.2 Methods

The PWVi device is based on a 12-bit RGB camera (Basler ac-A2000-165uc, Basler AG, Germany) capturing videos at a high frame rate to resolve the propagation of the pulse wave across the horizontal field of the camera, which was set in the direction of the pulse wave propagation. To verify the feasibility of the experimental setup, videos of the fingers taken from a single individual at various conditions were captured and processed.

62.2.1 Data Acquisition

All data were acquired in accordance with the Ryerson Research Ethics Board (Protocol # REB2014-077). Data were acquired from healthy volunteers ($n = 3$), between the ages of 20 and 28.

In each instance, the participant was seated, and their hands were placed on a table. The subject then waited 10 minutes in this position for blood pressure to equilibrate. The camera was suspended approximately 30 cm above the hand so that the rows of the camera sensor were parallel to the length of the fingers. Rows of the camera sensor were decimated to allow for higher frame rates, such that the width of the sensor, along the axial direction, was still full, but the height of the sensor was reduced, and remaining sensor rows centered on the index finger. Once in position, the horizontal field size was measured by placing a ruler on top of the hand before recording. Ten-second videos were acquired for each measurement. Figure 62.1a shows how the area of interest (AOI) would be positioned with respect to a full resolution image.

At 1000 fps, the exposure time was approximately 900 μs per frame. An image capturing optimization was used to reduce the Johnson-Nyquist (kTC) noise. Videos were then processed to assess pulse wave velocity and PPG signals.

62.2.2 Image Processing

The video binary files were processed in MATLAB. Because red light has relatively low absorption in hemoglobin, and so would change very little on each pulse, the red channel was used as a normalizing channel to correct for ambient lighting throughout the video in the green and blue channels. The green channel was then used to extract the PPG data, as the signal in the blue channel, in general, was too low. The green channel (G) data were subtracted from that of the red channel (R) to normalize for lighting changes and create a more physiologically relevant graph; increased blood volume during the systole leads to increased absorption due to hemoglobin, therefore lowering green and blue light reflectance intensities of each:

$$\text{PPG Signal} = R - G \tag{62.1}$$

The video was then separated spatially into several smaller segments (see Fig. 62.1b), of

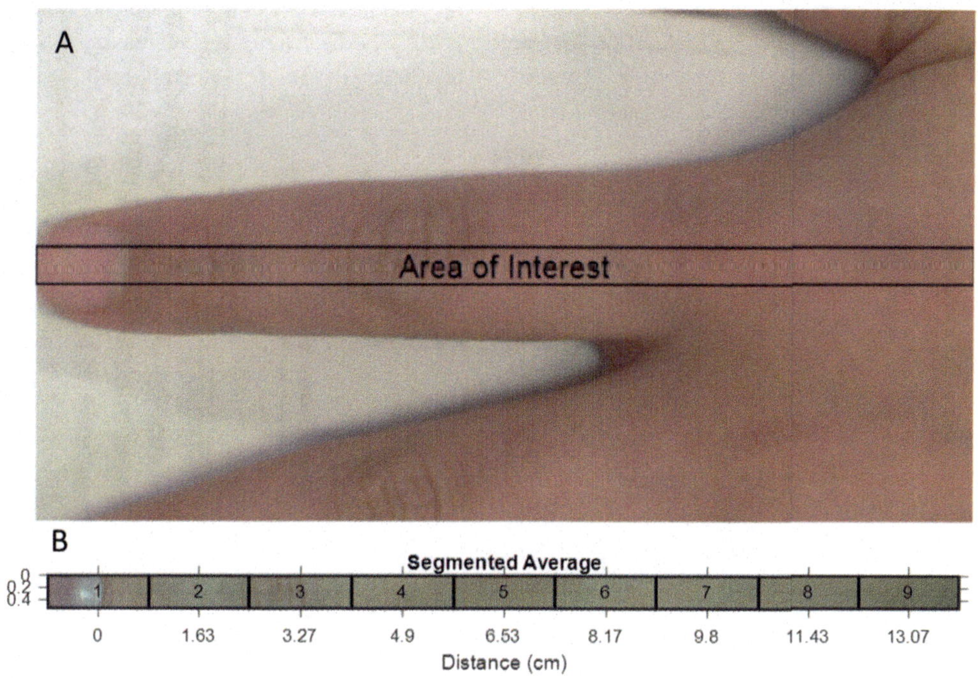

Fig. 62.1 Panel (**a**): A full resolution image of the hand, outlining the area of interest (AOI) that might be used to capture video at higher frame rates. Panel (**b**): AOI, split into several sections, each one averaged into individual time series

approximately 1 cm in length, each of which had its pixels averaged to increase the SNR.

The new spatially separated PPG signals were passed through MATLAB's cross-correlation function, "xcorr()," unscaled. Cross-correlation was used to determine where a PPG signal from a distal part of the frame aligned with the PPG signal at a more proximal (closer to the heart) part, thereby giving the delay in the pulse wave. A Savitsky-Golay filter was applied to the resulting cross-correlation to suppress any 60 or 120 Hz flicker due to room lighting, but still retain the shape of the cross-correlation. As well, any spike at zero, usually caused by ambient lighting changes, would be suppressed during this filtering. For signals corrupted with heavy power mains noise, the Savitsky-Golay filter would not be able to eliminate all the noise while still retaining the shape of the curve. A modest boxcar filter (7 sample window) was applied to smooth any remaining high-frequency noise.

A local maximum was searched for around zero lags of the resulting cross-correlation, which corresponds to the PTT of the pulse wave. The cross-correlation was performed on every combination of segment pairs, and the PTT for each pair was plotted against the separation distance of the segments (x). Linear regression was obtained from the resulting graph, where

$$PWV = x / PTT \tag{62.2}$$

62.3 Results and Discussion

The reliable PPG signal was extracted for each segment. The cross-correlation was applied to all combinations of segment pairs, and the PTT was calculated from each cross-correlation and plotted against the separation distance between segment pairs (see Fig. 62.2). A linear best fit line was applied to the result, and from Eq. (62.2), the reciprocal of the slope of the best fit line is the PWV. This process was repeated ten times on a single subject to determine the precision of the system.

The calculated PWV for volunteer 1 (341.3 cm/s) was in the physiological range; however, its standard deviation was relatively high (151.0 cm/s). This relatively broad variation in PWV can be due to several factors, including the balance between temporal resolution and noise. As the frame rate increases, the temporal resolution in the cross-correlation also increases.

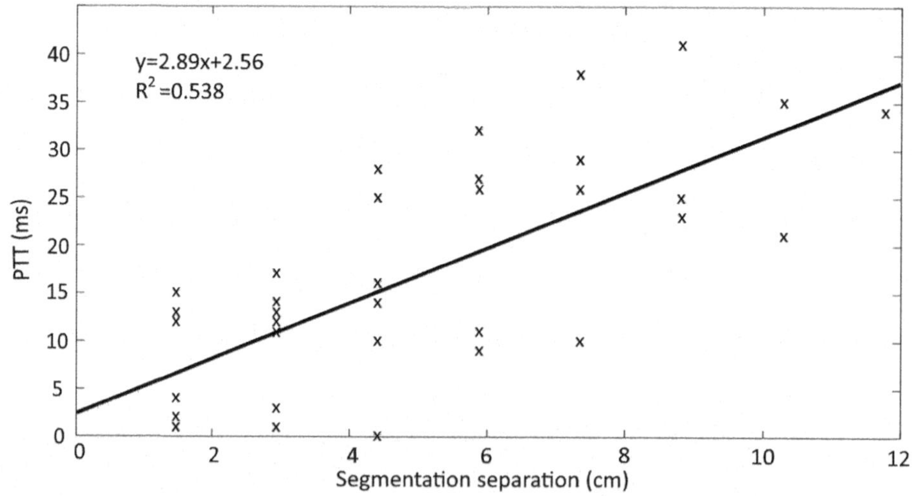

Fig. 62.2 The PTT is plotted for each segment pair against the distance between each segment pair for the trial under LED lighting for volunteer 1. The slope of the regression line is equal to the reciprocal of the PWV over the field of the video

At the same time, as exposure time decreases, read noise becomes overwhelming in the images. Thus, narrow band external illumination [18] (e.g., in the green range) can be helpful to improve the SNR.

The purpose of the present study was to assess the feasibility of PWV acquisition under generic lighting conditions. We performed assessment under LED and fluorescent lighting. Results are similar; however, fluorescent light requires more preprocessing (filtering). We limit our results and discussion to LED illumination only.

62.4 Conclusions

In summary, PWVi has the capacity to determine pulse wave velocity, pulse transit time, and perform plethysmographic waveform analysis within a single area. It is close to real-time (within 10–20 s) and can easily fit in clinical workflows. This proof-of-concept pilot study has shown that the technology is feasible; with a high frame rate RGB camera and a standard CCTV lens, it is shown to be possible to remotely obtain PPG waveforms and determine PWV in the skin under generic and even limited lighting situations.

Acknowledgments Authors would like to acknowledge the support of Dr. Douplik's NSERC Discovery grant, Ryerson Health Fund, NSERC Collaborative Health Research Project grant (CHRP). We appreciate Prof. Catherine Beauchemin (Ryerson University) for her helpful comments when designing the project.

References

1. Safar ME, O'Rourke MF (2006) Handbook of hypertension, volume 23: Arterial stiffness in hypertension. Elsevier, Edinburgh
2. Nichols WW, O'Rourke MF (2005) McDonald's blood flow in arteries, theoretical, experimental and clinical principles, 5th edn. Oxford University Press, Oxford
3. Hansen TW, Staessen JA, Torp-Pedersen C et al (2006) Prognostic value of aortic pulse wave velocity as index of arterial stiffness in the general population. Circulation 113(5):664–670
4. Sutton-Tyrrell K, Najjar SS, Boudreau RM et al (2005) Elevated aortic pulse wave velocity, a marker of arterial stiffness, predicts cardiovascular events in well-functioning older adults. Circulation 111(25):3384–3390
5. Weinman J, Hayat A, Raviv G (1977) Reflection photoplethysmography of arterial-blood-volume pulses. Med Biol Eng Comput 15(1):22–31
6. Verkruysse W, Svaasand LO, Nelson JS (2008) Remote plethysmographic imaging using ambient light. Opt Express 16(26):21434–21445
7. Scully CG, Lee J, Meyer J et al (2012) Physiological parameter monitoring from optical recordings with a mobile phone. IEEE Trans Biomed Eng 59(2):303–306
8. Beiderman Y, Horovitz I, Burshtein N et al (2010) Remote estimation of blood pulse pressure via temporal tracking of reflected secondary speckles pattern. J Biomed Opt 15(6):061707–061707
9. McDuff D, Gontarek S, Picard RW (2014) Remote detection of photoplethysmographic systolic and diastolic peaks using a digital camera. IEEE Trans Biomed Eng 61(12):2948–2954
10. Kumar M, Veeraraghavan A, Sabharwal A (2015) DistancePPG: Robust non-contact vital signs monitoring using a camera. Biomed Opt Express 6:1565–1588
11. Shao D, Yang Y, al LC (2014) Noncontact monitoring breathing pattern, exhalation flow rate and pulse transit time. IEEE Trans Biomed Eng 61(11):2760–2767
12. Mitchell GF, van Buchem MA, Sigurdsson S et al (2011) Arterial stiffness, pressure and flow pulsatility and brain structure and function: the Age, Gene/Environment Susceptibility–Reykjavik study. Brain 134(11):3398–3407
13. Katakami N, Osonoi T, Takahara M et al (2014) Clinical utility of brachial-ankle pulse wave velocity in the prediction of cardiovascular events in diabetic patients. Cardiovasc Diabetol 13:128
14. Chae MJ, Jung IH, Jang DH et al (2013) The brachial ankle pulse wave velocity is associated with the presence of significant coronary artery disease but not the extent. Korean Circ J 43(4):239–245
15. Durst F, Melling A, Whitelaw J (1981) Principles and practices of laser Doppler anemometry. Academic Press, London
16. Chandrasekaran V, Dantu R, Jonnada S et al (2013) Cuffless differential blood pressure estimation using smart phones. IEEE Trans Biomed Eng 60(4):1080–1089
17. Secerbegovic A, Bergsland J, Halvorsen PS et al (2016) Blood pressure estimation using video plethysmography, 2016 IEEE 13th international symposium on biomedical imaging (ISBI), Prague, pp. 461–464
18. Saiko G, Betlen A (2020) Optimization of band selection in multispectral and narrow-band imaging: an analytical approach. Adv Exp Med Biol 1232:361–367

Author Index

E. M. Nemoto et al. (eds.), *Oxygen Transport to Tissue XLII*, Advances in Experimental Medicine and Biology 1269, https://doi.org/10.1007/978-3-030-48238-1

Subject Index

E. M. Nemoto et al. (eds.), *Oxygen Transport to Tissue XLII*, Advances in Experimental Medicine and Biology 1269, https://doi.org/10.1007/978-3-030-48238-1

M

N

Printed by Printforce, the Netherlands